Clinical Neurogastroenterology

Clinical Neurogastroenterology

Editor: Kiersten Meyer

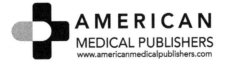

AMERICAN
MEDICAL PUBLISHERS
www.americanmedicalpublishers.com

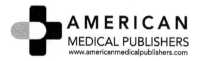

AMERICAN
MEDICAL PUBLISHERS
www.americanmedicalpublishers.com

Cataloging-in-Publication Data

Clinical neurogastroenterology / edited by Kiersten Meyer.
    p. cm.
Includes bibliographical references and index.
ISBN 978-1-63927-830-5
1. Gastroenterology. 2. Digestive organs--Diseases. 3. Gastrointestinal system--Innervation.
4. Neurology. 5. Gastrointestinal system--Diseases--Treatment. I. Meyer, Kiersten.
RC801 .C55 2023
616.33--dc23

© American Medical Publishers, 2023

American Medical Publishers,
41 Flatbush Avenue,
1st Floor, New York,
NY 11217, USA

ISBN 978-1-63927-830-5 (Hardback)

Contents

Preface

Neurogastroenterology is a subspecialty of gastroenterology which deals with the diseases wherein disordered interactions take place between the central nervous system (CNS) and the gastrointestinal (GI) system. Neurogastroenterology deals with alterations taking place along the gut-brain axis. The brain-gut axis refers to the two-way biochemical signaling that takes place between the GI tract and the CNS. Neurogastroenterology deals with the neurology of the GI tract, liver, gallbladder, and pancreas. It also focuses on the control of digestion through the enteric nervous system, the central nervous system, and integrative centers in sympathetic ganglia. The field of neurogastroenterology predominantly studies the diseases of the intrinsic enteric nervous system, i.e. the brain of the gut, which is a part of the nervous system and is responsible for controlling motility, endocrine secretions, and microcirculation of the gastrointestinal system. This book is a valuable compilation of topics, ranging from the basic to the most complex advancements in the field of neurogastroenterology. It is appropriate for students seeking detailed information on this area as well as for experts.

After months of intensive research and writing, this book is the end result of all who devoted their time and efforts in the initiation and progress of this book. It will surely be a source of reference in enhancing the required knowledge of the new developments in the area. During the course of developing this book, certain measures such as accuracy, authenticity and research focused analytical studies were given preference in order to produce a comprehensive book in the area of study.

This book would not have been possible without the efforts of the authors and the publisher. I extend my sincere thanks to them. Secondly, I express my gratitude to my family and well-wishers. And most importantly, I thank my students for constantly expressing their willingness and curiosity in enhancing their knowledge in the field, which encourages me to take up further research projects for the advancement of the area.

Editor

Mucosal Tuft Cell Density is Increased in Diarrhea-Predominant Irritable Bowel Syndrome Colonic Biopsies

Jessica Aigbologa[1†], Maeve Connolly[2†], Julliette M. Buckley[3,4] and Dervla O'Malley[1,2]*

[1] APC Microbiome Ireland, Cork, Ireland, [2] Department of Physiology, University College Cork, Cork, Ireland, [3] Department of Surgery, University College Cork, Cork, Ireland, [4] Mater Private Hospital, Cork, Ireland

*Correspondence:
Dervla O'Malley
d.omalley@ucc.ie

[†] These authors have contributed equally to this work

Tuft cells are rare chemosensory sentinels found in the gut epithelium. When triggered by helminth infection, tuft cells secrete interleukin-25 (IL-25) basolaterally and subsequently evoke an immune response. Irritable bowel syndrome (IBS) is a common and heterogeneous disorder characterized by bowel dysfunction and visceral pain sensitivity. Dysfunctional gut-brain communication and immune activation contribute to the pathophysiology of this disorder. The study aims were to investigate changes in tuft cell density in non-post-infectious IBS patients. Immunofluorescent labeling of DCLK1-positive tuft cells was carried out in mucosal biopsies from the distal colons of diarrhea and constipation-predominant IBS patients and healthy controls. Tuft cell numbers were also assessed in animal models. Concentrations of interleukin-25 (IL-25) secreted from colonic biopsies and in plasma samples were analyzed using an immunoassay. The density of tuft cells was increased in diarrhea—but not constipation-predominant IBS patient colonic biopsies. Biopsy secretions and plasma concentrations of IL-25 were elevated in diarrhea—but not constipation-predominant IBS participants. Tuft cell hyperplasia was detected in a rat model of IBS but not in mice exposed to chronic stress. Tuft cell hyperplasia is an innate immune response to helminth exposure. However, the patients with diarrhea-predominant IBS have not reported any incidents of enteric infection. Moreover, rats exhibiting IBS-like symptoms displayed increased tuft cell density but were not exposed to helminths. Our findings suggest that factors other than helminth exposure or chronic stress lead to tuft cell hyperplasia in IBS colonic biopsies.

Keywords: interleukin-25, irritable bowel syndrome, helminths, Wistar Kyoto, brush cells, Doublecortin Linked Kinase-1, DCAMKL1, chronic stress

INTRODUCTION

Tuft cells are rare differentiated epithelial cells, anatomically and functionally distinct from other border cells in the gastrointestinal (GI) tract (1). Characterized by long, blunt microvilli, pear-shaped tuft cells are scattered along the crypt-villus axis (2). Uniquely, they express a microtubule linked protein known as Doublecortin Linked Kinase-1 (3) (DCLK1, also known as DCAMK1 (4)] and contain axial bundles of actin filaments supporting the microvilli (5, 6). The chemosensory activity and intimate physical contact between tuft cells and enteric nerves (7, 8) suggests a role in regulating gut motility and absorpto-secretory function. Tuft cells could also act as cross-epithelial signal transducers (8), informing the host nervous system of changes in the luminal environment. Parasitic infections, in particular (9), uniquely stimulate release of immune cytokines, such as interleukin (IL)-25 (also known as IL-17E), from tuft cells (10–12). IL-25, in turn, induces secretion of IL-13 from stromal group 2 innate lymphoid cells (ILC2), which promote release of IgE, eosinophilia, goblet cell hyperplasia (13) and, in a feed forward circuit, tuft cell hyperplasia (14).

Irritable bowel syndrome (IBS), a prevalent, chronic and heterogeneous functional bowel disorder, is characterized by abdominal pain, bloating and altered bowel motility (15). Prevalence of IBS is ~7–18% of the worldwide population (16), and this includes a subset referred to as post-infectious IBS (PI-IBS) patients, who develop intestinal dysfunction following infectious enteritis (17). Indeed, prior GI infection is a strong predictor of developing IBS (18), with one in ten patients believing their IBS symptoms emerged subsequent to an infectious illness (17). Infection with protozoans as opposed to bacteria conferred a greater risk of developing IBS following resolution of the infection (19).

Although it is plausible that tuft cell numbers could be elevated in patients with PI-IBS, the majority of IBS patients do not report prior GI infection. Rather, a significant proportion of these patients, who may be sub-categorized with diarrhea (IBS-D), constipation (IBS-C) or alternating subtypes of IBS, experience co-morbid anxiety and depressive disorders (20). Thus, it is generally accepted that dysfunction of the bi-directional gut-brain axis underlies symptoms in these patient groups. This study aims to quantify expression of tuft cells in colonic samples from IBS patients who have not, to their knowledge, had prior intestinal enteritis. Tuft cell density was assessed in non-PI IBS patients, in a stress-sensitive rat model of IBS and in mice exposed to a chronic stressor to determine if stimuli other than exposure to parasites contributes to IBS pathophysiology.

MATERIALS AND METHODS

Ethical Approval

The protocol for collecting biopsies and blood samples from IBS patients and healthy control volunteers was approved by the University College Cork Clinical Research Ethics Committee (ECM 4 (r) 010316) and was carried out in the Mater Private Hospital, Cork. Informed consent was obtained from all participants.

Experiments using animal tissue were all in full accordance with the principles of the European Community Council Directive (86/609/EEC) as well as the local University College Cork animal ethical committee (#2011/015).

Human Colon Biopsy and Plasma Collection

Patients attending the General Surgery Clinic at the Mater Private Hospital, Cork, Ireland were recruited for the study. Males and females aged between 18 and 65 years of age and able to provide written informed consent were enrolled. Inclusion criteria for IBS patients included confirmed clinical diagnosis of IBS that satisfied Rome III criteria for IBS. No PI-IBS patients were included in this study. Biopsies from age and weight-matched healthy controls were taken from patients undergoing routine colonoscopies that were in good health and negative for bowel disease. Exclusion criteria for participation included acute or chronic co-existing illness, recent unexplained bleeding or prior GI surgery (apart from hernia repair and appendectomy), coeliac or other GI disease, psychiatric disease, immunodeficiency, bleeding disorder, coagulopathy, a malignant disease or any concomitant end-stage organ disease. Subjects were also excluded if they were taking any experimental drugs or if the subject had taken part in an experimental trial less than 30 days prior to this study. Mucosal biopsies from the distal colon were taken from fasting patients at the same time as obtaining a matched serum sample. Samples were assigned a study number, with the key held only by the treating surgeon, so as to preserve patient confidentiality in accordance with the study protocol. The secretory products from biopsies incubated in Dubellco's Modified Eagle Medium (Sigma Aldrich, UK, overnight, 37°C) were used to measure local tissue concentration of interleukin-25 (IL-25)/hu-17E. Mucosal biopsies were subsequently fixed overnight in 4% paraformaldehyde at 4°C, cryoprotected in 30% sucrose and stored at −80°C for immunofluorescent staining.

Animals and Tissue Collecting

Male Sprague Dawley (SD) and Wistar Kyoto (WKY) rats, > 8 weeks of age, were purchased from Envigo, Derbyshire, UK. Given that hormonal cycles in the female are associated with exacerbation of IBS-like symptoms, we used male rodents in this study such that the additional complexity of changing female hormone levels was not a factor in the studies. The Animals were group-housed four per cage and maintained on a 12/12-hour dark-light cycle with a room temperature of 22 ± 1°C with food and water *ad libitum*. Rats were euthanized by CO_2 overdose and perforation of the diaphragm.

Male adult mice (C57Bl/6J, The Jackson Laboratory, Maine, US) were bred in-house (Biological Service Unit, University College Cork, Ireland). Prior to social defeat sessions (~1 week) mice were singly housed. Singly-housed adult male CD1 mice (Envigo, UK) were used as aggressors for the chronic social defeat stress procedure. Mice were maintained on a 12/12-hour dark-light cycle with a room temperature of 22 ± 1°C with food and water *ad libitum*. Mice were sacrificed by cervical decapitation.

Chronic social defeat stress in these mice has been previously described (21). In brief, mice assigned to the chronic social defeat stress group underwent 10 consecutive days of stress. The same researcher carried out all interventions. All defeat sessions were carried out in the mornings during the light cycle. CD1 aggressor mice were selected based on the shortest latency to attack another CD1 mouse. Test mice were subjected to a different CD1 aggressor mouse each day over the study period. Exposure of the test mouse to the aggressive CD1 mouse lasted until the first attack, expression of submissive posturing or until 5 min had passed, whichever happened first. The test and CD1 aggressor mice were then separated by a perforated transparent barrier for 2 h. The separator was subsequently removed and, after another defeat, mice were transferred back to their home-cage. Control mice were handled but remained in their home-cages over the course of the stress.

The distal colon (< 4 cm from anus) from both rats and mice were isolated and placed in ice-cold 95% O_2/5% CO_2 bubbled Krebs saline solution consisting of (in mmol/L) NaCl, 117; KCl, 4.8; $CaCl_2$, 2.5; $MgCl_2$, 1.2; $NaHCO_3$, 25; NaH_2PO_4, 1.2; and D-glucose, 11. Colonic samples were fixed in 4% paraformaldehyde at 4°C overnight. The samples were then cryoprotected in 30% sucrose and snap frozen at −80°C.

Mesoscale Discovery Biomarker Assay

An immunoassay (U-PLEX Human IL-17E/IL-25 Assay, MesoScale Discovery, Gaithersburg, MD, USA) was carried out to determine the concentration of IL-17E/IL-25 in plasma and supernatant samples of IBS patients and healthy control samples (dynamic range: 0.58–9,200 pg/ml). The assay was run in triplicate and an electrochemiluminescent detection method was used to measure protein levels in the samples. The plates were read using MesoScale Discovery plate-reader (MESO QuickPlex SQ 120). A calibration curve was generated using standards, and cytokine concentrations were determined from the curve.

Immunofluorescence and Confocal Microscopy

Cross-sections of rat and mouse distal colon and human distal colonic biopsies, fixed in 4% paraformaldehyde (4°C, overnight), were cryo-sectioned (10 μm in thickness, Leica Biosystems, Wetzler, Germany) and mounted on glass slides (VWR, Dublin 15, Ireland). Rodent cross-sections or human mucosal biopsies were permeabilized with 0.1% Triton X-100 and blocked with 1% donkey serum (Sigma Aldrich, UK). Colonic tissue was immunolabeled with anti-DCLK1 (1:100, overnight at 4°C, anti-DCAMKL1 polyclonal rabbit antibody, Abcam, Cambridge, UK) and a complimentary TRITC-conjugated fluorophore (1:250, 2 h at room temperature, Jackson ImmunoResearch Europe Ltd., Cambridgeshire, UK). This primary antibody recognizes a protein of the predicted size and is blocked by using a DCAMKL1 peptide (22). No non-specific fluorescence was detected in control experiments where tissues were incubated with anti-DCLK1 in the absence of secondary antibodies or secondary antibodies alone. As tuft cells have a unique arrangement of cytoskeletal components, colonic samples were co-stained with a cytoskeletal marker, Phalloidin-iFluor 488-Cytopainter (1:1,000, Abcam, Cambridge, UK), which was prepared in 1% bovine serum albumin in phosphate buffered saline solution (PBS, (in mM): NaCl 137, KCl 2.7 and Na_2HPO_4

10 at pH 7.4). Tissue sections were mounted using Dako-fluorescent mounting medium containing DAPI (Agilent Pathology Solutions Santa Clara, California, USA) and a coverslip placed over all tissue. Images were captured using a FVl0i-Olympus-confocal microscope with Fluoview software (FV10i-SW, Olympus Europe, Hamburg, Germany). At least three different biopsy slices from six different participants per group were compared in the human study. In the animal studies, at least three different cross-section slices from three different animals per group were compared. Analysis was carried out independently by two different researchers and the mean number of cells from each was calculated.

Statistical Analyses

Data was analyzed using GraphPad prism for windows (version 7). Data were plotted as box and whisker plots with 95% confidence intervals. Data were compared using paired two-tailed Student's tests or One-way or repeated measures ANOVA with Tukey post-hoc test, as appropriate. P values of <0.05 were considered significant.

RESULTS

Tuft Cell Density Is Elevated in IBS-D Patient Biopsies

Samples from healthy controls (HC, n = 6 (three males, three females)) were compared with samples from diarrhea-predominant (IBS-D, n = 6 (one male, five females)) and constipation-predominant (IBS-C, n = 6, (two males, four females)) participants. HC and patient participants similar in terms of ethnicity (all Caucasian), age—(44.7 ± 4.56 (HCs) versus 40 ± 3.91 (IBS) years, p >0.05) and weight—(72.9 ± 13.95 (HCs) versus 71.83 ± 10.97 (IBS) kg, p >0.05). Gastrointestinal symptoms, such as bloating, abdominal pain and altered bowel habit were consistent with their categorization into the appropriate IBS subtype, as determined by Rome III criteria for diagnosing IBS. Mood disorders were reported in one IBS-D (depression), two IBS-C (depression and/or anxiety) but no HC participants.

Triple-labeling of human colonic biopsies with an antibody against the gastrointestinal tuft cell marker, doublecortin-like kinase 1 protein (DCLK1, red staining) (23), a cytoskeletal marker (green staining) and the nuclear stain, DAPI, facilitated counting of tuft cells as a percentage of total DAPI-labeled epithelial cells in the visual field. The total number of DAPI-labeled cells in biopsies (n = 5 sections from five biopsies) from HCs (476.7 ± 83.3), IBS-D (383.1 ± 17.47) and IBS-C (447.4 ± 60.23) were comparable (p = 0.31, one-way ANOVA F(2, 12) = 1.293). Labeled tuft cells in human biopsies displayed classic pear-shaped morphology (2) with a large central nucleus and strong Phalloidin-labeled cytoskeletal filaments (**Figure 1A**). The density of tuft cells in IBS-C biopsies (n = 18 sections from six biopsies) was not different to HC biopsies (p >0.05, n = 18 sections from six biopsies, **Figure 1A**). However, the prevalence

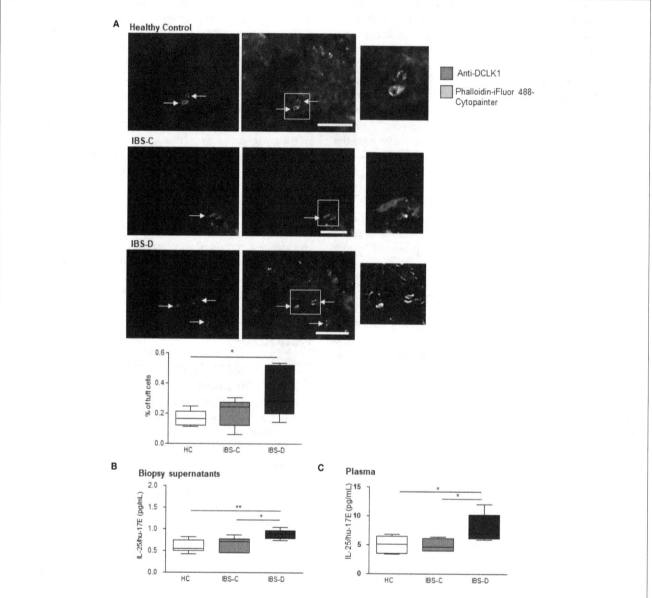

FIGURE 1 | Tuft cell density and IL-25 secretion is elevated in IBS-D colonic mucosa. **(A)** The representative immunofluorescent images and box and whisker plots of pooled data illustrate the density of DCLK1-labeled tuft cells as a percentage of the total DAPI-stained epithelial cells in mucosal biopsies from healthy patients and patients with constipation- (IBS-C) or diarrhea-predominant (IBS-D) IBS. Scalebar: 50 µm. **(B)** The pooled data shows that colonic biopsies and **(C)** plasma samples from human IBS-D patients secrete more IL-25 than other groups. * and ** indicate p <0.05 and p <0.01, respectively.

of tuft cells in IBS-D biopsies (n = 18 sections from six biopsies) was elevated as compared to HC samples (p <0.05, **Figure 1A**).

Biopsy Secretion of IL-25/hu-17E Is Elevated in IBS-D Samples

As activated tuft cells secrete IL-25 (10), we examined IL-25/hu-17E levels both in local secretions from human biopsies and in the matching plasma samples. IL-25/hu-17E was detected at sub-picomolar concentrations in supernatants from HC biopsies (n = 6) and concentrations were similar in IBS-C patient supernatants (n = 6, p >0.05). However, the concentration of secreted IL-25/hu-17E was elevated in IBS-D supernatants (n = 6, p <0.01, F(2,15) = 7.343, **Figure 1B**). Plasma

concentrations of IL-25/hu-17E were also increased in IBS-D samples (p = 0.02, F(2,14) = 5.36, **Figure 1C**).

Circulating Concentrations of IL-6 and IL-8 Are Altered in IBS Patients

Other inflammatory cytokines, such as IL-6 and IL-8 are reported to be elevated in IBS patients (24, 25). Thus, to confirm the findings from the previous studies, IL-6 was initially compared between plasma from HCs and pooled samples from both IBS-D and IBS-C. We found that circulating IL-6 was elevated in IBS patients (0.976 ± 0.17 pg ml^{-1}) as compared to HCs (0.398 ± 0.15 pg ml^{-1}, p = 0.06, Student's t-test). When examined by subtype, circulating IL-6 was elevated in IBS-D (1.343 ± 0.35 pg ml^{-1}, p = 0.04)) but not IBS-C

$(0.75 \pm 0.06$ pg ml^{-1}) as compared to HC samples $(0.504 \pm 0.16$ pg ml^{-1}, one-way ANOVA F(2,11) = 4.338). Circulating IL-8 concentrations were elevated in pooled IBS plasma samples $(12.27 \pm 1.06$ pg ml^{-1}) as compared to HC samples $(6.514 \pm 0.51$ pg ml^{-1}, Student's t-test, p = 0.004). However, when examined individually, IL-8 in IBS-C samples $(13.44 \pm 1.62$ pg ml^{-1}, p = 0.009) but not in IBS-D samples $(11.1 \pm 1.3$ pg ml^{-1}), was elevated by comparison to HC samples $(6.5 \pm 0.51$ pg ml^{-1}, one-way ANOVA F (2,14) = 6.799). IL-6 concentrations in secretions from colonic biopsies were not different between HCs $(57.87 \pm 23.6$ pg ml^{-1}), IBS-D $(40.16 \pm 11.45$ pg ml^{-1}) or IBS-C $(28.8 \pm 7.7$ pg ml^{-1}, one-way ANOVA F(2,14) = 0.86, p = 0.45) patients. Secretion of IL-8 from colonic biopsies was also similar in supernatants from HCs $(2617 \pm 1197$ pg ml^{-1}) and individuals with IBS-D $(926.7 \pm 358$ pg ml^{-1}) and IBS-C $(1570 \pm 571$ pg ml^{-1}, one-way ANOVA F(2,15) = 1.31, p = 0.304).

Colonic Tuft Cell Density Is Elevated in Stress-Sensitive Wistar Kyoto Rats

Immunofluorescence and confocal microscopy were used to determine the presence and prevalence of tuft cells in the colons of IBS-like Wistar Kyoto (WKY) rats as compared to Sprague Dawley (SD) controls. Triple-labeling with DAPI, anti-DCLK1 (red staining) and a cytoskeletal marker (green labeling) was carried out on colonic cross-sections from SD and WKY rats to determine the density of tuft cells in each rat strain. DCLK1-labeled tuft cells were readily identifiable in cross-sections of both SD and WKY colons (**Figure 2**, red staining, tuft cells indicated by arrows). However, in contrast to tuft cells in human colonic mucosa, rat DCLK1-labeled tuft cells did not strongly express phalloidin-labeled cytoskeletal proteins. They did however, exhibit similar flask shaped morphology (**Figure 2**). The overall number of DAPI-labeled cells was comparable

between SD $(197.7 \pm 49.3$, n = 3) and WKY $(219.3 \pm 22.7$, n = 3, p >0.05, Student's t-test) rats. However, the number of tuft cells in WKY rats (n = nine slices from three rats) was increased as compared to SD controls (n = nine slices from three rats; p <0.05, Student's t-test, **Figure 2**).

Tuft Cell Density Does Not Change in Response to Chronic Stress

As sensitivity to stress is a key trait of both WKY rats (26–28) and human IBS (29), we investigated if chronic stress alone impacted on numbers of tuft cells. Colons from male C57/BL6J control mice were compared to mice which had endured 10 consecutive days of chronic social defeat stress (21). The overall number of DAPI-stained epithelial cells in non-stressed control C57/BL6J mice $(452.8 \pm 109.6$, n = 4) was not different to stressed mice $(402.5 \pm 94.63$, n = 4, p >0.05, Student's t-test). DCLK1-labeled (red staining, tuft cells indicated by arrows, **Figure 3**) tuft cells were evident in the colonic mucosa of these mice, but similar to the rat tissue, strong actin labeling was not evident. The density of mucosal tuft cells did not differ between stressed C57/BL6J mice and their non-stressed comparators (n = 15 slices from five mice, p >0.05, Student's t-test, **Figure 3**).

DISCUSSION

Tuft cells have been proposed as chemosensory sentinels important in the host response to exposure to common eukaryotes, such as helminths and protists (11). Although not well elucidated, mechanisms involving basolateral release of immune or neuromodulatory factors from these cells may result in modulation of gut function (9) through interaction

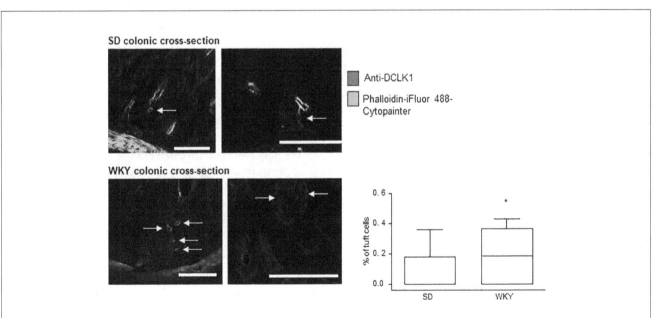

FIGURE 2 | Tuft cell density is increased in Wistar Kyoto (WKY) colons. The representative immunofluorescent images and box and whisker plots of pooled data show the density of DCLK1-labeled tuft cells as a percentage of the total DAPI-stained epithelial cells. Numbers of tuft cells are increased in stress-sensitive WKY rats, which have been validated as an animal model of IBS, as compared to Sprague Dawley control rats. * indicates p <0.05. Scalebar: 50 μm.

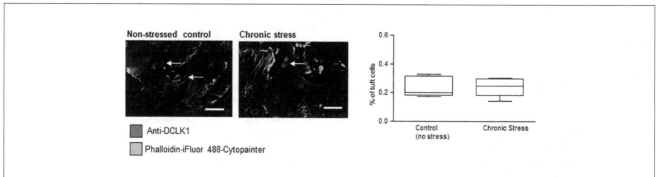

FIGURE 3 | Tuft cell density is not altered by chronic stress. The representative immunofluorescent images and box and whisker plots of pooled data show the density of DCLK1-labeled tuft cells as a percentage of the total DAPI-stained epithelial cells. No difference in the density of tuft cells was detected in colonic samples from mice which had undergone chronic stress. Scalebar: 50 µm.

with enteric neural plexi (7, 8). We have examined tuft cell density in colonic mucosal biopsies from patients with IBS, diagnosed in the absence of previous known enteric infection. Increased density of tuft cells was detected only in diarrhea-predominant IBS biopsies. Thus, tuft cell hyperplasia may represent a potential biomarker for this subtype of IBS.

The intestinal profile of IBS patients exhibits lower bacterial diversity that healthy individuals (30, 31). Moreover, transfer of faecal microbiota from IBS-D patients is sufficient to evoke changes in gut function, low-grade inflammation and the expression of anxiety-like behaviors in germ-free mice (32). However, studies focussed only on bacteria cannot explain the heterogeneity of IBS symptomology (33, 34). Given that the human microbiome includes many other non-bacterial microorganisms such as viruses, fungi, archaea and protozoans; other luminal residents have the potential to contribute to the pathophysiology of this functional bowel disorder. Indeed, the mycobiome differs in IBS patients (35) and viral infection has been linked to increased risk of developing IBS (36). The prevalence of protozoans is also increased in IBS patients (37) with some, such as *Dientamoeba fragilis* (38) and *Giardia intestinalis* (39) actually inducing IBS-like symptoms such as abdominal pain and looseness of stools. Chemosensory activation of tuft cells, which are in close proximity to the neuronal plexi that regulate gut function (7, 8), could therefore potentially contribute to IBS symptom manifestation.

Immunofluorescent labeling of tuft cells in mucosal biopsies revealed rare DCLK1-expressing cells which displayed classic pear-shaped morphology (2) and a strong cytoskeletal component. Similar to other studies (1), we found that these tuft cells made up less than 0.4% of DAPI-labeled epithelial cells in control subjects. Biopsies from the distal colon of patients with IBS-C had a similar prevalence of tuft cells to healthy study participants, however, in the absence of any change in total epithelial cell number, IBS-D patients exhibited tuft cell hyperplasia. Although an active helminth infection can induce more than ten-fold increase in tuft cell numbers in the upper intestine (12), our more modest results (< 2 fold) are present in the absence of any documented history of enteric infection.

Helminths and protists evoke a type 2 innate immune response, which is characterized by secretion of ILC2 cytokines. In particular, IL-25, which, in the intestine, is uniquely secreted by tuft cells, is a key signalling molecule secreted in responses to helminth infections (40, 41). IL-25 subsequently stimulates ILC2 to secrete IL-5, IL-9 and IL-13. IL-13 promotes goblet cell hyperplasia and in a feed-forward cycle, tuft cell hyperplasia. Increased goblet cell activity and mucus secretion has been reported in IBS patients (42) and we now provide evidence of tuft cell hyperplasia in IBS-D colonic mucosal samples.

Interestingly, in one study, biopsy-secreted IL-13 was decreased as compared to controls in PI-IBS patients, who had a history of acute gastroenteritis with diarrhea and/or vomiting, (43), although in contrasting results, stimulated lymphocytes from IBS patients secreted more IL-13 as compared to controls, leading the authors to conclude that exposure to bacterial products led to a shift from a Th1 to a Th2 type of cytokine production (44). Our study has detected increased epithelial tuft cell numbers in IBS-D colonic biopsies. Concentrations of local and circulating IL-25 are also elevated in IBS-D samples, which could be related to tuft cell hyperplasia, although no statistical correlation was detected. However, small sample sizes of each IBS subtype could underlie this finding, which is a recognized limitation of the study. Overall, plasma concentrations of IL-25 were notably higher than local secretions, which likely reflects cumulative tuft cell secretion throughout the gut.

We have previously reported changes in cytokine profiles in IBS patients from this geographical region (24, 25), with elevated concentrations of IL-6 and IL-8 in pooled plasma samples from all IBS subtypes. We were able to reproduce these findings in pooled samples, however, subtype-specific analysis determined that IL-6 was only significantly increased in IBS-D subtypes. In contrast, plasma concentrations of IL-8, was elevated only in IBS-C samples. No differences in local concentrations of IL-6 or IL-8 were detected in secretions from colonic biopsies and indeed, there was no statistical correlation between tuft cell density and concentrations of these cytokines. IL-6 and IL-8 both have neurostimulatory actions in the enteric nervous system and also modify gut function (27, 45, 46). While tuft cells have been linked with enteric neuronal function (7, 8), and IL-25 receptor immune-reactivity has been detected in central neurons (47), further studies are needed to explore if this cytokine can modify activity in enteric neurons or gut function. Indeed, if this is found to be the case, it could be through indirect mechanisms, such as through stimulation of mucosal mast cells (48) or other immune cells (10, 11, 49) which are activated by IL-25.

Validated animal models of IBS have been very useful in understanding the pathophysiological changes underlying bowel dysfunction. One such model is the WKY rat, which exhibits visceral hypersensitivity, raised corticosterone in response to a challenge (50) and increased stress-induced defecation (26, 27). Moreover, WKY rats exhibit altered colonic morphology including elevated levels of mucus-secreting goblet cells (26). We determined that distal colonic mucosal sections display DCLK1-immunostained tuft cells with a prevalence of <0.4% in control SD rats. In contrast to the human biopsies, these tuft cells did not express overly strong cytoskeletal proteins. Nonetheless, tuft cell hyperplasia was apparent in the WKY rat model of IBS. In contrast to the human study participants, who may have unknowingly been exposed to parasites resulting in altered bowel function and changes to mucosal cells, the controlled environment in which laboratory animals are maintained, allows us to say with confidence that these animals have not been exposed to helminths or protists. Thus, some other factor may contribute to the increase in tuft cell numbers in WKY rats.

It is generally accepted that psychological stressors are complicit in the onset (51), exacerbation and prolongation of IBS symptoms (52, 53). Stressors can also modify gut morphology and permeability (54). Sensitivity to stress is a key trait in WKY rats, but modified cytokine profiles indicate that immune activation (55), among other factors, also contribute to the overall phenotype. Two groups of C57/BL6J mice, reared under controlled conditions and protected from helminth exposure, were compared to explore if stress alone modifies expression of epithelial tuft cells. A control, non-stressed group was compared to mice which were susceptible to the stress associated with ten consecutive days of chronic social defeat stress. A previously published study using these mice demonstrated that susceptible mice exhibited elevated levels of corticosterone and adrenal gland weight, reflecting dysregulation of the hypothalamic–pituitary–adrenal axis (21). Stressed mice did not exhibit changes in the numbers of colonic epithelial tuft cells, suggesting that activation of the stress axis *per se* does not lead to tuft cell hyperplasia. However, as these mice did display some changes in innate immunity (21), the chronic stressor clearly impacts other systems apart from the stress response.

These studies have determined that tuft cell hyperplasia is evident in patients with IBS-D with no history of enteric infection. A parallel increase in secreted and circulating IL-25 was also observed. Although no statistical correlation was detected between tuft cell density and IL-25 concentrations, this may be detected with a larger sample size. Tuft cell hyperplasia was replicated in a rat model of IBS, which was not exposed to microbes such as helminths or protists. Activation of the stress response, which is central to symptom manifestation and prolongation in functional bowel disturbances, had no impact on tuft cell densities in mice, suggesting that stress, in of itself, does not contribute to tuft cell hyperplasia. The clinical diagnosis of IBS is hampered by the lack of specific biological biomarkers, necessitating a symptom-based diagnosis following exclusion of other organic diseases. Our findings contribute to gathering evidence of subtype-specific changes in intestinal epithelial morphology in IBS patients.

ETHICS STATEMENT

The studies involving human participants were reviewed and approved by University College Cork Clinical Research Ethics Committee (ECM 4 (r) 010316). The patients/participants provided their written informed consent to participate in this study. The animal study was reviewed and approved by University College Cork animal ethical committee (#2011/015).

AUTHOR CONTRIBUTIONS

JA and MC performed the research and analyzed the data. JB contributed human samples. DO'M designed the research study, sourced funding, prepared and reviewed the manuscript.

ACKNOWLEDGMENTS

We express our thanks to Rebecca O'Brien, UCC; Maria M. Buckley, UCC and Anand Gururajan, UCC for their help with this study.

REFERENCES

1. McKinley ET, Sui Y, Al-Kofahi Y, Millis BA, Tyska MJ, Roland JT, et al. Optimized multiplex immunofluorescence single-cell analysis reveals tuft cell heterogeneity. *JCI Insight* (2017) 2(11):e93487. doi: 10.1172/jci.insight.93487
2. Sato A. Tuft cells. *Anat. Sci Int* (2007) 82:187–99. doi: 10.1111/j.1447-073X.2007.00188.x
3. Gerbe F, Jay P. Intestinal tuft cells: epithelial sentinels linking luminal cues to the immune system. *Mucosal. Immunol* (2016) 9:1353–9. doi: 10.1038/mi.2016.68
4. Gerbe F, Legraverend C, Jay P. The intestinal epithelium tuft cells: specification and function. *Cell Mol Life Sci* (2012) 69:2907–17. doi: 10.1007/s00018-012-0984-7
5. Höfer D, Drenckhahn D. Identification of the taste cell G-protein, alpha-gustducin, in brush cells of the rat pancreatic duct system. *Histochem. Cell Biol* (1998) 110:303–9. doi: 10.1007/s004180050292
6. Gerbe F, van Es JH, Makrini L, Brulin B, Mellitzer G, Robine S, et al. Distinct ATOH1 and Neurog3 requirements define tuft cells as a new secretory cell type in the intestinal epithelium. *J Cell Biol* (2011) 192:767–80. doi: 10.1083/jcb.201010127

7. Bezencon C, Furholz A, Raymond F, Mansourian R, Metairon S, Le Coutre J, et al. Murine intestinal cells expressing Trpm5 are mostly brush cells and express markers of neuronal and inflammatory cells. *J Comp Neurol* (2008) 509:514–25. doi: 10.1002/cne.21768

8. Westphalen CB, Asfaha S, Hayakawa Y, Takemoto Y, Lukin DJ, Nuber AH, et al. Long-lived intestinal tuft cells serve as colon cancer-initiating cells. *J Clin Invest* (2014) 124:1283–95. doi: 10.1172/JCI73434

9. Schneider C, O'Leary CE, Locksley RM. Regulation of immune responses by tuft cells. *Nat Rev Immunol* (2019) 19(9):584–93. doi: 10.1038/s41577-019-0176-x

10. Howitt MR, Lavoie S, Michaud M, Blum AM, Tran SV, Weinstock JV, et al. Tuft cells, taste-chemosensory cells, orchestrate parasite type 2 immunity in the gut. *Science* (2016) 351:1329–33. doi: 10.1126/science.aaf1648

11. Gerbe F, Sidot E, Smyth DJ, Ohmoto M, Matsumoto I, Dardalhon V, et al. Intestinal epithelial tuft cells initiate type 2 mucosal immunity to helminth parasites. *Nature* (2016) 529:226–30. doi: 10.1038/nature16527

12. von Moltke J, Ji M, Liang HE, Locksley RM. Tuft-cell-derived IL-25 regulates an intestinal ILC2-epithelial response circuit. *Nature* (2016) 529:221–5. doi: 10.1038/nature16161

13. Fort MM, Cheung J, Yen D, Li J, Zurawski SM, Lo S, et al. IL-25 induces IL-4, IL-5, and IL-13 and Th2-associated pathologies in vivo. *Immunity* (2001) 15:985–95. doi: 10.1016/S1074-7613(01)00243-6

14. Grencis RK, Worthington JJ. Tuft Cells: A New Flavor in Innate Epithelial Immunity. *Trends Parasitol.* (2016) 32:583–5. doi: 10.1016/j.pt.2016.04.016

15. Quigley EMM. The Gut-Brain Axis and the Microbiome: Clues to Pathophysiology and Opportunities for Novel Management Strategies in Irritable Bowel Syndrome (IBS). *J Clin Med* (2018) 7(1):E6. doi: 10.3390/jcm7010006

16. Chey WD, Kurlander J, Eswaran S. Irritable bowel syndrome: a clinical review. *JAMA* (2015) 313:949–58. doi: 10.1001/jama.2015.0954

17. Spiller R, Garsed K. Postinfectious irritable bowel syndrome. *Gastroenterology* (2009) 136:1979–88. doi: 10.1053/j.gastro.2009.02.074

18. O'Malley D. Immunomodulation of enteric neural function in irritable bowel syndrome. *World J Gastroenterol* (2015) 21:7362–6. doi: 10.3748/wjg.v21.i24.7362

19. Klem F, Wadhwa A, Prokop LJ, Sundt WJ, Farrugia G, Camilleri M, et al. Prevalence, Risk Factors, and Outcomes of Irritable Bowel Syndrome After Infectious Enteritis: A Systematic Review and Meta-analysis. *Gastroenterology* (2017) 152:1042–1054 e1. doi: 10.1053/j.gastro.2016.12.039

20. Lackner JM, Ma CX, Keefer L, Brenner DM, Gudleski GD, Satchidanand N, et al. Type, rather than number, of mental and physical comorbidities increases the severity of symptoms in patients with irritable bowel syndrome. *Clin Gastroenterol Hepatol* (2013) 11:1147–57. doi: 10.1016/j.cgh.2013.03.011

21. Gururajan A, van de Wouw M, Boehme M, Becker T, O'Connor R, Bastiaanssen TFS, et al. Resilience to chronic stress is associated with specific neurobiological, neuroendocrine and immune responses. *Brain Behav Immun* (2019) 80:583–94. doi: 10.1016/j.bbi.2019.05.004

22. May R, Riehl TE, Hunt C, Sureban SM, Anant S, Houchen CW. Identification of a novel putative gastrointestinal stem cell and adenoma stem cell marker, doublecortin and CaM kinase-like-1, following radiation injury and in adenomatous polyposis coli/multiple intestinal neoplasia mice. *Stem Cells* (2008) 26:630–7. doi: 10.1634/stemcells.2007-0621

23. Gerbe F, Brulin B, Makrini L, Legraverend C, Jay P. DCAMKL-1 expression identifies Tuft cells rather than stem cells in the adult mouse intestinal epithelium. *Gastroenterology* (2009) 137:2179–80. doi: 10.1053/j.gastro.2009.06.072

24. Dinan TG, Quigley EM, Ahmed SM, Scully P, O'Brien S, O'Mahony L, et al. Hypothalamic-pituitary-gut axis dysregulation in irritable bowel syndrome: plasma cytokines as a potential biomarker? *Gastroenterology* (2006) 130:304–11. doi: 10.1053/j.gastro.2005.11.033

25. Dinan TG, Clarke G, Quigley EM, Scott LV, Shanahan F, Cryan J, et al. Enhanced cholinergic-mediated increase in the pro-inflammatory cytokine IL-6 in irritable bowel syndrome: role of muscarinic receptors. *Am J Gastroenterol* (2008) 103:2570–6. doi: 10.1111/j.1572-0241.2008.01871.x

26. O'Malley D, Julio-Pieper M, Gibney SM, Dinan TG, Cryan JF. Distinct alterations in colonic morphology and physiology in two rat models of enhanced stress-induced anxiety and depression-like behaviour. *Stress* (2010) 13:114–22. doi: 10.3109/10253890903067418

27. Buckley MM, O'Halloran KD, Rae MG, Dinan TG, O'Malley D. Modulation of enteric neurons by interleukin-6 and corticotropin-releasing factor contributes to visceral hypersensitivity and altered colonic motility in a rat model of irritable bowel syndrome. *J Physiol* (2014) 592(23):5235–50. doi: 10.1113/jphysiol.2014.279968

28. Braw Y, Malkesman O, Dagan M, Bercovich A, Lavi-Avnon Y, Schroeder M, et al. Anxiety-like behaviors in pre-pubertal rats of the Flinders Sensitive Line (FSL) and Wistar-Kyoto (WKY) animal models of depression. *Behav Brain Res* (2006) 167:261–9. doi: 10.1016/j.bbr.2005.09.013

29. Levy RL, Olden KW, Naliboff BD, Bradley LA, Francisconi C, Drossman DA, et al. Psychosocial aspects of the functional gastrointestinal disorders. *Gastroenterology* (2006) 130:1447–58. doi: 10.1053/j.gastro.2005.11.057

30. Raskov H, Burcharth J, Pommergaard HC, Rosenberg J. Irritable bowel syndrome, the microbiota and the gut-brain axis. *Gut Microbes* (2016) 7:365–83. doi: 10.1080/19490976.2016.1218585

31. Ohman L, Simren M. Intestinal microbiota and its role in irritable bowel syndrome (IBS). *Curr Gastroenterol Rep* (2013) 15:323. doi: 10.1007/s11894-013-0323-7

32. De Palma G, Lynch MD, Lu J, Dang VT, Deng Y, Jury J, et al. Transplantation of fecal microbiota from patients with irritable bowel syndrome alters gut function and behavior in recipient mice. *Sci Transl Med* (2017) 99(379): eaaf6397. doi: 10.1126/scitranslmed.aaf6397

33. Frost F, Kacprowski T, Ruhlemann MC, Franke A, Heinsen FA, Volker U, et al. Functional abdominal pain and discomfort (IBS) is not associated with faecal microbiota composition in the general population. *Gut* (2019) 68:1131–3 doi: 10.1136/gutjnl-2018-316502

34. Maharshak N, Ringel Y, Katibian D, Lundqvist A, Sartor RB, Carroll IM, et al. Fecal and Mucosa-Associated Intestinal Microbiota in Patients with Diarrhea-Predominant Irritable Bowel Syndrome. *Dig Dis Sci* (2018) 63:1890–9. doi: 10.1007/s10620-018-5086-4

35. Gu Y, Zhou G, Qin X, Huang S, Wang B, Cao H. The Potential Role of Gut Mycobiome in Irritable Bowel Syndrome. *Front Microbiol.* (2019) 10:1894 doi: 10.3389/fmicb.2019.01894

36. Zanini B, Ricci C, Bandera F, Caselani F, Magni A, Laronga AM, et al. Incidence of post-infectious irritable bowel syndrome and functional intestinal disorders following a water-borne viral gastroenteritis outbreak. *Am J Gastroenterol* (2012) 107:891–9. doi: 10.1038/ajg.2012.102

37. Jadallah KA, Nimri LF, Ghanem RA. Protozoan parasites in irritable bowel syndrome: A case-control study. *World J Gastrointest. Pharmacol Ther* (2017) 8:201–7. doi: 10.4292/wjgpt.v8.i4.201

38. Stark D, Beebe N, Marriott D, Ellis J, Harkness J. Prospective study of the prevalence, genotyping, and clinical relevance of Dientamoeba fragilis infections in an Australian population. *J Clin Microbiol* (2005) 43:2718–23. doi: 10.1128/JCM.43.6.2718-2723.2005

39. Grazioli B, Matera G, Laratta C, Schipani G, Guarnieri G, Spiniello E, et al. Giardia lamblia infection in patients with irritable bowel syndrome and dyspepsia: a prospective study. *World J Gastroenterol* (2006) 12:1941–4. doi: 10.3748/wjg.v12.i12.1941

40. Owyang AM, Zaph C, Wilson EH, Guild KJ, McClanahan T, Miller HR, et al. Interleukin 25 regulates type 2 cytokine-dependent immunity and limits chronic inflammation in the gastrointestinal tract. *J Exp Med* (2006) 203:843–9. doi: 10.1084/jem.20051496

41. Fallon PG, Ballantyne SJ, Mangan NE, Barlow JL, Dasvarma A, Hewett DR, et al. Identification of an interleukin (IL)-25-dependent cell population that provides IL-4, IL-5, and IL-13 at the onset of helminth expulsion. *J Exp Med* (2006) 203:1105–16. doi: 10.1084/jem.20051615

42. Cheng P, Yao J, Wang C, Zhang L, Kong W. Molecular and cellular mechanisms of tight junction dysfunction in the irritable bowel syndrome. *Mol Med Rep* (2015) 12:3257–64. doi: 10.3892/mmr.2015.3808

43. Sundin J, Rangel I, Repsilber D, Brummer RJ. Cytokine Response after Stimulation with Key Commensal Bacteria Differ in Post-Infectious Irritable Bowel Syndrome (PI-IBS) Patients Compared to Healthy Controls. *PloS One* (2015) 10:e0134836. doi: 10.1371/journal.pone.0134836

44. Kindt S, Van Oudenhove L, Broekaert D, Kasran A, Ceuppens JL, Bossuyt X, et al. Immune dysfunction in patients with functional gastrointestinal disorders. *Neurogastroent. Motil* (2009) 21:389–98. doi: 10.1111/j.1365-2982.2008.01220.x

45. O'Malley D, Cryan JF, Dinan TG. Crosstalk between interleukin-6 and corticotropin-releasing factor modulate submucosal plexus activity and colonic secretion. *Brain Behav Immun* (2013) 30:115–24. doi: 10.1016/j.bbi.2013.01.078

46. O'Malley D, Liston M, Hyland NP, Dinan TG, Cryan JF. Colonic soluble mediators from the maternal separation model of irritable bowel syndrome activate submucosal neurons via an interleukin-6-dependent mechanism. *Am J Physiol Gastrointest. Liver Physiol* (2011) 300:G241–52. doi: 10.1152/ ajpgi.00385.2010

47. Kan AA, de Jager W, de Wit M, Heijnen C, van Zuiden M, Ferrier C, et al. Protein expression profiling of inflammatory mediators in human temporal lobe epilepsy reveals co-activation of multiple chemokines and cytokines. *J Neuroinflamm* (2012) 9:207. doi: 10.1186/1742-2094-9-207

48. Gordon ED, Locksley RM, Fahy JV. Cross-Talk between Epithelial Cells and Type 2 Immune Signaling. The Role of IL-25. *Am J Respir Crit Care Med* (2016) 193:935–6. doi: 10.1164/rccm.201512-2534ED

49. Seyedmirzaee S, Hayatbakhsh MM, Ahmadi B, Baniasadi N, Rafsanjani AMB, Nikpoor AR, et al. Serum immune biomarkers in irritable bowel syndrome. *Clinics Res Hepatol Gastroenterol* (2016) 40:631–7. doi: 10.1016/ j.clinre.2015.12.013

50. O'Mahony SM, Clarke G, McKernan DP, Bravo JA, Dinan TG, Cryan JF. Differential visceral nociceptive, behavioural and neurochemical responses to an immune challenge in the stress-sensitive Wistar Kyoto rat strain. *Behav Brain Res* (2013) 253:310–7. doi: 10.1016/j.bbr.2013.07.023

51. Mayer EA, Naliboff BD, Chang L, Coutinho SV. V. Stress and irritable bowel syndrome. *Am J Physiol Gastrointest. Liver Physiol* (2001) 280:G519–24. doi: 10.1152/ajpgi.2001.280.4.G519

52. Saha L. Irritable bowel syndrome: pathogenesis, diagnosis, treatment, and evidence-based medicine. *World J Gastroenterol* (2014) 20:6759–73. doi: 10.3748/wjg.v20.i22.6759

53. Moloney RD, Johnson AC, O'Mahony SM, Dinan TG, Greenwood-Van Meerveld B, Cryan JF. Stress and the Microbiota-Gut-Brain Axis in Visceral Pain: Relevance to Irritable Bowel Syndrome. *CNS Neurosci Ther* (2016) 22:102–17. doi: 10.1111/cns.12490

54. Soderholm JD, Perdue MH. Stress and gastrointestinal tract. II. Stress and intestinal barrier function. *Am J Physiol Gastrointest. Liver Physiol* (2001) 280: G7–G13. doi: 10.1152/ajpgi.2001.280.1.G7

55. O'Malley D, Dinan TG, Cryan JF. Interleukin-6 modulates colonic transepithelial ion transport in the stress-sensitive wistar kyoto rat. *Front Pharmacol* (2012) 3:190. doi: 10.3389/fphar.2012.00190

2

The Role of Brain-Derived Neurotrophic Factor in Irritable Bowel Syndrome

Thomas Jan Konturek [1,2], Cristina Martinez [3,4], Beate Niesler [4,5], Ivo van der Voort [2,6], Hubert Mönnikes [2], Andreas Stengel [7] and Miriam Goebel-Stengel [2,7,8*]

[1] Division of Gastroenterology, Loyola University Medical Center, Stritch School of Medicine, Maywood, IL, United States, [2] Department of Internal Medicine, Institute of Neurogastroenterology, Martin Luther Hospital, Johannesstift Diakonie, Berlin, Germany, [3] Lleida Institute for Biomedical Research Dr. Pifarré Foundation (IRBLleida), Lleida, Spain, [4] Department of Human Molecular Genetics, University Hospital Heidelberg, Heidelberg, Germany, [5] nCounter Core Facility Heidelberg, Institute of Human Genetics, Heidelberg, Germany, [6] Department of Internal Medicine and Gastroenterology, Berlin Jewish Hospital, Berlin, Germany, [7] Department of Psychosomatic Medicine, University Hospital Tübingen, Tübingen, Germany, [8] Department of Internal Medicine and Gastroenterology, Helios Clinic Rottweil, Rottweil, Germany

*Correspondence:
Miriam Goebel-Stengel
miriam.stengel@helios-gesundheit.de

Several studies have implied a role of brain-derived neurotrophic factor (BDNF) in abdominal pain modulation in irritable bowel syndrome (IBS). The aim of this study was to establish BDNF protein expression in human colonic biopsies and to show variation in IBS compared to controls. BDNF protein and mRNA levels were correlated with IBS symptom severity based on the IBS-symptom severity score (IBS-SSS). Biopsies from the descending colon and IBS-SSS were obtained from 10 controls and 20 IBS patients. Total protein of biopsies was extracted and assessed by ELISA and Western Blot. Total mRNA was extracted and gene expression measured by nCounter analysis. In IBS patients, symptom severity scores ranged from 124 to 486 (mean ± sem: 314.2 ± 21.2, >300 represents severe IBS) while controls ranged from 0 to 72 (mean ± sem: 27.7 ± 9.0, <75 represents healthy subjects, $p < 0.001$). IBS patients reported significantly more food malabsorption, former abdominal surgery and psychiatric comorbidities. BDNF protein was present in all samples and did not differ between IBS and controls or sex. Subgroup analysis showed that female IBS patients expressed significantly more BDNF mRNA compared to male patients ($p < 0.05$) and male IBS-D patients had higher IBS symptom severity scores and lower BDNF mRNA and protein levels compared to male controls ($p < 0.05$). Scatter plot showed a significant negative correlation between IBS-SSS and BDNF mRNA levels in the cohort of male IBS-D patients and their male controls ($p < 0.05$). We detected a high proportion of gastrointestinal surgery in IBS patients and confirmed food intolerances and psychiatric diseases as common comorbidities. Although in a small sample, we demonstrated that BDNF is detectable in human descending colon, with higher BDNF mRNA levels in female IBS patients compared to males and lower mRNA and protein levels in male IBS-D patients compared to male controls. Further research should be directed toward subgroups of IBS since their etiologies might be different.

Keywords: comorbidities, colonic biopsy, hypersensitivity, IBS subgroup, symptom severity

INTRODUCTION

Irritable bowel syndrome (IBS) is a debilitating (but not life-threatening) disorder of brain-gut interaction characterized by abdominal pain and dysfunctional bowel habits based on the Rome IV criteria as the latest worldwide standard for the diagnosis of IBS (1).

The pathophysiology of IBS is based on a multifactorial and bidirectional dysfunction of the brain-gut-axis including genetics and epigenetics, visceral hypersensitivity, changes in the synthesis and release of neuropeptides and proinflammatory cytokines and altered gastrointestinal motility as well as psychosomatic predisposition (2).

The brain-derived neurotrophic factor (BDNF) belongs to the family of nerve growth factors (NGF). Through interaction with the tyrosine receptor kinase B (TrkB) (3) BDNF promotes the survival and differentiation of brain neurons, and participates in the modification of neurotransmission and synaptic plasticity of the central and peripheral nervous systems (4). Dysfunctions in epigenetic control, transport or signal cascades of BDNF were discussed on an emergence of various neurological and psychiatric diseases (5). There is also ample evidence of an important role played by BDNF in visceral pain and hypersensitivity conditions (6–11).

Studies in the murine colon showed that BDNF mRNA was expressed in epithelial cells and neurons of the myenteric plexus, and that BDNF levels in the colon were higher than in the brain (12, 13). Similar studies in rats showed that BDNF can be isolated in the distal colonic mucosa. In humans, BDNF has so far been established in the gastric corpus (14), dorsal root ganglia (15, 16), in enteric ganglion cells (17) and in blood (18). Four studies confirmed the presence of BDNF protein in human colonic mucosa of the rectosigmoid junction (11, 19–21).

There is growing evidence of the effects of BDNF on intestinal activity (6–9, 20, 22). Studies in human subjects showed that treatment with recombinant BDNF for several diseases was accompanied by changes in bowel activity. Patients reported a dose-dependent increase in stool frequency and changes in stool consistency, the related mechanism being unclear. In another study, administration of recombinant BDNF in healthy subjects showed an increase in total as well as proximal colonic transit time (23).

Four studies have specifically examined the involvement of BDNF in IBS and its correlation with symptom severity (11, 19–21). Recently, hypermethylated *BDNF* gene, an epigenetic modification, was described in human monocytes and sigmoid colon of IBS patients and was associated with early life stress and psychiatric as well as somatic symptoms (24). However, Videlock et al. performed gene microarray analysis in sigmoid biopsies of subtype-balanced IBS patients and found a multitude of differentially expressed genes, but not BDNF, and only in IBS-C vs. controls (25).

The aim of this study is to demonstrate that BDNF mRNA and protein are detectable in human colonic biopsies and to determine if these correlate with symptom predominance and severity in IBS.

MATERIALS AND METHODS

Study Location

The study was performed with patients with IBS and healthy control subjects at the Institute for Neurogastroenterology at Martin Luther Hospital, a teaching hospital of Charité-Universitätsmedizin in Berlin, Germany between 2011 and 2014. Molecular analysis was carried out at the research institution Charité-Universitätsmedizin Berlin, Campus Virchow Klinikum and Department of Human Molecular Genetics at University of Heidelberg.

Ethics Commission and Patient Selection

All experimental protocols for the human study were approved by the Clinical Ethical Committee of Charité Universitätsmedizin Berlin (ethical approval number EA1/108/11). All study subjects gave their informed written consent prior to enrollment. All methods used in the human study were carried out in accordance with the approved guidelines and according to standard procedures.

Healthy controls: Healthy subjects were recruited within the framework of preventive colonoscopy for colorectal cancer screening. They had no history of IBS.

IBS patients were newly diagnosed and subclassified according to the ROME III criteria on the basis of the predominant symptom and stool pattern (26). In addition, each subject was screened for organic diseases by medical history taking, physical examination, detailed blood and stool analysis and endoscopy.

Participants were age-matched but not gender-matched. A total of 30 participants were eligible to participate in the study.

Inclusion and Exclusion Criteria

The following inclusion criteria applied to all study participants: age between 18 and 65 years; body mass index (BMI) between 20 and 25 kg/m^2; good general condition.

The following criteria led to exclusion of study participants: unstable body weight (weight fluctuation of more than 3 kg within the last month, or weight fluctuation of more than 10 kg in the last 6 months prior to the study); alcohol consumption (>1 alcoholic drink per day); irregular nicotine consumption; pregnancy; use of psychotropic drugs within the last 3 months before the examination; inflammatory bowel disease (IBD); celiac disease; history of malignant tumors and abnormal laboratory values. Laboratory work-up in all study participants included infection parameters with CRP and blood count, INR, electrolytes including sodium and potassium, liver enzymes, kidney function and thyroid hormone TSH. Normal range was based on in-house laboratory standards. Except for sodium, a deviation of >10% (lower or higher) was considered abnormal. For sodium only a deviation of 5% was tolerated. Subjects that displayed parameters outside the normal range were advised to see their general practitioner and could interview again.

Endoscopy and Material Extraction

For every study subject a complete ileocolonoscopy (CF series, Olympus, Japan) was performed by an experienced gastroenterologist including stepwise biopsies from all sections of the ileocolon for routine histology to rule out pathologies.

During withdrawal of the endoscope, five biopsy specimens were removed from the descending colon of each study participant, ~40 to 50 cm above the anocutaneous line. Four colonic biopsy specimens were placed on dry ice and then stored at −80°C, while one biopsy specimen was fixed in formaldehyde at room temperature.

Questionnaire – IBS Symptom Severity Score (IBS-SSS)

All subjects were asked to answer part 1 of the IBS symptom severity score (IBS-SSS) (27). The questionnaire is meant to register complaint levels related to gastrointestinal symptoms in the form of four questions: (1) Do you suffer from abdominal pain? (2) Do you currently suffer from abdominal distention? (3) How satisfied are you with your bowel habits? (4) Please indicate on the line (visual analog scale) below how much your IBS is affecting or interfering with your life in general? A total of 500 points can be reached. A score of up to 75 points is considered as control, 75–175 points as mild IBS, 175–300 as moderate IBS, and more than 300 as severe IBS.

RNA Isolation and Quality Assessment

Total RNA was isolated from IBS and control samples. After disruption in TRIzol, the resulting aqueous phase was cleaned-up by the RNAqueous-Micro Total RNA isolation kit (AM1931, Thermo Fisher Scientific) according to the manufacturer's instructions. Quantity and quality of RNA were assessed by Agilent 2100 Bioanalyzer (Agilent Technologies, Waldbronn, Germany) taking into account the RNA integrity number (RIN) value with a cut off of RIN below 5. Samples were stored at −80°C until expression analysis.

nCounter Analysis

Expression analysis was performed from 100 ng total RNA using the nCounter system Gene 1 (NanoString Technologies, Seattle, USA). A customized codeset comprising 48 target genes including *BDNF* and 7 reference genes was hybridized as recommended by the manufacturer. Background correction and normalization of data was performed using the NanoString software nSolver 3.0 (NanoString Technologies). Stably expressed reference genes were chosen for normalization based on the geNorm method, a popular algorithm to determine the most stable reference genes from a set of tested candidate reference genes in a given sample panel. This algorithm calculates a gene expression normalization factor for each sample based on the geometric mean of a user-defined number of reference genes. The underlying principles and formulas are described in (28). Following this, the selected reference genes were *GAPDH, RPS17, TBP* and *UBC*.

Gel Electrophoresis and Western Blot Analysis

Ten milliliters of phosphate buffer saline solution (PBS) without calcium and magnesium (PAA Laboratories, Pasching, Austria) was first mixed with half a tablet of proteinase inhibitor cocktail (cOmplete™, Mini, 11836170001, EDTA-free Protease Inhibitor Cocktail, Roche, Mannheim, Germany) and processed in a vortex

for 3 s. The finished mixture was distributed in an amount of 400 μl each among lysing matrix tubes (D Matrix, 116913050-CF, MP Biomedicals, California, USA) and placed on ice.

The colonic biopsy specimens stored in the freezer at −80°C were weighed (two biopsies per control subject/patient) with a precision balance (Sartorius, Göttingen, Germany) and then transferred to the prepared matrix tubes, homogenized two times each at 4 m/s for 20 s using a homogenizer (MP Biomedicals, California, USA) and placed on ice for 3 min.

This was followed by centrifugation of the samples at 10 × 1,000 rpm (Eppendorf, Hamburg, Germany) in a cooling chamber at −4°C for 10 min to remove cell debris and nuclei, and subsequent pipetting of the supernatant from the matrix tubes. Final protein concentrations were determined using a BCA protein assay according to the manufacturer's protocol (23225, Pierce Biotechnology, Rockford, IL, USA).

For subsequent sodium dodecyl sulfate - polyacrylamide gel electrophoresis (SDS-PAGE) protein samples were mixed with a gel sample buffer comprising 4% sodium dodecyl sulfate (SDS), 0.05% bromophenol blue solution (w/v), 20% glycerol, 1% mercaptoethanol (v/v) in 0.1 tris(hydroxymethyl)aminomethane (TRIS). The gel samples were immersed for 1 min at 100°C in boiling water, and applied on a 4–12% SDS polyacrylamide gel (Bis-Tris Minigel, NP0321BOX, NuPage; Invitrogen, Carlsbad, CA, USA) with 30 μl of protein per lane. The first lane was filled with 10 μl of a marker (SeeBlue, LC5625, Invitrogen, Carlsbad, CA, USA). A 2-(N-morpholino) ethanesulfonic acid buffer was used as a running buffer. The SDS-PAGE ran for 2 h at 120 V, 300 W, and 350 mA.

After SDS-PAGE, a wet transfer of proteins was carried out by electrophoresis on a nitrocellulose membrane for 1.5 h at room temperature in a TRIS base methanol transfer buffer at pH 8.1–8.4. The membranes were then washed in glass containers using distilled water.

Subsequently, the membranes were stained with Ponceau S staining solution (0.1% Ponceau S and 5% ice acetic acid) to confirm protein transfer. For antibody staining, the membranes were washed twice with TRIS-Tween buffered saline solution (10 mM TRIS, 150 mM NaCl, 0.05% Tween, v/v). This was followed by incubation of the membranes in fat-free milk (Carnation instant skim milk powder, Nestlé, Glendale, CA, USA) for 30 min at room temperature. After removal of the milk, the membranes were washed additionally three times for 5 min each with 15 ml of TRIS-Tween buffered saline solution.

Polyclonal anti-BDNF antibody (ab 72439, Abcam, Cambridge, UK) or a polyclonal antibody against the housekeeping protein β-actin (Ab #4967, Cell Signaling Technology Inc., Danvers, MA, USA) were used in a dilution of 1:5,000 and 1:1,000, respectively, by means of TRIS-Tween buffered saline solution. Incubation took place for 60 min at room temperature on a shaker. This step was followed by a 4-fold washing process with TRIS-Tween buffered saline solution until the secondary antibody was used (alkaline phosphatase conjugated anti-rabbit IgG, S373B 30687401, dilution 1:2,000, Promega, Madison, WI, USA). This was followed by further washing with TRIS-Tween buffered saline solution and subsequent color development in an alkaline phosphatase buffer

(100 mM TRIS, 100 mM sodium chloride and 5 mM magnesium chloride, pH 9.5) according to the manufacturer's protocol. For initiation of the 5-min color reaction in the dark, 5 ml of the alkaline phosphatase buffer were added to each membrane, and the two substances nitro-blue tetrazolium (NBT, 0.3%, N6495, Thermo Scientific, Rockford, IL, USA) and 5-bromo-4-chloro-3-indoxyl phosphate (BCIP, 0.15%, 34040, Thermo Scientific, Rockford, IL, USA) were added.

ELISA

For quantitative determination of the concentration of BDNF protein in colonic biopsies, a commercial BDNF Human ELISA (enzyme-linked immunosorbent assay) Kit (ab99978, Abcam, Cambridge, MA, USA) was used that was based on mouse monoclonal IgG2A antibodies.

The minimum detectable amount of BDNF was 80 pg/ml. Each sample was analyzed in duplicate. The ELISA was run according to the manufacturer's protocol.

Statistics

Since this was a pilot study, no power analysis was included.

Data are presented as mean $\pm$ sem; alternatively, data are indicated as total number and percentage values. Normality was assessed using the Kolmogorow-Smirnov test. Differences were assessed using χ^2-tests, t-tests or the Mann-Whitney-U test depending on the distribution of the data.

Molecular data are presented as mean $\pm$ sem. Normality was assessed using the Kolmogorow-Smirnov test. Differences were assessed using t-tests or the Mann-Whitney-U test depending on the distribution of the data.

For statistical analysis of nCounter data two-tailed Mann-Whitney U test was used with GraphPad Prism 5.0 (Graph Pad Software, La Jolla, CA, USA). Data are summarized by mean $\pm$ standard deviation (SD) or median (range), unless otherwise stated. P-values < 0.05 were considered significant.

RESULTS

Study Population

Characteristics of the study population are outlined in **Table 1**. The IBS group comprised 20 patients (14 female, six male) while 10 healthy subjects participated (two female, eight male). The mean age in the IBS and control group was 55.6 and 49.5 years, respectively. No significant differences were noted in ethnicity (most subjects were Caucasian) and in socioeconomic status with most subjects having a university entrance diploma. It is to note that in the IBS group more incomplete data sets were obtained with regards to partnership, children, level of education and employment status.

Comparing comorbidities, 89% of subjects in the IBS group were suffering from an intestinal malabsorption compared to 0% in the control group ($p < 0.001$) with fructose malabsorption and lactose intolerance being most prevalent. Somatoform and psychiatric disorders which have been associated with IBS (29) were of a wide spectrum and could be found in 42% ($p = 0.048$) of subjects in the IBS group compared to 0% in the control group.

Diagnosis of gastritis and peptic ulcer disease (**Table 1**) was based on patient charts and history. Two controls reported nonspecific chronic gastritis. Of IBS patients, 2 had a history of Helicobacter pylori (H.pylori) positive antrum or corpus gastritis, respectively, while two had H. pylori negative antrum gastritis and one had a history of healing duodenal ulcer. Of those five patients, only one (H. pylori negative antrum gastritis) was on proton pump inhibitor medication at the time of study. Neither patients nor controls underwent diagnostics for functional dyspepsia.

There was also a significantly higher amount of prior abdominal surgeries noted in the IBS group (42 vs. 0% in control group, $p = 0.048$). Hysterectomy and cholecystectomy were the most frequent surgeries in the IBS group with 26 and 21%, respectively. Three women had undergone oophorectomies but were past menopause and not taking any hormonal supplements.

Overall, IBS patients tended to take more medications than control subjects ($p = 0.191$).

BDNF Is Detectable in Human Descending Colonic Tissue With Similar Levels in IBS Patients and Healthy Controls

Western blot analysis of human colonic biopsies containing mucosa and submucosa of the descending colon stained with anti-BDNF antibody indicated multiple prominent bands (**Figure 1**). The presence of different molecular weight forms of BDNF has been reported in prior studies using cultured neuronal and non-neuronal cells (30, 31) and represents differently glycosylated and glycosulfated forms of mature BDNF and proBDNF (32). BDNF was further successfully quantified using ELISA confirming the above Western Blot findings (**Figures 2B,E, Supplementary Figures 1B,E**) and by nCounter analysis (**Figure 2C**). No notable differences in BDNF protein and BDNF mRNA expression between healthy controls and IBS patients were detected.

Characterization of IBS in Patient Population

In the IBS group, 14 subjects met criteria for diarrhea-predominant IBS (IBS-D), 2 for constipation-predominant IBS (IBS-C), 3 for IBS with mixed bowel habits (IBS-M) and 1 for unsubtyped IBS. Mean duration of disease in the IBS group was 6.1 ± 1.5 (1–22) years.

Mean symptom severity was significantly higher in the IBS group as compared to controls (314.2 ± 20.7 vs. 27.7 ± 8.5, $p < 0.001$, **Figure 2A, Supplementary Figure 1A**). No differences in symptom severity were noted in men and women both within the IBS group and the control group (**Table 2**).

Based on the IBS-SSS, most subjects in the IBS group were classified as either having severity grade 2 (40%) or severity grade 3 (50%).

Women With IBS Show Higher BDNF Levels Than Men With IBS

Female IBS patients had significantly more BDNF mRNA expression compared to male IBS patients (13.2 ± 3.6 vs. 4.7 ± 1.1, $p < 0.05$).

BDNF protein tissue levels in women with IBS compared to men with IBS were not significantly different (2.0 ± 0.3 ng/mg vs.

TABLE 1 | Demographic and socioeconomic characteristics, comorbidities, and medication of study patients.

Parameter	Group		p
	Control ($n = 10$, ♀ = 2, ♂ = 8)	IBS ($n = 20$, ♀ = 14, ♂ = 6)	
Demographic characteristics			
Age (years)	55.6 ± 3.0 (38–65)	49.5 ± 3.8 (20–74)	0.301
Ethnicity			
Caucasian	10 (100%)	19 (95%)	0.719
Mediterranean	0 (0%)	1 (5%)	
Socioeconomic characteristics			
Living in a partnership (yes/no)	6/4	10/5 (5 missing data)	0.932
Children (yes/no)	5/5	11/4 (5 missing data)	0.444
Level of Education		5 missing data	0.870
- University entrance diploma	6 (60%)	9 (60%)	
- Secondary education certificate	2 (20%)	2 (13%)	
- Basic school qualification	2 (20%)	4 (27%)	
- Without school-leaving qualification	0 (0%)	0 (0%)	
Currently employed (yes/no)	5/5	8/7 (5 missing data)	0.806
Comorbidities			
Gastrointestinal	6 (60%)	13 (68%, 1 missing data)	0.996
- Reflux esophagitis	2 (20%)	2 (11%)	
- Diaphragmatic hernia	0 (0%)	1 (5%)	
- Gastritis	2 (20%)	4 (21%)	
- Duodenal ulcer	0 (0%)	1 (5%)	
- Diverticular disease	2 (20%)	3 (16%)	
- Hämorrhoids	0 (0%)	2 (11%)	
Malabsorption	0 (0%)	17 (89%, 1 missing data)	**<0.001**
- Fructose malabsorption	0 (0%)	10 (53%)	
- Lactose intolerance	0 (0%)	4 (21%)	
- Histamine intolerance	0 (0%)	1 (5%)	
- Bile acid malabsorption	0 (0%)	1 (5%)	
- Vitamin B12 deficiency	0 (0%)	1 (5%)	
IBS-associated	0 (0%)	8 (42%, 1 missing data)	**0.048**
Abdominal pain syndrome	0 (0%)	1 (5%)	
Somatoform disorder	0 (0%)	1 (5%)	
Anxiety disorder	0 (0%)	1 (5%)	
Dysthymia	0 (0%)	1 (5%)	
Insomnia	0 (0%)	1 (5%)	
Migraine	0 (0%)	1 (5%)	
Chronic pain syndrome	0 (0%)	1 (5%)	
Fibromyalgia	0 (0%)	1 (5%)	
Metabolic	3 (30%)	12 (63%, 1 missing data)	0.191
- Hyperuricemia	1 (10%)	0 (0%)	
- Diabetes mellitus Type 2	0 (0%)	1 (5%)	
- Fatty liver disease	0 (0%)	3 (16%)	
- Hypothyroidism	0 (0%)	3 (16%)	
- Hyperlipoproteinemia	1 (10%)	2 (11%)	
- Nephrolithiasis	1 (10%)	1 (5%)	
- Cholecystolithiasis	0 (0%)	1 (5%)	
- Pancreas divisum	0 (0%)	1 (5%)	
Cardiovascular	3 (30%)	6 (32%, 1 missing data)	0.738
- Arterial hypertension	2 (20%)	3 (16%)	
- Arteriosclerosis	0 (0%)	1 (5%)	
- Past stroke	0 (0%)	1 (5%)	
- Past embolism	1 (10%)	1 (5%)	

(Continued)

TABLE 1 | Continued

Parameter	Group		p
	Control (n = 10, ♀ = 2, ♂ = 8)	IBS (n = 20, ♀ = 14, ♂ = 6)	
Other	3 (30%)	7 (37%, 1 missing data)	0.966
- Gynecological disorder	0 (0%)	2 (11%)	
- Benign prostate hyperplasia	2 (20%)	0 (0%)	
- Degenerative orthopedic condition (e.g., arthrosis, disc etc.)	1 (10%)	5 (26%)	
Former surgery	0 (0%)	8 (42%, 1 missing data)	**0.048**
- Cholecystectomy	0 (0%)	4 (21%)	
- Appendectomy	0 (0%)	3 (16%)	
- Bowel surgery	0 (0%)	2 (11%)	
- Hernioplastic	0 (0%)	1 (5%)	
- Hysterectomy	0 (0%)	5 (26%)	
- Ovarectomy	0 (0%)	3 (16%)	
- Tonsillectomy	0 (0%)	1 (5%)	
Medication			
Medication use	3 (30%)	12 (63%, 1 missing data)	0.191
- Proton pump inhibitors	2 (20%)	2 (11%)	
- Antihypertensives	1 (10%)	4 (21%)	
- Vitamin B12	0 (0%)	1 (5%)	
- Thyroid supplementation	0 (0%)	3 (16%)	
- Gynecological hormone substitution	0 (0%)	1 (5%)	
- Statins	0 (0%)	2 (11%)	
- Antidiabetics	0 (0%)	1 (5%)	
- Sleep aids	0 (0%)	1 (5%)	
- Selective serotonine reuptake inhibitors	0 (0%)	1 (5%)	
- Tricyclic antidepressants	0 (0%)	2 (11%)	
- Neuroleptics	0 (0%)	1 (5%)	
- Budenoside	0 (0%)	1 (5%)	
- Mesalazine	0 (0%)	1 (5%)	
- Prostate medication	1 (10%)	0 (0%)	
- Laxatives	0 (0%)	1 (5%)	
- Antispasmodics	0 (0%)	1 (5%)	
- Antidiarrheals	0 (0%)	1 (5%)	

Data are presented as mean ± sem, the range is indicated in parentheses; alternatively, data are indicated as total number and percentage values in parentheses. Normality was assessed using the Kolmogorow-Smirnov test. Differences were assessed using χ2-tests, t-tests or the Mann-Whitney-U test depending on the distribution of the data. Significant differences are displayed in bold. IBS, irritable bowel syndrome.

1.2 ± 0.2; $p = 0.076$) when analyzed with ELISA (**Table 3**). Due to limited group size no comparison of female and male controls was performed.

Men With IBS-D Have Lower BDNF Levels Than Male Controls

Comparing the whole IBS-D group to controls, BDNF protein (1.5 ± 0.2 ng/mg vs. 1.74 ± 0.3; $p = 0.500$) or mRNA (7.0 ± 1.0 ng/ml vs. 1.74 ± 0.3; $p = 0.07$) levels were not different. IBS-SSS was significantly higher with 297.4 ± 21.0 points vs. 27.7 ± 9.0 (mean $\pm$ SEM; $p < 0.0001$).

Further dividing the IBS-D subgroup into male and female, five male IBS-D patients were compared to eight male controls. Here, the IBS-SSS was significantly higher in male IBS-D compared to male controls (346.6 ± 45.0 vs. 29.3 ± 10.1, $p < 0.001$). BDNF protein (1.0 ± 0.2 ng/mg vs. 1.5 ± 0.1, $p <$

0.05) and mRNA levels (5.3 ± 1.1 vs. 10.2 ± 1.2, $p < 0.05$) were significantly lower compared to controls (**Figures 2D–F, Supplementary Table 1, Supplementary Figures 1D–F**).

The female IBS-D subgroup was comprised of eight individuals compared to two female controls. Data are shown for completion in **Supplementary Table 1** but were not statistically analyzed.

BDNF Levels Do Not Differ in IBS Patients With Fructose Malabsorption

Except one, all patients with fructose malabsorption had IBS-D with a sex ratio of seven female and three male. Mean symptom severity was significantly higher in the IBS + fructose malabsorption group compared to IBS without fructose malabsorption (312.1 ± 28.6 vs. 316.2 ± 31.4, $p = 0.575$). In IBS with fructose malabsorption, BDNF protein levels (1.7

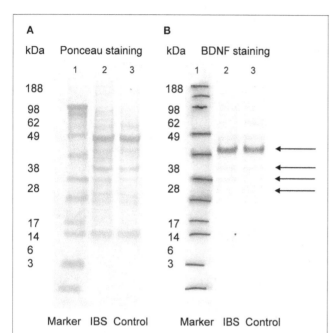

FIGURE 1 | Western blot for BDNF (1:5,000) in IBS patients and control subjects. Lane 1 contains the molecular weight standards. Lane 2 contains colonic wall protein obtained by deep tissue biopsy from mucosa/submucosa in patients with IBS (14 female and six male, pooled sample) and lane 3 colonic wall protein from control subjects (two female and eight male, pooled sample, **A**). Same blot after washout of ponceau staining solution and application of primary anti-BDNF antibody (1:5,000) and secondary antibody goat anti-rabbit AP (1:2,000). Lane 1 contains molecular standards highlighted with pen. Lane 2 and 3 show detection of multiple bands with similar intensity for patients with IBS and healthy controls, respectively. For BDNF (UniProt P23560) multiple Western Blot bands are possible and expected. The strongest band was found between 49 and 62 kDa most likely representing glycosylated prepro-/pro BDNF dimer. Weaker bands were detected at ~ 45, 38, and ~ 30 kDa likely related to prepro-/pro BDNF **(B)**.

$\pm$ 0.3 ng/mg vs. 1.8 $\pm$ 0.3; p = 0.904) and BDNF mRNA levels (10.8 $\pm$ 2.8 vs. 10.2 $\pm$ 4.4, p = 0.918) did not differ from IBS without fructose malabsorption. Data are shown in **Supplementary Table 2**.

Correlation of IBS-SSS and BDNF Levels

There was no significant correlation between BDNF protein or mRNA levels and the severity of IBS symptoms in the study cohort (r = −0.097, p = 0.611 and r = −0.123, p = 0.526, respectively, **Figures 3A,B**).

In male IBS-D patients (n = 5) and their male controls (n = 8), BDNF protein did not significantly correlate (p = 0.156) but mRNA levels showed a significant negative correlation (p = 0.023) with IBS symptom score (**Figures 3C,D**).

DISCUSSION

Over a century ago Sir William Osler introduced the term mucous colitis and described a disorder of mucorrhea and abdominal colic with a high incidence in patients presenting with psychopathology (33). Over the decades, IBS has been diagnosed by means of exclusion and at the present time it still remains a diagnostic challenge. The pathophysiology of this disorder remains unclear and may be different depending on the subtype. Nonetheless, a disturbed physiological interplay between colon motility, hormones and transmitters, visceral hyperalgesia and psychopathology results in this heterogeneous symptom complex (2).

BDNF is suspected to be involved in the regulation of colonic motility as well as in the control of visceral hyperalgesia (6–10, 23). The aim of our study was to detect and quantify BDNF levels in human biopsies from the descending colon in patients with IBS and healthy controls and correlate them with IBS symptoms and severity.

We were able to demonstrate that BDNF is present in human descending colon biopsies obtained by endoscopy. Similar observations, however in biopsies from the rectosigmoid, were made by Yu et al. (19), Wang et al. (20) (affiliated groups) and Zhang et al. (21). Only Wang et al. performed Western Blot in human rectosigmoid biopsies for BDNF showing a cut-out band between 20 and 30 kDa (20). Our Western Blot analysis revealed multiple molecular weight forms of BDNF. Interestingly, the strongest band was found between 49 and 62 kDa with weaker bands at 45, 38, and 30 kDa. The presence of different molecular weight forms of BDNF has been reported in prior studies using cultured neuronal and non-neuronal cells (30, 31). It has been suggested that the variety of bands is due to differently glycosylated and glycosulfated forms of proBDNF and mature BDNF (32). Analysis of adult rat spinal cord revealed that BDNF knockout mice showed a positive band at 55 kDa when stained with BDNF antibody suggestive of a non-specific finding (34). It can be speculated whether the presence of the strongest band between 49 and 62 kDa is also a non-specific finding and that the 45, 38, and 30 kDa bands represent real BDNF protein. Given that the mature form of BDNF monomer is usually found at 14 kDa as suggested by the manufacturer (ab 72439, Abcam, Cambridge, UK), we believe that our western blot findings represent the proBDNF form which is usually found at around 34 kDa likely depending on the degree of glycosylation/glycosulfation. ProBDNF is of importance for proper dimerization, folding as well as targeting of mature BDNF, however, it has been found that this form also elicits its own distinct effects opposing those of mature BDNF (35). It has been shown that proBDNF induces cellular apoptosis (36), whereas the mature form promotes neuroplasticity and cell differentiation (37). On the cellular level, after binding to the TrkB receptor, mature BDNF results in recruitment of proteins that activate three distinct signaling pathways: Ras/MAPK-ERK pathway, PI3-K pathway and PLC pathway (38). So far Fu et al. could demonstrate in a rodent model with bowel obstruction that peripheral up-regulation of BDNF expression may play a critical role in the abnormal hyper-excitability of primary sensory neurons. Intraperitoneal administration of a TrkB inhibitor resulted in blocked hyper-excitability of colon neurons, which was associated with attenuation of referred visceral hypersensitivity (39). More investigations are needed to further evaluate the cellular actions of BDNF in the gut.

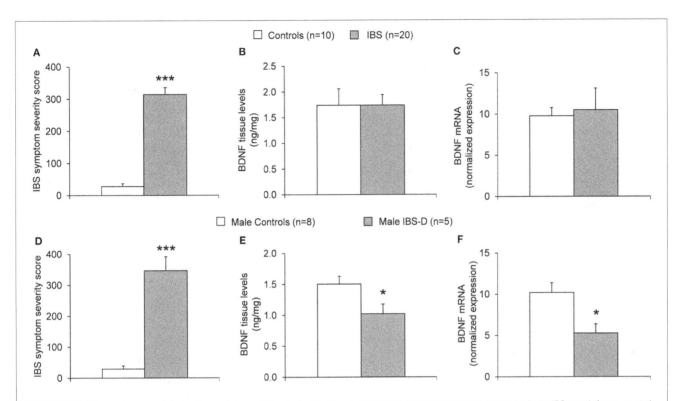

FIGURE 2 | **(A)** IBS symptom severity in healthy controls vs. IBS patients. Significantly higher symptom severity scores are notable in the IBS population vs. controls (***$p < 0.001$). **(B)** Measurement of BDNF protein tissue levels obtained from colonic biopsies of the descending colon by nCounter analysis in healthy controls ($n = 10$, two female and eight male) and IBS patients ($n = 20$, 14 female and six male). No notable difference is detected in BDNF protein levels in healthy controls vs. IBS patients. **(C)** Measurement of BDNF mRNA levels obtained from colonic biopsies of the descending colon by ELISA in healthy controls ($n = 10$) and IBS patients ($n = 20$) with no notable difference detected. **(D)** IBS symptom severity in healthy male controls vs. male IBS-D patients. Significantly higher symptom severity scores are notable in the male IBS-D population vs. male controls (***$p < 0.001$). **(E)** Measurement of BDNF protein tissue levels obtained from colonic biopsies of the descending colon by nCounter analysis in healthy male controls ($n = 8$) and male IBS-D patients ($n = 5$). BDNF protein levels in male IBS-D patients were significantly lower compared to male healthy controls (*$p < 0.05$). **(F)** Measurement of BDNF mRNA levels obtained from colonic biopsies of the descending colon by ELISA in healthy male controls ($n = 8$) and male IBS-D patients ($n = 5$). BDNF mRNA levels in male IBS-D patients were significantly lower compared to male healthy controls (*$p < 0.05$).

TABLE 2 | Characterization of irritable bowel syndrome in patient population.

Parameter	Group		p
	Control ($n = 10$, ♀ = 2, ♂ = 8)	IBS ($n = 20$, ♀ = 14, ♂ = 6)	
IBS subgroup			
Diarrhea	n.a.	14	n.a.
Constipation	n.a.	2	
Mixed	n.a.	3	
Unsubtyped	n.a.	1	
Duration of disease			
Duration (years)	n.a.	6.1 ± 1.5 (1–22)	n.a.
Severity			
IBS Symptom Severity Score	27.7 ± 9.0 (0–72)	314.2 ± 21.2 (124–486)	**<0.001**
IBS-SSS grade			**<0.001**
0	10	0 (0%)	
1	0	2 (10%)	
2	0	8 (40%)	
3	0	10 (50%)	
4	0	0 (0%)	

Data are presented as mean ± sem, the range is indicated in parentheses; alternatively, data are indicated as total number and percentage values in parentheses. Normality was assessed using the Kolmogorow-Smirnov test. Differences were assessed using χ2-tests or t-tests. Significant differences are displayed in bold. IBS, irritable bowel syndrome; IBS-SSS, IBS Symptom Severity Score; n.a., not applicable.

TABLE 3 | IBS symptom severity scores and BDNF levels according to sex.

Parameter	Group					
	Control (n = 10)			IBS (n = 20)		
	Women (n = 2)	Men (n = 8)	p	Women (n = 14)	Men (n = 6)	p
IBS-SSS	21.5 ± 19.5 (2–41)	29.3 ± 10.1 (0–72)	n.c.	293.7 ± 23.0 (124–439)	361.8 ± 39.8 (220–486)	0.133
BDNF mRNA (arbitrary unit)	8.1 ± 1.4 (6.7–9.4)	10.2 ± 1.2 (7.5–16.8)	n.c.	13.2 ± 3.6 (1.4–48.1)	4.7 ± 1.1 (1.9–8.6)	**0.048**
BDNF protein (ng/mg)	2.7 ± 1.6 (1.1–4.3)	1.5 ± 0.1 (0.9–1.9)	n.c.	2.0 ± 0.3 (0.6–3.4)	1.2 ± 0.2 (0.6–1.8)	0.076

BDNF levels were assessed using nCounter analysis and ELISA and corrected for housekeeping gene expression or total tissue protein, respectively. Data are presented as mean ± sem, the range is indicated in parentheses. Normality was assessed using the Kolmogorow-Smirnov test. Differences were assessed using t-tests or the Mann-Whitney-U test depending on the distribution of the data. Significant differences are displayed in bold. BDNF, brain-derived neurotrophic factor; IBS, irritable bowel syndrome; IBS-SSS, IBS Symptom Severity Score; n.c., not calculated.

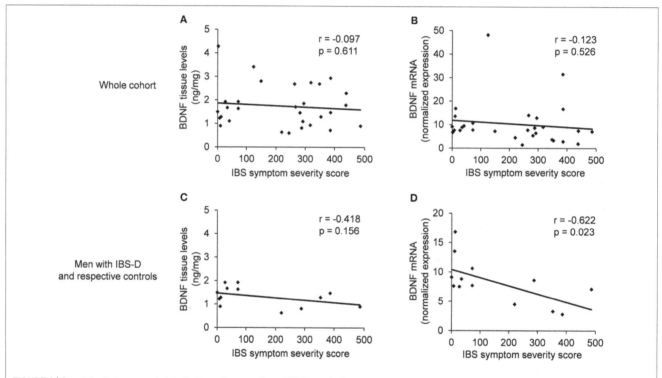

FIGURE 3 | Correlation between gastrointestinal symptom severity vs. BDNF protein tissue levels from the descending colon or BDNF mRNA levels. **(A,B)** shown the whole cohort (10 controls: eight female and two male; 20 IBS: 14 female and six male) and **(C,D)** show the subgroups of male IBS-D patients (n = 5) with their male controls (n = 8). Scatter plot showing **(A,B)** no significant correlation between IBS-SSS and BDNF protein or mRNA levels in the whole cohort (r = −0.097; p = 0.611 and r = −0.123; p = 0.526) and **(C)** no significant correlation between IBS-SSS and BDNF protein tissue levels in male IBS-D patients and respective control cohort (r = −0.418; p = 0.156) and **(D)** a significant negative correlation between IBS-SSS and BDNF mRNA levels in male IBS-D patients and male controls (r = −0.622; p = 0.023).

To our surprise in contrast to prior studies (11, 19–21), no significant differences in the concentration of BDNF protein and mRNA were found in the IBS cohort compared to controls. It can be speculated whether this is attributed to a different study population. Compared to Zhang et al. (21) we did include patients with carbohydrate malabsorption as well as patients with previous abdominal surgeries. Most of our patients were women while Zhang's study population consisted of more males. Our sample size is also smaller. However, in our opinion the reason for this discrepancy of

results may be mainly due to the different location in the colon the biopsies were taken from. In all prior investigations, biopsies were obtained from the rectosigmoid junction whereas our biopsies were taken from the descending colon (~40 to 50 cm above the anocutaneous line). In the physiological state the rectosigmoid colon is responsible for storage and eventually defecation while the more proximal parts of the colon are involved in mixing and propelling of the content and thus securing its optimal contact to the mucosal wall to absorb the water and eventually solidifying fecal contents (40). The different motility pattern of the rectosigmoid colon compared to the rest of the colon is a well-known phenomenon which has been previously attributed to a higher rate of the basic electrical rhythm (BER) probably resulting in occurrence of more intense motility observed in the rectosigmoid colon caused mainly by giant migrating contractions (40, 41). Our results showing no substantial difference between BDNF tissue concentration in healthy subjects and IBS patients suggest that the descending colon and probably parts of the ascending and transverse colon are not or at least to a lesser degree responsible for symptoms occurring in IBS mediated by BDNF. Unfortunately, there is no substantial clinical data on regional differences of visceral sensitivity of the colon and further investigations are needed to elucidate this phenomenon as well as regional BDNF expression, especially with regard to patients with IBS. Furthermore, our heterogeneous IBS group could be the reason why overall no differences in IBS vs. control were found. Analysis of the IBS-D subgroup showed that male IBS-D patients had significantly lower BDNF mRNA and protein levels compared to male controls. This supports the hypothesis that the subforms of IBS have many different etiologies and especially IBS-D may underlie a different pathology. As recently reviewed, NGFs together with mast cells modulate visceral sensitivity, intestinal barrier function, and motility in IBS-D (42). Unfortunately, due to limited subgroup size no further analyses of the other subgroups could be performed and one should keep in mind that the IBS-D subgroup is of small sample size as well. Thus, results should be interpreted with caution. Whether the differences found are exclusive to male IBS-D must be ascertained in future studies with higher numbers of sex-categorized and subgrouped IBS patients.

Our study reveals significantly higher levels of measurable BDNF mRNA in female IBS patients as compared to male IBS patients. A 2:1 female to male predominance of IBS is well known (43, 44) and could be reproduced in our study. Previous studies suggest that regulation of BDNF and its receptors is controlled by estrogen (45, 46). Recently, Ji et al. investigated the opposing roles of estradiol and testosterone on stress-induced visceral hypersensitivity (SIVH) in rats. It could be shown that estradiol injection in intact male rats increased both SIVH and BDNF levels in the spinal cord whereas testosterone injection in female rats attenuated SIVH and decreased BDNF levels. One rodent study looked at colonic BDNF levels after a single inflammatory insult to the distal colon and found strong up-regulation only in rats with concomitant high estrogen levels while the inflammation itself did not induce BDNF changes (47). Both studies support the hypothesis that estrogens seem to be involved in BDNF upregulation.

Our study included a total of 10 controls and 20 patients with IBS. Given the limited study size it is possible that our results could not reach significance. Furthermore, there was a disproportionate gender distribution within the two study groups without gender matching making results prone to bias. The IBS group included 14 women and six men whereas the control group consisted of mostly men ($n = 10$, ♀ $= 2$, ♂ $= 8$).

Our study population in many aspects represents typical demographic and epidemiologic findings as well as associated comorbidities of IBS. Interestingly, most of our patients in the IBS group owned a university entrance diploma or a secondary education certificate which supports data that a higher socioeconomic status is associated with IBS (48). We speculate if in a country like Germany with universal health care access, a possible reason for this phenomenon is a higher level of stress perceived by people working in the professional and managerial field.

Malabsorption, in particular fructose malabsorption, has been shown to be associated with IBS (49, 50). Our study population is representative in that regard as 53% of IBS patients had concurrent fructose malabsorption diagnosed prior to evaluation for IBS. No differences in BDNF levels in that subgroup could be detected. Except one, all patients with fructose malabsorption had IBS-D. The exact reason for this association remains unclear, however, possible suggested mechanisms include alteration of the enteric microbiome, changes in intestinal permeability, rapid small bowel transit, and immune responsiveness (51, 52). Education on nutrition in this subgroup of patients may be of benefit for better symptom control (49, 53). Similar associations were found with lactose intolerance and IBS (54).

IBS is further associated with a variety of somatic and psychiatric conditions which is reflected in our IBS study population in 42% of cases compared to 0% in the control group ($p = 0.048$). Recognition and treatment of these comorbidities is pertinent since it has been shown that there is a correlation with enhanced medical help seeking, worse prognosis and higher rates of depression and anxiety (29). These patients often undergo extensive diagnostic workup which may include surgical interventions (48). It needs to be emphasized that all of our IBS patients have a history of abdominal surgery. This association could raise suspicion that IBS is associated with intraabdominal/peritoneal adhesions, however, it could also reflect the poor diagnostic knowledge on IBS in the German healthcare setting leading to false diagnoses and common surgeries such as cholecystectomies or appendectomies.

IBS remains a debilitating disorder of brain-gut interaction. Although in a small sample, our study detected a high proportion of gastrointestinal surgery in IBS patients and confirmed food intolerances and psychiatric diseases as common comorbidities of IBS. We demonstrated that BDNF, a nerve growth factor suspected to be involved in the control of visceral hyperalgesia and colon motility, is detectable in human biopsies of the descending colon with lower levels in the small subgroup of male IBS-D patients suggesting that this subgroup may be different from the others. No difference was found between the whole IBS cohort and controls which could be due to the heterogeneous IBS subgroups. Regional differences in colonic BDNF expression could also account for these findings although this conclusion cannot be drawn from our current data that focused on BDNF expression in the descending colon only. A regional characterization of BDNF expression should thus be subject of future studies. The finding that female IBS patients show higher BDNF levels than male patients supports previous data that sex hormones are involved in the regulation of BDNF. Extrapolating from the current findings, female IBS patients as well as male IBS-D patients should be studied in a larger sample size to further characterize the role of BDNF in the pathophysiology of IBS.

ETHICS STATEMENT

The studies involving human participants were reviewed and approved by Clinical Ethical Committee of Charité Universitätsmedizin Berlin (ethical approval number EA1/108/11). The patients/participants provided their written informed consent to participate in this study.

AUTHOR CONTRIBUTIONS

TK performed experiments and wrote the manuscript. CM performed experiments. BN performed experiments and edited the manuscript. IV and HM performed experiments. HM provided some resources. AS edited the manuscript and provided some resources. MG-S performed experiments, reviewed the literature, wrote and edited the manuscript, and provided the resources. All authors contributed to the article and approved the submitted version.

SUPPLEMENTARY MATERIAL

Supplementary Figure 1 | Graphs are based on pooled data shown in **Figure 2**. The Supplementary Figure additionally shows individual data values. Details and levels of significance are displayed in **Figure 2**. **(A)** IBS symptom severity in healthy controls vs. IBS patients. **(B)** Measurement of BDNF protein tissue levels obtained from colonic biopsies of the descending colon by ELISA in healthy controls and IBS patients. **(C)** Measurement of BDNF mRNA levels obtained from colonic biopsies of the descending colon by ELISA in healthy controls and IBS patients. **(D)** IBS symptom severity in healthy male controls vs. male IBS-D patients. **(E)** Measurement of BDNF protein tissue levels obtained from colonic biopsies of the descending colon by ELISA in healthy male controls and male IBS-D patients. **(F)** Measurement of BDNF mRNA levels obtained from colonic biopsies of the descending colon by ELISA in healthy male controls and male IBS-D patients.

Supplementary Table 1 | IBS symptom severity scores and BDNF levels in IBS-D subgroup.

Supplementary Table 2 | IBS-SSS and BDNF levels in IBS patients without fructose malabsorption (IBS – FM) or with (IBS + FM).

REFERENCES

1. Drossman DA, Hasler WL. Rome IV-functional gi disorders: disorders of gut-brain interaction. *Gastroenterology*. (2016) 150:1257–61. doi: 10.1053/j.gastro.2016.03.035
2. Enck P, Aziz Q, Barbara G, Farmer AD, Fukudo S, Mayer EA, et al. Irritable bowel syndrome. *Nat Rev Dis Primers*. (2016) 2:16014. doi: 10.1038/nrdp.2016.14
3. Lewin GR, Barde YA. Physiology of the neurotrophins. *Annu Rev Neurosci*. (1996) 19:289–317. doi: 10.1146/annurev.ne.19.030196.001445
4. Leibrock J, Lottspeich F, Hohn A, Hofer M, Hengerer B, Masiakowski P, et al. Molecular cloning and expression of brain-derived neurotrophic factor. *Nature*. (1989) 341:149–52. doi: 10.1038/341149a0
5. Benarroch EE. Brain-derived neurotrophic factor: regulation, effects, and potential clinical relevance. *Neurology*. (2015) 84:1693–704. doi: 10.1212/WNL.0000000000001507
6. Zhu ZW, Friess H, Wang L, Zimmermann A, Buchler MW. Brain-derived neurotrophic factor. (BDNF) is upregulated and associated with pain in chronic pancreatitis. *Dig Dis Sci*. (2001) 46:1633–9. doi: 10.1023/A:1010684916863
7. Obata K, Noguchi K. BDNF in sensory neurons and chronic pain. *Neurosci Res*. (2006) 55:1–10. doi: 10.1016/j.neures.2006.01.005
8. Li CQ, Xu JM, Liu D, Zhang JY, Dai RP. Brain derived neurotrophic factor (BDNF) contributes to the pain hypersensitivity following surgical incision in the rats. *Mol Pain*. (2008) 4:27. doi: 10.1186/1744-8069-4-27
9. Yang J, Yu Y, Yu H, Zuo X, Liu C, Gao L, et al. The role of brain-derived neurotrophic factor in experimental inflammation of mouse gut. *Eur J Pain*. (2010) 14:574–9. doi: 10.1016/j.ejpain.2009.10.007
10. Joo YE. Increased expression of brain-derived neurotrophic factor in irritable bowel syndrome and its correlation with abdominal pain. (Gut 2012;61:685-694). *J Neurogastroenterol Motil*. (2013) 19:109–11. doi: 10.5056/jnm.2013.19.1.109
11. Qi Q, Chen F, Zhang W, Wang P, Li Y, Zuo X. Colonic N-methyl-d-aspartate receptor contributes to visceral hypersensitivity in irritable bowel syndrome. *J Gastroenterol Hepatol*. (2017) 32:828–36. doi: 10.1111/jgh.13588
12. Lommatzsch M, Braun A, Mannsfeldt A, Botchkarev VA, Botchkareva NV, Paus R, et al. Abundant production of brain-derived neurotrophic factor by adult visceral epithelia. Implications for paracrine and target-derived Neurotrophic functions. *Am J Pathol*. (1999) 155:1183–93. doi: 10.1016/S0002-9440(10)65221-2
13. Lucini C, Maruccio L, de Girolamo P, Vega JA, Castaldo L. Localisation of neurotrophin - containing cells in higher vertebrate intestine. *Anat Embryol*. (2002) 205:135–40. doi: 10.1007/s00429-002-0237-x
14. Cheung CKY, Lan LL, Kyaw M, Mak ADP, Chan A, Chan Y, et al. Up-regulation of transient receptor potential vanilloid (TRPV) and down-regulation of brain-derived neurotrophic factor (BDNF) expression in patients with functional dyspepsia (FD). *Neurogastroenterol Motil*. (2018) 30, 1–9. doi: 10.1111/nmo.13176
15. Yamamoto M, Sobue G, Yamamoto K, Terao S, Mitsuma T. Expression of mRNAs for neurotrophic factors (NGF, BDNF, NT-3, and GDNF) and their receptors (p75NGFR, trkA, trkB, and trkC) in the adult human peripheral nervous system and nonneural tissues. *Neurochem Res*. (1996) 21:929–38. doi: 10.1007/BF02532343
16. Pluchino N, Cubeddu A, Begliuomini S, Merlini S, Giannini A, Bucci F, et al. Daily variation of brain-derived neurotrophic factor and cortisol in women with normal menstrual cycles, undergoing oral contraception and in postmenopause. *Hum Reprod*. (2009) 24:2303–9. doi: 10.1093/humrep/dep119
17. Hoehner JC, Wester T, Pahlman S, Olsen L. Localization of neurotrophins and their high-affinity receptors during human enteric nervous system development. *Gastroenterology*. (1996) 110:756–67. doi: 10.1053/gast.1996.v110.pm8608885
18. Sen S, Duman R, Sanacora G. Serum brain-derived neurotrophic factor, depression, and antidepressant medications: meta-analyses and implications. *Biol Psychiatry*. (2008) 64:527–32. doi: 10.1016/j.biopsych.2008.05.005
19. Yu YB, Zuo XL, Zhao QJ, Chen FX, Yang J, Dong YY, et al. Brain-derived neurotrophic factor contributes to abdominal pain in irritable bowel syndrome. *Gut*. (2012) 61:685–94. doi: 10.1136/gutjnl-2011-300265

20. Wang P, Du C, Chen FX, Li CQ, Yu YB, Han T, et al. BDNF contributes to IBS-like colonic hypersensitivity via activating the enteroglia-nerve unit. *Sci Rep.* (2016) 6:20320. doi: 10.1038/srep20320

21. Zhang Y, Qin G, Liu DR, Wang Y, Yao SK. Increased expression of brain-derived neurotrophic factor is correlated with visceral hypersensitivity in patients with diarrhea-predominant irritable bowel syndrome. *World J Gastroenterol.* (2019) 25:269–81. doi: 10.3748/wjg.v25.i2.269

22. Wang P, Chen FX, Du C, Li CQ, Yu YB, Zuo XL, et al. Increased production of BDNF in colonic epithelial cells induced by fecal supernatants from diarrheic IBS patients. *Sci Rep.* (2015) 5:10121. doi: 10.1038/srep10121

23. Coulie B, Szarka LA, Camilleri M, Burton DD, McKinzie S, Stambler N, et al. Recombinant human neurotrophic factors accelerate colonic transit and relieve constipation in humans. *Gastroenterology.* (2000) 119:41–50. doi: 10.1053/gast.2000.8553

24. Mahurkar-Joshi S, Videlock EJ, Iliopoulos D, Pothoulakis C, Mayer EA, Chang L. 1090 - epigenetic changes in blood cells and colonic mucosa are associated with irritable bowel syndrome (IBS). *Gastroenterology.* (2018) 154:S-214. doi: 10.1016/S0016-5085(18)31105-3

25. Videlock EJ, Mahurkar-Joshi S, Hoffman JM, Iliopoulos D, Pothoulakis C, Mayer EA, et al. Sigmoid colon mucosal gene expression supports alterations of neuronal signaling in irritable bowel syndrome with constipation. *Am J Physiol Gastrointest Liver Physiol.* (2018) 315:G140–57. doi: 10.1152/ajpgi.00288.2017

26. Longstreth GF, Thompson WG, Chey WD, Houghton LA, Mearin F, Spiller RC. Functional bowel disorders. *Gastroenterology.* (2006) 130:1480–91. doi: 10.1053/j.gastro.2005.11.061

27. Francis CY, Morris J, Whorwell PJ. The irritable bowel severity scoring system: a simple method of monitoring irritable bowel syndrome and its progress. *Aliment Pharmacol Ther.* (1997) 11:395–402. doi: 10.1046/j.1365-2036.1997.142318000.x

28. Vandesompele J, De Preter K, Pattyn F, Poppe B, Van Roy N, De Paepe A, et al. Accurate normalization of real-time quantitative RT-PCR data by geometric averaging of multiple internal control genes. *Genome Biol.* (2002) 3:RESEARCH0034. doi: 10.1186/gb-2002-3-7-research0034

29. Riedl A, Schmidtmann M, Stengel A, Goebel M, Wisser AS, Klapp BF, et al. Somatic comorbidities of irritable bowel syndrome: a systematic analysis. *J Psychosom Res.* (2008) 64:573–82. doi: 10.1016/j.jpsychores.2008.02.021

30. Mowla SJ, Farhadi HF, Pareek S, Atwal JK, Morris SJ, Seidah NG, et al. Biosynthesis and post-translational processing of the precursor to brain-derived neurotrophic factor. *J Biol Chem.* (2001) 276:12660–6. doi: 10.1074/jbc.M008104200

31. Teng HK, Teng KK, Lee R, Wright S, Tevar S, Almeida RD, et al. ProBDNF induces neuronal apoptosis via activation of a receptor complex of p75NTR and sortilin. *J Neurosci.* (2005) 25:5455–63. doi: 10.1523/JNEUROSCI.5123-04.2005

32. Mowla SJ, Pareek S, Farhadi HF, Petrecca K, Fawcett JP, Seidah NG, et al. Differential sorting of nerve growth factor and brain-derived neurotrophic factor in hippocampal neurons. *J Neurosci.* (1999) 19:2069–80. doi: 10.1523/JNEUROSCI.19-06-02069.1999

33. Osler W. *The Principles and Practice of Medicine.* New York, NY: Appleton & Co. (1892).

34. Macias M, Dwornik A, Ziemlinska E, Fehr S, Schachner M, Czarkowska-Bauch J, et al. Locomotor exercise alters expression of pro-brain-derived neurotrophic factor, brain-derived neurotrophic factor and its receptor TrkB in the spinal cord of adult rats. *Eur J Neurosci.* (2007) 25:2425–44. doi: 10.1111/j.1460-9568.2007.05498.x

35. Lu B, Pang PT, Woo NH. The yin and yang of neurotrophin action. *Nat Rev Neurosci.* (2005) 6:603–14. doi: 10.1038/nrn1726

36. Lee R, Kermani P, Teng KK, Hempstead BL. Regulation of cell survival by secreted proneurotrophins. *Science.* (2001) 294:1945–8. doi: 10.1126/science.1065057

37. Egan MF, Kojima M, Callicott JH, Goldberg TE, Kolachana BS, Bertolino A, et al. The BDNF val66met polymorphism affects activity-dependent secretion of BDNF and human memory and hippocampal function. *Cell.* (2003) 112:257–69. doi: 10.1016/S0092-8674(03)00035-7

38. Bathina S, Das UN. Brain-derived neurotrophic factor and its clinical implications. *Arch Med Sci.* (2015) 11:1164–78. doi: 10.5114/aoms.2015.56342

39. Fu Y, Lin YM, Winston JH, Radhakrishnan R, Huang LM, Shi XZ. Role of brain-derived neurotrophic factor in the pathogenesis of distention-associated abdominal pain in bowel obstruction. *Neurogastroenterol Motil.* (2018) 30:e13373. doi: 10.1111/nmo.13373

40. Leung PS. *The Gastrointestinal System - Gastrointestinal, Nutritional and Hepatobiliary Physiology.* Dordrecht; Heidelberg; New York, NY; London: Springer (2014).

41. Sarna SK. Enteric descending and afferent neural signaling stimulated by giant migrating contractions: essential contributing factors to visceral pain. *Am J Physiol Gastrointest Liver Physiol.* (2007) 292:G572–81. doi: 10.1152/ajpgi.00332.2006

42. Xu XJ, Liang L, Yao SK, et al. Nerve growth factor and diarrhea-predominant irritable bowel syndrome (IBS-D): a potential therapeutic target? *Biomed Biotechnol.* (2016) 17:1–9. doi: 10.1631/jzus.B1500181

43. Hungin AP, Whorwell PJ, Tack J, Mearin F. The prevalence, patterns and impact of irritable bowel syndrome: an international survey of 40,000 subjects. *Aliment Pharmacol Ther.* (2003) 17:643–50. doi: 10.1046/j.1365-2036.2003.01456.x

44. Jung HK, Halder S, McNally M, Locke GR III, Schleck CD, Zinsmeister AR, et al. Overlap of gastro-oesophageal reflux disease and irritable bowel syndrome: prevalence and risk factors in the general population. *Aliment Pharmacol Ther.* (2007) 26:453–61. doi: 10.1111/j.1365-2036.2007.03366.x

45. Numakawa T, Yokomaku D, Richards M, Hori H, Adachi N, Kunugi H. Functional interactions between steroid hormones and neurotrophin BDNF. *World J Biol Chem.* (2010) 1:133–43. doi: 10.4331/wjbc.v1.i5.133

46. Karisetty BC, Joshi PC, Kumar A, Chakravarty S. Sex differences in the effect of chronic mild stress on mouse prefrontal cortical BDNF levels: a role of major ovarian hormones. *Neuroscience.* (2017) 356:89–101. doi: 10.1016/j.neuroscience.2017.05.020

47. Pan XQ, Malykhina AP. Estrous cycle dependent fluctuations of regulatory neuropeptides in the lower urinary tract of female rats upon colon-bladder cross-sensitization. *PLoS ONE.* (2014) 9:e94872. doi: 10.1371/journal.pone.0094872

48. Canavan C, West J, Card T. The epidemiology of irritable bowel syndrome. *Clin Epidemiol.* (2014) 6:71–80. doi: 10.2147/CLEP.S40245

49. Choi YK, Kraft N, Zimmerman B, Jackson M, Rao SS. Fructose intolerance in IBS and utility of fructose-restricted diet. *J Clin Gastroenterol.* (2008) 42:233–8. doi: 10.1097/MCG.0b013e31802cbc2f

50. Jung KW, Seo M, Cho YH, Park YO, Yoon SY, Lee J, et al. Prevalence of fructose malabsorption in patients with irritable bowel syndrome after excluding small intestinal bacterial overgrowth. *J Neurogastroenterol Motil.* (2018) 24:307–16. doi: 10.5056/jnm17044

51. Ohman L, Simren M. Pathogenesis of IBS: role of inflammation, immunity and neuroimmune interactions. *Nat Rev Gastroenterol Hepatol.* (2010) 7:163–73. doi: 10.1038/nrgastro.2010.4

52. Kennedy PJ, Clarke G, Quigley EM, Groeger JA, Dinan TG, Cryan JF. Gut memories: towards a cognitive neurobiology of irritable bowel syndrome. *Neurosci Biobehav Rev.* (2012) 36:310–40. doi: 10.1016/j.neubiorev.2011.07.001

53. Johlin FC Jr, Panther M, Kraft N. Dietary fructose intolerance: diet modification can impact self-rated health and symptom control. *Nutr Clin Care.* (2004) 7:92–7.

54. Yang J, Deng Y, Chu H, Cong Y, Zhao J, Pohl D, et al. Prevalence and presentation of lactose intolerance and effects on dairy product intake in healthy subjects and patients with irritable bowel syndrome. *Clin Gastroenterol Hepatol.* (2013) 11:262–8 e261. doi: 10.1016/j.cgh.2012.11.034

3

Association of the Salivary Microbiome with Animal Contact During Early Life and Stress-Induced Immune Activation in Healthy Participants

Dominik Langgartner[1‡], Cristian A. Zambrano[2‡], Jared D. Heinze[2], Christopher E. Stamper[2†], Till S. Böbel[1], Sascha B. Hackl[1], Marc N. Jarczok[3], Nicolas Rohleder[4], Graham A. Rook[5], Harald Gündel[3], Christiane Waller[3†], Christopher A. Lowry[2,6,7,8,9,10] and Stefan O. Reber[1*]

[1] Laboratory for Molecular Psychosomatics, Department of Psychosomatic Medicine and Psychotherapy, University of Ulm, Ulm, Germany, [2] Department of Integrative Physiology, University of Colorado Boulder, Boulder, CO, United States, [3] Department of Psychosomatic Medicine and Psychotherapy, University of Ulm, Ulm, Germany, [4] Department of Psychology, Friedrich-Alexander University, Erlangen, Germany, [5] Center for Clinical Microbiology, University College London (UCL), London, United Kingdom, [6] Center for Neuroscience and Center for Microbial Exploration, University of Colorado Boulder, Boulder, CO, United States, [7] Department of Physical Medicine and Rehabilitation and Center for Neuroscience, University of Colorado Anschutz Medical Campus, Aurora, CO, United States, [8] Veterans Health Administration, Rocky Mountain Mental Illness Research Education and Clinical Center (MIRECC), The Rocky Mountain Regional Medical Center (RMRMC), Aurora, CO, United States, [9] Military and Veteran Microbiome: Consortium for Research and Education (MVM-CoRE), Aurora, CO, United States, [10] inVIVO Planetary Health, Worldwide Universities Network (WUN), West New York, NJ, United States

*Correspondence:
Stefan O. Reber
stefan.reber@uni-ulm.de

†Present addresses:
Christopher E. Stamper,
Rocky Mountain Mental Illness
Research Education and Clinical
Center (MIRECC), Rocky Mountain
Regional VA Medical Center, Aurora,
CO, United States
Department of Physical Medicine &
Rehabilitation and Center for
Neuroscience, University of Colorado
Anschutz Medical Campus, Aurora,
CO, United States
Christiane Waller,
Department of Psychosomatic
Medicine and Psychotherapy,
Paracelsus Medical University,
Nuremberg General Hospital,
Nuremberg, Germany

‡These authors have contributed
equally to this work

The prevalence of stress-associated somatic and psychiatric disorders is increased in environments offering a narrow relative to a wide range of microbial exposure. Moreover, different animal and human studies suggest that an overreactive immune system not only accompanies stress-associated disorders, but might even be causally involved in their pathogenesis. In support of this hypothesis, we recently showed that urban upbringing in the absence of daily contact with pets, compared to rural upbringing in the presence of daily contact with farm animals, is associated with a more pronounced immune activation following acute psychosocial stressor exposure induced by the Trier Social Stress Test (TSST). Here we employed 16S rRNA gene sequencing to test whether this difference in TSST-induced immune activation between urban upbringing in the absence of daily contact with pets ($n = 20$) compared with rural upbringing in the presence of daily contact with farm animals ($n = 20$) is associated with differences in the composition of the salivary microbiome. Although we did not detect any differences in alpha or beta diversity measures of the salivary microbiome between the two experimental groups, statistical analysis revealed that the salivary microbial beta diversity was significantly higher in participants with absolutely no animal contact ($n = 5$, urban participants) until the age of 15 compared to all other participants ($n = 35$) reporting either daily contact with farm animals ($n = 20$, rural participants) or occasional pet contact ($n = 15$, urban participants).

Interestingly, when comparing these urban participants with absolutely no pet contact to the remaining urban participants with occasional pet contact, the former also displayed a significantly higher immune, but not hypothalamic-pituitary-adrenal (HPA) axis or sympathetic nervous system (SNS) activation, following TSST exposure. In summary, we conclude that only urban upbringing with absolutely no animal contact had long-lasting effects on the composition of the salivary microbiome and potentiates the negative consequences of urban upbringing on stress-induced immune activation.

Keywords: alpha diversity, animal contact, beta diversity, interleukin (IL)-6, salivary microbiome, Trier Social Stress Test (TSST), rural upbringing, urban upbringing

INTRODUCTION

Stress-related somatic and psychiatric disorders have been increasing in Western societies throughout the last decades (1, 2), with urban areas being more affected than rural ones (3, 4). Although the underlying mechanisms are not fully understood, recent studies promote the hypothesis that a compromised immunoregulatory capacity, due to diminished contact to microorganisms (i.e., "Old Friends") with which humans coevolved, might at least in part underlie the increased disease vulnerability of individuals living in urban compared with rural areas (5). Throughout human evolution, the interactions between the innate immune system and these ancestral microbiota promoted immunoregulation, as they were either part of host physiology (human microbiota), were harmless but inevitably contaminating air, food, and water (environmental microbiota), or were causing severe tissue damage when attacked by the host immune system (e.g., helminthic parasites) (6–8). However, microbial biodiversity and, thus, overall contact with environmental and commensal microorganisms that were present during mammalian evolution and that play a role in setting up regulatory immune pathways, is progressively diminishing in high-income countries, particularly in urban areas (5, 8). The latter is due to sanitation, drinking water treatment, excessive use of antibiotics, changes in diet, feeding of formula milk as a replacement for breast milk, increased caesarean section birth rates, as well as increased time spent within the built environment (6–10). In line with the hypothesis that immunoregulatory capacities of individuals raised in an environment offering a narrow range of microbial exposure are compromised, compared with immunoregulatory capacities of individuals raised in an environment offering a wide range of microbial exposure, we recently showed that young, physically and emotionally healthy, male participants raised during the first 15 years of life in a city with more than 100,000 residents and in the absence of daily contact with pets (urban; $n = 20$) show an increased stress-induced inflammatory response when exposed to the Trier Social Stress Test (TSST) (11), relative to respective participants raised on a farm in the presence of daily contact with farm animals (rural; $n = 20$). In detail, this was indicated by an aggravated stress-induced increase in peripheral blood mononuclear cell (PBMC) counts and plasma interleukin (IL)-6 concentrations, as well as an enhanced Concanavalin A

(ConA)-induced IL-6 response from *ex vivo* cultured PBMCs in urban participants with no daily animal contact (8). Importantly, there were no basal immunological differences between the groups before stressor exposure and stress-induced physiological responses also did not differ between the groups (8).

The microbiome data presented in the current study were collected in the identical cohort of participants recruited in our recent study (8) to test whether the increased TSST-induced immune activation in urban participants raised in the absence of daily pet contact, relative to rural participants raised in the presence of daily contact with farm animals, reported in this recent study (8), is accompanied by measureable differences in the composition of the salivary microbiome employing 16S rRNA gene sequencing. This hypothesis is based on recent findings that environment influences the human salivary microbiome, more so than host genetics (12), and the proposal that the oral microbiome may be useful in both the diagnosis and treatment of disease, including inflammatory disease (13, 14).

METHODS

Recruiting

Recruiting was performed as published recently (8). Briefly, all participants were male, between 20 and 40 years of age, and grew up (until the age of 15) either in a city with more than 100,000 residents and in the absence of daily contact with pets (urban: $n = 20$) or on a farm with daily contact with farm animals (rural: $n = 20$). All participants were physically (i.e., asked whether they suffered from chronic physical disorders) and emotionally healthy (i.e., based on responses to the Structured Clinical Interview for DSM-IV Disorders, SCID-I, administered during telephone screening) and asked to abstain from any kind of drugs (e.g., analgesics, sleep-inducing drugs, dietary supplements), exercise, caffeine, alcohol, and nicotine for a minimum of 3 days before the test day. Furthermore, participants were told to sleep at least 8 h during the night before the experiment and to drink at least 1 l of water on the experimental day itself. The detailed inclusion and exclusion criteria for participants of the current study are reported elsewhere (8). In cases of unforeseen illness, test persons were told to delay the experiment. All experiments were approved by the Ethics Committee of Ulm

University and the study is registered at the DRKS (German Clinical Trials Register, ID DRKS00011236). Moreover, a commuting accident insurance policy was installed for participating volunteers. Experimenters were covered by the employer's public liability insurance. All Data and Samples were collected between October 2016 and April 2017. Sociodemographic-, psychometric, physiological and immunological data from all participants of the present study have already been published recently (8).

Experimental Procedure

The detailed experimental procedures have already been described elsewhere (8). Briefly, sociodemographic features were assessed by questionnaire at the beginning of the experimental procedure. All participants were asked whether they had no animal contact at all, occasional animal contact, or daily animal contact until their 15th birthday, respectively. Importantly, while rural participants ($n = 20$) were only included in the study if they indicated daily contact with farm animals, urban participants ($n = 20$) were included when indicating either no daily animal contact or occasional animal contact until their 15th birthday (i.e., the requirement for enrollment in the study for urban participants was "no daily animal contact"). Five urban participants reported absolutely no animal contact until their 15th birthday. Following verification of emotional and physical health status by validated questionnaires (List of complaints for quantitative analysis of current bodily and general complaints (BL); State-(Trait-)Anxiety-Inventory (STAI-S) Questionnaire), the venous catheter (non-dominant arm), as well as the blood pressure and heart rate monitor (dominant arm) were placed (–60 min time point). Before (–5 min) and after (5, 15, 60, 90, and 120 min) the TSST, different parameters where assessed at each time point. In detail, heart rate and diastolic (D) and systolic (S) blood pressure (BP) were assessed (for calculation of mean arterial pressure (MAP) according to the formula: DBP + (SBP-DBP)/3), blood was drawn in ethylenediaminetetraacetic acid (EDTA) and lithium heparin-coated monovettes for collection of plasma and peripheral blood mononuclear cells (PBMCs), and saliva samples were collected for determination of cortisol concentration and microbiome analysis (for details see next section), respectively. After the 5th blood draw (90 min time point), STAI-S was used again to assess subjective strain induced by the TSST procedure. After the 6th blood draw (120 min) the catheter was removed and mental health status [Hospital Anxiety and Depression Scale - German Version, HADS-D; SCID-I (affective part)], early life (Childhood Experience of Care and Abuse Questionnaire, CECA-Q; Childhood Trauma Questionnaire, CTQ), and perceived life stress (Perceived Stress Scale-4, PSS-4) were assessed using validated questionnaires.

TSST

Acute psychosocial stress was induced using the TSST. For a detailed description of the testing procedure, see (8).

Blood Pressure and Heart Rate

BP and heart rate of the participants were determined at time points –5, 5, 15, 60, 90, and 120 min. For details, see (8). As TSST-induced changes in MAP in the original study (8) were most pronounced between time point 1 (baseline; –5 min) and 3 (+15 min), we used the respective area under the curve with respect to the ground (AUC) to compare urban participants who grew up with absolutely no animal contact with urban participants who grew up with occasional animal contact (**Figure 3**) in the present study.

Blood Draw

Blood was drawn as previously described (8). Briefly, blood (7.5 ml at each time point) was collected from an indwelling venous catheter in the non-dominant arm (inserted at –60 min) at time points –5 (5 min before the start of the TSST), 5 (5 min after termination of the TSST), 15, 60, 90, and 120 min into chilled EDTA-coated monovettes. Additionally, 9 ml of blood were collected at each time point into lithium-heparin-coated monovettes. For details about the processing of the blood samples, see (8).

PBMC Isolation

For a detailed description of the procedure, see (8). Briefly, nine ml blood were transferred from lithium-heparin-coated monovettes into Leucosep™ tubes (Greiner Bio-One GmbH, Frickenhausen, Germany), which were prepared beforehand with Ficoll® Paque (GE Healthcare Life Sciences, Freiburg, Germany) according to the manufacturer's instructions. The number of viable PBMCs was determined using an automated cell counter. As TSST-induced differences in blood PBMC counts between urban and rural participants in the original study (8) were most pronounced between time point 1 (baseline; –5 min) and 3 (+15 min), we used the respective AUC to compare urban participants who grew up with absolutely no animal contact with urban participants with who grew up with occasional animal contact (**Figure 3**) in the present study.

Enzyme-Linked Immunosorbent Assay (ELISA)

Plasma samples and supernatants from PBMC stimulations were analyzed using commercially available ELISA kits according to the manufacturers' instructions. In detail, plasma samples were analysed for IL-6 (Quantikine HS ELISA; R&D Systems Europe, Wiesbaden, Germany), and cortisol (IBL International, Hamburg, Germany). As TSST-induced changes in plasma cortisol in the original study (8) were most pronounced between time point 1 (baseline; –5 min) and 3 (+15 min), we used the respective AUC to compare urban participants who grew up with absolutely no animal contact with urban participants who grew up with occasional animal contact (**Figure 3**) in the present study. Accordingly, we calculated AUC between time point 5 (90 min) and 6 (120 min) for plasma IL-6 levels in the current study to compare urban participants who grew up with absolutely no animal contact with urban participants who grew up with occasional animal contact (**Figure 3**), as TSST-induced differences between urban and rural participants in plasma IL-6 levels were only detectable at these late stages.

Collection and Preparation of Salivary Samples

Salivary samples were collected at the –5, 5, 15, 60, 90, and 120 min time points. For salivary sample collection, a salivette® (Cat. No. 51.1534.500; Sarstedt, Nuernberg, Germany) was used. In detail, each participant was advised to chew a salivette® swab thoroughly for approximately one minute at each time point, then to spit the swab into a sterile tube. Subsequently, samples were centrifuged (1,000 g, 2 min, RT) and stored at –80°C until further processing. For microbiome analysis, salivary samples taken at the –5 min time point were used. 100 µl of saliva was used for the DNA extraction. DNA was extracted using the PowerSoil DNA extraction kit (Cat No. 12888-100 & 12955-4, MoBio Laboratories, Carlsbad, CA, USA) according to the manufacturer's instructions. Marker genes in isolated DNA were PCR-amplified using HotStarTaq Master Mix (Cat No. 203433, Qiagen, Valencia, CA, USA) and the 515 F (5'-GTGCCAGCMGCCGCGGTAA-3')/806 R (5'-GGACTACHVGGGTWTCTAAT-3') primer pair (Integrated DNA Technologies, Coralville, IA, USA) targeting the V4 hypervariable region of the 16S rRNA gene modified with a unique 12-base sequence identifier for each sample and the Illumina adapter, as previously described (15). The thermal cycling program consisted of an initial step at 94°C for 3 min followed by 35 cycles (94°C for 45 sec, 55°C for 1 min, and 72°C for 1.5 min), and a final extension at 72°C for 10 min. PCR reactions were run in duplicate and the products from the duplicate reactions were pooled and visualized on an agarose gel to ensure successful amplification. PCR products were cleaned and normalized using a SequalPrep Normalization Kit (Cat. No. A1051001, ThermoFisher, Waltham, MA, USA) following manufacturer's instructions. The normalized amplicon pool was sequenced on an Illumina MiSeq run using V3 chemistry, 600 cycles, and 2 x 300-bp paired-end sequencing. All sequencing and library preparation were conducted at the University of Colorado Boulder BioFrontiers Next-Gen Sequencing core facility.

Microbiome Analysis

Microbiome bioinformatics were performed with QIIME2-2019.7 (http://qiime2.org) (16, 17). Briefly, raw sequence data were demultiplexed and quality filtered using the q2-demux plugin followed by denoising with DADA2 via q2-dada2 (18) to identify all observed amplicon sequence variants (ASVs) [i.e., 100% operational taxonomic units (OTUs)]. All ASVs were aligned with mafft (19) (via q2-alignment) and used to construct a phylogeny with fasttree2 (20) (via q2-phylogeny). Alpha-diversity metrics [observed OTUs, Faith's Phylogenetic Diversity (21), and Shannon diversity index], and beta diversity metrics [weighted UniFrac (22), unweighted UniFrac (23)] were

estimated using q2-diversity after samples were rarefied (i.e., subsampled without replacement). A total of 9,280 sequences per sample were chosen as our rarefaction depth to retain all paired samples, as samples with fewer sequences than the rarefaction depth are excluded from downstream diversity analyses. PCoA plots were generated using the weighted UniFrac distance matrix in R Studio1.2.1335 [RStudio Team (2018). RStudio: Integrated Development for R. RStudio, Inc., Boston, MA URL http://www.rstudio.com/] and Phyloseq package 1.28.0 (24). The differentially abundant features between saliva samples of participants with or without animal contact until their 15th birthday were determined through the analysis of composition of microbiomes (ANCOM) pipeline (25). The microbiome data assessed in the present study are available in the NCBI SRA public repository (accession number: PRJNA606354).

Statistics

Significant differences in alpha diversity were calculated using the non-parametric Kruskal-Wallis ANOVA on ranks test (26); two-tailed p values < 0.05 were considered as statistically significant. Differences in beta diversity were calculated using a generalized UniFrac distance model (27). PERMANOVA pseudo p values < 0.05 were considered statistically different. For statistical analysis and graphical illustration of the area under the curve with respect to the ground (AUC) data, the software package Prism (version 8) was used. Raw data sets used for AUC calculation were already corrected for outliers (28) and thus identical to our previously published study (8). Within AUC datasets, Kolmogorov-Smirnov test using Lilliefors' significance was employed to test normal distribution of all acquired data sets. Normally distributed data sets were subsequently analyzed using parametric statistics (Student's t-test). Non-normally distributed data sets were analyzed using non-parametric statistics [Mann-Whitney U test (MWU)]. Normally distributed data are presented as bars (mean + SEM). Non-normally distributed data are presented as box plots (median; min, max, 25th and 75th percentile). The two-tailed level of significance was set at $p < 0.05$.

RESULTS

Salivary Microbial α- and/or β-Diversity Does Not Differ Between Participants Raised in Rural Areas in the Presence of Daily Contact With Farm Animals Compared With Participants Raised in Urban Areas in the Absence of Daily Animal Contact in Adulthood

Statistical analysis using Kruskal-Wallis-H-Test (KWH) revealed no significant difference in the α-diversity of the salivary microbiome as measured by Shannon diversity index between participants raised in urban areas without daily animal contact with animals vs. participants raised in rural areas in the presence of daily contact with farm animals

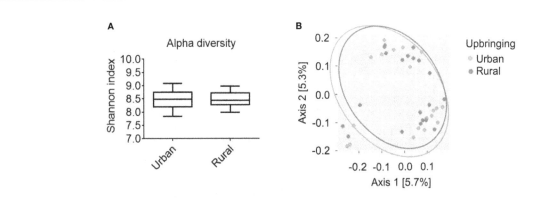

FIGURE 1 | Alpha and beta diversity analysis of the salivary microbiome composition for participants raised in urban areas in the absence of daily animal contact compared to individuals raised in rural areas in the presence of daily contact with farm animals. **(A)** Shannon diversity index representing richness and evenness within samples was not significantly different between urban ($n = 20$) and rural ($n = 20$) populations (Kruskal-Wallis, $p = 0.935$). Solid line represents the median. Lower box indicates 25th, upper box indicates 75th percentile. 10th and 90th percentile are indicated by lower and upper error bar, respectively. **(B)** Weighted UniFrac principal coordinates analysis (PCoA) plot represents beta diversity as phylogenetic distances among samples for both urban (turquoise; $n = 20$) and rural (orange; $n = 20$) populations. PCoA axes 1 and 2 explain 5.7 and 5.3% of the variation, respectively.

($p = 0.935$; **Figure 1A**). Consistent with the results observed with Shannon index, the analysis of Faith's Phylogenetic Diversity and observed OTUs alpha diversity indexes displayed no differences between urban and rural groups (Faith's PD, $p = 0.999$; observed OTUs, $p = 0.840$). There was also no association between salivary β-diversity and the factor urban-rural upbringing (pseudo-$F = 0.635$; $p = 0.908$). The latter is visualized using a weighted UniFrac principal component analysis (PCoA) plot presenting phylogenetic distances among all of the samples (**Figure 1B**).

Growing Up With Absolutely No Animal Contact Until the 15th Birthday Affects Salivary β-Diversity in Adulthood

The microbial β-diversity in "urban" participants raised with absolutely no animal contact until the 15th birthday ($n = 5$) was significantly increased compared with participants reporting either occasional ($n = 15$) or daily ($n = 20$) animal contact during upbringing. This is indicated by a PERMANOVA analysis (pseudo-$F = 1.988$; $p = 0.038$; **Figure 2A**) calculating the distances of each sample to all samples with a minimum of

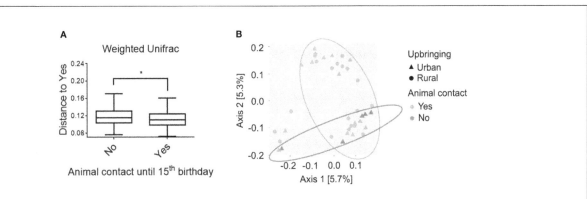

FIGURE 2 | Beta diversity analysis of salivary microbiome composition for participants with absolutely no animal contact compared to participants that were at minimum exposed to occasional animal contact until the 15th birthday, respectively. **(A)** Analysis of beta diversity using weighted-UniFrac distance metrics revealed differences in the microbial community structure of participants with no animal contact at all (red, $n = 5$) compared to participants with at least occasional animal contact until the 15th birthday (blue, $n = 35$), respectively. Distances to subjects with animal contact (Yes = animal contact; No = No animal contact) are represented by a PERMANOVA analysis with a total of 999 permutations, pseudo-$F = 1.988$, $p = 0.038$. Solid line represents the median. Lower box indicates 25th, upper box indicates 75th percentile. 10th and 90th percentile are indicated by lower and upper error bar, respectively. **(B)** Weighted-UniFrac principal coordinates analysis (PCoA) plot shows participants raised in rural areas in the presence of daily contact with farm animals (circles; $n = 20$) and participants raised in urban areas in the absence of daily animal contact (triangles; $n = 20$). Participants were further subdivided into the groups with "absolutely no animal contact until the 15th birthday" (orange, $n = 5$) or "occasional to daily animal contact until the 15th birthday" (turquoise, $n = 35$). PCoA axes 1 and 2 explain 5.7 and 5.3% of the variation, respectively. *$p < 0.05$.

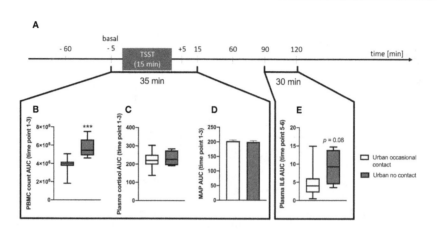

FIGURE 3 | Analysis of Trier Social Stress Test (TSST)-induced alterations on immunological and physiological parameters between urban participants growing up with no animal contact at all vs. urban participants growing up with "occasional" animal contact until the 15th birthday, respectively. **(A)** Timeline of the experimental procedure. At –60 min time point, the venous catheter as well as the blood pressure and heart rate monitor were placed. Before (–5 min) and after (5, 15, 60, 90, and 120 min) the TSST, different immunological and physiological parameters where assessed. **(B)** Area under the curve with respect to ground (AUC) analysis indicates that urban participants growing up with no animal contact at all ($n = 5$) vs. urban subjects growing up with "occasional" animal contact until the 15th birthday ($n = 15$), respectively showed significantly higher counts of plasma peripheral blood mononuclear cells (PBMCs) between time point 1 and 3. This effect was also by trend visible in plasma interleukin (IL)-6 levels between time point 5 and 6 **(E)**. There were no significant differences between both groups in the AUC between time point 1 and 3 of plasma cortisol levels **(C)** and the mean arterial pressure (MAP; **D**), respectively. Normally distributed data are presented as bars (mean + SEM). Non-normally distributed data are presented as box plots (Median, min, max, 25th and 75th percentile) ***$p < 0.001$.

"occasional" animal contact. The latter is further visualized by a weighted-UniFrac PCoA Plot showing the calculated distances between all samples assessed (**Figure 2B**).

Urban Participants Growing Up With Absolutely No Animal Contact Showed an Increased TSST-Induced Inflammatory Response Compared With Urban Participants Growing Up With Occasional Animal Contact

Statistical analysis revealed that urban participants reporting absolutely no animal contact during their first 15 years of life showed a significantly greater stress-induced increase in blood PBMC counts between time point 1 (baseline; –5 min) and 3 (+15 min) (AUC; $p < 0.001$; MWU; **Figures 3A, B**) than did respective urban participants reporting occasional animal contact. A comparable effect was also by trend detectable in plasma IL-6 levels between time point 5 (+90 min) and 6 (+120 min) (AUC; $p = 0.08$; MWU, **Figures 3A, E**). No significant differences between these two groups were found in plasma cortisol levels (AUC; **Figures 3A, C**) and MAP (AUC; **Figures 3A, D**), both assessed between time point 1 and 3.

DISCUSSION

In the present study, we showed that urban upbringing in the absence of pets compared to rural upbringing in the presence of farm animals is not associated with specific patterns in the α- or β-diversity of the salivary microbiome. In contrast, we were able

to reveal that the salivary microbial β-diversity is significantly different in individuals with no animal contact at all compared to all other participants with at least occasional animal contact until the age of 15, respectively—a finding that was further associated with a more pronounced immune activation within the group of urban participants following acute psychosocial stressor exposure induced by the TSST.

In line with the hypothesis that an overreactive immune system is causally involved in the pathogenesis (29, 30) and increased prevalence (3–5) of stress-associated disorders in urban vs. rural environments, we recently showed that healthy male individuals raised in urban areas without daily animal contact vs. individuals raised in rural areas in the presence of daily contact with farm animals respond with increased systemic immune activation towards the TSST (8), a standardized laboratory stressor in humans (11). Given that a modern urban lifestyle is associated with less contact to biodiversity (31), and that a reduced exposure to microbial antigens (32, 33) and immunoregulatory "Old Friends" microorganisms (6, 7, 34, 35), especially during early life (36), promotes development of inflammatory disorders later in life (37, 38), a role of the human microbiome in the accumulation (4, 39) of stress-associated disorders in urban vs. rural environments is very likely. Surprisingly and against our hypothesis, neither α- nor β-diversity measures were significantly different between the two experimental groups in the present study, suggesting the composition of the salivary microbiome in adulthood is not a reliable marker of the environment that an individual was raised in. A possible reason for this finding might be that differences in the salivary microbial composition between "urban" and "rural" individuals at a young age are just not surviving into an individual's adulthood. In support of this hypothesis, the mouth cavity is a rapidly changing environment for bacteria, affected by diet and sanitation (40), the currently prevailing environment, and host age (12, 41). In line with this possibility, C-section-induced differences in gut microbial composition are only present throughout the neonatal period, but largely disappear within the first years (42).

As the overall extent of animal contact during upbringing has been shown recently to affect the composition of the human gut microbiome (43, 44), we investigated in a next step if the salivary microbial diversity in adulthood is different between participants who reported absolutely no contact with pets compared to participants who reported occasional or daily contact with pets or farm animals. Notably, whereas the main criterion for rural participants ($n = 20$) to be included into the study was to have had daily contact with farm animals until the age of 15, urban participants ($n = 20$) were included when indicating either no animal contact at all or occasional animal contact until their 15th birthday. Interestingly, and in support of the above-reported hypothesis, comparing participants with no animal contact at all ($n = 5$; exclusively urban participants) to participants exposed to occasional ($n = 15$; urban participants) or daily ($n = 20$; rural participants) animal contact until the age of 15 (overall $n = 35$), respectively, revealed a significant difference in β-diversity of the salivary microbiome, indicating that, in contrast to the environment that an individual is brought up in, the extent of animal contact during childhood potentially has long-lasting effects on an individual's salivary microbiome. Our finding that microbial β-diversity was significantly higher in urban participants reporting absolutely no animal contact until the age of 15 years compared to all other participants reporting either daily contact to farm animals (rural) or occasional pet contact (urban) is in line with the fact that Westernization has been consistently associated with lower α-diversity but higher β-diversity (9). As microbiome alterations associated with Westernization are hypothesized to be mainly driven by dispersal limitation in combination with high inter-individual differences in selective environments, our findings suggest that a reduction in animal contact might be at least one factor contributing to the overall dispersal limitation in Western societies and the consequently increased risk to develop non-communicable diseases (9).

Of particular interest in the context of these results is a study showing that living on single-family dairy farms with regular contact with farm animals in Amish farm children goes along with a lower asthma and allergy risk and innate immune system activation compared to living on highly industrialized farms with little contact with farm animals in Hutterite farm children (38). In accordance with these findings, other studies revealed that early exposure to both pets and farm animals reduces the risk of childhood asthma and other inflammatory disorders (45, 46). Strikingly, comparing TSST-induced changes in blood PBMC counts at the initial phase of stress [urban vs. rural differences were most pronounced between time point 1–3 (8)] and plasma IL-6 levels at the late phase [urban vs. rural differences were most

pronounced between time point 5–6 (8)] between urban individuals with absolutely no animal contact vs. occasional animal contact during upbringing, revealed that the former showed a significantly greater stress-induced increase in blood PBMC counts and by trend increased plasma IL-6 levels, both quantified as area under the curve between respective time points. In contrast to the effects on stress-induced immune activation and in contrast to the hypothesis that increased hypothalamic–pituitary–adrenal (HPA) axis activity is associated with the development of stress-related psychiatric disorders (47), the overall animal contact during upbringing did not affect TSST-reactivity of the HPA axis and the cardiovascular system. This was indicated by comparable stress-induced increases in plasma cortisol levels and mean arterial pressure at the initial phase after TSST between urban participants raised with no vs. occasional animal contact, respectively. However, given that these parameters were also comparable between rural vs. urban participants raised in the presence or absence of animals, respectively (8), an exaggerated HPA axis and sympathetic nervous system activity seem to only play a minor role in mediating the increased prevalence of stress-associated disorders in urban vs. rural environments.

Nevertheless, our study has some limitations that have to be taken into consideration. One limitation in the current study is that the sample size in the urban group raised without any pet contact is small, clearly indicating the rather preliminary character of our findings and the need for confirmation in adequately powered future studies. Of note, statistical analysis employing partial least squares discriminant analysis (PLSDA) as a supervised learning approach (48, 49) did not reveal that the salivary microbiome was predictive of urban status with or without animal contact. However, as discerning subtle variations in community configurations along the pet-contact/urban or rural living categories would add important mechanistic knowledge on the involved bacterial species mediating these beneficial long-term effects of animal contact, these type of analyses should be repeated employing larger cohorts of participants. Additional limitations are that we did not take into account possible differences in participants' mode of delivery at birth, antibiotic usage during the first years of life, feeding of formula milk as a replacement for breast milk, or exposure to kindergarten, which are all known to affect the composition of the microbiome (38, 50–52).

Together with our previous work (8), the results of the present study suggest that the complete absence of animal contact in early life during urban upbringing promotes life-long differences in the composition of the salivary microbiome and potentiates the negative consequences of urban vs. rural upbringing on stress-induced immune activation. As urban participants in the present study reporting animal contact were only included if this contact was occasional and not daily, we are convinced that future studies comparing urban participants raised in the absolute absence vs. daily presence of pets will reveal even more prominent differences in TSST-induced immune activation between the groups.

ETHICS STATEMENT

The studies involving human participants were reviewed and approved by Ethics Committee of Ulm University. The participants provided their written informed consent to participate in this study.

AUTHOR CONTRIBUTIONS

GR, CL, HG, CW, and SR designed the study. DL, CZ, TB, SH, MJ, NR, CS, JH, CW, and SR performed experiments. DL, CZ, CL, and SR analyzed data. DL, CZ, CL, and SR wrote the manuscript.

ACKNOWLEDGMENTS

The authors gratefully thank P. Hornischer and U. Binder (both from the Laboratory for Molecular Psychosomatics, Clinic for Psychosomatic Medicine and Psychotherapy, University Ulm, 89081 Ulm, Germany) for their excellent technical assistance and help in performing the experiments. The authors further are grateful to L. Hackl, B. Schembera, P. Marquardt, A. Bauer, B. Häringer, T. Richter, L. Hermann, M. Tisch, M. Zeh, F. Weinreich, H. Holzrichter, and J. Kunze for participating as jury members in the TSST. Furthermore, the authors would like to thank Prof. Dr. M. Wirsching (University of Freiburg) for his critical and helpful project discussions.

REFERENCES

1. M'Koma AE. Inflammatory bowel disease: an expanding global health problem. *Clin Med Insights Gastroenterol* (2013) 6:33–47. doi: 10.4137/CGast.S12731

2. Twenge JM, Cooper AB, Joiner TE, Duffy ME, Binau SG. Age, period, and cohort trends in mood disorder indicators and suicide-related outcomes in a nationally representative dataset, 2005-2017. *J Abnorm Psychol* (2019) 128(3):185–99. doi: 10.1037/abn0000410

3. Ekbom A, Adami HO, Helmick CG, Jonzon A, Zack MM. Perinatal risk factors for inflammatory bowel disease: a case-control study. *Am J Epidemiol* (1990) 132(6):1111–9. doi: 10.1093/oxfordjournals.aje.a115754

4. Peen J, Schoevers RA, Beekman AT, Dekker J. The current status of urban-rural differences in psychiatric disorders. *Acta Psychiatr Scand* (2010) 121(2):84–93. doi: 10.1111/j.1600-0447.2009.01438.x

5. Langgartner D, Lowry CA, Reber SO. Old Friends, immunoregulation, and stress resilience. *Pflugers Arch* (2019) 471(2):237–69. doi: 10.1007/s00424-018-2228-7

6. Blaser MJ. The theory of disappearing microbiota and the epidemics of chronic diseases. *Nat Rev Immunol* (2017) 17(8):461–3. doi: 10.1038/nri.2017.77

7. Rook GA, Lowry CA, Raison CL. Microbial 'Old Friends', immunoregulation and stress resilience. *Evol Med Public Health* (2013) 2013(1):46–64. doi: 10.1093/emph/eot004

8. Böbel TS, Hackl SB, Langgartner D, Jarczok MN, Rohleder N, Rook GA, et al. Less immune activation following social stress in rural vs. urban participants raised with regular or no animal contact, respectively. *Proc Natl Acad Sci U S A* (2018) 115(20):5259–64. doi: 10.1073/pnas.1719866115

9. Martínez I, Stegen James C, Maldonado-Gómez Maria X, Eren AM, Siba Peter M, Greenhill Andrew R, et al. The gut microbiota of rural Papua New Guineans: composition, diversity patterns, and ecological processes. *Cell Rep* (2015) 11(4):527–38. doi: 10.1016/j.celrep.2015.03.049

10. Stamper CE, Hoisington AJ, Gomez OM, Halweg-Edwards AL, Smith DG, Bates KL, et al. The microbiome of the built environment and human behavior: implications for emotional health and well-being in postmodern western societies. *Int Rev Neurobiol* (2016) 131:289–323. doi: 10.1016/bs.irn.2016.07.006

11. Kirschbaum C, Pirke KM, Hellhammer DH. The 'Trier Social Stress Test'–a tool for investigating psychobiological stress responses in a laboratory setting. *Neuropsychobiology* (1993) 28(1-2):76–81. doi: 119004

12. Shaw L, Ribeiro ALR, Levine AP, Pontikos N, Balloux F, Segal AW, et al. The human salivary microbiome is shaped by shared environment rather than genetics: Evidence from a large family of closely related individuals. *MBio* (2017) 8(5):1–13. doi: 10.1128/mBio.01237-17

13. Kodukula K, Faller DV, Harpp DN, Kanara I, Pernokas J, Pernokas M, et al. Gut microbiota and salivary diagnostics: The mouth is salivating to tell us something. *Biores Open Access* (2017) 6(1):123–32. doi: 10.1089/biores.2017.0020

14. Said HS, Suda W, Nakagome S, Chinen H, Oshima K, Kim S, et al. Dysbiosis of salivary microbiota in inflammatory bowel disease and its association with oral immunological biomarkers. *DNA Res* (2014) 21(1):15–25. doi: 10.1093/dnares/dst037

15. Caporaso JG, Lauber CL, Walters WA, Berg-Lyons D, Huntley J, Fierer N, et al. Ultra-high-throughput microbial community analysis on the Illumina HiSeq and MiSeq platforms. *ISME J* (2012) 6(8):1621–4. doi: 10.1038/ismej.2012.8

16. Bolyen E, Rideout JR, Dillon MR, Bokulich NA, Abnet CC, Al-Ghalith GA, et al. Reproducible, interactive, scalable and extensible microbiome data science using QIIME 2. *Nat Biotechnol* (2019) 37(8):852–7. doi: 10.1038/s41587-019-0209-9

17. Pearson T, Caporaso JG, Yellowhair M, Bokulich NA, Padi M, Roe DJ, et al. Effects of ursodeoxycholic acid on the gut microbiome and colorectal adenoma development. *Cancer Med* (2019) 8(2):617–28. doi: 10.1002/cam4.1965

18. Callahan BJ, McMurdie PJ, Rosen MJ, Han AW, Johnson AJA, Holmes SP. DADA2: High-resolution sample inference from Illumina amplicon data. *Nat Methods* (2016) 13(7):581–3. doi: 10.1038/nmeth.3869

19. Katoh K, Misawa K, Ki K, Miyata T. MAFFT: a novel method for rapid multiple sequence alignment based on fast Fourier transform. *Nucleic Acids Res* (2002) 30(14):3059–66. doi: 10.1093/nar/gkf436

20. Price MN, Dehal PS, Arkin AP. FastTree 2–approximately maximum-likelihood trees for large alignments. *PloS One* (2010) 5(3):e9490–e. doi: 10.1371/journal.pone.0009490

21. Faith DP. Conservation evaluation and phylogenetic diversity. *Biol Conserv* (1992) 61(1):1–10. doi: 10.1016/0006-3207(92)91201-3

22. Lozupone CA, Hamady M, Kelley ST, Knight R. Quantitative and qualitative β diversity measures lead to different insights into factors that structure microbial communities. *Appl Environ Microbiol* (2007) 73(5):1576–85. doi: 10.1128/aem.01996-06

23. Lozupone C, Knight R. UniFrac: a new phylogenetic method for comparing microbial communities. *Appl Environ Microbiol* (2005) 71(12):8228–35. doi: 10.1128/aem.71.12.8228-8235.2005

24. McMurdie PJ, Holmes S. phyloseq: An R Package for reproducible interactive analysis and graphics of microbiome census data. *PloS One* (2013) 8(4):e61217. doi: 10.1371/journal.pone.0061217

25. Mandal S, Van Treuren W, White RA, Eggesbo M, Knight R, Peddada SD. Analysis of composition of microbiomes: a novel method for studying microbial composition. *Microb Ecol Health Dis* (2015) 26:27663. doi: 10.3402/mehd.v26.27663

26. Kruskal WH, Wallis WA. Use of ranks in one-criterion variance analysis. *J Am Stat Assoc* (1952) 47(260):583–621. doi: 10.1080/01621459.1952.10483441

27. Chen J, Bittinger K, Charlson ES, Hoffmann C, Lewis J, Wu GD, et al. Associating microbiome composition with environmental covariates using generalized UniFrac distances. *Bioinformatics* (2012) 28(16):2106–13. doi: 10.1093/bioinformatics/bts342

28. Grubbs FE. Procedures for detecting outlying observations in samples. *Technometrics* (1969) 11: (1):1–21. doi: 10.2307/1266761

29. Khandaker GM, Pearson RM, Zammit S, Lewis G, Jones PB. Association of serum interleukin 6 and C-reactive protein in childhood with depression and psychosis in young adult life: a population-based longitudinal study. *JAMA Psychiatry* (2014) 71(10):1121–8. doi: 10.1001/jamapsychiatry.2014.1332

30. Kivimaki M, Shipley MJ, Batty GD, Hamer M, Akbaraly TN, Kumari M, et al. Long-term inflammation increases risk of common mental disorder: a cohort study. *Mol Psychiatry* (2014) 19(2):149–50. doi: 10.1038/mp.2013.35

31. Sonnenburg JL, Sonnenburg ED. Vulnerability of the industrialized microbiota. *Science* (2019) 366(6464):aaw9255. doi: 10.1126/science.aaw9255

32. Braun-Fahrlander C, Riedler J, Herz U, Eder W, Waser M, Grize L, et al. Environmental exposure to endotoxin and its relation to asthma in school-age children. *N Engl J Med* (2002) 347(12):869–77. doi: 10.1056/NEJMoa020057

33. Riedler J, Braun-Fahrlander C, Eder W, Schreuer M, Waser M, Maisch S, et al. Exposure to farming in early life and development of asthma and allergy: a cross-sectional survey. *Lancet* (2001) 358(9288):1129–33. doi: 10.1016/S0140-6736(01)06252-3

34. Rook GAW. The hygiene hypothesis and the increasing prevalence of chronic inflammatory disorders. *Trans R Soc Trop Med Hygiene* (2007) 101(11):1072–4. doi: 10.1016/j.trstmh.2007.05.014

35. Rook GA, Raison CL, Lowry CA. Microbiota, immunoregulatory old friends and psychiatric disorders. *Adv Exp Med Biol* (2014) 817:319–56. doi: 10.1007/978-1-4939-0897-4_15

36. Lynch SV, Boushey HA. The microbiome and development of allergic disease. *Curr Opin Allergy Clin Immunol* (2016) 16(2):165–71. doi: 10.1097/ACI.0000000000000255

37. Ege MJ, Mayer M, Normand AC, Genuneit J, Cookson WO, Braun-Fahrlander C, et al. Exposure to environmental microorganisms and childhood asthma. *N Engl J Med* (2011) 364(8):701–9. doi: 10.1056/NEJMoa1007302

38. Stein MM, Hrusch CL, Gozdz J, Igartua C, Pivniouk V, Murray SE, et al. Innate immunity and asthma risk in amish and hutterite farm children. *N Engl J Med* (2016) 375(5):411–21. doi: 10.1056/NEJMoa1508749

39. Vassos E, Agerbo E, Mors O, Pedersen CB. Urban-rural differences in incidence rates of psychiatric disorders in Denmark. *Br J Psychiatry* (2016) 208(5):435–40. doi: 10.1192/bjp.bp.114.161091

40. The Human Microbiome Project Consortium. Structure, function and diversity of the healthy human microbiome. *Nature* (2012) 486(7402):207–14. doi: 10.1038/nature11234

41. Stahringer SS, Clemente JC, Corley RP, Hewitt J, Knights D, Walters WA, et al. Nurture trumps nature in a longitudinal survey of salivary bacterial communities in twins from early adolescence to early adulthood. *Genome Res* (2012) 22(11):2146–52. doi: 10.1101/gr.140608.112

42. Shao Y, Forster SC, Tsaliki E, Vervier K, Strang A, Simpson N, et al. Stunted microbiota and opportunistic pathogen colonization in caesarean-section birth. *Nature* (2019) 574(7776):117–21. doi: 10.1038/s41586-019-1560-1

43. Azad MB, Konya T, Maughan H, Guttman DS, Field CJ, Sears MR, et al. Infant gut microbiota and the hygiene hypothesis of allergic disease: impact of household pets and siblings on microbiota composition and diversity. *Allergy Asthma Clin Immunol* (2013) 9(1):15. doi: 10.1186/1710-1492-9-15

44. Tun HM, Konya T, Takaro TK, Brook JR, Chari R, Field CJ, et al. Exposure to household furry pets influences the gut microbiota of infant at 3-4 months following various birth scenarios. *Microbiome* (2017) 5(1):40. doi: 10.1186/s40168-017-0254-x

45. Fall T, Lundholm C, Ortqvist AK, Fall K, Fang F, Hedhammar A, et al. Early exposure to dogs and farm animals and the risk of childhood asthma. *JAMA Pediatr* (2015) 169(11):e153219. doi: 10.1001/jamapediatrics.2015.3219

46. Mubanga M, Byberg L, Nowak C, Egenvall A, Magnusson PK, Ingelsson E, et al. Dog ownership and the risk of cardiovascular disease and death - a nationwide cohort study. *Sci Rep* (2017) 7(1):15821. doi: 10.1038/s41598-017-16118-6

47. Holsboer F. The corticosteroid receptor hypothesis of depression. *Neuropsychopharmacology* (2000) 23(5):477–501. doi: 10.1016/S0893-133X(00)00159-7

48. Perez-Enciso M, Tenenhaus M. Prediction of clinical outcome with microarray data: a partial least squares discriminant analysis (PLS-DA) approach. *Hum Genet* (2003) 112(5-6):581–92. doi: 10.1007/s00439-003-0921-9

49. Rohart F, Gautier B, Singh A, Le Cao KA. mixOmics: An R package for 'omics feature selection and multiple data integration. *PloS Comput Biol* (2017) 13(11):e1005752. doi: 10.1371/journal.pcbi.1005752

50. Stilling RM, Dinan TG, Cryan JF. Microbial genes, brain & behaviour - epigenetic regulation of the gut-brain axis. *Genes Brain Behav* (2014) 13(1):69–86. doi: 10.1111/gbb.12109

51. Cryan JF, Dinan TG. Mind-altering microorganisms: the impact of the gut microbiota on brain and behaviour. *Nat Rev Neurosci* (2012) 13(10):701–12. doi: 10.1038/nrn3346

52. Nygaard AB, Charnock C. Longitudinal development of the dust microbiome in a newly opened Norwegian kindergarten. *Microbiome* (2018) 6(1):159. doi: 10.1186/s40168-018-0553-x

4

Animal Models for Functional Gastrointestinal Disorders

Alison Accarie[1] and Tim Vanuytsel[1,2]*

[1] Department of Chronic Diseases, Metabolism and Ageing (ChroMetA), Translational Research Center for Gastrointestinal Disorders (TARGID), KU Leuven, Leuven, Belgium, [2] Department of Gastroenterology and Hepatology, University Hospitals Leuven, Leuven, Belgium

*Correspondence:
Tim Vanuytsel
tim.vanuytsel@uzleuven.be

Functional gastrointestinal disorders (FGID), such as functional dyspepsia (FD) and irritable bowel syndrome (IBS) are characterized by chronic abdominal symptoms in the absence of an organic, metabolic or systemic cause that readily explains these complaints. Their pathophysiology is still not fully elucidated and animal models have been of great value to improve the understanding of the complex biological mechanisms. Over the last decades, many animal models have been developed to further unravel FGID pathophysiology and test drug efficacy. In the first part of this review, we focus on stress-related models, starting with the different perinatal stress models, including the stress of the dam, followed by a discussion on neonatal stress such as the maternal separation model. We also describe the most commonly used stress models in adult animals which brought valuable insights on the brain-gut axis in stress-related disorders. In the second part, we focus more on models studying peripheral, i.e., gastrointestinal, mechanisms, either induced by an infection or another inflammatory trigger. In this section, we also introduce more recent models developed around food-related metabolic disorders or food hypersensitivity and allergy. Finally, we introduce models mimicking FGID as a secondary effect of medical interventions and spontaneous models sharing characteristics of GI and anxiety-related disorders. The latter are powerful models for brain-gut axis dysfunction and bring new insights about FGID and their comorbidities such as anxiety and depression.

Keywords: functional gastrointestinal disorders, animal models, stress, irritable bowel syndrome, functional dyspepsia, intestinal permeability, visceral pain, mast cells

INTRODUCTION

Functional gastrointestinal disorders (FGID), such as functional dyspepsia (FD) and irritable bowel syndrome (IBS) are highly prevalent, occurring in 10–30% of the general population depending on the criteria used, and represent an important part of the workload of gastroenterology and primary care clinical practice. Those syndromes are characterized by chronic abdominal symptoms in the absence of an organic, metabolic or systemic cause that readily explains these complaints. Based on the Rome IV criteria, FD is defined as bothersome postprandial fullness, early satiation, epigastric pain and/or epigastric burning (1) while IBS is characterized by recurrent abdominal pain or discomfort in association with altered defecation patterns (2, 3). The etiology and pathophysiology remain incompletely understood, which is reflected in the paucity and limited effectiveness of the available treatment options. Moreover, in the last years, FGIDs have been conceptualized as disorders of brain-gut interaction, highlighting the bidirectional interplay between central and peripheral mechanisms and opening new possibilities for anxiety and depression animal models to study FGID.

Over the last 20 years, many animal models, which originally focused on one particular pathophysiological factor, have been developed for FGID. These models have contributed a lot to the understanding of the pathophysiological mechanisms behind the symptoms and were also used to test and validate therapeutic targets and potential therapies (4). However, many aspects of functional disorders remain poorly understood and unsolved in these unidimensional models. An animal model is considered suitable for a disorder, when the etiology of the disease is as close as possible to what is known in humans. Several conditions must be fulfilled, among them (1) the construct validity, i.e., the experimental conditions used to produce the animal model should replicate the cause of the disease in human, (2) the face validity, i.e., the symptoms observed in the animal should replicate the clinical features observed in the patients and (3) the predictive validity where the response to drugs in the animal models can predict reliably the potential response in the human counterpart. It is clear that unidimensional models for FGID do not fulfill these criteria. To overcome the weaknesses of the classic models, more recently, several new models have been introduced, either combining several of the putative factors involved in FGID pathophysiology or using new insights such as the impact of nutrition to try and represent the large panel of symptoms and complex interactions between the pathophysiological factors found in FGID (4).

In this review, we will summarize the state of the art concerning the most relevant and most commonly used pre-clinical models that have been developed for FGID and highlight their contribution to the understanding of FGID pathophysiology. Most of the published studies use rodent models, due to the possibility of genetic manipulations and the quick turnover of the models through fast reproduction and a large number of pups in one litter, in comparison to larger animal models such as pig models. Therefore, this review will largely focus on rodent models.

Abbreviations: 5HT, serotonin; 5HT1A/1B/2A/2B, serotonin receptor type 1A, 1B, 2A, 2B; ACTH, adreno cortico trophic hormone; AMPA, α-amino-3-hydroxy-5-methyl-4-isoxazolepropionic acid; BB-DP, biobreeding diabetes prone; BDNF, brain-derived neurotrophic factor; CCL2, chemokine ligand 2; CEACAM6, CEA cell adhesion molecule 6; CNS, central nervous system; COX-2, cyclo-oxygenase 2; CGRP, calcitonin gene-related peptide; CRF, corticotropin-releasing factor; CRFR, corticotropin-releasing factor receptor; DSS, dextran sodium sulfate; ELS, early life stress; FD, functional dyspepsia; FGID, functional gastrointestinal disorders; FODMAP, Fermentable Oligo-, Di-, Mono-saccharides And Polyols; FSL, Findler sensitive line; GC-C/cGMP, guanylate cyclase C/cyclic guanylin monophosphate; GI, gastro intestinal; GR, Glucocorticoid receptor; HPA, hypothalamus-pituitary-adrenal; HSHF, high fat high sugar; IFN, interferon; IgE, immune globulin E; IL, interleukin; IBS, irritable bowel syndrom; IBD, inflammatory bowel disease; KO, knock out; MS, maternal separation; MPO, myeloperoxidase activity; MUC2, Mucin 2; NGF, nerve growth factor; NMDA, N-methyl-D-aspartate; P2X, purinergic receptor; PAR2, Protease-activated receptor 2; PI, post infectious; PND, post-natal day; POI, post-operative ileus; SCFA, short chain fatty acids; SERT, serotonin transporter; SHR, spontaneously hypertensive rat; SIS, social isolation stress; TFF3, rail fold factor 3; TLR, toll like receptor; TNBS, Trinitrobenzene sulfonic acid; TNF, tumor necrosis factor; TRH, thyrotropin-releasing hormone; TRPV1, transient receptor potentiate vanilloid 1; VNS, vagal nerve stimulation; WAS, water avoidance stress; WKY, wistar kyoto; ZO-1, Zona occludens 1.

PATHOPHYSIOLOGY OF FGID

Functional gastrointestinal disorders have long been regarded as purely psychosomatic conditions. In the last decade, however, evidence for a low-grade mucosal inflammation, dominated by mast cells, eosinophils, and T-lymphocytes (5–8), as well as impaired epithelial barrier function (9) and neuronal hyperexcitability (10) leading to visceral hypersensitivity (11) and dysmotility has accumulated in FGID, challenging the traditional paradigm of a purely functional disorder. Mast cells represent a crucial link in colonic neuro-immune interaction as they communicate with both the intrinsic; i.e., enteric, and extrinsic nervous system in the gut and release mediators such as tryptase and nerve growth factor, which are involved in visceral hypersensitivity and mucosal permeability in FGID patients (12). A commonly cited hypothesis is based on the concept that luminal antigens, originating from food components, microbiota or other noxious substances such as bile and acid can induce a mast cell and eosinophil predominant immune activation through a failing mucosal barrier which has been found in FD and IBS (13, 14). Nevertheless, it is still unclear whether the mucosal barrier function has any causal role in the pathogenesis of immune activation or whether it is a consequence of the inflammatory response or an unimportant epiphenomenon without a role in disease pathogenesis. Another potentially important player, the microbiota, have been studied intensively in the last years (15). While alterations in colonic and fecal microbiota have been described by several groups in IBS (16), disruption in microbial homeostasis in FD is still largely uncharted territory. Only a limited number of studies have reported alterations in gastric (17) and duodenal microbiota composition in FD (15).

As mentioned above, FGIDs are currently understood as disorders of the brain-gut axis, i.e., the neurohumoral communication system between the brain and the gastrointestinal tract, leading to gastrointestinal hypersensitivity and dysmotility (18). However, central alterations have been mostly studied in the context of visceral hypersensitivity, and the anterior cingulate gyrus, the prefrontal cortex, and the insular cortex have been found to be abnormally activated in IBS patients with visceral hypersensitivity (19). Other structures such as the amygdala or hippocampus have an altered functionality in FGID patients (20). Furthermore, these brain areas are also strongly implicated in psychiatric disorders such as depression and anxiety, two co-morbidities highly represented in FGID patients and associated with visceral hypersensitivity (11, 21, 22).

STRESS-RELATED MODELS OF FGID

Stress is biologically defined as a physiological response to a stimulus that allows organisms to adapt to their environment (23). However, when stress becomes chronic or occurs whilst important development processes are ongoing, the consequences can be harmful and lead to a predisposition for several diseases, including cardiovascular diseases (24), metabolic disorders (25, 26), depression (27), neurodegenerative diseases (28), drug abuse

TABLE 1 | Effect of stress on the Gastrointestinal tract and brain in animal models.

Stress models	Stomach	Small intestine	Colon	Central nervous system
Prenatal stress			Hypersensitivity (66) Dysbiosis (67) Decreased innervation & increase colonic secretory response to adrenaline (68)	Overactivation of the HPA axis in adulthood with female predominance Epigenetic changes BDNF (SC-female predominance) (67)
Maternal separation	Susceptibility to erosion (83) Delayed gastric emptying (84)		Hyperpermeability during separation At weaning, fecal dysbiosis (74) & hyperpermeability (75) Adult hyperpermeability, mostly transcellular pathway associated with abnormal cholinergic regulation (81) Hypersensitivity (76, 78) Immune cells infiltration (MC Eo) (77) Hypersensitivity of neurons from myenteric plexus to IL6 modulation of secretory and motility functions (79) Increased number of enterochromaffin cells & Increased expression SERT (92)	Decreased activity of glucocorticoid negative feedback (85) increased ACTH response to stressors (86) Increased serotonin concentration in frontal cortex Increased expression 5HT1A/1B/2A in parietal cortex & hippocampus Increased activation of 5HT neuron in raphe magnus and spinal cord (60, 89) Increased sympathetic activity and decreased of parasympathetic activity (94) Increased release of glutamate & AMPA/NMDA receptors involved in remodeling of synapses in hippocampus (95, 96)
Limited bedding			At weaning, fecal dysbiosis (female predominance) & hyperpermeability (69, 74) In adulthood hypersensitivity (male predominance) (102–104)	Decreased social/exploratory behavior & impaired learning and memory (102, 103). Decreased dendritic branching hippocampus Altered thalamo-cortico-amygdala pathway Increased connectivity in locus coeruleus (females) (102) Acts on neuronal development of dentate gyrus (105)
Odor shock conditioning			Hyperpermeability and hypersensitivity through estrogen and GC-C/cGMP pathway; female predominance (104)	Increased expression CRF & GR receptors in central nucleus amygdala (109)
Water Avoidance Stress	Impaired gastric accommodation at D2 via peripheral 5HT2B signaling (119) Increased postprandial gastric contractions at D2 (120)	Hyperpermeability at D1 (112, 113) Structural changes mucus layer at D4 (115) Dysbiosis at D8 (117, 118)	Hyperpermeability at D1 (112, 113) Hypersensitivity at D3 (114) Structural changes mucus layer at D4 (115) Dysbiosis at D10 (117, 118)	Increased glial, neuronal activation in hypothalamus and amygdala & synaptogenesis in the hippocampus (121, 123)
Restrain stress			Increased fecal output CRFR1-dependent manner (37)	Neuronal activation over several brain structures and nuclei including the supraoptic nucleus, locus coeruleus, the ventrolateral medulla, the medial division of the central amygdaloid nucleus, nucleus of the solitary tract and even the dorsal nucleus of the vagus nerve, structures involved in food intake and stress response. Neurons also expressing phoexinin and/or nesfatin (127, 128)
Partial restraint stress	Delayed gastric emptying through sympathetic activation (36, 137) Increased active ghrelin concentration (137, 139, 140)		Hypersensitivity (134–136) Hyperpermeability through re-organization of the cytoskeleton (134) Changes in mucosal morphology and decrease of glial cells in the submucosa plexus Increased immune cells infiltration (MC Eo) (135)	Overactivation of the insular cortex related with colonic hypersensitivity (19)

(Continued)

TABLE 1 | Continued

Stress models	Stomach	Small intestine	Colon	Central nervous system
Crowding stress		Hyperpermeability In WKY rat, activated mast cells (146)	Increased mast cells density (145) In WKY rat activated mast cells, MPO level & transient hyperpermeability, alteration of mitochondrial activity (146)	Anxiety-like and depression-like symptoms Early transient changes (Day 3) in the nitrergic expression in the PFC, hippocampus, hypothalamus (147)
Social isolation			Alterations in the IL-18 pathway and MUC2/TFF3 expression (149)	Anxiety-like and depression-like symptoms Reduced BDNF levels & increased reactivity of the HPA axis (148) Changes in the nitrergic expression in the PFC, hippocampus, hypothalamus (147)
Abdominal surgery	Impaired gastric emptying Low ghrelin concentration (249, 251, 252)	Impaired motility through the activation of the inhibitory reflex pathway increased cytokines expression (TNFa, IL1α, IL6, IL1β, CCL2) (241) infiltration resident macrophages (245)	Impaired motility, delayed transit increased cytokines expression in muscular layers (240) (241) Increased permeability non-related to TLR2/4 (244)	Activation of nuclei (supraoptic nucleus, locus coeruleus, paraventricular nucleus of the hypothalamus & rostral raphe pallidus) expressing nucleobindin2/nefastin complex involved in the decrease of food intake and GI transit (253)

5HT, serotonin; 5HT1A/1B/2A/2B, serotonin receptor type 1A, 1B, 2A, 2B; ACTH, adreno cortico trophic hormone; AMPA, α-amino-3-hydroxy-5-methyl-4-isoxazolepropionic acid; BDNF, brain-derived neurotrophic factor; CCL2, chemokine ligand 2; CRH, corticotropin-releasing hormone; CRHR1 corticotropin-releasing hormone receptor type 1; D1/2/3/4/8/10, day 1/2/3/4/8/10; Eo, eosinophils; GC-C/cGMP, guanylate cyclase C/cyclic guanylin monophosphate; GI, Gastrointestinal; GR, Glucocorticoid receptor; HPA, hypothalamus-pituitary-adrenal; IL, interleukin; MC, mast cell; MPO, myeloperoxidase activity; MUC2, Mucin 2; NMDA, N-methyl-D-aspartate; PFC, prefrontal cortex; SC, spinal cord; SERT, serotonin transporter; TFF3, rail fold factor 3; WKY, wistar kyoto.

(29), etc. Over the last decade, the incidence of the stress-related disease has increased, especially in societies where socio-economic pressure plays a crucial role in daily life (30). Physical and psychological stress have been documented intensively as decisive factors in the clinical course of several disorders including FGID (31). The hypothalamus-pituitary-adrenal gland (HPA) axis is the endocrine effector of the stress response, with a central role for corticotropin-releasing hormone (CRH), secreted in the hypothalamus, but also locally in the GI tract (32). By binding to its receptors, CRH stimulates the production and the release of glucocorticoids including cortisol in humans and corticosterone in rodents (33), key regulators of the physiological adaptation to stress (34). In normal conditions, the HPA axis is under rigorous regulation, at both the neuronal and hormonal level, since the glucocorticoid and mineralocorticoid receptors are part of a negative feedback loop which protects organisms against the harmful effect of prolonged exposure to stressors. Nonetheless, a combination of repeated environmental stressors may lead to a maladaptive response resulting in altered brain structure and function (35), predisposing to disease. CRH receptors are found to be expressed in both the GI tract and the central nervous system (CNS) suggesting a crucial role for this factor in the stress-induced disruption of gut homeostasis (36) including transit (37–39), visceral sensitivity (40–42), intestinal permeability (36, 43, 44) and gastric inflammation (45).

Psychological stress and anxiety, often reported by FGID patients, influence the onset of symptoms and predict the clinical outcome (46). Recently, data from our group identified

a crucial role for CRH and mast cells in this response, translating previous rodent studies to the human situation (47). Intriguingly, also in inflammatory bowel disease (IBD), longitudinal studies of patients in clinical remission have indicated that stress increases the risk of disease relapse, although the underlying mechanism remains elusive (48). It is still unclear whether stress induces inflammatory changes or whether it is a modulator of symptom perception independent of gut inflammation. Recent studies found that stress influenced the composition of the microbiota, associated with mood disorders and alterations in neurotransmitter pathways (49). Several stress-related animal models have been developed to elucidate the role of stress in the observed changes in the altered sensorimotor function of the gastrointestinal tract in patients with FGID.

In this section, we made a distinction between models of stress applied to adult animals and those involving stress around birth (pre- and post-natal models), i.e., early life stress (ELS). The stress models presented in this section are summarized in **Table 1**. Evidence from literature indicates that a similar stress paradigm has different effects depending on whether it occurs while the brain is still under development or when the neuronal circuits are already fully developed. Indeed, several studies in humans found that stressors in early life are more likely to result in psychiatric and functional disorders, including FGID (50, 51). Post-natal ELS models use this strategy to induce an increased corticosterone concentration in pups during a period in which they are normally only exposed to low corticosterone levels due to the continuous maternal care (52, 53). The two first weeks of life in rodents (from PND2 til 14) correspond to an insensitive period to environmental stimuli for the HPA axis called stress hyporesponsiveness period (SHRP) (54). During this SHRP, the HPA axis is quiescent and circulating corticosterone, ACTH and CRH levels are very low (55). During this period, stimuli that normally induce corticosterone increase in adults, do not affect pups and the reduced adrenal sensitivity observed is illustrated by the fact that pups do not show a significant elevation of corticosterone concentration following injections of high doses of ACTH (56). The HPA axis maturation mechanisms have not been fully uncovered. Part of these involves enhanced negative feedback due to the low expression of transcortin at the pituitary level (57, 58) and also the decreased expression or transport of hypothalamic secretagogues (59) further supported by the fact that the glucocorticoid regulation of hypothalamic CRH gene expression is not mature during the SHRP (60). Moreover, the regulation of the hypothalamic expression of the arginine vasopressin gene - that occurs at very early stages (61)—which is involved in the ACTH stress response in young rats has a key role for the control of ACTH release from the pituitary (62). Furthermore, it is also the most critical period in the development of central structures such as the amygdala (63) and hippocampus (64). In those two structures, neurodevelopment is very active with neurogenesis, cell differentiation, and migration (65). The existence of such a hyporesponsiveness period suggests that high-stress level might be harmful to the normal development of the brain and could affect the maturation of behavior dependent on those brain systems that are normally developing at that time like the emotional learning systems (57).

Prenatal Stress

In the last decade, data coming from clinical psychiatry showed that women's health status before and during pregnancy is a determining factor for the development of psychiatric disorders, including schizophrenia and depression, socio-emotional problems or altered stress response of the children later in life (49). History of a poor socio-economic context, malnutrition, obesity, metabolic disease, depression, and anxiety in the mother, has been linked to the development of FGID in the child (51). Several paradigms have been used in rodent mothers, including repeated daily immobilization, exposure to noise, sleep deprivation or an alternation of unpredictable stressors to mimic the human situation (49). The effect of those maternal stressors on the development of psychiatric disorders in the offspring is well described, and their effect on the GI tract have been studied in a couple of them. Winston et al. demonstrated that unpredictable chronic stress, i.e., a random sequence of twice daily application of either water avoidance stress, cold restraint stress or forced swimming stress, applied from mid-gestation until delivery in pregnant Sprague Dawley rats induced colonic hypersensitivity in both male and female offspring. Besides, when the animals were re-exposed to the same pattern of stress as their dam at 8–12 weeks of age, they displayed an increased response compared to the offspring of non-stressed dams with a more pronounced effect in females (66). The observed effect in females correlated with epigenetic modifications of the brain-derived neurotrophic factor (BDNF)

gene in the dorsal horn of the lumbosacral spinal cord. Using the same stress model in mice, Jasnarevic et al. could point out a strong link between the stress-altered maternal microbiota and neurodevelopmental alterations and microbiota composition in the offspring (67). This important finding was further confirmed in another study that demonstrated long-lasting changes in the intestinal microbiota composition, associated with a deficiency in the innervation of the distal colon and an increased colonic secretory response to adrenergic stimulation and an exaggerated response of the HPA axis to stress (68).

Neonatal Stress
Maternal Separation

The most frequently studied and used model of ELS is the maternal separation (MS) model in which pups are separated from the dam and the rest of the nest every day during their first weeks of life. Multiple variations of the MS procedure have been described, with changes in the duration of the separation and the number of days of separation. Variations include MS until weaning whereas other protocols use a 24 h separation between post-natal day 3 (PND3) and PND4 (69). The most common protocol consists of about 12 days of separation, 3 h per day, starting from PND2 till PND14. This daily separation induces anxiety in the mother (70) leading to a discontinuity in maternal care and an abnormal mother-pups relationship (70, 71) and initiates the premature end of the hypo-responsiveness period through a rise of corticosterone in the pups (72). Short separation (< 60 min) is not harmful and separation of 15 min even diminishes anxiety-related behavior and the pup's response to stress later in life (73). Repetitive, short separations are reminiscent of the natural behavior of the mother who needs to gather food. However, longer separation mirrors caregivers neglect and physical and psychological abuse during childhood.

Pups who underwent the maternal separation, display an increased intestinal permeability as well as changes in the microbiota composition at the time of weaning which are associated with an increase in the basal level of corticosterone (74). Changes in the microbiota included a lower diversity of the microbiome with a decrease of the fiber-digesting bacteria, mucus-resident and butyrate-producing bacteria (74). Another study showed that, during the maternal separation (at PND9) in mice, the separated pups had an enhanced permeability with a decreased trans-epithelial electrical resistance and an increased transcellular permeability in the colon while the small intestine was not affected (75). In adulthood, at 2 to 3 months, animals who underwent the maternal separation protocol (12 days of separation 3 h/day) have an increased response to colorectal distension, which was more pronounced in mice than in rats (76). In fact, in rats, the MS protocol alone does not change visceral sensitivity but rather induces a susceptibility to develop visceral hypersensitivity when animals are re-exposed to an acute stressor later on during adulthood. Interestingly, this susceptibility is transmitted across generations through a mast cell-dependent mechanism (77). The latter is an important part of the immune cell infiltration characterized after MS in the intestinal mucosa. When activated, mast cells released mediators such as histamine and other inflammatory factors including IL6 and nerve growth factor (NGF), which are able to sensitize the nerve endings located in the colonic mucosa which express ionic channels including the transient receptor potentiate vanilloid 1 (TRPV1). The modulation of this ion channel has been shown to be an important factor in the maternal separation stress-induced visceral hypersensitivity (78). O'Malley et al. also demonstrated an IL6-dependent hypersensitivity of the neurons from the submucous plexus, which are involved in the secretory and motility function of the colon (79). Local inflammatory mediators such as the myeloperoxidase activity (MPO), IL4, IL1β, or IFNγ are also associated with intestinal barrier dysfunction and to an alteration in morphology of the colon of adult rats (80). The increased permeability described in maternally deprived animals mainly involves the transcellular pathway and seems to involve an abnormal cholinergic regulation of the epithelial permeability (81). As previously mentioned, CRH receptors are expressed along the GI tract and CRH is one of the mediators of the GI effects of maternal separation. However, the two receptors for CRH have a differential effect on the intestinal physiology. Indeed, while maternally separated adult rats treated with CRH Receptor1 (CRHR1) antagonists displayed a decreased inflammation, the group treated with a CRH Receptor2 (CRHR2) antagonist showed an inhibited stem cell activity and injury repair. CRHR1 contributes to intestinal injury and modulation of the microbiota while CRHR2 promotes healing and repair of the intestine (82). Besides the well-documented colonic injury in animals submitted to maternal separation, studies also showed an alteration in gastric function characterized by enhanced susceptibility to gastric erosion (83) and a delayed gastric emptying associated with structural changes in the glial cells (84).

The separated pups develop an increased reactivity of the HPA axis in response to stress during adulthood (71), as shown by a decreased activity of the glucocorticoid negative feedback loop (85) and an increased adreno cortico trophic hormone (ACTH) response to a stressor (86). Several central neurotransmitter pathways are also affected by MS including the serotonergic (87), cholinergic (81) and glutamatergic (88) pathway. The serotoninergic pathway is altered with an increased 5-hydroxytryptamine (5HT, serotonin) concentration in the frontal cortex and increased expression of the 5HT 1A, 1B, and 2A receptors in the parietal cortex and the hippocampus (60, 89). Furthermore, MS rats showed increased activation of serotoninergic neurons in the raphe nucleus and the spinal cord. Rat studies have demonstrated the involvement of the 5-HT1A receptor in the pathophysiology of stress-induced visceral hypersensitivity as a treatment with the mast cell blocker Resveratrol was potentiated by a pre-treatment with a 5-HT1A agonist (90). In the same way, a therapeutic effect of anti-depressants targeting the monoaminergic system has been reported in this model (91). At the enteric nervous system (ENS) level, an increased number of enterochromaffin cells producing 5HT and increased expression of the serotonin transporter (SERT) were observed in MS rats (92). These findings may contribute to the observed altered sensorimotor function in FGID patients with a childhood abuse history, although the role of enterochromaffin cells and SERT has not

been studied in particular context. Increased noradrenaline levels, the main neurotransmitter of the sympathetic branch of the autonomic nervous system, in the cingulate cortex was associated with fear and anxiety in the MS model (93). In IBS patients, studies measuring heart rate variability confirmed an increased sympathetic nervous system activity and a decreased parasympathetic nervous system activity (94). Alterations have also been described in the glutamergic pathway, which is involved in emotion and cognitive behavior. Maternal separation induced a release of glutamate in the hippocampus which activated receptors leading to neuronal excitotoxicity (95). In the hippocampus of the MS rat, an increased expression of the α-amino-3-hydroxy-5-methyl-4-isoxazolepropionic acid (AMPA) and the N-methyl-D-aspartate (NMDA) receptors have been found to be associated with a remodeling of the synaptic plasticity (95, 96). Alterations in the hippocampus also concerns neurogenesis which explains the long-term consequences in adult behavior. Maternal separation affects the neurogenes which is very active during the SHRP and leads to impaired coping behavior in adulthood and the learning process (97).

Limited Bedding

As mentioned above, the socio-economic status of caregivers affects the onset of FGID in children. To mimic poverty and precarious conditions in humans and also to limit the intervention of an external experimenter which is subject to variability, a model of limited cage bedding, mostly applied between the PND2 and PND9, was developed first in rats and later also in mice (98, 99). Some recent studies have proposed a variation by applying intermittent limited bedding from PND1 to PND7 or limited bedding from PND8 to PND12 (100). In this model, the female does not have access to any form of enrichment to build a nest. This altered environment is stressful for the mother and leads to a fragmentation of maternal care without changing the overall duration. The periods of maternal care are shorter and the behavior is more frequently shifted from one to another e.g., grooming, nursing, going in or out of the nest, self-licking, self-grooming... (101). The mother's stress can be modulated by varying the amount of nesting material introduced in the cage. With this protocol, the stress applied to the pups is chronic, unpredictable and uncontrollable which has good construct validity for stress-related disruption of parental care in a context of economic difficulties (69). The profound chronic stress induced by this protocol leads to a transient increase of the corticosterone concentration and hypertrophy of the adrenal glands, increased intestinal permeability and a fecal dysbiosis in 21-day old pups while these effects had disappeared at 12 months (69, 74). Although the concentration of corticosterone was strongly correlated with the hypertrophy of the adrenal glands, the elevated concentration of corticosterone was associated neither with the observed dysbiosis (lower diversity and increased abundance of genera of Gram positive cocci) nor intestinal permeability, for which a sex difference was observed with the females being more affected than the males (74). However, in adulthood, the rats submitted to this early life stress showed a reduction in social and exploratory behavior, impaired learning and memory processes, a decreased dendritic branching in the hippocampus, an increased response to a stress challenge and visceral hypersensitivity (102, 103). The latter, depending on the method used for the colonic pain assessment, showed no sex difference or a higher colonic sensitivity in males (104). Similar results were observed for anxiety-like behavior. Moreover, differences in the brain connectivity of the thalamo-cortico-amygdala pathway during a painful stimulus have been reported to be altered in rats submitted to this protocol of ELS. The authors pointed out a sex difference with increased brain connectivity in the locus coeruleus/lateral parabrachial nucleus in females only (102). A recent finding showed that limited bedding affects the neuronal development of the dentate gyrus and depletes the stem cell pool in adult animals but does not influence neurogenesis (105).

Odor Shock Conditioning

Many mammals including rodents are born blind and deaf, and to stay warm and obtain the food and care needed to survive, they need to learn the odor of their caregiver, e.g., their mother. For this purpose, during the first 9 days of their life, pups display an enhanced capacity for odor preference learning through a stimulated release of norepinephrine, produced in the locus coeruleus, which binds to its receptors in the olfactory bulb (53). This allows the pups to learn the odor of their caregivers without associating it to fear or aversion. Furthermore, during this period, the pups display an inability to initiate a stress response. Once this period ends, the level of secreted norepinephrine decreases, associated with the development of the α2 inhibitory auto-receptors functionality and the downregulation of the α1 excitatory auto-receptors (53). In a second phase, called the conditional sensitive period, from PND10 till PND15, pups start to explore their environment and learn avoidance and fear for aversive stimuli in the absence of the mother. As we described earlier, the maturation of the HPA axis and maturation of fear behavior happens during the time-window in which neuronal circuits are located on the trajectory of the HPA axis maturation. Several studies showed that the rise of corticosterone levels starts during this period and is critical for the engagement of the amygdala and the learning of aversion and fear in response to a stimulus such as the odor of a predator (106). Interestingly, during this period, the presence of the mother can reengage the fear learning process (107).

Developed by and mostly used in the Greenwood-Van Meerveld lab, the model of odor shock-conditioning consists of predictable and unpredictable odor-shock pairings which mimic attachment to an abusive caregiver. This model uses the association between an odor and a modest electrical shock to the tail to reproduce the pup-dam interaction and creates an olfactory attachment to the conditioned odor in response to predictable or paired odor/shock. In practice, pups are exposed from PND8 to PND12 to an odor associated with an electrical shock 2 minutes after the odor exposition while controls are only exposed to the odor (104, 107–109). During adulthood, only female Long-Evans rats displayed an increased colonic permeability and a colonic hypersensitivity which persisted later in life and seemed to be directly linked to estrogen concentrations, as an ovariectomy in females subjected to

the odor shock conditioning model, rescued this phenotype (108). Moreover, increased expression of the CRF and the glucocorticoid receptor was found in the central nucleus of the amygdala which was involved in the maintenance of the colonic hypersensitivity (104). The use of linaclotide, a guanylate cyclase C (GC-C) agonist used in clinical practice to treat constipation-predominant IBS, restored both colonic hypersensitivity and permeability, proposing the GC-C/cGMP pathway as an important player in the peripheral regulation of the persistent visceral pain in adults exposed to this form of ELS (109).

Adult Stress
Physical Stress

Water avoidance stress (WAS) is one of the most frequently used models of stress in adult rodents either alone or combined with the maternal separation model. Several studies over the last decade have used it to characterize acute and chronic stress-induced GI symptoms and to study the effect of treatment, including nutritional and probiotic interventions (110, 111). During this protocol, the animal is placed on a platform (usually 10 × 10 for rats and 3 × 3 cm for mice) surrounded by water, either cold or at room temperature, until 1 cm below the platform. The water reservoir should be large enough to avoid the animal to jump out and thus give the animal the impression that no escape is possible. This protocol can serve as either an acute or a chronic stressor and mimics resilience to an uncomfortable situation. A large number of variations on the protocol have been described in the literature and often differ by their duration. WAS induces a robust activation of the HPA axis which transiently alters gut physiology (110). One day of stress induces an increased intestinal permeability (112, 113) while 3 days of stress are needed for colonic hypersensitivity to appear (114). Morphological changes, including the composition and the structure of the mucus layer, were present from the fourth day (115). Interestingly, the follicle-associated epithelium in the ileum seemed to be more affected than the colon (116). A fecal dysbiosis, including an altered composition and function of the microbiota, has been described after 10 days of stress in rats while in mice it already appears after 8 days in the small intestine (117, 118). Gastric contractions after a meal were increased in rats after two sessions of WAS, through the activation of the peripheral CRH1 receptors (119). Impaired gastric accommodation occurred after 2 days of stress and was mediated through the peripheral serotoninergic receptors 5HT2B (120). In mice, after four sessions, alterations in the brain occurred with an increase of the neuronal and glial activation in the hypothalamus, hippocampus, and amygdala. These structures are not only involved in the stress response but also in memory, pain and emotion pathways which are often found to be altered in IBS patients (121–123). A sex-difference has been described in the processing of emotional signals in healthy humans (124), in patients with FGID (125) and stress-related visceral hypersensitivity in rats (126).

As for the maternal separation, several models of physical constraint have been developed over the years, among them three versions of physical constraint: the partial restraint stress, full restraint stress and cold restraint stress. The extent and the duration of the stressor differ amongst the protocols. With a full body restraint stress applied in rats for 30 min, studies have shown neuronal activation over several brain structures and nuclei including the supraoptic nucleus, locus coeruleus, the ventrolateral medulla, the medial division of the central amygdaloid nucleus, nucleus of the solitary tract and even the dorsal nucleus of the vagus nerve, structures involved in food intake and the stress response (127, 128). Interestingly, in those nuclei and structures, the activated neurons also expressed nesfatin-1 and/or phoenixin, two peptides involved in the regulation of food intake and anxiety behavior (129, 130). Nesfatin-1 is mainly expressed in the hypothalamus and brainstem where it colocalized with CRF (131). When administered directly into mice brain, nesfatin-1 led to an increase of plasmatic ACTH and corticosterone levels, as well as an activation of neurons expressing CRH, noradrenalin and serotonin, indicating both a central and a peripheral response to stress. Furthermore, the nesfatin-1 system is activated when rats are submitted to restraint stress for 1 h (132). In mice, a protocol of 60 min of full restraint stress showed a CRF-dependent increase of pellet output which was abolished by central injection of a specific CRFR1 antagonist—while a CRFR2 specific antagonist had no effect—(37) and also by a systemic injection of peptide YY (133). Partial restraint stress is another common form of the model which consists of restriction of the upper body movements. In this model, the shoulders, upper forelimbs, and thoracic trunk of the animal are wrapped in a confining harness of paper tape or cloth to restrict, but not to prevent, body movements (134). This protocol is mostly used as an acute stressor with a 1 to 2 h period of restraint. However, this short exposure already promoted (1) colonic hypersensitivity (134–136), (2) an increased influx of immune cells in the mucosa, mostly consisting of mast cells and eosinophils (135), (3) an intestinal hyperpermeability through the reorganization of the cytoskeleton in epithelial cells (134), (4) a delayed gastric emptying associated with the stress-induced sympathetic activation, increased CRF (36, 137) and associated peptides (138) as well as active ghrelin concentration (137, 139, 140), and (5) changes in colonic morphology and a decrease of enteric glial cells especially in the submucosa plexus (135). By using this model for 14 days, Yi et al. could demonstrate the implication of the insular cortex in stress-induced visceral hypersensitivity, a region found to be abnormally activated in FGID patients (19) and more in general in patients with chronic pain (141).

Social Stress

One of the important findings of the last century in the field of psychobiology is the stress-buffering effect of social relationships, with an important role for oxytocin (142). Social buffering conceptualizes the idea that social support can attenuate the stress response and reduce the release of stress hormones (143). As we discussed in the previous section, the more powerful demonstration of this concept is the mother's social buffering of the offspring in which the mother and the pups can influence each other's corticosterone concentration (144).

However, the positive effect of this social buffering depends on the nature of the relationship between individuals as well as on the social organization of the species and/or gender. Many species, including humans and rodents, live for almost their entire life in a group with a strong hierarchy. As a result, any disturbance in this social order or abuse is a potential source of stress. In rodents, stress models used either the isolation of one animal from the rest of the group, i.e., social isolation stress, or, at the other end of the spectrum, an overpopulation within a small area, i.e., crowding stress. Often used as models for anxiety and depression-related disorders alterations of the GI physiology have also been studied in rodents submitted either to the social isolation stress or the crowding stress models. Crowding induces a strong competition for space, food, and water and leads to a strong increase of the corticosterone concentration in the first days associated with early transient alterations in the nitrergic system in the hippocampus, prefrontal cortex and hypothalamus, an increase of iNOS expression in all structures and increased of nNOS in the hippocampus and hypothalamus. These changes are normalized over time through a habituation process but remains higher than in normal housing conditions. This protocol is used for 2 to 9 weeks depending on the strain and type of rodent and is often combined with other types of a stressor to simulate the combination of chronic and (sub)acute stressors that naturally occurs in humans. Work from our group demonstrated that 14 days of crowding stress in Wistar rats induced increased permeability in the jejunum which correlated with plasma corticosterone levels. However, mast cell density was only increased in the colon (145). In Wistar Kyoto rats, a strain sensitive to anxiety, a crowding stress protocol applied for 15 days induced a transient increase of the small intestine and colon permeability associated with a transient rise of MPO activity and altered mitochondrial activity (146) as well as mast cell infiltration (colon) and activation in the GI tract (small intestine and colon) (146).

Conversely, in the social isolation stress (SIS) model, the animal is isolated from the rest of the cage. Often applied just after the weaning, SIS modifies the development of the brain and influences the nitrergic system in several brain areas such as the hippocampus, the frontal cortex by increasing the nNOS expression in the hippocampus and hypothalamus and iNOS in the prefrontal cortex (147). A decrease production of BDNF, and an activation of the HPA axis which produce more corticosterone.. Mice exposed to SIS, have an impaired reactivity to stress with an overreaction to another stressor together with increased anxiety- and depression-like symptoms (148). In the GI tract, regional differences have been pointed out between the colon and the rectum concerning MUC2/TFF3 expression and in the IL-18 pathway in mice exposed to 16 days of SIS (149).

Combined Stress and Chronic Mild Unpredictable Stress

Although the various animal stress models developed over the last years have provided critical information about the influence of stress on physiology, humans are usually not exposed to only one stressor during their life and a combination of stressors is often present in patients with FGID. Also, physiology can adapt to one homotypic stressor in humans and rodents, leading to habituation and absence of effect after repeated exposure. As a variety of animal models of stress are available, a wide range of stress combinations can be used to better understand the pathophysiological mechanisms behind stress-induced FGID symptoms. Combinations of unpredictable mild stress are also often used with a rotation between different stressors such as light/dark cycle, isolation, crowding, predator odor exposure, shock, cold environment, restraint stress....

An often-used combination in rats is the maternal separation combined with one session of water avoidance stress in adult rats. In contrast to mice, maternal separation is not always sufficient to induce GI symptoms in rats (76) but increases the susceptibility for GI symptoms upon subsequent exposure to stress (150) which is transmitted to the next generation (77). In another type of combination of early life stress, i.e., odor shock conditioning, and water avoidance, a sex-difference was observed with a more pronounced female susceptibility to develop visceral hypersensitivity, which is in line with the female predominance in FGID (151).

With the use of unpredictable stress models, which consist of applying a stressor (SIS, restrain, WAS...) at unpredictable moments of the day for a few days, the involvement of nerve growth factor, endorphin, beta-adrenergic pathway, BDNF and mast cells mediators and the toll-like receptor 4 (TLR4) pathways have been demonstrated in stress-induced visceral hypersensitivity (107). Recent studies suggested a role of an altered microbiota in the anxiety and depression-like behavior in animals exposed to unpredictable mild stress with a strong correlation between the alterations in the microbiota and colonic serotonin concentrations (152, 153).

LOW GRADE INFLAMMATORY, POST-INFECTIOUS AND POST-INFLAMMATORY MODELS OF FGID

Infections and inflammation are among the best-characterized triggers for FGID symptoms. Although the pathophysiological mechanisms are not yet fully understood, a low-grade inflammation is considered as the main explanation for the symptoms in so-called post-infectious (PI) IBS and FD (154). Evidence from IBD patients in remission has also brought some more arguments for this mechanism of persistent low-grade inflammation triggering IBS-like symptoms (155). Psychological factors have been shown to be associated with the prevalence of PI-IBS as well as somatization which, when happening during the infectious period, is positively correlated with the incidence of IBS symptoms (156).

Low Grade Inflammatory Models
Low dose injections of inflammatory factors like the bacteria-derived lipopolysaccharide (LPS), injected systemically at the dose of 1 mg/kg can also trigger FGID features such as rectal allodynia and colonic hyperpermeability. Visceral allodynia appears 3 h after injection last up to 12 h and is mediated by mast cell degranulation, IL1β and TNFa (157). When

Authors performed a subdiaphragmatic vagotomy, they observed an increased allodynia compared to sham animal which suggest that the rectal allodynia seen after LPS injection is controlled by the vagus nerve (158). In another study, both the hyperpermeability and allodynia observed 3 h after injection, were normalized with antagonist of TLR4 and IL1β as well as with a CRFR2 specific agonist and Astressin a non-selective CRFRs antagonist suggesting an important role of the CRF in the effect of LPS injection on visceral sensitivity and permeability (159). Moreover, allodynia and hyperpermeability were abolished with peripheral injection of a selective CRFR2 agonist and with an non-selective inhibitor of CRF receptors (157). Losartan, an angiotensin II blocker, and lovastatin reversed the permeability and allodynia, dependent on the macrophage peroxisome proliferator-activated receptor gamma (PPARγ) and the endogenous opioid, dopaminergic and nitrergic system, potentially opening the door for novel therapeutic strategies of FGID (160, 161). Similarly, the tricyclic antidepressant imipramine reversed LPS-induced allodynia and colonic hyperpermeability (162).

Several models have also been developed using a low concentration of dextran sodium sulfate (DSS) to induce low-grade inflammatory changes (163). This model contrasts with the post-inflammatory model of high-dose DSS followed by a recovery period, discussed in the next paragraph. An overexpression of the T-type calcium channel cav3.2 in this model, which was also observed in colonic biopsies of IBS patients, was associated with colonic hypersensitivity in this model (163, 164).

Post-inflammatory Models
Rodent models of post-inflammatory GI disorders attempt to simulate a post-inflammatory situation mostly represented by the resolution of an acute infection. Most of the models presented below originally are models for IBD but can be instrumental to study certain aspects of the development of GI symptoms after resolution of the acute inflammation. The development of post-inflammatory GI disorders occurs in 25 to 100% of the treated animals depending on the trigger used. Furthermore, the severity of symptoms and functional alterations developed in the post-inflammatory period—except for the visceral hypersensitivity—seems to be independent of the severity of the initial inflammation (165).

An acute treatment with a high percentage of DSS followed by a DSS-free period (166) creates a remaining low-grade inflammation which is associated with visceral hypersensitivity and SERT downregulation leading to gut dysmotility. The expression of TRPV1, another ionic channel, has been shown to be increased in the recovery phase only in the colonic mucosa and linked to the persistent visceral hypersensitivity (167). However, other studies have shown a quick restoration of the original phenotype without colonic hypersensitivity to mechanical stimuli (152).

Trinitrobenzene sulfonic acid (TNBS), leads to a Th1 immune response with ulcers in rodents within the first 3 days after instillation. Two weeks after instillation, the inflammation is resolved, but a visceral hypersensitivity, motility dysfunction due to a persistent long-term smooth muscle hyperactivity to acetylcholine, an increased mast cell infiltration in the mucosa, an upregulation of the NMDA-NR1, as well as galanin and tachykinin expression in the mucosa and myenteric plexus, a barrier hyperpermeability and a decreased secretory function through a cyclooxygenase-2 (COX-2) dependent mechanism can be demonstrated (168). The long-lasting symptoms, such as visceral hypersensitivity, are present up to 17 weeks after the induction and involve overexpression of the NMDA receptor NR1 in the spinal cord as well as changes in the distribution and the sensitivity of the colonic afferents. A TRPV1 antagonist, a guanylate cyclase agonist, melatonin and a probiotic (*Bifidobacterium infantis* 35624) were able to rescue this phenotype (169). Mast cells, through their main mediator histamine and its receptors H4R and H1A, play a substantial role in post-inflammatory visceral hypersensitivity (170). Recently, Winston et al. demonstrated a gastric hypersensitivity in 8 weeks-old rats previously exposed to TNBS (171) which positioned this model as a general model for FGID and a good model for patients with FD and IBS overlap symptoms, which is common in clinical practice (172).

Acid acetic, Zymosan and mustard oil are irritants administered directly into the colon of adult or neonatal animals by enema. When administered in pups, long-lasting visceral hypersensitivity has been reported for 8 to 10 weeks for Zymosan and mustard oil and up to 12 weeks for acid acetic (168) without histological damage in adult rats (173). Seven days after acid acetic induction in adult rats, when the inflammatory phase has subsided, a defect of the intestinal barrier function was reported with altered occludin and ZO-1 protein expression in a miR-144-dependent manner (174). The same barrier defect was also observed in rats submitted to the neonatal protocol. When administered directly into the submucosal layer of the stomach using 15 to 20 injections in adult rats, acid acetic promoted gastric hypersensitivity (175). Zymosan and mustard oil sensitized the mechanoreceptor and other neurons present in the colonic wall which persisted after the inflammatory phase (176, 177). Both Zymosan and mustard oil, induced neuronal changes in the spinal cord and the brain by increasing the neuronal excitability as shown by an increased presence of c-FOS positive neurons (178). The latter was associated with an altered expression pattern in the NMDA receptors in females which might be responsible for the female predominance in visceral sensitization following the mustard oil model (179). The stimulating effect of mustard oil on GI motility has been documented in both the upper and lower GI tract (180). Although the increased neuronal activation in the central nervous system in those models would suggest behavioral changes, anxiety-like symptoms have only been described in the zymosan model in which these behavioral symptoms were present during the inflammatory phase and remained present for 2 weeks after the induction, associated with increased c-FOS expression in different brain regions such as the amygdala, prefrontal cortex, periaqueductal gray... and increased TNF-α levels in the colonic mucosa (181).

Iodoacetamide is an alkylating agent administered by gavage in neonate rodents to induce a mild inflammation of the gastric mucosa that is associated with acute changes in sensory and motor function. Inhibition of the glucocorticoid receptors, adrenergic receptors, BDNF or the nerve growth factor (NGF) during the neonatal period suppressed the induced gastric hypersensitivity (171). The inflammation phase in pups is characterized by a thickening of the neuromuscular layer without increased MPO levels. During adulthood, histology and inflammation levels are comparable to control animals while the gastric sensory and motor dysfunction remained present up to 8 weeks after the treatment (182).

Post-infectious Models

Within the GI tract, the host and billions of micro-organisms are co-existing, creating a unique symbiosis. Products secreted by the microflora influence the gut function by their effect on neurotransmitters, epithelial function, secretion, or muscle contraction (183). The composition of the gut microflora depends on different factors such as diet, geographic position, genetics, and gender. The balance is strongly influenced by changes in the diet, travel or bacterial and parasitic gastrointestinal infections. The occurrence of FGID symptoms after an infectious episode has been found in a range of 3 to 36% of an infected population (156, 184, 185). The latter has been found to alter gut physiology through different mechanisms including the triggering of an inflammatory reaction, alterations at the neurochemical level and immune function, and alterations of the nerve distribution (186). Some of the parasites and bacteria that can infect the human GI tract, can also infect rodents and trigger symptoms or GI abnormalities reminiscent of human FGID.

Trichinella spiralis is an intestinal parasite found in humans, rodents, and pigs and is used as a model of post-infectious IBS in mice. For this purpose, mice are infected with 200 to 300 larvae in one gavage. During the acute phase, parasites are evacuated from the organism triggering a Th2 inflammatory phase in both the mucosa and muscular layers (187, 188). The post-infectious phase is defined at 4 weeks post-infection when the inflammatory phase has subsided (188). However, Akiho et al. found that transforming growth factor (TGF)-β remained overexpressed during this post-inflammatory phase and the smooth muscle cells were still hyperreactive to an immune challenge (primary culture of smooth muscle cells incubated with Th2 cytokines TGF-β1 and COX2) in a COX-2 dependent manner (187). Moreover, the long-lasting effects of the infection, such as visceral hyperalgesia which has been reported up to 70 days after infection, were inhibited by selective and non-selective COX-2 inhibitors (187, 189). Data on the effect of COX-2 inhibitors in humans are still lacking. In the post-infectious phase, the small intestine smooth muscle contractility, as well as the mucosal transport, remained altered. The latter shifted from a predominantly cholinergic in normal conditions to a non-cholinergic regulation (188).

Other animal models used infections with *Nippostrongylus brasiliensis* and *Cryptosporidium parvum*, which are both characterized by mast cell hyperplasia, visceral hypersensitivity, motility dysfunction with an increased motor response to excitatory agonists due to a remodeling of the nerve pattern as found in PI-IBS patients long after the infection. Other bacteria have been used including *Campylobacter rodentium*, *Campylobacter jejuni* or *Salmonella enterica*. However, those infections are less well-characterized regarding their FGID features or have a low success rate in rodents (168).

Overgrowth of *Escherichia coli* in the ileum of IBS and IBD patients has been associated with the expression of the human bacterial colonizing receptor CEACAM6 (190). Expression of the human CEACAM6 in the murine GI tract induced colonization and growth of pathogenic Escherichia coli upon gavage and led to an infection. In this model, mice are treated with the bacteria for 3 days, leading to a transient inflammation, intestinal hyperpermeability, and colonic hypersensitivity. The latter was present until 3 weeks after infection and was associated with a remaining low-grade inflammation and overexpression of the purinergic receptors P2X receptors in the colon (191).

FOOD-RELATED MODELS OF FGID

Food indigestion, intolerance or allergy are major triggers for abdominal symptoms. Due to genetic predisposition, infection or stress, oral tolerance, which is critical in avoiding immune reactions against food antigens, may be disrupted, leading to FGID symptoms. In IBS patients, the ingestion of certain food compounds triggers FGID symptoms (192) and elimination diet strategies, such as low FODMAP or gluten-free diets, are effective in some patients (193).

Food allergy represents a break in the oral tolerance and the consumption of allergens trigger a Th2 response and the activation of mast cells through the IgE pathway. FGID manifestations such as low-grade inflammation, visceral hypersensitivity, increased permeability, have been reported in rodent models of food allergy (194, 195). In those models as well as in humans, gender differences have been described. However, studies are diverging on the effect of the gender with female rodents being more affected than males while in children the prevalence is higher in males. Those differences might be related to the difference in the immune system response to allergens which is strongly influenced by sex hormones (102, 195). Those models differ by the allergen used, which can be egg proteins, peanut components, milk or seafood extracts, but all follow the same pattern with a phase of allergy-induction and a re-challenge with the same allergen several days or weeks after the induction (195). Many of the validation criteria for a rodent allergy model are comparable to the evaluation of the FGID related changes, e.g., presence of histological changes with local and systemic inflammation and activation of eosinophils and mast cells (195). In an elegant study, Aguilera-Lizarraga and Florens demonstrated that the establishment of oral tolerance can be impaired due to stress or intestinal infection, two major triggers of FGID symptoms, without triggering a systemic allergic reaction. Their results showed that this impaired tolerance triggered a mast cell activation through local (but not systemic) IgE, leading to colonic hypersensitivity and hyperpermeability (196, 197).

Obesity is one of the main health problems of our society and affects an increasing number of people over the world. Obesity is often associated with metabolic disorders such as diabetes or hypertension and also with FGID (198). IBS is three times more frequent in obese patients compared to the general population (199) and patients report both upper and lower GI complaints (200). Moreover, studies have reported an increased incidence of GI symptoms among fast-food and western-diet consumers (201, 202). Although, no animal model of FGID includes eating habits or genetic background leading to obesity, several observations in obesity models have pointed out a chronic GI low-grade inflammation and hyperpermeability induced by high fat, high sugar diet (HFHS) (203) which is associated with changes in the microbiota composition (204). Therapeutic strategies targeting the microbiota (205) as well as dietary strategies (204, 206) have shown some promising results in this model on the immune dysfunction and colonic hyperpermeability. Although the effect of obesity on low-grade inflammation, neuropathy, and hyperpermeability is not specific to the gut—some studies reported epigenetic changes in several organs (207)—it will be interesting to further investigate the effect of obesity on the gastro-intestinal features of FGID and on how it affects the outcome and/or the development of FGID.

The imbalance between some bacterial phyla such as Firmicutes/Bacteroidetes has been reported in IBS patients (208). The firmicutes are the predominant butyrate and other short-chain fatty acids (SCFA)-synthesizing bacteria within the colon. Although the benefits of SCFA has been demonstrated, rectal butyrate instillation in animals has been linked to visceral hypersensitivity (209, 210). This hypersensitivity without inflammation involved the enteric glial cells-derived NGF pathway which sensitized the nerve fibers within the colonic wall (211).

SPONTANEOUS MODELS OF FGID

Spontaneous animal models sharing key characteristics with human FGID are of great value to unravel the complex chain of events ultimately leading to symptoms and to aid in preclinical drug development. Only a few spontaneous models for FGID have been described (212–214) often sharing common features for FD and IBS, mostly in rats.

The BioBreeding rat (BB-rat) is an inbred colony originating from Wistar rats and have been selected for their ability to spontaneously develop type 1 diabetes (215). The BB-rat consists of a diabetes-resistant (control) and a diabetes-prone (BB-DP) strain of which about 50 to 90% develops hyperglycemia depending on their environment (216). Originally mostly used as a model for type 1 diabetes, several groups have demonstrated GI alterations closely mimicking FGID. Indeed, Neu et al. have described changes in intestinal morphology and intestinal permeability before the onset of diabetes (217). In the last 5 years, our lab has described a gastrointestinal phenotype in those BB-DP animals which did not develop diabetes, at all levels of the GI tract. The intestinal changes closely resemble the alterations found in patients with FD and IBS (213, 218–220). Based on these observations, we proposed the normoglycemic BB-DP rat as a spontaneous animal model for FGID. A natural history study of the small intestine demonstrated that the earliest abnormality was an increased intestinal permeability at 50 days of age, followed by an immune cell infiltration, progressing from the mucosa to the myenteric plexus in animals from 110 days onwards (213). This myenteric plexitis is associated with a loss of nitrergic neurons and disturbed motility (213, 220). Concomitantly, an impaired gastric accommodation, like in functional dyspepsia, has been observed in young normoglycemic rats (220). The immune infiltration is affecting the stomach, the small intestine, and the colon and is characterized by activated mast cells and eosinophils (221). Although the barrier defect precedes the infiltration of the immune cells in the small intestine, we observed that in the colon, the infiltration of the immune cells, which is present at the same age as in the jejunum, precedes the hyperpermeability suggesting a different mechanism in both locations. At both levels, we found a positive correlation between mast-cells density and mucosal permeability. Following this immune activation, we also demonstrated colonic hypersensitivity to colorectal distention and anxiety-like behavior in older BB-DP rats, which, however, was not associated with the increased permeability or immune infiltration in the colon (219). Altogether, the BB-rat model is a valid spontaneous animal model for FGID, recapitulating the permeability defect, eosinophil and mast cell predominant immune activation, motility disturbances at different levels of the GI tract, visceral hypersensitivity and behavioral alterations, similar to human FGID.

The Wistar Kyoto (WKY) rat, originally used as a control normotensive strain for the spontaneously hypertensive rats (SHR), has been studied in the last decades as a model of brain-gut dysfunction. Those rats display an exaggerated response to chronic stress compared to Sprague Dawley rats (222–224), associated with a higher susceptibility to develop anxiety-like and depression-like symptoms (225). Regional differences in monoamines concentration within the brain may explain their susceptibility to anxiety and depression (226). As described above, stress is a potent trigger for alterations in gut physiology, especially through the central expression of CRH in key structures involved in stress but also in pain and emotion regulation. Wistar Kyoto rats have an increased response to colorectal distension associated with increased neuronal activation in the cortex (227). Specific inhibition of the CRH pathway in the central amygdala and inhibition of central and peripheral 5HT2B inhibits the increased response to colorectal distension (87, 228). Besides the well-described colonic hypersensitivity (87, 228, 229) and impaired intestinal permeability (223, 224), the WKY rats also display gastric alterations such as an impaired gastric accommodation and a higher sensitivity to gastric distension (230). Interestingly, O'Malley et al. have compared the WKY to Sprague Dawley in a maternal separation paradigm and showed that the susceptibility to gastrointestinal dysfunction in stressed Sprague Dawley is comparable to what is found in non-stressed WKY (231).

The Flinders Sensitive Line (FSL) rat originates from selective breeding from Sprague Dawley and has been selected for their resistance to the choline esterase inhibitor, diisopropyl fluorophosphate (232). Used first as a model of cholinergic-adrenergic hypothesis depression (233), they are now more generally used as a model of depression without comorbidity of anxiety and with a female predominance (234). The effect of the microbiota composition has been studied in those rats showing that their microbiota composition is different (235) and might represent a target to improve the depression phenotype (236). However, only a few studies have investigated the gastrointestinal features in those rats. Some characteristics of functional dyspepsia including a delayed gastric emptying but not an impairment of the gastric accommodation have been described (214). Taking into consideration the link between depression and FGID, a more detailed study of the GI features in the FSL rats may bring some new insights for the link between GI symptoms and depression in FGID.

INTERVENTIONAL MODELS OF FGID

During abdominal surgery, the opening of the skin and the abdominal cavity triggers adrenergic reflexes involving a spinal loop which temporarily blocks GI motility. Considered as an iatrogenic disorder, postoperative ileus (POI) occurs in most patients undergoing abdominal surgery and is characterized by a transiently impaired GI motility. However, when recovery of bowel function is delayed for more than 3–7 days, this disorder is defined as an illness (237). Several rodent models exist to induce POI: briefly, either the abdominal cavity is opened and exposed to room temperature air for 3 h (238) or the intestinal tract is gently manipulated during 5–10 min (239). In both cases, an impaired GI motility affecting the stomach, small intestine, and colon, an intestinal inflammatory response, and hyperpermeability have been reported. The inflammatory response is associated with increased production of TNFα, IL1α, and IL6 in the early stage, followed by an increase of myeloid cell-derived cytokines, e.g., IL1β and CCL2. During this early stage, the inhibitory reflex pathway is activated, inhibiting gut motility. The transit time is delayed from 12 h up to 1 week after the surgery (240). At 24 h after the surgery, small intestine and colonic transit were delayed and associated with increased cytokine expression within the smooth muscle layer. The role of mast cells in the POI is still controversial as some studies found a mast cell-dependent mechanism in the POI-induced intestinal hyperpermeability and bacterial translocation (241) while other studies found no involvement of these cells by using another type of mast cell knockout (KO) mice (242). While intestinal permeability to bacteria is increased in this model, the TLR2/4 pathway does not seem to be involved (243). Although the role of mast cells is still unsure, the infiltration of resident macrophages through their expression of the alpha7 nicotinic acetylcholine receptors plays a critical role (244). The early cytokines released from the drop of temperature and dry stimulation due to the opening of the abdominal cavity, are potent activators of the macrophages. Furthermore, the afferent nerves activated by the manipulation of the intestine may also activate the resident macrophages and trigger an inflammatory response. In this context, pharmacological or electrical stimulation of the cholinergic anti-inflammatory pathway has been presented as an attractive option to reduce POI (245). Moreover, stimulation of the vagal nerve has been shown to reduce the severity of the POI in animal models (246). As mentioned before, the decrease of the ambient temperature plays an important role in the inflammatory response and also for the activation the thyrotropin-releasing hormone (TRH) in the brain which stimulates gastric motility and secretion for the activation of gastric myenteric cholinergic neurons (247). Several hormones expressed both in the brain and the GI tract are involved in the pathophysiology of POI, including ghrelin, nesfastin-1, somatostatin, TRH, CRF and calcitonin gene-related peptide (CGRP). In the POI model, lower ghrelin concentrations were observed which—like CRF and CGRP—leads to a delayed gastric emptying (248–250). Pharmacological inhibition of somatostatin, a hormonal modulator, in the POI model induced elevated ghrelin levels (251). Centrally, POI activates brain nuclei (supraoptic nucleus, locus coeruleus, paraventricular nucleus of the hypothalamus & rostral raphe pallidus) expressing the nucleobindin2/nesfatin-1 complex which contribute to the decrease in food intake and intestinal transit (252).

Manipulations of the central nervous system have also been described as potential models of GI disorders associated with anxiety-like symptoms. As described before, the limbic system and especially the amygdala are strongly involved in stress-induced colonic hypersensitivity associated with anxiety-like symptoms and the manipulation of this brain region is sufficient to induce colonic pain (253). Direct delivery of corticosterone through a surgically implanted cannula in the central nucleus of the amygdala (CeA) induces a persistent colonic hypersensitivity, which is dependent on CRH, mineralocorticoid and glucocorticoid receptors (169). The activation with a specific agonist of one of those receptors in the CeA, has the same effect on colonic sensitivity as stress (254, 255). Furthermore, the infusion of corticosterone directly into the amygdala leads to epigenetic modifications that enhance the expression of those receptors in a long-term and transmissible manner (256).

MISCELLANEOUS MODELS OF FGID

Genetic models of FGID include specific KO animals for several receptors, ion channels, and cellular pathways. These models have provided important knowledge of FGID pathophysiology. Mostly used to better understand the pathophysiology of colonic pain, they have demonstrated the importance of BDNF, guanylate cyclase, serotonin transporters, and ion channels. The latter have been extensively described in the literature to be involved in the intestinal mechanoreception and inflammation (257, 258). Therefore, all compounds capable of activation/inhibition of those channels can trigger IBS-like symptoms and especially colonic pain (169), the full description of which is beyond the scope of the current review. Studies in mice deficient for the protease-activated receptor 2 (PAR2) highlighted the importance of this receptor in colonic sensitivity (259), and immune response, notably against *Trichinella spiralis* (260). Other key components of innate immunity, e.g., the TLRs, such as TLR4, are expressed in the intestinal tract and the CNS (261). The activation of TLR4 leads to the activation of inflammatory

cascade but also pain behavior through its expression in the spinal cord. Furthermore, TLR4 has been found to be upregulated in the GI tract of patients with IBS (262, 263). Studies in TLR4 KO mice demonstrated a role of the central expression of TLR4 in visceral hypersensitivity following maternal separation stress (264). More generally, in the CRH-induced colonic hypersensitivity and hyperpermeability, TLR4 is a pivotal factor for CRH-mediated modulation of the immune system (159).

Several studies have demonstrated a cross-sensitization between different abdominal organs. In the spinal cord and the brain, the convergence of the sensory neuronal pathways of the different organs is one of the mechanisms underlying this sensory visceral crosstalk (265). Furthermore, within the abdominal cavity, all organs are linked to each other through physical contact and blood circulation. The best-documented model of cross-sensitization is the interaction between the bladder and the colon, in which inflammation in one of the two will affect the other partner as well. Similar to FGID, bladder pain syndrome and bladder hyperactivity syndrome has a female predominance and is often associated with IBS (266). Animal models of bladder irritation, e.g., triggered by protamine sulfate, display an increased colonic hypersensitivity and permeability (267, 268).

NON-RODENT MODELS

Although most of the research focuses on rodent models, some other species have been used to investigate the FGID pathophysiology. The guinea pig is a good model to study intestinal motility and the enteric nervous system. The models used are similar to what we previously described in rodents, with the use of stress models such as water avoidance and CRH injection (269, 270). As a model of altered GI transit, several chemical approaches have been used in guinea pigs such as the gavage with mustard oil and serotonin or the injection of TRH. Mustard oil, given orally, induces elongation of the transit time in the upper GI (esophagus) and a decreased transit time in the lower GI part (colon) (271). Ricinoleic acid-induced defecation in the guinea pig is suppressed by a specific tachykinin receptor NK2 antagonist (272).

In rabbits, intracolonic infusion of Zymosan leads to colonic hypersensitivity (272) which is reduced by a tachykinin NK2 receptor antagonist.

Pigs have a comparable GI system to humans, with an equivalent size, anatomy, development and diet preference, which are evidently very different in rodents (273). Also, the enteric nervous system phenotype is comparable to the human counterpart with more complex inter-neuronal connections and plexi compared to rodents (274). It has been shown that pigs have a more highly developed CNS with a complex behavior response to psychosocial stimuli (275) and therefore are more suitable as a model for the response of the GI tract to early life stress in humans. In pigs, the weaning itself is considered a very stressful event (both psychological and physical) which promotes an intestinal barrier defect (276). In a model of early weaning, the piglets are separated from their sow 1 week earlier

TABLE 2 | Strengths and limitations for common models of Functional GI disorders.

Model	Strengths	Limitations	Part of the GI tract studied
Pre-natal stress	Allows to study epigenetic changes	Individual variation among animals, around 80 to 95% of animals are sensitized by the stress applied	Small bowel and colon
Maternal separation	Reproduces maternal neglect and mistreatment of FGID patients		Colon
Limited bedding	Non-interventional model, avoids experimenter influence		Colon
Odor shock conditioning	Specifically mimics alterations in learning and fear conditioning		colon
Water avoidance	Strong acute models reproducing a strong stressor and mimicking resilience in an uncomfortable situation	Limited construct validity: physical constraint is not a factor commonly encountered in the etiology of FGID in patients	Stomach Ileum (more affected) colon
Partial restraint stress			Stomach and colon
Crowding stress	Models capture the social component in stress-induced FGID	Social organization, and individual reactions to stress are obviously less standardized and more complicated in humans	Small intestine and colon
Social isolation			Colon
Combined stress	Good model to reproduce anetiology commonly found in human	Because of the more complex interaction of stressors and depending on the protocol used, results tend to be more difficult to reproduce	Colon
Post-inflammatory	Reproduces low-grade inflammation often found in FGID e.g., after infection or in IBD in remission	Limited construct validity: interventional models using irritants/chemicals	Local effect depending on the targeted organ: mainly Stomach and colon
Post-infectious	Model for post-infectious FGID which allow a detailed study of dysbiosis involved in FGID	Different infectious agents compared to humans; most models have used parasitic infections which is uncommon in human FGID	Depending on the infection, small bowel or colon
Food allergy	Murine immune response in case of loss of oral tolerance closely resembles the human counterpart	The nutritional pattern differs between rodents and humans; evidence for immune reaction to food is still limited in human FGID	Colon
Spontaneous models	Non-interventional models, good face and construct validity	Sensitivity to environmental factors (food, stressors…) which makes these model more difficult to reproduce	Stomach, small bowel, colon
Postoperative Ileus	Good construct validity. Allows to study of the mechanisms of interventional surgery as a trigger of intestinal alterations	Intervention is highly operator and experimental condition dependent	Small bowel
Manipulation central nervous system	Suitable for mechanistic studies of the involvement of the central nervous system	Limited construct validity: far from human etiology	Mainly colon
Genetic model	Ideal models to study a specific genetic target and its role in FGID	Compensation phenomena; human FGID is not monogenetic	If KO: all levels of the GI tract If conditional KO: organ targeted
Cross sensitization	Understanding of the overlap in neuronal pathways which is common in human FGID	Interventional models using irritants	Depending on the organs targeted (mainly bladder and colon)

KO, knockout; FGID, functional gastrointestinal disorders; IBD, inflammatory bowel disease.

than usual. In this model, adult pigs display a defect in the small intestinal and colon mucosal barrier function with an elevated electrogenic transport activity, chronic diarrhea associated with an enhanced mast cell activation and an upregulation of the enteric cholinergic population (277, 278) Pretreatment of the stressed animals with a CRH antagonist abolished the stress-induced elevated secretory activity and increased intestinal permeability in jejunum and colon (279). *Ex-vivo* experiments demonstrated that CRH increased permeability via a TNF-α dependent mechanism (280). Similar to rodent models and

humans, female pigs are more affected than males by this stress paradigm (276). Despite the differences listed above, pig and rodent models reach the same conclusions on the effect of stress on the GI tract, confirming the critical and harmful effect of early life stress across species.

SUMMARY AND CONCLUSION

Functional gastrointestinal disorders are complex and multifactorial disorders involving a complex interaction between biological, psychological and social variables that none of the current animal models can reproduce perfectly. The strengths and limitations of the varied models are listed in **Table 2**. The main limitation of those models remains the societal component of the FGID pathophysiology that is extremely difficult to reproduce in animals. Nevertheless, animal models have brought pivotal insights into the pathophysiology of FGID, including the complex interaction between the gut and the central nervous system, and represent essentials tools for identifying novel therapeutic targets and testing of new generations of pharmaceutical and non-pharmaceutical therapies. Over the years, the improved understanding of the FGID pathophysiology has stimulated the conception of new animal models, which are now more complex and include a combination of causes triggering FGID features, which more closely resembles the human condition. However, with the development of those new multidimensional models using a multitude of slightly different protocols—sometimes not explained in detail in the literature—comes a lack of reproducibility hampering further progression. Several guidelines have been created to address this problem and to enhance scientific rigor (281, 282).

Most of the published studies still suffer from two limitations which weaken their translational relevance. First, most of the available studies focus on the lower GI tract (**Table 2**), while increasing evidence points out the overlap between the different FGIDs. Many of the models described above are characterized as IBS models but might also be suitable as FD models if alterations in the upper GI tract would be investigated. The second limitation is that the large majority of the pre-clinical studies are performed in male animals to avoid the "hormonal fluctuation" problem although FGID are mainly affecting women. Moreover, recent findings about the impact of sex hormones on the immune response suggest that estrogen is an important player in the onset and development of FGID. For each model presented in this review, at least one study performed in females was available, but often studies comparing both genders were lacking. The early life stress models more frequently addressed the impact of gender because of their methodology, since the stress is applied to pups in a stage when the sex is more difficult to determine. Although the field is slowly changing, studies including females are still underrepresented and those taking the hormonal parameters into account are even fewer. In order to improve the construct validity of the animal models capturing the female predominance of human FGID these studies are awaited in the near future.

AUTHOR CONTRIBUTIONS

All authors contributed to the first draft of the manuscript, critically revised subsequent drafts, and approved the final version.

REFERENCES

1. Tack J, Talley NJ, Camilleri M, Holtmann G, Hu P, Malagelada JR, et al. Functional gastroduodenal disorders. *Gastroenterology.* (2006) 130:1466–79. doi: 10.1053/j.gastro.2005.11.059
2. Longstreth GF, Thompson WG, Chey WD, Houghton LA, Mearin F, Spiller RC. Functional bowel disorders. *Gastroenterology.* (2006) 130:1480–91. doi: 10.1053/j.gastro.2005.11.061
3. Drossman DA. Functional gastrointestinal disorders: history, pathophysiology, clinical features and Rome IV. *Gastroenterology.* (2016) 150:1262–79. doi: 10.1053/j.gastro.2016.02.032
4. Camilleri M, Bueno L, Andresen V, de Ponti F, Choi MG, Lembo A. Pharmacological, pharmacokinetic, and pharmacogenomic aspects of functional gastrointestinal disorders. *Gastroenterology.* (2016) 150:1319–31. doi: 10.1053/j.gastro.2016.02.029
5. Vanheel H, Farre R. Changes in gastrointestinal tract function and structure in functional dyspepsia. *Nat Rev Gastroenterol Hepatol.* (2013) 10:142–9. doi: 10.1038/nrgastro.2012.255
6. Matricon J, Meleine M, Gelot A, Piche T, Dapoigny M, Muller E, et al. Review article: associations between immune activation, intestinal permeability and the irritable bowel syndrome. *Aliment Pharmacol Ther.* (2012) 36:1009–31. doi: 10.1111/apt.12080
7. vanheel H, Vicario M, Boesmans W, Vanuytsel T, Salvo-Romero E, Tack J, et al. Activation of eosinophils and mast cells in functional dyspepsia: an ultrastructural evaluation. *Sci Rep.* (2018) 8:5383. doi: 10.1038/s41598-018-23620-y
8. Robles A, Perez Ingles D, Myneedu K, Deoker A, Sarosiek I, Zuckerman MJ, et al. Mast cells are increased in the small intestinal mucosa of patients with irritable bowel syndrome: a systematic review and meta-analysis. *Neurogastroenterol Motil.* (2019) 31:e13718. doi: 10.1111/nmo.13718
9. Farre R, Vicario M. Abnormal barrier function in gastrointestinal disorders. *Handb Exp Pharmacol.* (2017) 239:193–217. doi: 10.1007/164_2016_107

10. Balemans D, Boeckxstaens GE, Talavera K, Wouters MM. Transient receptor potential ion channel function in sensory transduction and cellular signaling cascades underlying visceral hypersensitivity. *Am J Physiol Gastrointest Liver Physiol.* (2017) 312:G635–48. doi: 10.1152/ajpgi.00401.2016
11. Simren M, Tornblom H, Palsson OS, van Oudenhove L, Whitehead WE, Tack J. Cumulative effects of psychologic distress, visceral hypersensitivity, and abnormal transit on patient-reported outcomes in irritable bowel syndrome. *Gastroenterology.* (2019) 157:391–402.e2. doi: 10.1053/j.gastro.2019.04.019
12. Barbara G, Stanghellini V, de Giorgio R, Corinaldesi R. Functional gastrointestinal disorders and mast cells: implications for therapy. *Neurogastroenterol Motil.* (2006) 18:6–17. doi: 10.1111/j.1365-2982.2005.00685.x
13. Holtmann G, Shah A, Morrison M. Pathophysiology of functional gastrointestinal disorders: a holistic overview. *Dig Dis.* (2017) 35(Suppl. 1):5–13. doi: 10.1159/000485409
14. Beeckmans D, Riethorst D, Augustijns P, Vanuytsel T, Farre R, Tack J, et al. Altered duodenal bile salt concentration and receptor expression in functional dyspepsia. *United Eur Gastroenterol J.* (2018) 6:1347–55. doi: 10.1177/2050640618799120
15. Zhong L, Shanahan ER, Raj A, Koloski NA, Fletcher L, Morrison M, et al. Dyspepsia and the microbiome: time to focus on the small intestine. *Gut.* (2017) 66:1168–9. doi: 10.1136/gutjnl-2016-312574
16. Pittayanon R, Lau JT, Yuan Y, Leontiadis GI, Tse F, Surette M, et al. Gut microbiota in patients with irritable bowel syndrome-a systematic review. *Gastroenterology.* (2019) 157:97–108. doi: 10.1053/j.gastro.2019.03.049
17. Igarashi M, Nakae H, Matsuoka T, Takahashi S, Hisada T, Tomita J, et al. Alteration in the gastric microbiota and its restoration by probiotics in patients with functional dyspepsia. *BMJ Open Gastroenterol.* (2017) 4:e000144. doi: 10.1136/bmjgast-2017-000144
18. Mayer EA, Tillisch K. The brain-gut axis in abdominal pain syndromes. *Annu Rev Med.* (2011) 62:381–96. doi: 10.1146/annurev-med-012309-103958

19. Yi L, Sun H, Ge C, Chen Y, Peng H, Jiang Y, et al. Role of insular cortex in visceral hypersensitivity model in rats subjected to chronic stress. *Psychiatry Res.* (2014) 220:1138–43. doi: 10.1016/j.psychres.2014.09.019

20. Pinto-Sanchez MI, Hall GB, Ghajar K, Nardelli A, Bolino C, Lau JT, et al. Probiotic Bifidobacterium longum NCC3001 reduces depression scores and alters brain activity: a pilot study in patients with irritable bowel syndrome. *Gastroenterology.* (2017) 153:448–59.e8. doi: 10.1053/j.gastro.2017.05.003

21. van Oudenhove L, Aziz Q. The role of psychosocial factors and psychiatric disorders in functional dyspepsia. *Nat Rev Gastroenterol Hepatol.* (2013) 10:158–67. doi: 10.1038/nrgastro.2013.10

22. van Oudenhove L, vandenberghe J, Vos R, Fischler B, Demyttenaere K, Tack J. Abuse history, depression, and somatization are associated with gastric sensitivity and gastric emptying in functional dyspepsia. *Psychosom Med.* (2011) 73:648–55. doi: 10.1097/PSY.0b013e31822f32bf

23. Ulrich-Lai YM, Herman JP. Neural regulation of endocrine and autonomic stress responses. *Nat Rev Neurosci.* (2009) 10:397–409. doi: 10.1038/nrn2647

24. Song H, Fang F, Arnberg FK, Mataix-Cols D, Fernández de la Cruz L, Almqvist C, et al. Stress related disorders and risk of cardiovascular disease: population based, sibling controlled cohort study. *BMJ.* (2019) 365:l1255. doi: 10.1136/bmj.l1255

25. Kelly RR, McDonald LT, Jensen NR, Sidles SJ, LaRue AC. Impacts of psychological stress on osteoporosis: clinical implications and treatment interactions. *Front Psychiatry.* (2019) 10:200. doi: 10.3389/fpsyt.2019.00200

26. Afrisham R, Paknejad M, Soliemanifar O, Sadegh-Nejadi S, Meshkani R, Ashtary-Larky D. The influence of psychological stress on the initiation and progression of diabetes and cancer. *Int J Endocrinol Metab.* (2019) 17:e67400. doi: 10.5812/ijem.67400

27. Yang L, Zhao Y, Wang Y, Liu L, Zhang X, Li B, et al. The effects of psychological stress on depression. *Curr Neuropharmacol.* (2015) 13:494–504. doi: 10.2174/1570159X1304150831150507

28. Austin KW, Ameringer SW, Cloud LJ. An integrated review of psychological stress in Parkinson's disease: biological mechanisms and symptom and health outcomes. *Parkinsons Dis.* (2016) 2016:9869712. doi: 10.1155/2016/9869712

29. Haass-Koffler CL, Bartlett SE. Stress and addiction: contribution of the corticotropin releasing factor (CRF) system in neuroplasticity. *Front Mol Neurosci.* (2012) 5:91. doi: 10.3389/fnmol.2012.00091

30. Tamashiro KL, Nguyen MM, Sakai RR. Social stress: from rodents to primates. *Front Neuroendocrinol.* (2005) 26:27–40. doi: 10.1016/j.yfrne.2005.03.001

31. Bhatia V, Tandon RK. Stress and the gastrointestinal tract. *J Gastroenterol Hepatol.* (2005) 20:332–9. doi: 10.1111/j.1440-1746.2004.03508.x

32. Bunnett NW. The stressed gut: contributions of intestinal stress peptides to inflammation and motility. *Proc Natl Acad Sci USA.* (2005) 102:7409. doi: 10.1073/pnas.0503092102

33. Smith SM, Vale WW. The role of the hypothalamic-pituitary-adrenal axis in neuroendocrine responses to stress. *Dialogues Clin Neurosci.* (2006) 8:383–95.

34. Munck A, Guyre PM, Holbrook NJ. Physiological functions of glucocorticoids in stress and their relation to pharmacological actions. *Endocr Rev.* (1984) 5:25–44. doi: 10.1210/edrv-5-1-25

35. McEwen BS. Brain on stress: how the social environment gets under the skin. *Proc Natl Acad Sci USA.* (2012) 109(Suppl. 2):17180–5. doi: 10.1073/pnas.1121254109

36. Tache Y, Perdue MH. Role of peripheral CRF signalling pathways in stress-related alterations of gut motility and mucosal function. *Neurogastroenterol Motil.* (2004) 16(Suppl. 1):137–42. doi: 10.1111/j.1743-3150.2004.00490.x

37. Martinez V, Wang L, Rivier J, Grigoriadis D, Tache Y. Central CRF, urocortins and stress increase colonic transit via CRF1 receptors while activation of CRF2 receptors delays gastric transit in mice. *J Physiol.* (2004) 556:221–34. doi: 10.1113/jphysiol.2003.059659

38. Martinez V, Wang L, Rivier JE, Vale W, Tache Y. Differential actions of peripheral corticotropin-releasing factor (CRF), urocortin II, and urocortin III on gastric emptying and colonic transit in mice: role of CRF receptor subtypes 1 and 2. *J Pharmacol Exp Ther.* (2002) 301:611–7. doi: 10.1124/jpet.301.2.611

39. Yin Y, Dong L, Yin D. Peripheral and central administration of exogenous urocortin 1 disrupts the fasted motility pattern of the small intestine in rats via the corticotrophin releasing factor receptor 2 and a cholinergic mechanism. *J Gastroenterol Hepatol.* (2008) 23:e79–87. doi: 10.1111/j.1440-1746.2007.05142.x

40. Larauche M, Gourcerol G, Wang L, Pambukchian K, Brunnhuber S, Adelson DW, et al. Cortagine, a CRF1 agonist, induces stresslike alterations of colonic function and visceral hypersensitivity in rodents primarily through peripheral pathways. *Am J Physiol Gastrointest Liver Physiol.* (2009) 297:G215–27. doi: 10.1152/ajpgi.00072.2009

41. Trimble N, Johnson AC, Foster A, Greenwood-van Meerveld B. Corticotropin-releasing factor receptor 1-deficient mice show decreased anxiety and colonic sensitivity. *Neurogastroenterol Motil.* (2007) 19:754–60. doi: 10.1111/j.1365-2982.2007.00951.x

42. Million M, Wang L, Wang Y, Adelson DW, Yuan PQ, Maillot C, et al. CRF2 receptor activation prevents colorectal distension induced visceral pain and spinal ERK1/2 phosphorylation in rats. *Gut.* (2006) 55:172–81. doi: 10.1136/gut.2004.051391

43. la Fleur SE, Wick EC, Idumalla PS, Grady EF, Bhargava A. Role of peripheral corticotropin-releasing factor and urocortin II in intestinal inflammation and motility in terminal ileum. *Proc Natl Acad Sci USA.* (2005) 102:7647–52. doi: 10.1073/pnas.0408531102

44. Barreau F, Cartier C, Ferrier L, Fioramonti J, Bueno L. Nerve growth factor mediates alterations of colonic sensitivity and mucosal barrier induced by neonatal stress in rats. *Gastroenterology.* (2004) 127:524–34. doi: 10.1053/j.gastro.2004.05.019

45. Hagiwara SI, Kaushal E, Paruthiyil S, Pasricha PJ, Hasdemir B, Bhargava A. Gastric corticotropin-releasing factor influences mast cell infiltration in a rat model of functional dyspepsia. *PLoS ONE.* (2018) 13:e0203704. doi: 10.1371/journal.pone.0203704

46. Nicholl BI, Halder SL, Macfarlane GJ, Thompson DG, O'Brien S, Musleh M, et al. Psychosocial risk markers for new onset irritable bowel syndrome-results of a large prospective population-based study. *Pain.* (2008) 137:147–55. doi: 10.1016/j.pain.2007.08.029

47. Vanuytsel T, van Wanrooy S, Vanheel H, Vanormelingen C, Verschueren S, Houben E, et al. Psychological stress and corticotropin-releasing hormone increase intestinal permeability in humans by a mast cell-dependent mechanism. *Gut.* (2014) 63:1293–9. doi: 10.1136/gutjnl-2013-305690

48. Martin TD, Chan SS, Hart AR. Environmental factors in the relapse and recurrence of inflammatory bowel disease: a review of the literature. *Dig Dis Sci.* (2015) 60:1396–405. doi: 10.1007/s10620-014-3437-3

49. O'Mahony SM, Clarke G, Dinan TG, Cryan JF. Early-life adversity and brain development: is the microbiome a missing piece of the puzzle? *Neuroscience.* (2017) 342:37–54. doi: 10.1016/j.neuroscience.2015.09.068

50. Mayer EA, Naliboff BD, Chang L, Coutinho SV. Stress and irritable bowel syndrome. *Am J Physiol Gastrointest Liver Physiol.* (2001) 280:G519–24. doi: 10.1152/ajpgi.2001.280.4.G519

51. Klooker TK, Braak B, Painter RC, de Rooij SR, van Elburg RM, van den Wijngaard RM, et al. Exposure to severe wartime conditions in early life is associated with an increased risk of irritable bowel syndrome: a population-based cohort study. *Am J Gastroenterol.* (2009) 104:2250–6. doi: 10.1038/ajg.2009.282

52. Camp LL, Rudy JW. Changes in the categorization of appetitive and aversive events during postnatal development of the rat. *Dev Psychobiol.* (1988) 21:25–42. doi: 10.1002/dev.420210103

53. Moriceau S, Sullivan RM. Corticosterone influences on Mammalian neonatal sensitive-period learning. *Behav Neurosci.* (2004) 118:274–81. doi: 10.1037/0735-7044.118.2.274

54. Macri S. Neonatal corticosterone administration in rodents as a tool to investigate the maternal programming of emotional and immune domains. *Neurobiol Stress.* (2017) 6:22–30. doi: 10.1016/j.ynstr.2016.12.001

55. Walker CD, Perrin M, Vale W, Rivier C. Ontogeny of the stress response in the rat: role of the pituitary and the hypothalamus. *Endocrinology.* (1986) 118:1445–51. doi: 10.1210/endo-118-4-1445

56. Levine S, Glick D, Nakane PK. Adrenal and plasma corticosterone and vitamin A in rat adrenal glands during postnatal development. *Endocrinology.* (1967) 80:910–4. doi: 10.1210/endo-80-5-910

57. Sapolsky RM, Meaney MJ. Maturation of the adrenocortical stress response: neuroendocrine control mechanisms and the stress hyporesponsive period. *Brain Res.* (1986) 396:64–76. doi: 10.1016/0165-0173(86)90010-X

58. Levine S. Primary social relationships influence the development of the hypothalamic–pituitary–adrenal axis in the rat. *Physiol Behav.* (2001) 73:255–60. doi: 10.1016/S0031-9384(01)00496-6

59. Suchecki D, Mozaffarian D, Gross G, Rosenfeld P, Levine S. Effects of maternal deprivation on the ACTH stress response in the infant rat. *Neuroendocrinology.* (1993) 57:204–12. doi: 10.1159/000126361

60. Vazquez DM, Lopez JF, van Hoers H, Watson SJ, Levine S. Maternal deprivation regulates serotonin 1A and 2A receptors in the infant rat. *Brain Res.* (2000) 855:76–82. doi: 10.1016/S0006-8993(99)02307-0

61. Muret L, Priou A, Oliver C, Grino M. Stimulation of adrenocorticotropin secretion by insulin-induced hypoglycemia in the developing rat involves arginine vasopressin but not corticotropin-releasing factor. *Endocrinology.* (1992) 130:2725–32. doi: 10.1210/endo.130.5.1315256

62. Zelena D, Domokos A, Barna I, Mergl Z, Haller J, Makara GB. Control of the hypothalamo-pituitary-adrenal axis in the neonatal period: adrenocorticotropin and corticosterone stress responses dissociate in vasopressin-deficient brattleboro rats. *Endocrinology.* (2008) 149:2576–83. doi: 10.1210/en.2007–1537

63. Opendak M, Robinson-Drummer P, Blomkvist A, Zanca RM, Wood K, Jacobs L, et al. Neurobiology of maternal regulation of infant fear: the role of mesolimbic dopamine and its disruption by maltreatment. *Neuropsychopharmacology.* (2019) 44:1247–57. doi: 10.1038/s41386-019-0340-9

64. Claflin DI, Schmidt KD, Vallandingham ZD, Kraszpulski M, Hennessy MB. Influence of postnatal glucocorticoids on hippocampal-dependent learning varies with elevation patterns and administration methods. *Neurobiol Learn Mem.* (2017) 143:77–87. doi: 10.1016/j.nlm.2017.05.010

65. Daun KA, Fuchigami T, Koyama N, Maruta N, Ikenaka K, Hitoshi S. Early maternal and social deprivation expands neural stem cell population size and reduces hippocampus/amygdala-dependent fear memory. *Front Neurosci.* (2020) 14:22. doi: 10.3389/fnins.2020.00022

66. Winston JH, Li Q, Sarna SK. Chronic prenatal stress epigenetically modifies spinal cord BDNF expression to induce sex-specific visceral hypersensitivity in offspring. *Neurogastroenterol Motil.* (2014) 26:715–30. doi: 10.1111/nmo.12326

67. Jasarevic E, Howerton CL, Howard CD, Bale TL. Alterations in the vaginal microbiome by maternal stress are associated with metabolic reprogramming of the offspring gut and brain. *Endocrinology.* (2015) 156:3265–76. doi: 10.1210/en.2015–1177

68. Golubeva AV, Crampton S, Desbonnet L, Edge D, O'Sullivan O, Lomasney KW, et al. Prenatal stress-induced alterations in major physiological systems correlate with gut microbiota composition in adulthood. *Psychoneuroendocrinology.* (2015) 60:58–74. doi: 10.1016/j.psyneuen.2015.06.002

69. Molet J, Maras PM, Avishai-Eliner S, Baram TZ. Naturalistic rodent models of chronic early-life stress. *Dev Psychobiol.* (2014) 56:1675–88. doi: 10.1002/dev.21230

70. Orso R, Wearick-Silva LE, Creutzberg KC, Centeno-Silva A, Glusman Roithmann L, Pazzin R, et al. Maternal behavior of the mouse dam toward pups: implications for maternal separation model of early life stress. *Stress.* (2018) 21:19–27. doi: 10.1080/10253890.2017.1389883

71. Plotsky PM, Meaney MJ. Early, postnatal experience alters hypothalamic corticotropin-releasing factor (CRF) mRNA, median eminence CRF content and stress-induced release in adult rats. *Brain Res Mol Brain Res.* (1993) 18:195–200. doi: 10.1016/0169-328X(93)90189-V

72. McCormick CM, Kehoe P, Kovacs S. Corticosterone release in response to repeated, short episodes of neonatal isolation: evidence of sensitization. *Int J Dev Neurosci.* (1998) 16:175–85. doi: 10.1016/S0736-5748(98)00026-4

73. Plotsky PM, Thrivikraman KV, Nemeroff CB, Caldji C, Sharma S, Meaney MJ. Long-term consequences of neonatal rearing on central corticotropin-releasing factor systems in adult male rat offspring. *Neuropsychopharmacology.* (2005) 30:2192–204. doi: 10.1038/sj.npp.1300769

74. Moussaoui N, Jacobs JP, Larauche M, Biraud M, Million M, Mayer E, et al. Chronic early-life stress in rat pups alters basal corticosterone, intestinal permeability, and fecal microbiota at weaning: influence of sex. *J Neurogastroenterol Motil.* (2017) 23:135–43. doi: 10.5056/jnm16105

75. Li B, Lee C, Zani A, Zani-Ruttenstock E, Ip W, Chi L, et al. Early maternal separation induces alterations of colonic epithelial permeability and morphology. *Pediatr Surg Int.* (2014) 30:1217–22. doi: 10.1007/s00383-014-3611-x

76. Meleine M, Boudieu L, Gelot A, Muller E, Lashermes A, Matricon J, et al. Comparative effects of alpha2delta-1 ligands in mouse models of colonic hypersensitivity. *World J Gastroenterol.* (2016) 22:7111–23. doi: 10.3748/wjg.v22.i31.7111

77. van den Wijngaard RM, Stanisor OI, van Diest SA, Welting O, Wouters MM, Cailotto C, et al. Susceptibility to stress induced visceral hypersensitivity in maternally separated rats is transferred across generations. *Neurogastroenterol Motil.* (2013) 25:e780–90. doi: 10.1111/nmo.12202

78. van Den Wijngaard RM, Klooker TK, Welting O, Stanisor OI, Wouters MM, van Der Coelen D, et al. Essential role for TRPV1 in stress-induced (mast cell-dependent) colonic hypersensitivity in maternally separated rats. *Neurogastroenterol Motil.* (2009) 21:1107–94. doi: 10.1111/j.1365-2982.2009.01339.x

79. O'Malley D, Liston M, Hyland NP, Dinan TG, Cryan JF. Colonic soluble mediators from the maternal separation model of irritable bowel syndrome activate submucosal neurons via an interleukin-6-dependent mechanism. *Am J Physiol Gastrointest Liver Physiol.* (2011) 300:G241–52. doi: 10.1152/ajpgi.00385.2010

80. Barreau F, Ferrier L, Fioramonti J, Bueno L. Neonatal maternal deprivation triggers long term alterations in colonic epithelial barrier and mucosal immunity in rats. *Gut.* (2004) 53:501–6. doi: 10.1136/gut.2003.024174

81. Gareau MG, Jury J, Perdue MH. Neonatal maternal separation of rat pups results in abnormal cholinergic regulation of epithelial permeability. *Am J Physiol Gastrointest Liver Physiol.* (2007) 293:G198–203. doi: 10.1152/ajpgi.00392.2006

82. Li B, Lee C, Filler T, Hock A, Wu RY, Li Q, et al. Inhibition of corticotropin-releasing hormone receptor 1 and activation of receptor 2 protect against colonic injury and promote epithelium repair. *Sci Rep.* (2017) 7:46616. doi: 10.1038/srep46616

83. Ackerman SH, Hofer MA, Weiner H. Predisposition to gastric erosions in the rat: behavioral and nutritional effects of early maternal separation. *Gastroenterology.* (1978) 75:649–54. doi: 10.1016/S0016-5085(19)31674-9

84. Tominaga K, Fujikawa Y, Tanaka F, Kamata N, Yamagami H, Tanigawa T, et al. Structural changes in gastric glial cells and delayed gastric emptying as responses to early life stress and acute adulthood stress in rats. *Life Sci.* (2016) 148:254–9. doi: 10.1016/j.lfs.2016.02.025

85. Biagini G, Pich EM, Carani C, Marrama P, Agnati LF. Postnatal maternal separation during the stress hyporesponsive period enhances the adrenocortical response to novelty in adult rats by affecting feedback regulation in the CA1 hippocampal field. *Int J Dev Neurosci.* (1998) 16:187–97. doi: 10.1016/S0736-5748(98)00019-7

86. Daniels WM, Pietersen CY, Carstens ME, Stein DJ. Maternal separation in rats leads to anxiety-like behavior and a blunted ACTH response and altered neurotransmitter levels in response to a subsequent stressor. *Metab Brain Dis.* (2004) 19:3–14. doi: 10.1023/B:MEBR.0000027412.19664.b3

87. O'Mahony SM, Bulmer DC, Coelho AM, Fitzgerald P, Bongiovanni C, Lee K, et al. 5-HT(2B) receptors modulate visceral hypersensitivity in a stress-sensitive animal model of brain-gut axis dysfunction. *Neurogastroenterol Motil.* (2010) 22:573–8.e124. doi: 10.1111/j.1365-2982.2009.01432.x

88. Martisova E, Solas M, Horrillo I, Ortega JE, Meana JJ, Tordera RM, et al. Long lasting effects of early-life stress on glutamatergic/GABAergic circuitry in the rat hippocampus. *Neuropharmacology.* (2012) 62:1944–53. doi: 10.1016/j.neuropharm.2011.12.019

89. Matthews K, Dalley JW, Matthews C, Tsai TH, Robbins TW. Periodic maternal separation of neonatal rats produces region- and gender-specific effects on biogenic amine content in postmortem adult brain. *Synapse.* (2001) 40:1–10. doi: 10.1002/1098-2396(200104)40:1<1::AID-SYN1020>3.0.CO;2-E

90. Yu Y-C, Li J, Zhang M, Pan J-C, Yu Y, Zhang J-B, et al. Resveratrol improves brain-gut axis by regulation of 5-HT-dependent signaling in the rat model of irritable bowel syndrome. *Front Cell Neurosci.* (2019) 13:30. doi: 10.3389/fncel.2019.00030

91. Ford AC, Talley NJ, Schoenfeld PS, Quigley EM, Moayyedi P. Efficacy of antidepressants and psychological therapies in irritable bowel syndrome: systematic review and meta-analysis. *Gut.* (2009) 58:367–78. doi: 10.1136/gut.2008.163162

92. Bian ZX, Zhang M, Han QB, Xu HX, Sung JJ. Analgesic effects of JCM-16021 on neonatal maternal separation-induced visceral pain in rats. *World J Gastroenterol.* (2010) 16:837–45. doi: 10.3748/wjg.v16.i7.837

93. Arborelius L, Eklund MB. Both long and brief maternal separation produces persistent changes in tissue levels of brain

monoamines in middle-aged female rats. *Neuroscience.* (2007) 145:738–50. doi: 10.1016/j.neuroscience.2006.12.007

94. Manabe N, Tanaka T, Hata J, Kusunoki H, Haruma K. Pathophysiology underlying irritable bowel syndrome–from the viewpoint of dysfunction of autonomic nervous system activity. *J Smooth Muscle Res.* (2009) 45:15–23. doi: 10.1540/jsmr.45.15

95. Pickering C, Gustafsson L, Cebere A, Nylander I, Liljequist S. Repeated maternal separation of male Wistar rats alters glutamate receptor expression in the hippocampus but not the prefrontal cortex. *Brain Res.* (2006) 1099:101–8. doi: 10.1016/j.brainres.2006.04.136

96. Ryan B, Musazzi L, Mallei A, Tardito D, Gruber SH, El Khoury A, et al. Remodelling by early-life stress of NMDA receptor-dependent synaptic plasticity in a gene-environment rat model of depression. *Int J Neuropsychopharmacol.* (2009) 12:553–9. doi: 10.1017/S1461145708009607

97. Lajud N, Roque A, Cajero M, Gutierrez-Ospina G, Torner L. Periodic maternal separation decreases hippocampal neurogenesis without affecting basal corticosterone during the stress hyporesponsive period, but alters HPA axis and coping behavior in adulthood. *Psychoneuroendocrinology.* (2012) 37:410–20. doi: 10.1016/j.psyneuen.2011.07.011

98. Baram TZ, Davis EP, Obenaus A, Sandman CA, Small SL, Solodkin A, et al. Fragmentation and unpredictability of early-life experience in mental disorders. *Am J Psychiatry.* (2012) 169:907–15. doi: 10.1176/appi.ajp.2012.11091347

99. Gilles EE, Schultz L, Baram TZ. Abnormal corticosterone regulation in an immature rat model of continuous chronic stress. *Pediatr Neurol.* (1996) 15:114–9. doi: 10.1016/0887–8994(96)00153–1

100. Walker CD, Bath KG, Joels M, Korosi A, Larauche M, Lucassen PJ, et al. Chronic early life stress induced by limited bedding and nesting (LBN) material in rodents: critical considerations of methodology, outcomes and translational potential. *Stress.* (2017) 20:421–48. doi: 10.1080/10253890.2017.1343296

101. Ivy AS, Brunson KL, Sandman C, Baram TZ. Dysfunctional nurturing behavior in rat dams with limited access to nesting material: a clinically relevant model for early-life stress. *Neuroscience.* (2008) 154:1132–42. doi: 10.1016/j.neuroscience.2008.04.019

102. Holschneider DP, Guo Y, Mayer EA, Wang Z. Early life stress elicits visceral hyperalgesia and functional reorganization of pain circuits in adult rats. *Neurobiol Stress.* (2016) 3:8–22. doi: 10.1016/j.ynstr.2015.12.003

103. Guo Y, Wang Z, Mayer EA, Holschneider DP. Neonatal stress from limited bedding elicits visceral hyperalgesia in adult rats. *Neuroreport.* (2015) 26:13–6. doi: 10.1097/WNR.0000000000000292

104. Prusator DK, Greenwood-van Meerveld B. Gender specific effects of neonatal limited nesting on viscerosomatic sensitivity and anxiety-like behavior in adult rats. *Neurogastroenterol Motil.* (2015) 27:72–81. doi: 10.1111/nmo.12472

105. Youssef M, Atsak P, Cardenas J, Kosmidis S, Leonardo ED, Dranovsky A. Early life stress delays hippocampal development and diminishes the adult stem cell pool in mice. *Sci Rep.* (2019) 9:4120. doi: 10.1038/s41598-019-40868-0

106. Moriceau S, Sullivan RM. Maternal presence serves as a switch between learning fear and attraction in infancy. *Nat Neurosci.* (2006) 9:1004–6. doi: 10.1038/nn1733

107. Greenwood-van Meerveld B, Johnson AC. Stress-induced chronic visceral pain of gastrointestinal origin. *Front Syst Neurosci.* (2017) 11:86. doi: 10.3389/fnsys.2017.00086

108. Chaloner A, Greenwood-van Meerveld B. Sexually dimorphic effects of unpredictable early life adversity on visceral pain behavior in a rodent model. *J Pain.* (2013) 14:270–80. doi: 10.1016/j.jpain.2012.11.008

109. Ligon C, Mohammadi E, Ge P, Hannig G, Higgins C, Greenwood-Van Meerveld B. Linaclotide inhibits colonic and urinary bladder hypersensitivity in adult female rats following unpredictable neonatal stress. *Neurogastroenterol Motil.* (2018) 30:e13375. doi: 10.1111/nmo.13375

110. Takada M, Nishida K, Kataoka-Kato A, Gondo Y, Ishikawa H, Suda K, et al. Probiotic Lactobacillus casei strain Shirota relieves stress-associated symptoms by modulating the gut–brain interaction in human and animal models. *Neurogastroenterol Motil.* (2016) 28:1027–36. doi: 10.1111/nmo.12804

111. Lee JY, Kim N, Nam RH, Sohn SH, Lee SM, Choi D, et al. Probiotics reduce repeated water avoidance stress-induced colonic microinflammation in Wistar rats in a sex-specific manner. *PLoS ONE.* (2017) 12:e0188992. doi: 10.1371/journal.pone.0188992

112. Keita AV, Soderholm JD, Ericson AC. Stress-induced barrier disruption of rat follicle-associated epithelium involves corticotropin-releasing hormone, acetylcholine, substance P, and mast cells. *Neurogastroenterol Motil.* (2010) 22:770–8.e221–2. doi: 10.1111/j.1365–2982.2010.01471.x

113. Keita AV, Carlsson AH, Cigehn M, Ericson AC, McKay DM, Soderholm JD. Vasoactive intestinal polypeptide regulates barrier function via mast cells in human intestinal follicle-associated epithelium and during stress in rats. *Neurogastroenterol Motil.* (2013) 25:e406–17. doi: 10.1111/nmo.12127

114. Nozu T, Miyagishi S, Nozu R, Takakusaki K, Okumura T. Repeated water avoidance stress induces visceral hypersensitivity: role of interleukin-1, interleukin-6, and peripheral corticotropin-releasing factor. *J Gastroenterol Hepatol.* (2017) 32:1958–65. doi: 10.1111/jgh.13787

115. Da Silva S, Robbe-Masselot C, Ait-Belgnaoui A, Mancuso A, Mercade-Loubiere M, Salvador-Cartier C, et al. Stress disrupts intestinal mucus barrier in rats via mucin O-glycosylation shift: prevention by a probiotic treatment. *Am J Physiol Gastrointest Liver Physiol.* (2014) 307:G420–9. doi: 10.1152/ajpgi.00290.2013

116. Zhang L, Song J, Bai T, Qian W, Hou XH. Stress induces more serious barrier dysfunction in follicle-associated epithelium than villus epithelium involving mast cells and protease-activated receptor-2. *Sci Rep.* (2017) 7:4950. doi: 10.1038/s41598–017–05064-y

117. Zhang J, Song L, Wang Y, Liu C, Zhang L, Zhu S, et al. Beneficial effect of butyrate-producing Lachnospiraceae on stress-induced visceral hypersensitivity in rats. *J Gastroenterol Hepatol.* (2019) 34:1368–76. doi: 10.1111/jgh.14536

118. Yoshikawa K, Kurihara C, Furuhashi H, Takajo T, Maruta K, Yasutake Y, et al. Psychological stress exacerbates NSAID-induced small bowel injury by inducing changes in intestinal microbiota and permeability via glucocorticoid receptor signaling. *J Gastroenterol.* (2017) 52:61–71. doi: 10.1007/s00535-016-1205-1

119. Nozu T, Kumei S, Takakusaki K, Okumura T. Water-avoidance stress enhances gastric contractions in freely moving conscious rats: role of peripheral CRF receptors. *J Gastroenterol.* (2014) 49:799–805. doi: 10.1007/s00535–013–0828-8

120. Miwa H, Koseki J, Oshima T, Hattori T, Kase Y, Kondo T, et al. Impairment of gastric accommodation induced by water-avoidance stress is mediated by 5-HT2B receptors. *Neurogastroenterol Motil.* (2016) 28:765–78. doi: 10.1111/nmo.12775

121. Llorca-Torralba M, Suarez-Pereira I, Bravo L, Camarena-Delgado C, Garcia-Partida JA, Mico JA, et al. Chemogenetic silencing of the locus coeruleus-basolateral amygdala pathway abolishes pain-induced anxiety and enhanced aversive learning in rats. *Biol Psychiatry.* (2019) 85:1021–35. doi: 10.1016/j.biopsych.2019.02.018

122. Larsson MB, Tillisch K, Craig AD, Engstrom M, Labus J, Naliboff B, et al. Brain responses to visceral stimuli reflect visceral sensitivity thresholds in patients with irritable bowel syndrome. *Gastroenterology.* (2012) 142:463–72.e3. doi: 10.1053/j.gastro.2011.11.022

123. Labus JS, Hubbard CS, Bueller J, Ebrat B, Tillisch K, Chen M, et al. Impaired emotional learning and involvement of the corticotropin-releasing factor signaling system in patients with irritable bowel syndrome. *Gastroenterology.* (2013) 145:1253–61.e1–3. doi: 10.1053/j.gastro.2013.08.016

124. Kret ME, de Gelder B. A review on sex differences in processing emotional signals. *Neuropsychologia.* (2012) 50:1211–21. doi: 10.1016/j.neuropsychologia.2011.12.022

125. Labus JS, Gupta A, Coveleskie K, Tillisch K, Kilpatrick L, Jarcho J, et al. Sex differences in emotion-related cognitive processes in irritable bowel syndrome and healthy control subjects. *Pain.* (2013) 154:2088–99. doi: 10.1016/j.pain.2013.06.024

126. Hubbard CS, Karpowicz JM, Furman AJ, da Silva JT, Seminowicz DA, Traub RJ. Estrogen-dependent visceral hypersensitivity following stress in rats: an fMRI study. *Mol Pain.* (2016) 12:1744806916654145. doi: 10.1177/1744806916654145

127. Friedrich T, Schalla MA, Lommel R, Goebel-Stengel M, Kobelt P, Rose M, et al. Restraint stress increases the expression of

phoenixin immunoreactivity in rat brain nuclei. *Brain Res.* (2020) 1743:146904. doi: 10.1016/j.brainres.2020.146904

128. Goebel M, Stengel A, Wang L, Taché Y. Restraint stress activates nesfatin-1-immunoreactive brain nuclei in rats. *Brain Res.* (2009) 1300:114–24. doi: 10.1016/j.brainres.2009.08.082

129. Schalla MA, Stengel A. The role of phoenixin in behavior and food intake. *Peptides.* (2019) 114:38–43. doi: 10.1016/j.peptides.2019.04.002

130. Weibert E, Hofmann T, Stengel A. Role of nesfatin-1 in anxiety, depression and the response to stress. *Psychoneuroendocrinology.* (2019) 100:58–66. doi: 10.1016/j.psyneuen.2018.09.037

131. Foo KS, Brismar H, Broberger C. Distribution and neuropeptide coexistence of nucleobindin-2 mRNA/nesfatin-like immunoreactivity in the rat CNS. *Neuroscience.* (2008) 156:563–79. doi: 10.1016/j.neuroscience.2008.07.054

132. Yoshida N, Maejima Y, Sedbazar U, Ando A, Kurita H, Damdindorj B, et al. Stressor-responsive central nesfatin-1 activates corticotropin-releasing hormone, noradrenaline and serotonin neurons and evokes hypothalamic-pituitary-adrenal axis. *Aging.* (2010) 2:775–84. doi: 10.18632/aging.100207

133. Wang L, Gourcerol G, Yuan PQ, Wu SV, Million M, Larauche M, et al. Peripheral peptide YY inhibits propulsive colonic motor function through Y2 receptor in conscious mice. *Am J Physiol Gastrointest Liver Physiol.* (2010) 298:G45–56. doi: 10.1152/ajpgi.00349.2009

134. Ait-Belgnaoui A, Han W, Lamine F, Eutamene H, Fioramonti J, Bueno L, et al. Lactobacillus farciminis treatment suppresses stress induced visceral hypersensitivity: a possible action through interaction with epithelial cell cytoskeleton contraction. *Gut.* (2006) 55:1090–4. doi: 10.1136/gut.2005.084194

135. Traini C, Evangelista S, Girod V, Faussone-Pellegrini MS, Vannucchi MG. Changes of excitatory and inhibitory neurotransmitters in the colon of rats underwent to the wrap partial restraint stress. *Neurogastroenterol Motil.* (2016) 28:1172–85. doi: 10.1111/nmo.12816

136. Boulete IM, Thadi A, Beaufrand C, Patwa V, Joshi A, Foss JA, et al. Oral treatment with plecanatide or dolcanatide attenuates visceral hypersensitivity via activation of guanylate cyclase-C in rat models. *World J Gastroenterol.* (2018) 24:1888–900. doi: 10.3748/wjg.v24.i17.1888

137. Nakade Y, Tsuchida D, Fukuda H, Iwa M, Pappas TN, Takahashi T. Restraint stress delays solid gastric emptying via a central CRF and peripheral sympathetic neuron in rats. *Am J Physiol Regul Integr Comp Physiol.* (2005) 288:R427–32. doi: 10.1152/ajpregu.00499.2004

138. Million M, Maillot C, Saunders P, Rivier J, Vale W, Tache Y. Human urocortin II, a new CRF-related peptide, displays selective CRF(2)-mediated action on gastric transit in rats. *Am J Physiol Gastrointest Liver Physiol.* (2002) 282:G34–40. doi: 10.1152/ajpgi.00283.2001

139. Seto K, Sasaki T, Katsunuma K, Kobayashi N, Tanaka K, Tack J. Acotiamide hydrochloride (Z-338), a novel prokinetic agent, restores delayed gastric emptying and feeding inhibition induced by restraint stress in rats. *Neurogastroenterol Motil.* (2008) 20:1051–9. doi: 10.1111/j.1365-2982.2008.01135.x

140. Ye Y, Wang XR, Zheng Y, Yang JW, Yang NN, Shi GX, et al. Choosing an animal model for the study of functional dyspepsia. *Can J Gastroenterol Hepatol.* (2018) 2018:1531958. doi: 10.1155/2018/1531958

141. Bliss TV, Collingridge GL, Kaang BK, Zhuo M. Synaptic plasticity in the anterior cingulate cortex in acute and chronic pain. *Nat Rev Neurosci.* (2016) 17:485–96. doi: 10.1038/nrn.2016.68

142. Hostinar CE, Sullivan RM, Gunnar MR. Psychobiological mechanisms underlying the social buffering of the hypothalamic-pituitary-adrenocortical axis: a review of animal models and human studies across development. *Psychol Bull.* (2014) 140:256–82. doi: 10.1037/a0032671

143. Levine S, Johnson DF, Gonzalez CA. Behavioral and hormonal responses to separation in infant rhesus monkeys and mothers. *Behav Neurosci.* (1985) 99:399–410. doi: 10.1037/0735-7044.99.3.399

144. Hennessy MB, Kaiser S, Sachser N. Social buffering of the stress response: diversity, mechanisms, and functions. *Front Neuroendocrinol.* (2009) 30:470–82. doi: 10.1016/j.yfrne.2009.06.001

145. Lauffer A, Vanuytsel T, Vanormelingen C, Vanheel H, Salim Rasoel S, Toth J, et al. Subacute stress and chronic stress interact to decrease intestinal barrier function in rats. *Stress.* (2016) 19:225–34. doi: 10.3109/10253890.2016.1154527

146. Vicario M, Guilarte M, Alonso C, Yang P, Martinez C, Ramos L, et al. Chronological assessment of mast cell-mediated gut dysfunction and mucosal inflammation in a rat model of chronic psychosocial stress. *Brain Behav Immun.* (2010) 24:1166–75. doi: 10.1016/j.bbi.2010.06.002

147. Gadek-Michalska A, Tadeusz J, Bugajski A, Bugajski J. Chronic isolation stress affects subsequent crowding stress-induced brain nitric oxide synthase (NOS) Isoforms and hypothalamic-pituitary-adrenal (HPA) axis responses. *Neurotox Res.* (2019) 36:523–39. doi: 10.1007/s12640-019-00067-1

148. Berry A, Bellisario V, Capoccia S, Tirassa P, Calza A, Alleva E, et al. Social deprivation stress is a triggering factor for the emergence of anxiety- and depression-like behaviours and leads to reduced brain BDNF levels in C57BL/6J mice. *Psychoneuroendocrinology.* (2012) 37:762–72. doi: 10.1016/j.psyneuen.2011.09.007

149. Nishida K, Kamizato M, Kawai T, Masuda K, Takeo K, Teshima-Kondo S, et al. Interleukin-18 is a crucial determinant of vulnerability of the mouse rectum to psychosocial stress. *FASEB J.* (2009) 23:1797–805. doi: 10.1096/fj.08-125005

150. Stanisor OI, van Diest SA, Yu Z, Welting O, Bekkali N, Shi J, et al. Stress-induced visceral hypersensitivity in maternally separated rats can be reversed by peripherally restricted histamine-1-receptor antagonists. *PLoS ONE.* (2013) 8:e66884. doi: 10.1371/journal.pone.0066884

151. Prusator DK, Greenwood-van Meerveld B. Sex differences in stress-induced visceral hypersensitivity following early life adversity: a two hit model. *Neurogastroenterol Motil.* (2016) 28:1876–89. doi: 10.1111/nmo.12891

152. Jianguo L, Xueyang J, Cui W, Changxin W, Xuemei Q. Altered gut metabolome contributes to depression-like behaviors in rats exposed to chronic unpredictable mild stress. *Transl Psychiatry.* (2019) 9:40. doi: 10.1038/s41398-019-0645-9

153. Li H, Wang P, Huang L, Li P, Zhang D. Effects of regulating gut microbiota on the serotonin metabolism in the chronic unpredictable mild stress rat model. *Neurogastroenterol Motil.* (2019) 31:e13677. doi: 10.1111/nmo.13677

154. Lee YY, Annamalai C, Rao SSC. Post-infectious irritable bowel syndrome. *Curr Gastroenterol Rep.* (2017) 19:56. doi: 10.1007/s11894-017-0595-4

155. Teruel C, Garrido E, Mesonero F. Diagnosis and management of functional symptoms in inflammatory bowel disease in remission. *World J Gastrointest Pharmacol Ther.* (2016) 7:78–90. doi: 10.4292/wjgpt.v7.i1.78

156. Klem F, Wadhwa A, Prokop LJ, Sundt WJ, Farrugia G, Camilleri M, et al. Prevalence, risk factors, and outcomes of irritable bowel syndrome after infectious enteritis: a systematic review and meta-analysis. *Gastroenterology.* (2017) 152:1042–54.e1. doi: 10.1053/j.gastro.2016.12.039

157. Nozu T, Miyagishi S, Nozu R, Takakusaki K, Okumura T. Lipopolysaccharide induces visceral hypersensitivity: role of interleukin-1, interleukin-6, and peripheral corticotropin-releasing factor in rats. *J Gastroenterol.* (2017) 52:72–80. doi: 10.1007/s00535-016-1208-y

158. Coelho AM, Fioramonti J, Buéno L. Systemic lipopolysaccharide influences rectal sensitivity in rats: role of mast cells, cytokines, and vagus nerve. *Am J Physiol Gastrointest Liver Physiol.* (2000) 279:G781–90. doi: 10.1152/ajpgi.2000.279.4.G781

159. Nozu T, Miyagishi S, Nozu R, Takakusaki K, Okumura T. Altered colonic sensory and barrier functions by CRF: roles of TLR4 and IL-1. *J Endocrinol.* (2018) 239:241–52. doi: 10.1530/JOE-18-0441

160. Nozu T, Miyagishi S, Nozu R, Takakusaki K, Okumura T. Losartan improves visceral sensation and gut barrier in a rat model of irritable bowel syndrome. *Neurogastroenterol Motil.* (2020) 32:e13819. doi: 10.1111/nmo.13819

161. Nozu T, Miyagishi S, Kumei S, Nozu R, Takakusaki K, Okumura T. Lovastatin inhibits visceral allodynia and increased colonic permeability induced by lipopolysaccharide or repeated water avoidance stress in rats. *Eur J Pharmacol.* (2018) 818:228–34. doi: 10.1016/j.ejphar.2017.10.056

162. Nozu T, Miyagishi S, Ishioh M, Takakusaki K, Okumura T. Imipramine improves visceral sensation and gut barrier in rat models of irritable bowel syndrome. *Eur J Pharmacol.* (2020) 887:173565. doi: 10.1016/j.ejphar.2020.173565

163. Scanzi J, Accarie A, Muller E, Pereira B, Aissouni Y, Goutte M, et al. Colonic overexpression of the T-type calcium channel Cav 3.2 in a mouse model of visceral hypersensitivity and in irritable bowel syndrome patients. *Neurogastroenterol Motil.* (2016) 28:1632–40. doi: 10.1111/nmo.12860

164. Picard E, Carvalho FA, Agosti F, Bourinet E, Ardid D, Eschalier A, et al. Inhibition of Cav3.2 calcium channels: a new target for colonic hypersensitivity associated with low-grade inflammation. *Br J Pharmacol.* (2019) 176:950–63. doi: 10.1111/bph.14608

165. Adam B, Liebregts T, Gschossmann JM, Krippner C, Scholl F, Ruwe M, et al. Severity of mucosal inflammation as a predictor for alterations of visceral sensory function in a rat model. *Pain.* (2006) 123:179–86. doi: 10.1016/j.pain.2006.02.029

166. Tada Y, Ishihara S, Kawashima K, Fukuba N, Sonoyama H, Kusunoki R, et al. Downregulation of serotonin reuptake transporter gene expression in healing colonic mucosa in presence of remaining low-grade inflammation in ulcerative colitis. *J Gastroenterol Hepatol.* (2016) 31:1443–52. doi: 10.1111/jgh.13268

167. Lapointe TK, Basso L, Iftinca MC, Flynn R, Chapman K, Dietrich G, et al. TRPV1 sensitization mediates postinflammatory visceral pain following acute colitis. *Am J Physiol Gastrointest Liver Physiol.* (2015) 309:G87–99. doi: 10.1152/ajpgi.00421.2014

168. Qin HY, Wu JC, Tong XD, Sung JJ, Xu HX, Bian ZX. Systematic review of animal models of post-infectious/post-inflammatory irritable bowel syndrome. *J Gastroenterol.* (2011) 46:164–74. doi: 10.1007/s00535-010-0321-6

169. Johnson AC, Greenwood-van Meerveld B. Critical evaluation of animal models of gastrointestinal disorders. *Handb Exp Pharmacol.* (2017) 239:289–317. doi: 10.1007/164_2016_120

170. Fabisiak A, Włodarczyk J, Fabisiak N, Storr M, Fichna J. Targeting histamine receptors in irritable bowel syndrome: a critical appraisal. *J Neurogastroenterol Motil.* (2017) 23:341–8. doi: 10.5056/jnm16203

171. Winston JH, Sarna SK. Developmental origins of functional dyspepsia-like gastric hypersensitivity in rats. *Gastroenterology.* (2013) 144:570–9.e3. doi: 10.1053/j.gastro.2012.11.001

172. Stanghellini V. Functional dyspepsia and irritable bowel syndrome: beyond Rome IV. *Dig Dis.* (2017) 35(Suppl. 1):14–7. doi: 10.1159/000485408

173. Winston J, Shenoy M, Medley D, Naniwadekar A, Pasricha PJ. The vanilloid receptor initiates and maintains colonic hypersensitivity induced by neonatal colon irritation in rats. *Gastroenterology.* (2007) 132:615–27. doi: 10.1053/j.gastro.2006.11.014

174. Hou Q, Huang Y, Zhu S, Li P, Chen X, Hou Z, et al. MiR-144 increases intestinal permeability in IBS-D rats by targeting OCLN and ZO1. *Cell Physiol Biochem.* (2017) 44:2256–68. doi: 10.1159/000486059

175. Dai F, Lei Y, Li S, Song G, Chen JD. Desvenlafaxine succinate ameliorates visceral hypersensitivity but delays solid gastric emptying in rats. *Am J Physiol Gastrointest Liver Physiol.* (2013) 305:G333–9. doi: 10.1152/ajpgi.00224.2012

176. Jones RC 3rd, Otsuka E, Wagstrom E, Jensen CS, Price MP, Gebhart GF. Short-term sensitization of colon mechanoreceptors is associated with long-term hypersensitivity to colon distention in the mouse. *Gastroenterology.* (2007) 133:184–94. doi: 10.1053/j.gastro.2007.04.042

177. Banvolgyi A, Pozsgai G, Brain SD, Helyes ZS, Szolcsanyi J, Ghosh M, et al. Mustard oil induces a transient receptor potential vanilloid 1 receptor-independent neurogenic inflammation and a non-neurogenic cellular inflammatory component in mice. *Neuroscience.* (2004) 125:449–59. doi: 10.1016/j.neuroscience.2004.01.009

178. Chun E, Yoon S, Parveen A, Jin M. Alleviation of irritable bowel syndrome-like symptoms and control of gut and brain responses with oral administration of Dolichos lablab L. in a mouse model. *Nutrients.* (2018) 10:1475. doi: 10.3390/nu10101475

179. Ji Y, Tang B, Cao DY, Wang G, Traub RJ. Sex differences in spinal processing of transient and inflammatory colorectal stimuli in the rat. *Pain.* (2012) 153:1965–73. doi: 10.1016/j.pain.2012.06.019

180. Kimball ES, Palmer JM, D'Andrea MR, Hornby PJ, Wade PR. Acute colitis induction by oil of mustard results in later development of an IBS-like accelerated upper GI transit in mice. *Am J Physiol Gastrointest Liver Physiol.* (2005) 288:G1266–73. doi: 10.1152/ajpgi.00444.2004

181. Zhang MM, Liu SB, Chen T, Koga K, Zhang T, Li YQ, et al. Effects of NB001 and gabapentin on irritable bowel syndrome-induced behavioral anxiety and spontaneous pain. *Mol Brain.* (2014) 7:47. doi: 10.1186/1756-6606-7-47

182. Liu LS, Winston JH, Shenoy MM, Song GQ, Chen JD, Pasricha PJ. A rat model of chronic gastric sensorimotor dysfunction resulting from transient neonatal gastric irritation. *Gastroenterology.* (2008) 134:2070–9. doi: 10.1053/j.gastro.2008.02.093

183. Heiss CN, Olofsson LE. The role of the gut microbiota in development, function and disorders of the central nervous system and the enteric nervous system. *J Neuroendocrinol.* (2019) 31:e12684. doi: 10.1111/jne.12684

184. Spiller R, Garsed K. Postinfectious irritable bowel syndrome. *Gastroenterology.* (2009) 136:1979–88. doi: 10.1053/j.gastro.2009.02.074

185. Schwille-Kiuntke J, Mazurak N, Enck P. Systematic review with meta-analysis: post-infectious irritable bowel syndrome after travellers' diarrhoea. *Aliment Pharmacol Ther.* (2015) 41:1029–37. doi: 10.1111/apt.13199

186. Halliez MC, Buret AG. Gastrointestinal parasites and the neural control of gut functions. *Front Cell Neurosci.* (2015) 9:452. doi: 10.3389/fncel.2015.00452

187. Akiho H, Deng Y, Blennerhassett P, Kanbayashi H, Collins SM. Mechanisms underlying the maintenance of muscle hypercontractility in a model of postinfective gut dysfunction. *Gastroenterology.* (2005) 129:131–41. doi: 10.1053/j.gastro.2005.03.049

188. Venkova K, Greenwood-van Meerveld B. Long-lasting changes in small intestinal transport following the recovery from *Trichinella spiralis* infection. *Neurogastroenterol Motil.* (2006) 18:234–42. doi: 10.1111/j.1365-2982.2005.00753.x

189. Bercik P, Wang L, Verdu EF, Mao YK, Blennerhassett P, Khan WI, et al. Visceral hyperalgesia and intestinal dysmotility in a mouse model of postinfective gut dysfunction. *Gastroenterology.* (2004) 127:179–87. doi: 10.1053/j.gastro.2004.04.006

190. Barnich N, Carvalho FA, Glasser AL, Darcha C, Jantscheff P, Allez M, et al. CEACAM6 acts as a receptor for adherent-invasive *E. coli*, supporting ileal mucosa colonization in Crohn disease. *J Clin Invest.* (2007) 117:1566–74. doi: 10.1172/JCI30504

191. Lashermes A, Boudieu L, Barbier J, Sion B, Gelot A, Barnich N, et al. Adherent-Invasive *E. coli* enhances colonic hypersensitivity and P2X receptors expression during post-infectious period. *Gut Microbes.* (2018) 9:26–37. doi: 10.1080/19490976.2017.1361091

192. Bohn L, Storsrud S, Tornblom H, Bengtsson U, Simren M. Self-reported food-related gastrointestinal symptoms in IBS are common and associated with more severe symptoms and reduced quality of life. *Am J Gastroenterol.* (2013) 108:634–41. doi: 10.1038/ajg.2013.105

193. Fritscher-Ravens A, Schuppan D, Ellrichmann M, Schoch S, Rocken C, Brasch J, et al. Confocal endomicroscopy shows food-associated changes in the intestinal mucosa of patients with irritable bowel syndrome. *Gastroenterology.* (2014) 147:1012–20.e4. doi: 10.1053/j.gastro.2014.07.046

194. Smit JJ, Noti M, O'Mahony L. The use of animal models to discover immunological mechanisms underpinning sensitization to food allergens. *Drug Discov Today.* (2015) 17–18:63–9. doi: 10.1016/j.ddmod.2016.09.001

195. Liu T, Navarro S, Lopata AL. Current advances of murine models for food allergy. *Mol Immunol.* (2016) 70:104–17. doi: 10.1016/j.molimm.2015.11.011

196. Florens M, Aguilera-Lizarraga J, Theofanous S, Bosmans G, Balemans D, Perna E, et al. Food antigen-specific antibodies and mast cell activation in post-infectious visceral hypersensitivity. *Gastroenterology.* (2017) 152:S721. doi: 10.1016/S0016-5085(17)32508-8

197. Aguilera-Lizarraga J, Balemans D, Lopez CDL, Polanco JOJ, Florens M, Perna E, et al. 1092 - Food antigen-specific sensitization of nociceptive nerves as an underlying mechanism of visceral pain in Ibs. *Gastroenterology.* (2018) 154:S-214-S-5. doi: 10.1016/S0016-5085(18)31107-7

198. Bouchoucha M, Fysekidis M, Julia C, Airinei G, Catheline J-M, Reach G, et al. Functional gastrointestinal disorders in obese patients. The importance of the enrollment source. *Obes Surg.* (2015) 25:2143–52. doi: 10.1007/s11695-015-1679-6

199. Aasbrenn M, Høgestøl I, Eribe I, Kristinsson J, Lydersen S, Mala T, et al. Prevalence and predictors of irritable bowel syndrome in patients with morbid obesity: a cross-sectional study. *BMC Obes.* (2017) 4:22. doi: 10.1186/s40608-017-0159-z

200. Fysekidis M, Bouchoucha M, Bihan H, Reach G, Benamouzig R, Catheline JM. Prevalence and co-occurrence of upper and lower functional gastrointestinal symptoms in patients eligible for bariatric surgery. *Obes Surg.* (2012) 22:403–10. doi: 10.1007/s11695-011-0396-z

201. Shau JP, Chen PH, Chan CF, Hsu YC, Wu TC, James FE, et al. Fast foods—are they a risk factor for functional gastrointestinal disorders? *Asia Pac J Clin Nutr.* (2016) 25:393–401. doi: 10.6133/apjcn.2016.25.2.28

202. Buscail C, Sabate JM, Bouchoucha M, Kesse-Guyot E, Hercberg S, Benamouzig R, et al. Western dietary pattern is associated with irritable

bowel syndrome in the French NutriNet cohort. *Nutrients.* (2017) 9:986. doi: 10.3390/nu9090986

203. Brun P, Castagliuolo I, Leo VD, Buda A, Pinzani M, Palù G, et al. Increased intestinal permeability in obese mice: new evidence in the pathogenesis of nonalcoholic steatohepatitis. *Am J Physiol Gastrointest Liver Physiol.* (2007) 292:G518–25. doi: 10.1152/ajpgi.00024.2006

204. Luo Q, Cheng D, Huang C, Li Y, Lao C, Xia Y, et al. Improvement of colonic immune function with Soy isoflavones in high-fat diet-induced obese rats. *Molecules.* (2019) 24:1139. doi: 10.3390/molecules24061139

205. Thiennimitr P, Yasom S, Tunapong W, Chunchai T, Wanchai K, Pongchaidecha A, et al. Lactobacillus paracasei HII01, xylooligosaccharides, and synbiotics reduce gut disturbance in obese rats. *Nutrition.* (2018) 54:40–7. doi: 10.1016/j.nut.2018.03.005

206. Chen M, Hou P, Zhou M, Ren Q, Wang X, Huang L, et al. Resveratrol attenuates high-fat diet-induced non-alcoholic steatohepatitis by maintaining gut barrier integrity and inhibiting gut inflammation through regulation of the endocannabinoid system. *Clin Nutr.* (2019) 39:1264–75. doi: 10.1016/j.clnu.2019.05.020

207. Ouni M, Schurmann A. Epigenetic contribution to obesity. *Mamm Genome.* (2020) 31:134–45. doi: 10.1007/s00335-020-09835-3

208. Rajilic-Stojanovic M, Biagi E, Heilig HG, Kajander K, Kekkonen RA, Tims S, et al. Global and deep molecular analysis of microbiota signatures in fecal samples from patients with irritable bowel syndrome. *Gastroenterology.* (2011) 141:1792–801. doi: 10.1053/j.gastro.2011.07.043

209. Bourdu S, Dapoigny M, Chapuy E, Artigue F, Vasson MP, Dechelotte P, et al. Rectal instillation of butyrate provides a novel clinically relevant model of noninflammatory colonic hypersensitivity in rats. *Gastroenterology.* (2005) 128:1996–2008. doi: 10.1053/j.gastro.2005.03.082

210. Xu D, Wu X, Grabauskas G, Owyang C. Butyrate-induced colonic hypersensitivity is mediated by mitogen-activated protein kinase activation in rat dorsal root ganglia. *Gut.* (2013) 62:1466–74. doi: 10.1136/gutjnl-2012-302260

211. Long X, Li M, Li LX, Sun YY, Zhang WX, Zhao DY, et al. Butyrate promotes visceral hypersensitivity in an IBS-like model via enteric glial cell-derived nerve growth factor. *Neurogastroenterol Motil.* (2018) 30:e13227. doi: 10.1111/nmo.13227

212. Nielsen MA, Bayati A, Mattsson H. Wistar Kyoto rats have impaired gastric accommodation compared to Sprague Dawley rats due to increased gastric vagal cholinergic tone. *Scand J Gastroenterol.* (2006) 41:773–81. doi: 10.1080/00365520500483215

213. Vanuytsel T, Vanormelingen C, Vanheel H, Masaoka T, Salim Rasoel S, Toth J, et al. From intestinal permeability to dysmotility: the biobreeding rat as a model for functional gastrointestinal disorders. *PLoS ONE.* (2014) 9:e111132. doi: 10.1371/journal.pone.0111132

214. Mattsson H, Arani Z, Astin M, Bayati A, Overstreet DH, Lehmann A. Altered neuroendocrine response and gastric dysmotility in the flinders sensitive line rat. *Neurogastroenterol Motil.* (2005) 17:166–74. doi: 10.1111/j.1365-2982.2005.00665.x

215. Like AA, Butler L, Williams RM, Appel MC, Weringer EJ, Rossini AA. Spontaneous autoimmune diabetes mellitus in the BB rat. *Diabetes.* (1982) 31:7–13. doi: 10.2337/diab.31.1.S7

216. Visser JT, Lammers K, Hoogendijk A, Boer MW, Brugman S, Beijer-Liefers S, et al. Restoration of impaired intestinal barrier function by the hydrolysed casein diet contributes to the prevention of type 1 diabetes in the diabetes-prone BioBreeding rat. *Diabetologia.* (2010) 53:2621–8. doi: 10.1007/s00125-010-1903-9

217. Neu J, Reverte CM, Mackey AD, Liboni K, Tuhacek-Tenace LM, Hatch M, et al. Changes in intestinal morphology and permeability in the biobreeding rat before the onset of type 1 diabetes. *J Pediatr Gastroenterol Nutr.* (2005) 40:589–95. doi: 10.1097/01.MPG.0000159636.19346.C1

218. Demedts I, Masaoka T, Kindt S, de Hertogh G, Geboes K, Farre R, et al. Gastrointestinal motility changes and myenteric plexus alterations in spontaneously diabetic biobreeding rats. *J Neurogastroenterol Motil.* (2013) 19:161–70. doi: 10.5056/jnm.2013.19.2.161

219. Meleine M, Accarie A, Wauters L, Toth J, Gourcerol G, Tack J, et al. Colonic hypersensitivity and low-grade inflammation in a spontaneous animal model for functional gastrointestinal disorders. *Neurogastroenterol Motil.* (2019) 31:e13614. doi: 10.1111/nmo.13614

220. Vanormelingen C, Vanuytsel T, Masaoka T, de Hertogh G, Vanheel H, Vanden Berghe P, et al. The normoglycaemic biobreeding rat: a spontaneous model for impaired gastric accommodation. *Gut.* (2016) 65:73–81. doi: 10.1136/gutjnl-2014-308154

221. Vanuytsel T, Di Giovangiulio M, Vanormelingen C, Vanheel H, Rasoel SS, Tóth JG, et al. Mo2045 the normoglycemic BB-DP rat as a model for functional gastrointestinal disorders: the implication of mast cells and eosinophils. *Gastroenterology.* (2015) 148:778. doi: 10.1016/S0016-5085(15)32654-8

222. Rittenhouse PA, Lopez-Rubalcava C, Stanwood GD, Lucki I. Amplified behavioral and endocrine responses to forced swim stress in the Wistar-Kyoto rat. *Psychoneuroendocrinology.* (2002) 27:303–18. doi: 10.1016/S0306-4530(01)00052-X

223. Vicario M, Alonso C, Guilarte M, Serra J, Martinez C, Gonzalez-Castro AM, et al. Chronic psychosocial stress induces reversible mitochondrial damage and corticotropin-releasing factor receptor type-1 upregulation in the rat intestine and IBS-like gut dysfunction. *Psychoneuroendocrinology.* (2012) 37:65–77. doi: 10.1016/j.psyneuen.2011.05.005

224. Hyland NP, O'Mahony SM, O'Malley D, O'Mahony CM, Dinan TG, Cryan JF. Early-life stress selectively affects gastrointestinal but not behavioral responses in a genetic model of brain-gut axis dysfunction. *Neurogastroenterol Motil.* (2015) 27:105–13. doi: 10.1111/nmo.12486

225. Pare WP, Tejani-Butt SM. Effect of stress on the behavior and 5-HT system in Sprague-Dawley and Wistar Kyoto rat strains. *Integr Physiol Behav Sci.* (1996) 31:112–21. doi: 10.1007/BF02699783

226. Scholl JL, Renner KJ, Forster GL, Tejani-Butt S. Central monoamine levels differ between rat strains used in studies of depressive behavior. *Brain Res.* (2010) 1355:41–51. doi: 10.1016/j.brainres.2010.08.003

227. Gibney SM, Gosselin RD, Dinan TG, Cryan JF. Colorectal distension-induced prefrontal cortex activation in the Wistar-Kyoto rat: implications for irritable bowel syndrome. *Neuroscience.* (2010) 165:675–83. doi: 10.1016/j.neuroscience.2009.08.076

228. Greenwood-Van Meerveld B, Johnson AC, Cochrane S, Schulkin J, Myers DA. Corticotropin-releasing factor 1 receptor-mediated mechanisms inhibit colonic hypersensitivity in rats. *Neurogastroenterol Motil.* (2005) 17:415–22. doi: 10.1111/j.1365-2982.2005.00648.x

229. Gunter WD, Shepard JD, Foreman RD, Myers DA, Greenwood-van Meerveld B. Evidence for visceral hypersensitivity in high-anxiety rats. *Physiol Behav.* (2000) 69:379–82. doi: 10.1016/S0031-9384(99)00254-1

230. Martinez V, Ryttinger M, Kjerling M, Astin-Nielsen M. Characterisation of colonic accommodation in Wistar Kyoto rats with impaired gastric accommodation. *Naunyn Schmiedebergs Arch Pharmacol.* (2007) 376:205–16. doi: 10.1007/s00210-007-0195-1

231. O'Malley D, Julio-Pieper M, Gibney SM, Dinan TG, Cryan JF. Distinct alterations in colonic morphology and physiology in two rat models of enhanced stress-induced anxiety and depression-like behaviour. *Stress.* (2010) 13:114–22. doi: 10.3109/10253890903067418

232. Overstreet DH, Russell RW. Selective breeding for diisopropyl fluorophosphate-sensitivity: behavioural effects of cholinergic agonists and antagonists. *Psychopharmacology.* (1982) 78:150–5. doi: 10.1007/BF00432254

233. Janowsky DS, el-Yousef MK, Davis JM, Sekerke HJ. A cholinergic-adrenergic hypothesis of mania and depression. *Lancet.* (1972) 2:632–5. doi: 10.1016/S0140-6736(72)93021-8

234. Overstreet DH, Wegener G. The flinders sensitive line rat model of depression—25 years and still producing. *Pharmacol Rev.* (2013) 65:143–55. doi: 10.1124/pr.111.005397

235. Tillmann S, Abildgaard A, Winther G, Wegener G. Altered fecal microbiota composition in the flinders sensitive line rat model of depression. *Psychopharmacology.* (2019) 236:1445–57. doi: 10.1007/s00213-018-5094-2

236. Tillmann S, Wegener G. Probiotics reduce risk-taking behavior in the elevated plus maze in the flinders sensitive line rat model of depression. *Behav Brain Res.* (2019) 359:755–62. doi: 10.1016/j.bbr.2018.08.025

237. Wolthuis AM, Bislenghi G, Fieuws S, de Buck van Overstraeten A, Boeckxstaens G, D'Hoore A. Incidence of prolonged postoperative ileus after colorectal surgery: a systematic review and meta-analysis. *Colorectal Dis.* (2016) 18:1–9. doi: 10.1111/codi.13210

238. Tan S, Yu W, Lin Z, Chen Q, Shi J, Dong Y, et al. Peritoneal air exposure elicits an intestinal inflammation resulting in postoperative ileus. *Mediators Inflamm.* (2014) 2014:924296. doi: 10.1155/2014/924296

239. Lyu JH, Lee H-T. Effects of dried Citrus unshiu peels on gastrointestinal motility in rodents. *Arch Pharm Res.* (2013) 36:641–8. doi: 10.1007/s12272-013-0080-z

240. Goetz B, Benhaqi P, Müller MH, Kreis ME, Kasparek MS. Changes in beta-adrenergic neurotransmission during postoperative ileus in rat circular jejunal muscle. *Neurogastroenterol Motil.* (2013) 25:154–84. doi: 10.1111/nmo.12020

241. Snoek SA, Dhawan S, van Bree SH, Cailotto C, van Diest SA, Duarte JM, et al. Mast cells trigger epithelial barrier dysfunction, bacterial translocation and postoperative ileus in a mouse model. *Neurogastroenterol Motil.* (2012) 24:172–91. doi: 10.1111/j.1365-2982.2011.01820.x

242. Gomez-Pinilla PJ, Farro G, Di Giovangiulio M, Stakenborg N, Nemethova A, de Vries A, et al. Mast cells play no role in the pathogenesis of postoperative ileus induced by intestinal manipulation. *PLoS ONE.* (2014) 9:e85304. doi: 10.1371/journal.pone.0085304

243. Stoffels B, Hupa KJ, Snoek SA, van Bree S, Stein K, Schwandt T, et al. Postoperative ileus involves interleukin-1 receptor signaling in enteric glia. *Gastroenterology.* (2014) 146:176–87.e1. doi: 10.1053/j.gastro.2013.09.030

244. Matteoli G, Gomez-Pinilla PJ, Nemethova A, Di Giovangiulio M, Cailotto C, van Bree SH, et al. A distinct vagal anti-inflammatory pathway modulates intestinal muscularis resident macrophages independent of the spleen. *Gut.* (2014) 63:938–48. doi: 10.1136/gutjnl-2013–304676

245. The FO, Boeckxstaens GE, Snoek SA, Cash JL, Bennink R, LaRosa GJ, et al. Activation of the cholinergic anti-inflammatory pathway ameliorates postoperative ileus in mice. *Gastroenterology.* (2007) 133:1219–28. doi: 10.1053/j.gastro.2007.07.022

246. Stakenborg N, Wolthuis AM, Gomez-Pinilla PJ, Farro G, Di Giovangiulio M, Bosmans G, et al. Abdominal vagus nerve stimulation as a new therapeutic approach to prevent postoperative ileus. *Neurogastroenterol Motil.* (2017) 29:e13075. doi: 10.1111/nmo.13075

247. Taché Y, Yang H, Miampamba M, Martinez V, Yuan PQ. Role of brainstem TRH/TRH-R1 receptors in the vagal gastric cholinergic response to various stimuli including sham-feeding. *Auton Neurosci.* (2006) 125:42–52. doi: 10.1016/j.autneu.2006.01.014

248. Falkén Y, Webb DL, Abraham-Nordling M, Kressner U, Hellström PM, Näslund E. Intravenous ghrelin accelerates postoperative gastric emptying and time to first bowel movement in humans. *Neurogastroenterol Motil.* (2013) 25:474–80. doi: 10.1111/nmo.12098

249. Luckey A, Wang L, Jamieson PM, Basa NR, Million M, Czimmer J, et al. Corticotropin-releasing factor receptor 1-deficient mice do not develop postoperative gastric ileus. *Gastroenterology.* (2003) 125:654–9. doi: 10.1016/S0016-5085(03)01069-2

250. Zittel TT, Lloyd KC, Rothenhöfer I, Wong H, Walsh JH, Raybould HE. Calcitonin gene-related peptide and spinal afferents partly mediate postoperative colonic ileus in the rat. *Surgery.* (1998) 123:518–27. doi: 10.1067/msy.1998.88090

251. Stengel A, Goebel-Stengel M, Wang L, Shaikh A, Lambrecht NW, Rivier J, et al. Abdominal surgery inhibits circulating acyl ghrelin and ghrelin-O-acyltransferase levels in rats: role of the somatostatin receptor subtype 2. *Am J Physiol Gastrointest Liver Physiol.* (2011) 301:G239–48. doi: 10.1152/ajpgi.00018.2011

252. Stengel A, Goebel M, Wang L, Taché Y. Abdominal surgery activates nesfatin-1 immunoreactive brain nuclei in rats. *Peptides.* (2010) 31:263–70. doi: 10.1016/j.peptides.2009.11.015

253. Greenwood-Van Meerveld B, Gibson M, Gunter W, Shepard J, Foreman R, Myers D. Stereotaxic delivery of corticosterone to the amygdala modulates colonic sensitivity in rats. *Brain Res.* (2001) 893:135–42. doi: 10.1016/S0006-8993(00)03305-9

254. Johnson AC, Greenwood-van Meerveld B. Knockdown of steroid receptors in the central nucleus of the amygdala induces heightened pain behaviors in the rat. *Neuropharmacology.* (2015) 93:116–23. doi: 10.1016/j.neuropharm.2015.01.018

255. Johnson AC, Tran L, Greenwood-Van Meerveld B. Knockdown of corticotropin-releasing factor in the central amygdala reverses persistent viscerosomatic hyperalgesia. *Transl Psychiatry.* (2015) 5:e517. doi: 10.1038/tp.2015.16

256. Tran L, Schulkin J, Ligon CO, Greenwood-van Meerveld B. Epigenetic modulation of chronic anxiety and pain by histone deacetylation. *Mol Psychiatry.* (2014) 20:1219–31. doi: 10.1038/mp.2014.122

257. Sekiguchi F, Tsubota M, Kawabata A. Involvement of voltage-gated calcium channels in inflammation and inflammatory pain. *Biol Pharm Bull.* (2018) 41:1127–34. doi: 10.1248/bpb.b18–00054

258. Holzer P. Acid-sensing ion channels in gastrointestinal function. *Neuropharmacology.* (2015) 94:72–9. doi: 10.1016/j.neuropharm.2014.12.009

259. Kawabata A, Kawao N, Kitano T, Matsunami M, Satoh R, Ishiki T, et al. Colonic hyperalgesia triggered by proteinase-activated receptor-2 in mice: involvement of endogenous bradykinin. *Neurosci Lett.* (2006) 402:167–72. doi: 10.1016/j.neulet.2006.03.074

260. Park MK, Cho MK, Kang SA, Park H-K, Kim YS, Kim KU, et al. Protease-activated receptor 2 is involved in Th2 responses against *Trichinella spiralis* infection. *Korean J Parasitol.* (2011) 49:245–43. doi: 10.3347/kjp.2011.49.3.235

261. Yuan B, Tang W-H, Lu L-J, Zhou Y, Zhu H-Y, Zhou Y-L, et al. TLR4 upregulates CBS expression through NF-κB activation in a rat model of irritable bowel syndrome with chronic visceral hypersensitivity. *World J Gastroenterol.* (2015) 21:8615–28. doi: 10.3748/wjg.v21.i28.8615

262. McKernan DP, Gaszner G, Quigley EM, Cryan JF, Dinan TG. Altered peripheral toll-like receptor responses in the irritable bowel syndrome. *Aliment Pharmacol Ther.* (2011) 33:1045–52. doi: 10.1111/j.1365-2036.2011.04624.x

263. Brint EK, MacSharry J, Fanning A, Shanahan F, Quigley EMM. Differential expression of Toll-like receptors in patients with irritable bowel syndrome. *American J Gastroenterol.* (2011) 106:329–36. doi: 10.1038/ajg.2010.438

264. Tang H-L, Zhang G, Ji N-N, Du L, Chen B-B, Hua R, et al. Toll-like receptor 4 in paraventricular nucleus mediates visceral hypersensitivity induced by maternal separation. *Front Pharmacol.* (2017) 8:309. doi: 10.3389/fphar.2017.00309

265. Bielefeldt K, Lamb K, Gebhart GF. Convergence of sensory pathways in the development of somatic and visceral hypersensitivity. *Am J Physiol Gastrointest Liver Physiol.* (2006) 291:G658–65. doi: 10.1152/ajpgi.00585.2005

266. Ustinova EE, Fraser MO, Pezzone MA. Colonic irritation in the rat sensitizes urinary bladder afferents to mechanical and chemical stimuli: an afferent origin of pelvic organ cross-sensitization. *Am J Physiol Renal Physiol.* (2006) 290:F1478–87. doi: 10.1152/ajprenal.00395.2005

267. Greenwood-van Meerveld B, Mohammadi E, Tyler K, van Gordon S, Parker A, Towner R, et al. Mechanisms of visceral organ crosstalk: importance of alterations in permeability in rodent models. *J Urol.* (2015) 194:804–11. doi: 10.1016/j.juro.2015.02.2944

268. Winnard KP, Dmitrieva N, Berkley KJ. Cross-organ interactions between reproductive, gastrointestinal, and urinary tracts: modulation by estrous stage and involvement of the hypogastric nerve. *Am J Physiol Regul Integr Comp Physiol.* (2006) 291:R1592–601. doi: 10.1152/ajpregu.004 55.2006

269. Hussain Z, Jung DH, Lee YJ, Park H. The effect of Trimebutine on the overlap syndrome model of guinea pigs. *J Neurogastroenterol Motil.* (2018) 24:669–75. doi: 10.5056/jnm18049

270. Hussain Z, Kim HW, Huh CW, Lee YJ, Park H. The effect of peripheral CRF peptide and water avoidance stress on colonic and gastric transit in guinea pigs. *Yonsei Med J.* (2017) 58:872–7. doi: 10.3349/ymj.2017.58.4.872

271. Park JJ, Chon NR, Lee YJ, Park H. The effects of an extract of atractylodes Japonica Rhizome, SKI3246 on gastrointestinal motility in guinea pigs. *J Neurogastroenterol Motil.* (2015) 21:352–60. doi: 10.5056/jnm14112

272. Tanaka T, Tanaka A, Nakamura A, Matsushita K, Imanishi A, Matsumoto-Okano S, et al. Effects of TAK-480, a novel tachykinin NK(2)-receptor antagonist, on visceral hypersensitivity in rabbits and ricinoleic acid-induced defecation in guinea pigs. *J Pharmacol Sci.* (2012) 120:15–25. doi: 10.1254/jphs.12085FP

273. Brown DR, Timmermans JP. Lessons from the porcine enteric nervous system. *Neurogastroenterol Motil.* (2004) 16:50–4. doi: 10.1111/j.1743-3150.2004.00475.x

274. Timmermans J-P, Hens J, Adriaensen D. Outer submucous plexus: an intrinsic nerve network involved in both secretory and motility processes in the intestine of large mammals and humans. *Anat Rec.* (2001) 262:71–

8. doi: 10.1002/1097–0185(20010101)262:1<;71::AID-AR1012>;3.0.CO;2-A

275. Gieling ET, Schuurman T, Nordquist RE, van der Staay FJ. The pig as a model animal for studying cognition and neurobehavioral disorders. In: Hagan JJ, editor. *Molecular and Functional Models in Neuropsychiatry*. Berlin, Heidelberg: Springer Berlin Heidelberg (2011). p. 359–83. doi: 10.1007/7854_2010_112

276. Medland JE, Pohl CS, Edwards LL, Frandsen S, Bagley K, Li Y, et al. Early life adversity in piglets induces long-term upregulation of the enteric cholinergic nervous system and heightened, sex-specific secretomotor neuron responses. *Neurogastroenterol Motil.* (2016) 28:1317–29. doi: 10.1111/nmo.12828

277. Moeser AJ, Ryan KA, Nighot PK, Blikslager AT. Gastrointestinal dysfunction induced by early weaning is attenuated by delayed weaning and mast cell blockade in pigs. *Am J Physiol Gastrointest Liver Physiol.* (2007) 293:G413–21. doi: 10.1152/ajpgi.00304.2006

278. Smith F, Clark JE, Overman BL, Tozel CC, Huang JH, Rivier JE, et al. Early weaning stress impairs development of mucosal barrier function in the porcine intestine. *Am J Physiol Gastrointest Liver Physiol.* (2010) 298:G352–63. doi: 10.1152/ajpgi.00081.2009

279. Moeser AJ, Klok CV, Ryan KA, Wooten JG, Little D, Cook VL, et al. Stress signaling pathways activated by weaning mediate intestinal dysfunction in the pig. *Am J Physiol Gastrointest Liver Physiol.* (2007) 292:G173–81. doi: 10.1152/ajpgi.00197.2006

280. Overman EL, Rivier JE, Moeser AJ. CRF induces intestinal epithelial barrier injury via the release of mast cell proteases and TNF-α. *PLoS ONE.* (2012) 7:e39935. doi: 10.1371/journal.pone.0039935

281. Clayton JA. Studying both sexes: a guiding principle for biomedicine. *FASEB J.* (2016) 30:519–24. doi: 10.1096/fj.15–279554

282. Miller LR, Marks C, Becker JB, Hurn PD, Chen WJ, Woodruff T, et al. Considering sex as a biological variable in preclinical research. *FASEB J.* (2017) 31:29–34. doi: 10.1096/fj.201600781r

5

Psychotherapeutic Interventions in Irritable Bowel Syndrome

Larissa Hetterich[1] and Andreas Stengel[1,2]*

[1] Department of Psychosomatic Medicine and Psychotherapy, University Hospital Tübingen, Tübingen, Germany,
[2] Department for Psychosomatic Medicine—Germany, Charité Center for Internal Medicine and Dermatology, Corporate Member of Freie Universität Berlin, Berlin Institute of Health, Charité - Universitätsmedizin Berlin, Humboldt-Universität zu Berlin, Berlin, Germany

*Correspondence:
Andreas Stengel
andreas.stengel@med.
uni-tuebingen.de

Irritable bowel syndrome (IBS) is a frequent functional gastrointestinal disorder. The patients complain about various symptoms like change in bowel habits, constipation or diarrhea, abdominal pain, and meteorism leading to a great reduction in quality of life. The pathophysiology is complex and best explained using the biopsychosocial model encompassing biological, psychological as well as (psycho)social factors. In line with the multitude of underlying factors, the treatment is comprised of a multitude of components. Often, patients start with lifestyle changes and dietary advice followed by medical treatment. However, also psychotherapy is an important treatment option for patients with IBS and should not be restricted to those with psychiatric comorbidities. Several evidence-based psychotherapeutic treatment options exist such as psychoeducation, self-help, cognitive behavioral therapy, psychodynamic psychotherapy, hypnotherapy, mindfulness-based therapy, and relaxation therapy which will be discussed in the present review.

Keywords: brain-gut axis, hypnotherapy, psychodynamic, psychoeducation, psychosomatic

INTRODUCTION

Irritable bowel syndrome (IBS) is a functional disorder of the large bowel (1). In the ICD-10 it is categorized within the functional disorders, in the ICD-11 it will be found in the section of bodily distress disorders. Patients with IBS can present with a wide array of symptoms such as abdominal distension, meteorism and flatulence, abdominal pain as well as a change in bowel habits such as constipation or diarrhea (2). The prevalence of IBS varies greatly with 1 to 45%—most likely due to different diagnostic criteria applied—with an average worldwide prevalence of 11.2% (3), well reflecting the prevalence in western countries with 10–20% (4).

IBS can be diagnosed worldwide using the Rome criteria (last revised in 2016 and termed Rome IV) when the patient complains of the main symptom being recurring abdominal pain that occurred during the last 3 months not less than once per week (2). Additionally, two of the following three criteria have to be fulfilled:

- The complaints are associated with defecation,
- The complaints are associated with change in frequency of defecation and
- The complaints are associated with change in consistency of stool (2).

According to the Rome IV criteria IBS can be classified into four different subgroups:

- IBS-D (diarrhea): >25% of the stool is fluid, without solid components, <25% are solid components,
- IBS-C (constipation): >25% of the stool are separate solid clots, <25% fluid, without solid components,
- IBS-M (mixed): >25% of the stool are fluid, without solid components and >25% are separate solid clots,
- IBS-U (unclassified): not clearly allocable (2).

These complaints are very often associated with a great reduction in quality of life. A study from 2014 showed that quality of life in patients with IBS depends on different parameters such as clinical variables (24%), fear of gastrointestinal symptoms (14%) or demographics (10%). Also psychiatric disorders may be a consequence of the disease (5). This underlines the need for a proper treatment offer (6).

In the present review we evaluated the state-of-knowledge on psychological treatment options for patients with IBS and as well discussed gaps in knowledge in order to foster further research. We employed the following databases: PubMed and ScienceDirect using these keywords: brain-gut axis, cognitive behavioral therapy, hypnotherapy, IBS, irritable bowel syndrome, mindfulness-based therapy, psychodynamic, psychoeducation, psychosomatic, relaxation therapy, and self-help. Only human studies were considered for the review, while animal studies were excluded. The search was conducted for articles from 1983 to 2019, the discussion highlights recent developments.

PATHOPHYSIOLOGY

The pathogenesis of IBS is complex and best explained using the biopsychosocial model encompassing biological, psychological, and (psycho)social factors (7) that can all contribute to the development and maintenance of the disease. In line with this model, genetic and environmental factors can affect the disorder as well as special personality traits (8). These traits can contribute to coping strategies which, when not sufficient anymore, might also facilitate development of the disease. Various psychosocial factors are important for IBS e.g., early life experiences, infections, trauma, stress, cultural background, and also the level of support the individual receives. Negative life experiences are considered an important risk factor for the development of IBS. People who experienced more (severe or frequent) negative life events show a higher prevalence of IBS and might have a more severe progress of the disorder (9).

The gut-brain-axis is a bidirectional communication system between the gut and the central nervous system (10). Afferent nerve pathways as well as humoral signals transmit information from the gastrointestinal tract to the central nervous system. The information gets processed in various brain areas and often feedbacks back to the gut. A dysregulated gut-brain-axis can lead to e.g., altered bowel motility, intestinal immune reaction, or intestinal permeability which may drive inflammatory responses that may contribute to visceral hypersensitivity (11). Also, the microbiome may likely play a role in the pathophysiology of IBS since the microbiome of patients with IBS seems to be less variable (12) and might be located in other parts of the gut as seen in small intestinal bacterial overgrowth (13). Due to the impact of the microbiome on gastrointestinal as well as central processes, the term microbiome-gut-brain axis was introduced. The importance of the gut-brain axis in the pathophysiology of IBS is also reflected in the Rome IV criteria where IBS has been allocated to diseases with discorded gut-brain interaction (14). The intimate interaction between gut and brain also explains the high overlap between IBS and psychiatric diseases which also has an impact on the selection of the treatment components. Most frequent psychiatric comorbidities are anxiety disorders (30–50%), depression (70%), but also—although less frequent—eating disorders (5).

PSYCHOTHERAPY

Besides lifestyle changes, dietary advice, and drug treatment, psychotherapy is an important column in the treatment of IBS. Not every patient has to undergo psychotherapy but especially in patients with insufficient social support, traumatic events in their history, or dysfunctional relations, psychotherapy should be considered early on (15). Moreover, patients with psychiatric comorbidities (5) or those that do not show significant improvement after treatment with other treatment options (e.g., drugs) (16) should be considered for psychotherapy. The National Institute of Health and Care Excellence (NICE) guidelines recommend a psychological therapy for patients who do not respond to pharmacological treatments after 12 months and develop refractory IBS. Psychotherapy options contain psychoeducation, self-help, cognitive behavioral therapy, psychodynamic psychotherapy, hypnotherapy, mindfulness-based-therapy, and relaxation therapy (17) which will be discussed in this review. The likelihood for a psychological intervention to be successful is greater in patients that are motivated and open for psychotherapy (18), although this should be the prerequisite for offering this therapy.

A meta-analysis showed the benefit of pooled psychological interventions in patients with IBS with a very low number needed to treat (NNT) of 2 (18). Similarly, a recent meta-analysis calculated a NNT of 4 (95% confidence interval, CI, 3.5–5.5) (19). While the NNT suggests a very prominent effect of psychotherapy, a systematic review reported that the psychotherapy-induced positive effects on symptoms did not last longer than the positive effects induced by other treatment options such as medication (20). A more recent meta-analysis included 41 trials with overall 2,290 individuals and compared psychological interventions with a mix of control conditions. It was shown that psychotherapeutic interventions decreased the symptoms immediately after the treatment, while 1–6 months (short-term) and 6–12 months (long-term) after start of the treatment the reduction remained significant compared to the control group(s) (21). Additionally, another meta-analysis analyzed the effect of psychotherapeutic interventions on mental health and the daily functioning of patients. All psychotherapeutic interventions showed a greater improvement of mental health and daily functioning of IBS patients compared to a mixed group of control conditions (22). The next paragraphs will provide an overview on the effects of different psychotherapeutic techniques in the treatment of IBS.

Psychoeducation

It is important that the physician takes time to explain the medical condition. This contains the name of the disease, development, pathophysiology, prognosis, and various treatment options (23). If this information is provided according to the biopsychosocial model, it would be referred to as psychoeducation (7). Moreover, psychoeducation is key for a trustful doctor-patient-relationship which greatly impacts on the course of the disease and reduction of symptoms, respectively (24). Psychoeducation can also help to reduce/avoid unnecessary repetitive (and sometimes invasive) examinations and/or non-suited therapeutic interventions as this could increase the probability of an incorrect concept of the disorder and potentially harm the patient (25). Therefore, the world gastroenterology organization mentions in its global guidelines that educating the patients about IBS has a positive effect on the treatment outcome (26).

A study used psychoeducation with information about pathophysiology in combination with elements of cognitive behavioral therapy (CBT) and progressive muscle relaxation for 5 weeks. After this psychoeducation, patients reported a significant reduction of somatic complaints and depressive symptoms and an improvement in quality of life compared to the control group. These effects persisted after a follow-up of 3 months (27).

Another study used a group education based on the biopsychosocial model with aspects of CBT compared to a control group that used an IBS manual. The group-educated patients reported a significant increase of knowledge after 3 and 6 months compared to the group using the manual. There was a reduction of symptom-specific anxiety in the group education group, while no significant differences between groups were seen with regards to quality of life, anxiety symptoms, and depressive complaints. Nevertheless, there was an increase of quality of life and reduction of anxiety in the group-educated group compared to the beginning of the treatment (28) (**Table 1**).

Self-Help

Self-help can be supported by detailed consultation and information about IBS e.g., with manuals or guidebooks. The patients can learn about experiences, coping strategies, or treatment options. This encourages the patients' self-management (29).

A randomized, controlled trial studied the effect of different self-help methods on the frequency of doctor's appointments and on symptom severity. One group received a self-help-manual, the other additionally visited a self-help group once per week. These groups were compared to a control group with routine outpatient care. Compared to the control group, the group with the self-help-manual reduced doctor's appointments (60% less in 1 year) associated with a reduction in health costs (40% less). The intervention group showed a significant improvement of complaints compared to the start of the study (Cohen's d=0.51). However, there was no difference related to symptom severity and quality of life between groups (30). Another trial studied the effect of a self-help manual on health-associated quality of life. After 6 months of intervention there was a significant improvement in quality of life. This effect was also observed in patients with psychiatric comorbidities like depression, anxiety, or somatization disorders. The severity of

---

TABLE 1 | Randomized controlled studies investigating the effects of psychoeducation in patients with irritable bowel syndrome.

Study	Population	Variables	Intervention	Results
Ringström et al. (2010) Structured patient education is superior to written information in the management of patients with irritable bowel syndrome: a randomized controlled study. *Eur J Gastroenterol Hepatol.* (28)	143 (87% female)	Quality of life Anxiety Depressive symptoms	Group education *vs.* IBS-manual	Group education: Increase of knowledge after 3 and 6 months, reduction of symptom-specific anxiety. No difference in groups: quality of life, anxiety, depressive complaints.
Labus et al. (2013) Randomised clinical trial: symptoms of the irritable bowel syndrome are improved by a psychoeducation group intervention. *Aliment Pharmacol Ther.* (27)	69 (72% female)	Somatic symptoms Depressive symptoms Quality of life	5 weeks: psychoeducation + elements of CBT + progressive muscle relaxation *vs.* control group	After treatment: significant reduction of somatic complaints, depressive symptoms, and improvement of quality of life.

TABLE 2 | Randomized controlled study investigating the effects of self-help in patients with irritable bowel syndrome.

Study	Population	Variables	Intervention	Results
Robinson et al. (2006) A randomised controlled trial of self-help interventions in patients with a primary care diagnosis of irritable bowel syndrome. *Gut.* (30)	420 (89% female)	Symptom severity Frequency of doctor's appointments	Self-help manual *vs.* self-help manual + 1x/week self-help group *vs.* control group (outpatient care)	No difference between self-help groups; reduction of doctor's appointments (60% less) and health costs (40%) compared to control group; improvement of symptoms compared to beginning.

the psychiatric comorbidity was reduced over time (31) (**Table 2**).

A meta-analysis examined the effect of self-help and self-management methods. There was a medium effect size (d=0.72) for the reduction of symptom severity and a large effect size (d=0.84) for the improvement of quality of life (32). Online interventions were especially suited to reduce somatic complaints and improve quality of life (32). However, it is to note that several studies do not have adequate control groups, the study population is often very small and blinding often not possible.

Cognitive Behavioral Therapy

Most of the psychological interventions in the treatment of IBS are based on CBT aiming at the reduction of irrational fears and the modulation of behavioral patterns. The NNT with CBT was 4 (95% CI 3–9) (32). However, although CBT shows good results, it is not always available and labor-intensive. Therefore, the application also depends on the patient's intention, the expertise of the professional and the resources available (26).

A meta-analysis from 2019 studied nine randomized controlled trials (RCTs) compared to control groups with 610 patients in total. In 145 of 349 (41.5%) patients undergoing CBT the symptoms did not improve, compared to 166 of 261 (63.6%) patients in the control groups (19) indicating a beneficial effect of CBT.

A trial showed a 50% reduction of gastrointestinal symptoms, anxiety, and depression in the CBT group compared to symptom scores assessed at baseline (33). Another study investigated a combination of progressive muscle relaxation, cognitive behavioral strategies, and problem-solving approaches in comparison to a standardized medical treatment with drugs and regular appointments with a gastroenterologist. The group with the extended psychological treatment showed a decrease of bowel symptoms and an increase of well-being, quality of life and control of disease after 3 and 6 months compared to the control group whose symptoms remained unchanged (34). This study showed that the combination of drug therapy and psychological interventions is superior to medical treatment alone.

A more recent RCT used an online program based on CBT. A total of 86 patients were included and randomized to the control (an online discussion forum) or treatment group. The main measures were IBS symptom severity, quality of life, anxiety, depression, and general functioning. Patients in the treatment group reported a 42% decrease in IBS symptoms in comparison to the control group that reported a 12% increase in IBS symptoms (35). The follow-up after 15 and 18 months also showed that the group with the psychological intervention benefited with regards to symptoms, quality of life and anxiety (d=0.78–1.11) (36). Similarly, an internet-based treatment with CBT exerted positive effect in adolescents with IBS. A controlled study showed after an intervention of 10 weeks a decrease of gastrointestinal symptoms (d=0.45, NNT 4) and an improvement in quality of life (d=0.40) in the group with online psychotherapy in comparison to the control group (37). The symptoms of anxiety and depression also decreased in the course of the intervention but there was no significant difference between the therapy group and the control group (37). The follow-up after 6 months showed that the effects remained constant. Fear-characteristics, quality of life and frequency of pain further decreased during the follow-up (37).

A large study in 436 IBS patients allocated to either standard CBT (10 weekly sessions, 60 min/session with information on brain-gut interaction, self-monitoring symptoms, muscle-relaxation), four sessions of primarily home-based CBT with minimal therapist contact (MC-CBT), or four sessions of IBS education (EDU). After 12 weeks, a higher proportion of patients with MC-CBT reported an improvement in gastrointestinal symptoms (61%) than patients with EDU (43%), while 55% patients in the CBT group showed an improvement (16). At 6 months after the end of treatment, a significant difference was observed between MC-CBT (58.4%) and EDU (44.8%) with regards to improvement of bowel symptoms. Both CBT methods (CBT and MC-CBT) showed significantly higher patient satisfaction than EDU (d for MC-CBT = 0.53). The results showed that MC-CBT is as efficacious as standard CBT (16). Therefore, CBT might be offered also on a telemedical basis with minimal therapist contact, probably in an (even more) cost effective manner. In line with this assumption, another study investigated telephone-delivered CBT (TCBT) and web-based CBT (WCBT) in comparison to treatment as usual (TAU). The study showed that both CBT methods led to an improvement in IBS severity and coping strategies compared to TAU (38). Both methods were cost-effective.

A recent trial from 2019 with 60 IBS patients with diarrhea-predominant IBS and 30 healthy controls studied the effect of CBT and exercise on the coping styles and cognitive bias of patients (**Table 3**). The patients were divided into two groups: experimental group (CBT + exercise) and control group (conventional drugs). After 6–24 weeks there was an improvement of neglect and pain behavior along with a difference in perfectionism, dependence and vulnerability (47). This study shows that CBT in combination with exercise can help to change the cognitive bias and coping styles of patients with diarrhea-predominant IBS. Lastly, a study using rectal barostat showed that although CBT did not alter visceral discomfort, urge, and pain during barostat testing, self-rated visceral sensitivity did improve after CBT (48).

Psychodynamic Psychotherapy

Psychodynamic psychotherapy focuses on intra- and interpersonal conflicts and how they contribute to the development and maintenance of symptoms. Psychodynamic psychotherapy leads to an improvement in IBS symptoms with a NNT of 4 (95% CI 2–20) (19). Therefore, also psychodynamic psychotherapy is recommended by the world gastroenterology organization (26).

A study from 1983 studied the impact of psychodynamic interventions on symptoms of IBS. A group received, additionally to a medical therapy, a psychodynamic intervention. Compared to the control group with medical therapy only, the intervention group showed a more pronounced improvement of symptoms after 3 months. The improvement was still observed after 1 year (49).

TABLE 3 | Randomized controlled studies investigating the effects of cognitive behavioral therapy in patients with irritable bowel syndrome.

Study	Population	Variables	Intervention	Results
Greene & Blanchard (1994) Cognitive therapy for irritable bowel syndrome. *J Consult Clin Psychol.* (39)	20 (75% female)	GI symptoms	2 weeks: 2x 1 h intervention/week, 6 weeks: 1x 1 h intervention/week *vs.* control group with symptom monitoring	Post treatment: 80% of CBT group and 10% of control group with significant improvement of GI symptoms.
Payne & Blanchard (1995) A controlled comparison of cognitive therapy and self-help support groups in the treatment of irritable bowel syndrome. *J Consult Clin Psychol.* (33)	22 (82% female)	Individual GI symptoms Composite index for GI symptoms	2 weeks: 2x 1 h intervention/week, 6 weeks: 1x1 h intervention/ week *vs.* symptom-monitoring waiting-list control	50% reduction of gastrointestinal symptoms, anxiety, and depression in the CBT-group compared to baseline symptom score.
Vollmer & Blanchard (1998) Controlled comparison of individual *versus* group cognitive therapy for irritable bowel syndrome. *Behav Ther.* (40)	34 (76% female)	Clinical symptoms	10 weeks: 1 h individual CBT session/ week or 10 weeks: 90 min group CBT session/week or monitoring (control group)	Post treatment: improvement of clinical symptoms: 64% in group CBT, 55% in individual CBT, 10% in control group.
Heymann-Mönnikes et al. (2000) The combination of medical treatment plus multicomponent behavioral therapy is superior to medical treatment alone in the therapy of irritable bowel syndrome. *Am J Gastroenterol.* (34)	21 (87.5% female)	IBS symptoms Well-being Quality of life	10 weeks: 1x1 h session multicomponent behavioral therapy/ week + medication *vs.* control group: medication only	Improvement in the behavioral therapy group (well-being, quality of life, symptoms; no change in the control group).
Boyce et al. (2003) A randomized controlled trial of cognitive behavior therapy, relaxation training, and routine clinical care for the irritable bowel syndrome. *Am J Gastroenterol.* (41)	105 (81% female)	General health Pain Physical functioning Anxiety Depression	8 weeks: 1x 1 h CBT/week *vs.* 8 weeks: 1x 30 min relaxation therapy/ week	Reduction in anxiety, depression, improvement of general health, pain and physical functioning, no difference between groups.
Drossman et al. (2003) Cognitive-behavioral therapy *versus* education and desipramine *versus* placebo for moderate to severe functional bowel disorders. *Gastroenterology.* (42)	169 (100% female)	Clinical, physiological, and psychosocial assessment	12 weeks: 1x 1 h CBT/week *vs.* control group (education)	CBT was more beneficial over Education for all parameters except for depressiveness.
Tkachuk et al. (2003) Randomized controlled trial of cognitive-behavioral group therapy for irritable bowel syndrome in a medical setting. *J Clin Psychol Med Settings.* (43)	28 (96% female)	Global symptoms	1 week: 2x 90 min group CBT intervention, 8 weeks: 1x 90 min group CBT intervention/week *vs.* home-based symptom monitoring	Better improvement in global symptoms, daily pain, psychological distress, and quality of life in CBT group.
Kennedy et al. (2003) Cognitive behaviour therapy in addition to antispasmodic treatment for irritable bowel syndrome in primary care: randomised controlled trial. *BMJ.* (29)	149 (n.s.)	Work and social adjustment scale Symptom severity	6 weeks: 1x 50 min CBT/week + mebeverine *vs.* control group (mebeverine only)	CBT showed better reduction of symptom severity, benefit on work, and social adjustment scale compared to control group; effects persisted after 6–12 months.
Lackner et al. (2008) Self-administered cognitive behavior therapy for moderate to severe irritable bowel syndrome: clinical efficacy, tolerability, feasibility. *Clin Gastroenterol Hepatol.* (44)	75 (87% female)	IBS symptom severity Quality of life Global symptoms	10 weeks: 1x 1 h CBT/week *vs.* 10 weeks: 1x 1 h CBT on four occasions *vs.* control group (waiting list)	Both CBT methods were superior to control group and induced adequate relief of global symptoms.
Ljótsson et al. (2010) Internet-delivered exposure and mindfulness based therapy for irritable bowel syndrome—a randomized controlled trial. *Behav Res Ther.* (35)	85 (85% female)	IBS symptom severity Quality of life Anxiety Depression General functioning	CBT *via* Internet *vs.* control group (online discussion forum)	CBT group: 42% decrease in IBS symptoms, control group: 12% increase in IBS symptoms.
Craske et al. (2011) A cognitive-behavioral treatment for irritable bowel syndrome using interoceptive exposure to visceral sensations. *Behav Res Ther.* (45)	110 (74% female)	Clinical symptoms	10 sessions of CBT or stress reduction training or attention control	CBT was superior to stress reduction training and attention control with regards to several domains; no difference between stress reduction training and attention control.
Bonnert et al. (2017) Internet-delivered cognitive behavior therapy for adolescents with irritable bowel syndrome: a randomized controlled trial. *Am J Gastroenterol.* (37)	101 (61% female)	Gastrointestinal symptoms Quality of life	10 weeks internet CBT *vs.* control group (wait list)	Greater improvement of gastrointestinal symptoms and quality of life in CBT compared to control group.

(Continued)

TABLE 3 | Continued

Study	Population	Variables	Intervention	Results
Lackner et al. (2018) Improvement in gastrointestinal symptoms after cognitive behavior therapy for refractory irritable bowel syndrome. *Gastroenterology.* (46)	436 (80% female)	Gastrointestinal symptoms	Standard CBT: 10 weeks: 1x 60 min/week or minimal therapist contact CBT: four sessions or education (four sessions)	Minimal contact CBT was more effective than education and as effective as standard CBT.
Everitt et al. (2019) Therapist telephone-delivered CBT and web-based CBT compared with treatment as usual in refractory irritable bowel syndrome: the ACTIB three-arm RCT. *Health Technol Assess.* (38)	558 (76% female)	IBS severity score Work and social adjustment scale	Telephone-delivered CBT: 9 weeks: 6x 1 h sessions + 2 x 1 h at months 4+8 *vs.* web-delivered CBT: 9 weeks: 3x 30 min telephone sessions + 2x 30 min at months 4+8 *vs.* treatment as usual	CBT increased capacity to cope with symptoms and negative emotions; both CBT arms induced improvement in IBS severity score at 3, 6, 12 months compared to TAU.
Zhao et al. (2019) Effect of cognitive behavior therapy combined with exercise intervention on the cognitive bias and coping styles of diarrhea-predominant irritable bowel syndrome patients. *World J Clin Cases.* (47)	57 (75% female)	Cognitive bias Coping styles	CBT + exercise *vs.* control group (drug therapy)	Greater improvement of cognitive bias and coping styles in CBT + exercise compared to control group.

CBT, cognitive behavioral therapy; GI, gastrointestinal; IBS, irritable bowel syndrome; n.s., not specified; TAU, treatment as usual; RCT, randomized controlled trial.

An RCT showed that a psychodynamic intervention is related to a reduction of interpersonal conflicts (**Table 4**). The reduction of interpersonal conflicts was a predictor for an improvement of health status in comparison to medical therapy (52). Nonetheless, also the control group with antidepressant medication showed a reduction of somatic symptoms.

Another study compared the effects of a psychodynamic intervention with a treatment with paroxetin (selective serotonin reuptake inhibitor, SSRI). There was no significant difference related to pain reduction after 3 months. After 1 year both interventions improved the somatic component of quality of life. Overall, psychodynamic psychotherapy is a cost-effective alternative for a drug therapy of IBS (51).

Hypnotherapy

Hypnotherapy is a method to focus on the perception of intestinal symptoms. The therapist is trying to impart bowel

control to the patient and to achieve a change of the individual reaction on somatic symptoms (53). It was shown that the NNT with hypnotherapy is 5 (95% CI 3.5–10) (19). The world gastroenterology organization recommends hypnotherapy for patients with IBS refractory to drug treatment. However, although it shows more safety and tolerability compared to drug therapy, it may be labor-intensive and not always available (26).

A study from 1984 investigated the effect of hypnotherapy in patients with hard-to-treat IBS in comparison to supportive psychotherapy. The group with hypnotherapy showed a significant improvement of pain, flatulencies, changes in bowel habit, and general well-being. The follow-up after 3 months showed a persistence of the improvement (54). Another study showed that both hypnotherapy one-to-one sessions and group sessions induced a subjective relief associated with an improvement in quality of life, somatic and psychological symptoms (**Table 5**). The improvement continued for 12

TABLE 4 | Randomized controlled studies investigating the effects of psychodynamic psychotherapy in patients with irritable bowel syndrome.

Study	Population	Variables	Intervention	Results
Svedlund et al. (1983) Controlled study of psychotherapy in irritable bowel syndrome. *Lancet.* (49)	101 (69% female)	Somatic symptoms	3 months: 10x 1 h session psychodynamic psychotherapy + medical treatment *vs.* control group (medical treatment)	Greater improvement of somatic symptoms in psychodynamic group; difference between both groups more pronounced after 1 year follow-up.
Guthrie et al. (1991) A controlled trial of psychological treatment for the irritable bowel syndrome. *Gastroenterology.* (50)	102 (74% female)	IBS symptoms	3 months: eight sessions psychodynamic therapy (plus relaxation plus medication) *vs.* control (medical treatment)	At 3 months greater improvement in diarrhea and abdominal pain in psychodynamic group compared to control.
Creed et al. (2003) The cost-effectiveness of psychotherapy and paroxetine for severe irritable bowel syndrome. *Gastroenterology* (51)	252 (80% female)	IBS symptoms Quality of life Health care costs	3 months: eight sessions of psychodynamic psychotherapy *vs.* paroxetine *vs.* control group (routine care)	Psychodynamic and paroxetine improved in global symptoms; during follow up psychotherapy was more cost efficient than paroxetine and control.
Hyphantis et al. (2009) Psychodynamic interpersonal therapy and improvement in interpersonal difficulties in people with severe irritable bowel syndrome. *Pain.* (52)	247 (80% female)	Interpersonal problems Abdominal pain Bowel symptoms Psychological distress Health status	Psychodynamic psychotherapy *vs.* antidepressant *vs.* control group (routine care)	Psychodynamic therapy induced a reduction of interpersonal conflicts; medical treatment improved somatic symptoms.

IBS, irritable bowel syndrome.

TABLE 5 | Randomized controlled studies investigating the effects of hypnotherapy in patients with irritable bowel syndrome.

Study	Population	Variables	Intervention	Results
Whorwell et al. (1984) Controlled trial of hypnotherapy in the treatment of severe refractory irritable-bowel syndrome. *Lancet.* (55)	30 (87% female)	Gastrointestinal symptoms General well-being	Hypnotherapy *vs.* control (supportive psychotherapy)	Hypnotherapy group: significant improvement of gastrointestinal symptoms, no change in control group; benefit persisted after 3 months follow-up.
Galovski & Blanchard (1998) The treatment of irritable bowel syndrome with hypnotherapy. *Appl Psychophysiol Biofeedback.* (56)	12 (83% female)	IBS symptoms Anxiety	6 weeks: 1x 30 min to 1 h gut directed hypnotherapy/week *vs.* control group: symptom watching waiting list	Greater improvement of gastrointestinal symptoms in hypnotherapy group, decrease of anxiety.
Simrén et al. (2004) Treatment with hypnotherapy reduces the sensory and motor component of the gastrocolonic response in irritable bowel syndrome. *Psychosom Med.* (57)	26 (68% female)	IBS symptoms Barostat measurements	12 weeks: 1x 1 h session gut-directed hypnotherapy/week *vs.* control (supportive therapy)	More frequent improvement in global symptoms in hypnotherapy *vs.* control group; hypnotherapy reduced the sensory and motor component gastrocolonic response.
Lindfors et al. (2012) Effects of gut-directed hypnotherapy on IBS in different clinical settings—results from two randomized, controlled trials. *Am J Gastroenterol.* (58)	Study 1: 90 (79% female) Study 2: 48 (81% female)	IBS symptoms	Study 1: 12 weeks: 1x 1 h hypnotherapy/week + audiotapes for exercising at home *vs.* supportive therapy Study 2: hypnotherapy sessions in hospital *vs.* waiting list controls	Improvement of IBS symptoms in 3 months in both studies; greater improvement in hypnotherapy groups.
Moser G et al. (2013) Long-term success of gut-directed group hypnosis for patients with refractory irritable bowel syndrome: a randomized controlled trial. *Am J Gastroenterol.* (59)	90 (79% female)	Quality of life Psychological status IBS symptoms	12 weeks: 10x 45 min gut-directed hypnotherapy sessions + exercise at home + medical treatment *vs.* control group (medical treatment)	Gut-directed hypnotherapy was superior to medication therapy and showed a long-term effect.
Rutten et al. (2017) Home-based hypnotherapy self-exercises *vs.* individual hypnotherapy with a therapist for treatment of pediatric irritable bowel syndrome, functional abdominal pain, or functional abdominal pain syndrome: a randomized clinical trial. *JAMA Pediatr.* (60)	260 (72% female)	Pain frequency Intensity score	Cd group: 3 months hypnotherapy with 3 exercises/week *vs.* therapist group: 3 months hypnotherapy with six sessions	Cd hypnotherapy is not inferior to therapist hypnotherapy.
Flik et al. (2019) Efficacy of individual and group hypnotherapy in irritable bowel syndrome (IMAGINE): a multicentre randomised controlled trial. *Lancet Gastroenterol Hepatol.* (61)	354 (76% female)	Quality of life IBS symptoms	Individual hypnotherapy *vs.* group hypnotherapy *vs.* control group (education)	Improvement in life quality, somatic and psychological symptoms by hypnotherapy; no difference between individual or group therapies.

Cd, compact disc; IBS, irritable bowel syndrome.

months and there was no difference between the different types of sessions (61).

In a study from 2003, 23 patients with IBS and rectal hyper-/hypo- or normal sensitivity were treated with hypnotherapy for 12 weeks and the sensory perception was compared with a healthy control group. The study showed that hypnotherapy can improve abnormal sensory perception in patients with IBS (62). Another study from 2004 investigated the gastrocolonic response of patients with IBS undergoing hypnotherapy and showed a reduction of the sensory and motor component of the gastrocolonic response (57). Hypnotherapy has also an effect on the processing and perception of visceral stimuli in patients with IBS. A study using fMRI suggested that hypnotherapy is able to normalize altered perception (63).

Lastly, a study showed that children with IBS benefit from a Cd-based therapy to the same extent as from therapeutic one-to-one sessions (60). Therefore, also hypnotherapy can be applied in a highly cost-efficient manner.

Mindfulness-Based Therapy

Mindfulness-based therapy combines stress reduction and elements from CBT. The patients learn to perceive the complaints and to better cope with them (64). Due to the small number of studies investigating mindfulness-based therapies, no NNT has been calculated yet.

A prospective study investigated the effects from a stress reduction program on parameters like bowel complaints, quality of life, and gastrointestinal symptom-specific anxiety in patients with IBS. No effect was seen after 2 months, but after 6 months there was an improvement in quality of life and a reduction of symptom-specific anxiety. However, bowel-associated complaints did not change significantly (65). A randomized, controlled trial with 75 female IBS patients showed a reduction of gastrointestinal symptoms after 8 weeks of mindfulness-based therapy in comparison to the control group with social support only. The follow-up after 3 months showed that the reduction persisted associated with an improvement in quality of life and reduction of stress (64). Other studies with female IBS patients reported a significant improvement of symptom severity and quality of life after 8 weeks of mindfulness-based therapy compared to a control group. Mindfulness-based therapy reduced visceral sensitivity, mental stress, or over-evaluation of stress. Moreover, patients with IBS undergoing mindfulness training showed a nonreactivity to gut-focused anxiety and

TABLE 6 | Randomized controlled studies investigating the effects of mindfulness-based therapy in patients with irritable bowel syndrome.

Study	Population	Measured variable	Intervention	Results
Gaylord et al. (2011) Mindfulness training reduces the severity of irritable bowel syndrome in women: results of a randomized controlled trial. *Am J Gastroenterol.* (64)	75 (100% female)	Quality of life Visceral sensitivity index Treatment credibility scale	8 weeks: 1x 2 h mindfulness training/ week *vs.* support group	Greater reductions in IBS symptom severity after treatment and at 3 months follow up in mindfulness compared to support group.
Garland et al. (2012) Therapeutic mechanisms of a mindfulness-based treatment for IBS: effects on visceral sensitivity, catastrophizing, and affective processing of pain sensations. *J Behav Med.* (66)	75 (100% female)	IBS severity Quality of life	8 weeks: mindfulness training *vs.* social support	Mindfulness training promoted nonreactivity to IBS-associated anxiety and catastrophic appraisals.
Zernicke et al. (2013) Mindfulness-based stress reduction for the treatment of irritable bowel syndrome symptoms: a randomized wait-list controlled trial. *Int J Behav Med.* (67)	90 (90% female)	IBS symptom severity Quality of life Stress Mood	8 weeks: 1x 90 min/week mindfulness-based stress reduction *vs.* control group (waiting list)	Greater decrease in symptom severity in mindfulness group; benefit for overall symptoms persisted at 6 months follow-up.

IBS, irritable bowel syndrome.

catastrophic appraisals compared to a social support control group (66).

Lastly, in a study population of 90% women and 10% men a mindfulness-based therapy was applied for 8 weeks (**Table 6**). The bowel complaints showed a significant reduction in comparison to control patients on the waiting list. The level of stress was reduced, but there was no significant difference in quality of life and mood between the two groups. The outcome after 6 months showed no difference between both groups due to a rebound of complaints (67). Therefore, mindfulness-based therapy might have to be supplemented by other treatments in order to exert a more sustained effect.

Relaxation Therapy

Relaxation therapies like progressive muscle relaxation or autogenic training aim to reduce perceived stress since stress can lead to a physiological arousal further increasing the somatic complaints and negatively influencing the communication between gut and brain (68). These therapies were shown to have a NNT of 6, however, with a broad range (95% CI 3–60) (19). This broad range likely also contributed to the assessment that relaxation therapy (alone) is not more effective than usual care in the relief of global IBS symptoms (26).

A randomized controlled trial showed the effect of a stress management program in comparison to peppermint oil. These patients learned different relaxation methods and 2/3 of them were able to reduce their pain attacks as well as their complaints. The reduction persisted up to 1 year follow-up (69). A comparison between medical therapy and progressive muscle relaxation showed that the relaxation method could reduce anxiety more effectively; however, there was no significant difference in reducing the somatic symptoms (70). A program of progressive muscle relaxation for 2 months at home led to an improvement of gastrointestinal symptoms compared to symptom control only. However, the study size was very small with 16 patients only (71).

A more recent trial studied the effects of relaxation methods (progressive muscle relaxation, breathing techniques) and training of emotional awareness and expression compared to

waiting list patients. At the beginning the patients frequently showed a low emotional reaction to stress events and relationship conflicts. This can lead to avoidance behavior and chronic arousal. The emotional awareness and expression training reduced IBS symptom severity after 2 and 10 weeks compared to the control group. There was an improvement of quality of life in the emotional training group as well as in the group with relaxation methods. After 10 weeks the positive effects persisted; however, only in the relaxation group there was a significantly lower level of depressive and anxious symptoms (72).

A trial on young patients studied the effect of yoga exercises on IBS symptoms. The patients exercised yoga at home for 4 weeks. In comparison to patients on a waiting list, there was a reduced functional limitation, a lower avoidance behavior, and less anxiety symptoms (**Table 7**). However, there was no effect on depressive symptoms and on somatic symptoms (60). A recent trial compared the effect of yoga with the effect of a low-FODMAP diet. After 12 weeks yoga exercise at home and nutritional counselling in the control group, there was a significant reduction of the severity of gastrointestinal symptoms in both groups which persisted in the following year. It is to note that yoga also reduced anxiety symptoms (61).

SUMMARY

IBS patients often report a great burden of disease associated with a significant impairment in quality of life. Psychotherapy is an important treatment column for patients with IBS with different procedures available, all of which are well to very well evidence-based by now. Consequently, the world gastroenterology organization states that CBT, hypnotherapy, and psychodynamic therapy are more effective in improving global symptoms than usual care (26).

It is to note that the current review also has limitations. First of all, only few studies were at low risk of bias which should be taken into account when interpreting the data. Moreover, some psychotherapeutic techniques were tested in few randomized

TABLE 7 | Randomized controlled studies investigating the effects of relaxation therapy in patients with irritable bowel syndrome.

Study	Population	Measured variable	Intervention	Results
Bennett & Wilkinson (1985) A comparison of psychological and medical treatment of the irritable bowel syndrome. *Br J Clin Psychol.* (70)	33 (70% female)	IBS symptoms Anxiety	Progressive muscle relaxation *vs.* medical treatment	Reduction of initial high anxiety levels in relaxation group only; IBS symptoms were reduced in both groups.
Lynch & Zamble (1989) A controlled behavioral treatment study of irritable bowel syndrome. *Behav Ther.* (73)	21 (67% female)	IBS symptoms Mood Self perception	8 weeks: 1x 2 h relaxation therapy /week and audio material for practicing twice at home *vs.* control group (waiting period)	Improvement of measured variables after treatment; benefit persisted for 5 months.
Shaw et al. (1991) Stress management for irritable bowel syndrome: a controlled trial. *Digestion.* (69)	35 (57% female)	IBS symptoms	6x 40 min sessions stress management program *vs.* control group (conventional therapy including antispasmodic)	2/3 of patients attending the stress program showed relief in symptoms and fewer attacks of less severity; benefit maintained for 12 months.
Blanchard et al. (1993) Relaxation training as a treatment for irritable bowel syndrome. *Biofeedback Self Regul.* (71)	23 (78% female)	Gastrointestinal symptoms	2 weeks: two sessions progressive muscle relaxation/ week, 6 weeks: one session progressive muscle relaxation/ week with regular home training *vs.* control group (monitoring)	Relaxation showed greater improvement in gastrointestinal symptoms than the symptom monitoring group.
Keefer & Blanchard (2001) The effects of relaxation response meditation on the symptoms of irritable bowel syndrome: results of a controlled treatment study. *Behav Res Ther.* (74)	13 (69% female)	IBS symptoms	6 weeks: 1x 30 min relaxation response meditation/week *vs.* control group (waiting list)	Meditation was superior to control.
Kuttner et al. (2006) A randomized trial of yoga for adolescents with irritable bowel syndrome. *Pain Res Manag.* (75)	28 (71% female)	Gastrointestinal symptoms Pain Functional disability Anxiety Depression	Yoga intervention: 1 h instruction, daily home practice over 4 weeks *vs.* control group (wait list)	Yoga group showed lower levels of functional disability, lower avoidance behavior and less anxiety symptoms compared to control.
van der Veek et al. (2007) Clinical trial: short- and long-term benefit of relaxation training for irritable bowel syndrome. *Aliment Pharmacol Ther.* (76)	98 (73% female)	IBS symptom severity Quality of life Frequency of doctor visits	4x 90 min sessions of relaxation therapy in small groups *vs.* control group (standard medical care)	Improvement in the measured variables by relaxation therapy compared to control; number needed to treat for long-term improvement was 5.
Shinozaki et al. (2010) Effect of autogenic training on general improvement in patients with irritable bowel syndrome: a randomized controlled trial. *Appl Psychophysiol Biofeedback.* (77)	21 (52% female)	IBS symptoms Anxiety Depression	8 weeks: 1x 30–40 min session autogenic training/week *vs.* control group (discussions)	Improvement of social functioning and bodily pain by autogenic training.
Boltin et al. (2015) Gut-directed guided affective imagery as an adjunct to dietary modification in irritable bowel syndrome. *J Health Psychol.* (78)	34 (76% female)	Symptom severity Quality of life	8 weeks: 1x 3 h session psychotherapy + guided affective imagery *vs.* control (no psychotherapy)	Reduction of symptom severity and improvement of quality of life by affective imagination.
Thakur et al. (2017) Emotional awareness and expression training improves irritable bowel syndrome: a randomized controlled trial. *Neurogastroenterol Motil,* (72)	106 (80% female)	Symptom severity Quality of life	2 weeks: 3x 50 min sessions relaxation therapy or emotional awareness/expression training or control (wait list)	Relaxation training reduced depressive symptoms; emotional awareness/ expression training reduced IBS symptom severity and improved quality of life after 10 weeks follow-up while it did not reduce somatic symptoms.
Schumann et al. (2018) Randomised clinical trial: yoga *vs.* 6low-FODMAP diet in patients with irritable bowel syndrome. *Aliment Pharmacol Ther.* (79)	59 (n.s.)	Gastrointestinal symptoms Quality of life	12 weeks: two sessions/week yoga + exercise at home *vs.* control group (FODMAP)	Reduction of gastrointestinal symptoms in both groups; yoga reduced anxiety symptoms.

FODMAP, fermentable, oligo-, di-, monosaccharides and polyols; IBS, irritable bowel syndrome; n.s., not specified.

studies so far; therefore, conclusions should be drawn with caution. Lastly, IBS is a heterogeneous disease which should be considered when performing a study and also when extrapolating the results to "real life" patients, especially those presenting to tertiary care centers which very often report (psychiatric) comorbidities.

Future perspectives of psychotherapy in IBS have also been investigated in few studies. A recent study showed that tele-hypnotherapy also leads to a reduction of pain, anxiety, and IBS severity in patients with IBS (80). Moreover, CBT offered *via* computer or telephone was superior to treatment as usual (38). Future studies should further explore these media as well as options for e-health interventions.

Taken together, it seems to be important to offer a multicomponent therapeutic strategy including psychoeducation, other psychotherapeutic interventions in addition to basal/drug therapy. These multicomponent approaches should be further investigated in controlled trials.

AUTHOR CONTRIBUTIONS

LH performed the literature search and wrote the first draft of the paper, AS planned and supervised the project as well as thoroughly revised the paper.

ACKNOWLEDGMENTS

We further acknowledge support from the German Research Foundation (DFG) and the Open Access Publication Fund of the Tübingen University.

REFERENCES

1. Holtmann GJ, Ford AC, Talley NJ. Pathophysiology of irritable bowel syndrome. *Lancet Gastroenterol Hepatol* (2016) 1(2):133–46. doi: 10.1016/S2468-1253(16)30023-1

2. Mearin F, Lacy BE, Chang L, Chey WD, Lembo AJ, Simren M, et al. Bowel disorders. *Gastroenterology* (2016) 150:1393–1407. doi: 10.1053/j.gastro.2016.02.031

3. Enck P, Aziz Q, Barbara G, Farmer AD, Fukudo S, Mayer EA, et al. Irritable bowel syndrome. *Nat Rev Dis Primers* (2016) 2:16014. doi: 10.1038/nrdp.2016.14

4. Thompson WG. The treatment of irritable bowel syndrome. *Aliment Pharmacol Ther* (2002) 16(8):1395–406. doi: 10.1046/j.1365-2036.2002.01312.x

5. Creed F, Ratcliffe J, Fernandes L, Palmer S, Rigby C, Tomenson B, et al. Outcome in severe irritable bowel syndrome with and without accompanying depressive, panic and neurasthenic disorders. *Br J Psychiatry* (2005) 186:507–15. doi: 10.1192/bjp.186.6.507

6. Lackner JM, Gudleski GD, Ma CX, Dewanwala A, Naliboff B. Fear of GI symptoms has an important impact on quality of life in patients with moderate-to-severe IBS. *Am J Gastroenterol* (2014) 109(11):1815–23. doi: 10.1038/ajg.2014.241

7. Tanaka Y, Kanazawa M, Fukudo S, Drossman DA. Biopsychosocial model of irritable bowel syndrome. *J Neurogastroenterol Motil* (2011) 17(2):131–9. doi: 10.5056/jnm.2011.17.2.131

8. Van Oudenhove L, Crowell MD, Drossman DA, Halpert AD, Keefer L, Lackner JM, et al. Biopsychosocial aspects of functional gastrointestinal disorders. *Gastroenterology* (2016) 150:1355–1367. doi: 10.1053/j.gastro.2016.02.027

9. Drossman DA. Abuse, trauma, and GI illness: is there a link? *Am J Gastroenterol* (2011) 106(1):14–25. doi: 10.1038/ajg.2010.453

10. Mayer EA, Savidge T, Shulman RJ. Brain-gut microbiome interactions and functional bowel disorders. *Gastroenterology* (2014) 146(6):1500–12. doi: 10.1053/j.gastro.2014.02.037

11. Soares RL. Irritable bowel syndrome: a clinical review. *World J Gastroenterol* (2014) 20(34):12144–60. doi: 10.1053/j.gastro.2014.02.037

12. Pigrau M, Rodino-Janeiro BK, Casado-Bedmar M, Lobo B, Vicario M, Santos J, et al. The joint power of sex and stress to modulate brain-gut-microbiota axis and intestinal barrier homeostasis: implications for irritable bowel syndrome. *Neurogastroenterol Motil* (2016) 28(4):463–86. doi: 10.1111/nmo.12717

13. Ghoshal UC, Ghoshal U. Small intestinal bacterial overgrowth and other intestinal disorders. *Gastroenterol Clin North Am* (2017) 46(1):103–20. doi: 10.1016/j.gtc.2016.09.008

14. Drossman DA, Hasler WL. Rome IV-Functional GI disorders: Disorders of gut-brain interaction. *Gastroenterology* (2016) 150(6):1257–61. doi: 10.1053/j.gastro.2016.03.035

15. Drossman DA, Chang L, Schneck S, Blackman C, Norton WF, Norton NJ. A focus group assessment of patient perspectives on irritable bowel syndrome and illness severity. *Dig Dis Sci* (2009) 54(7):1532–41. doi: 10.1007/s10620-009-0792-6

16. Lackner JM, Jaccard J, Keefer L, Brenner DM, Firth RS, Gudleski GD, et al. Improvement in gastrointestinal symptoms after cognitive behavior therapy for refractory irritable bowel syndrome. *Gastroenterology* (2018) 155(1):47–57. doi: 10.1053/j.gastro.2018.03.063

17. Dalrymple J, Bullock I. Diagnosis and management of irritable bowel syndrome in adults in primary care: summary of NICE guidance. *BMJ* (2008) 336(7643):556–8. doi: 10.1136/bmj.39484.712616.AD

18. Lackner JM, Mesmer C, Morley S, Dowzer C, Hamilton S. Psychological treatments for irritable bowel syndrome: a systematic review and meta-analysis. *J Consult Clin Psychol* (2004) 72(6):1100–13. doi: 10.1037/0022-006X.72.6.1100

19. Ford AC, Lacy BE, Harris LA, Quigley EMM, Moayyedi P. Effect of antidepressants and psychological therapies in irritable bowel syndrome: an updated systematic review and meta-analysis. *Am J Gastroenterol* (2019) 114(1):21–39. doi: 10.1038/s41395-018-0222-5

20. Zijdenbos IL, de Wit NJ, van der Heijden GJ, Rubin G, Quartero AO. Psychological treatments for the management of irritable bowel syndrome. *Cochr Database Syst Rev* (2009), CD006442. doi: 10.1002/14651858.CD006442.pub2

21. Laird KT, Tanner-Smith EE, Russell AC, Hollon SD, Walker LS. Short-term and long-term efficacy of psychological therapies for irritable bowel syndrome: A systematic review and meta-analysis. *Clin Gastroenterol Hepatol* (2016) 14(7):937–47.e4. doi: 10.1016/j.cgh.2015.11.020

22. Laird KT, Tanner-Smith EE, Russell AC, Hollon SD, Walker LS. Comparative efficacy of psychological therapies for improving mental health and daily functioning in irritable bowel syndrome: A systematic review and meta-analysis. *Clin Psychol Rev* (2017) 51:142–52. doi: 10.1016/j.cpr.2016.11.001

23. Drossman DA. 2012 David Sun lecture: helping your patient by helping yourself—how to improve the patient-physician relationship by optimizing communication skills. *Am J Gastroenterol* (2013) 108(4):521–8. doi: 10.1038/ajg.2013.56

24. Di Palma JA, Herrera JL. The role of effective clinician-patient communication in the management of irritable bowel syndrome and chronic constipation. *J Clin Gastroenterol* (2012) 46(9):748–51. doi: 10.1097/MCG.0b013e31825a2ff2

25. Longstreth GF, Drossman DA. Severe irritable bowel and functional abdominal pain syndromes: managing the patient and health care costs.

Clin Gastroenterol Hepatol (2005) 3(4):397–400. doi: 10.1016/S1542-3565(05)00084-4

26. Quigley EMM, Fried M, Gwee K-A, Khalif I, Hungin APS, Lindberg G, et al. World Gastroenterology Organisation global guidelines irritable bowel syndrome: a global perspective update September 2015. *J Clin Gastroenterol* (2016) 50(9):704–13. doi: 10.1097/MCG.0000000000000653

27. Labus J, Gupta A, Gill HK, Posserud I, Mayer M, Raeen H, et al. Randomised clinical trial: symptoms of the irritable bowel syndrome are improved by a psycho-education group intervention. *Aliment Pharmacol Ther* (2013) 37(3):304–15. doi: 10.1111/apt.12171

28. Ringström G, Störsrud S, Posserud I, Lundqvist S, Westman B, Simrén M. Structured patient education is superior to written information in the management of patients with irritable bowel syndrome: a randomized controlled study. *Eur J Gastroenterol Hepatol* (2010) 22(4):420–8. doi: 10.1097/MEG.0b013e3283333b61

29. Kennedy A, Robinson A, Rogers A. Incorporating patients' views and experiences of life with IBS in the development of an evidence based self-help guidebook. *Patient Educ Couns* (2003) 50(3):303–10. doi: 10.1016/S0738-3991(03)00054-5

30. Robinson A, Lee V, Kennedy A, Middleton L, Rogers A, Thompson DG, et al. A randomised controlled trial of self-help interventions in patients with a primary care diagnosis of irritable bowel syndrome. *Gut* (2006) 55(5):643–8. doi: 10.1136/gut.2004.062901

31. Schneider A, Rosenberger S, Bobardt J, Bungartz-Catak J, Atmann O, Haller B, et al. Self-help guidebook improved quality of life for patients with irritable bowel syndrome. *PloS One* (2017) 12(7):e0181764. doi: 10.1371/journal.pone.0181764

32. Liegl G, Plessen CY, Leitner A, Boeckle M, Pieh C. Guided self-help interventions for irritable bowel syndrome: a systematic review and meta-analysis. *Eur J Gastroenterol Hepatol* (2015) 27(10):1209–21. doi: 10.1097/MEG.0000000000000428

33. Payne A, Blanchard EB. A controlled comparison of cognitive therapy and self-help support groups in the treatment of irritable bowel syndrome. *J Consult Clin Psychol* (1995) 63(5):779–86. doi: 10.1037/0022-006X.63.5.779

34. Heymann-Mönnikes I, Arnold R, Florin I, Herda C, Melfsen S, Mönnikes H. The combination of medical treatment plus multicomponent behavioral therapy is superior to medical treatment alone in the therapy of irritable bowel syndrome. *Am J Gastroenterol* (2000) 95(4):981–94. doi: 10.1111/j.1572-0241.2000.01937.x

35. Ljótsson B, Falk L, Vesterlund AW, Hedman E, Lindfors P, Rück C, et al. Internet-delivered exposure and mindfulness based therapy for irritable bowel syndrome–a randomized controlled trial. *Behav Res Ther* (2010) 48(6):531–9. doi: 10.1016/j.brat.2010.03.003

36. Ljótsson B, Hedman E, Lindfors P, Hursti T, Lindefors N, Andersson G, et al. Long-term follow-up of internet-delivered exposure and mindfulness based treatment for irritable bowel syndrome. *Behav Res Ther* (2011) 49(1):58–61. doi: 10.1016/j.brat.2010.10.006

37. Bonnert M, Olén O, Lalouni M, Benninga MA, Bottai M, Engelbrektsson J, et al. Internet-delivered cognitive behavior therapy for adolescents with irritable bowel syndrome: a randomized controlled trial. *Am J Gastroenterol* (2017) 112(1):152–62. doi: 10.1038/ajg.2016.503

38. Everitt H, Landau S, Little P, Bishop FL, O'Reilly G, Sibelli A, et al. Therapist telephone-delivered CBT and web-based CBT compared with treatment as usual in refractory irritable bowel syndrome: the ACTIB three-arm RCT. *Health Technol Assess* (2019) 23(17):1–154. doi: 10.3310/hta23170

39. Greene B, Blanchard EB. Cognitive therapy for irritable bowel syndrome. *J Consult Clin Psychol* (1994) 62(3):576–82.

40. Vollmer A, Blanchard EB. Controlled comparison of individual versus group cognitive therapy for irritable bowel syndrome. *Behav Ther* (1998) 29(1):19–33.

41. Boyce PM, Talley NJ, Balaam B, Koloski NA, Truman G. A randomized controlled trial of cognitive behavior therapy, relaxation training, and routine clinical care for the irritable bowel syndrome. *Am J Gastroenterol* (2003) 98(10):2209–18.

42. Drossman DA, Toner BB, Whitehead WE, Diamant NE, Dalton CB, Duncan S, et al. Cognitive-behavioral therapy versus education and desipramine versus placebo for moderate to severe functional bowel disorders. *Gastroenterology* (2003) 125(1):19_31.

43. Tkachuk GA, Graff LA, Martin GL, Bernstein CN. Randomized controlled trial of cognitive behavioral group therapy for irritable bowel syndrome in a medical setting. *J Clin Psychol Med Settings* (2003) 10:57–69.

44. Lackner JM, Jaccard J, Krasner SS, Katz LA, Gudleski GD. Self-administered cognitive behavior therapy for moderate to severe irritable bowel syndrome: clinical efficacy, tolerability, feasibility. *Clin Gastroenterol Hepatol* (2008) 6(8):899–906. doi: 10.1016/j.cgh.2008.03.004

45. Craske MG, Wolitzky-Taylor KB, Labus J, Wu S, Frese M, Mayer EA, et al. A cognitive-behavioral treatment for irritable bowel syndrome using interoceptive exposure to visceral sensations. *Behav Res Ther* (2011) 49(6-7):413–21. doi: 10.1016/j.brat.2011.04.001

46. Lackner JM, Jaccard J, Keefer L, Brenner DM, Firth RS, Gudleski GD, et al. Improvement in gastrointestinal symptoms after cognitive behavior therapy for refractory irritable bowel syndrome. *Gastroenterology* (2018) 155(1):47–57. doi: 10.1053/j.gastro.2018.03.063

47. Zhao S-R, Ni X-M, Zhang X-A, Tian H. Effect of cognitive behavior therapy combined with exercise intervention on the cognitive bias and coping styles of diarrhea-predominant irritable bowel syndrome patients. *World J Clin Cases* (2019) 7(21):3446–62. doi: 10.12998/wjcc.v7.i21.3446

48. Edebol-Carlman H, Ljótsson B, Linton SJ, Boersma K, Schrooten M, Repsilber D, et al. Face-to-cace cognitive-behavioral therapy for irritable bowel syndrome: the effects on gastrointestinal and psychiatric symptoms. *Gastroenterol Res Pract* (2017) 2017:8915872. doi: 10.1155/2017/8915872

49. Svedlund J, Sjödin I, Ottosson JO, Dotevall G. Controlled study of psychotherapy in irritable bowel syndrome. *Lancet* (1983) 2(8350):589–92. doi: 10.1016/S0140-6736(83)90678-5

50. Guthrie E, Creed F, Dawson D, Tomenson B. A controlled trial of psychological treatment for the irritable bowel syndrome. *Gastroenterology* (1991) 100(2):450–7.

51. Creed F, Fernandes L, Guthrie E, Palmer S, Ratcliffe J, Read N, et al. The cost-effectiveness of psychotherapy and paroxetine for severe irritable bowel syndrome. *Gastroenterology* (2003) 124(2):303–17. doi: 10.1053/gast.2003.50055

52. Hyphantis T, Guthrie E, Tomenson B, Creed F. Psychodynamic interpersonal therapy and improvement in interpersonal difficulties in people with severe irritable bowel syndrome. *Pain* (2009) 145(1-2):196–203. doi: 10.1016/j.pain.2009.07.005

53. Gonsalkorale WM, Toner BB, Whorwell PJ. Cognitive change in patients undergoing hypnotherapy for irritable bowel syndrome. *J Psychosom Res* (2004) 56(3):271–8. doi: 10.1016/S0022-3999(03)00076-X

54. Whorwell PJ, Prior A, Faragher EB. Controlled trial of hypnotherapy in the treatment of severe refractory irritable-bowel syndrome. *Lancet* (1984) 2(8414):1232–4. doi: 10.1016/S0140-6736(84)92793-4

55. Whorwell PJ, Prior A, Faragher EB. Controlled trial of hypnotherapy in the treatment of severe refractory irritable-bowel syndrome. *Lancet* (1984) 2(8414):1232–4.

56. Galovski TE, Blanchard EB. The treatment of irritable bowel syndrome with hypnotherapy. *Appl Psychophysiol Biofeedback* (1998) 23(4):219–32.

57. Simrén M, Ringström G, Björnsson ES, Abrahamsson H. Treatment with hypnotherapy reduces the sensory and motor component of the gastrocolonic response in irritable bowel syndrome. *Psychosom Med* (2004) 66(2):233–8. doi: 10.1097/01.psy.0000116964.76529.6e

58. Lindfors P, Unge P, Arvidsson P, Nyhlin H, Björnsson E, Abrahamsson H, et al. Effects of gut-directed hypnotherapy on IBS in different clinical settings-results from two randomized, controlled trials. *Am J Gastroenterol* (2012) 107(2):276–85. doi: 10.1038/ajg.2011.340

59. Moser G, Trägner S, Gajowniczek EE, Mikulits A, Michalski M, Kazemi-Shirazi L, et al. Long-term success of gut-directed group hypnosis for patients with refractory irritable bowel syndrome: a randomized controlled trial. *Am J Gastroenterol* (2013) 108(4):602–9. doi: 10.1038/ajg.2013

60. Rutten JMTM, Vlieger AM, Frankenhuis C, George EK, Groeneweg M, Norbruis OF, et al. Home-based hypnotherapy self-exercises vs individual hypnotherapy with a therapist for treatment of pediatric irritable bowel syndrome, functional abdominal pain, or functional abdominal pain syndrome: a randomized clinical trial. *JAMA Pediatr* (2017) 171(5):470–7. doi: 10.1001/jamapediatrics.2017.0091

61. Flik CE, Laan W, Zuithoff NPA, van Rood YR, Smout AJPM, Weusten BLAM, et al. Efficacy of individual and group hypnotherapy in irritable bowel

syndrome (IMAGINE): a multicentre randomised controlled trial. *Lancet Gastroenterol Hepatol* (2019) 4(1):20–31. doi: 10.1016/S2468-1253(18)30310-8

62. Lea R, Houghton LA, Calvert EL, Larder S, Gonsalkorale WM, Whelan V, et al. Gut-focused hypnotherapy normalizes disordered rectal sensitivity in patients with irritable bowel syndrome. *Aliment Pharmacol Ther* (2003) 17 (5):635–42. doi: 10.1046/j.1365-2036.2003.01486.x

63. Lowén MBO, Mayer EA, Sjöberg M, Tillisch K, Naliboff B, Labus J, et al. Effect of hypnotherapy and educational intervention on brain response to visceral stimulus in the irritable bowel syndrome. *Aliment Pharmacol Ther* (2013) 37 (12):1184–97. doi: 10.1111/apt.12319

64. Gaylord SA, Palsson OS, Garland EL, Faurot KR, Coble RS, Mann JD, et al. Mindfulness training reduces the severity of irritable bowel syndrome in women: results of a randomized controlled trial. *Am J Gastroenterol* (2011) 106(9):1678–88. doi: 10.1038/ajg.2011.184

65. Kearney DJ, McDermott K, Martinez M, Simpson TL. Association of participation in a mindfulness programme with bowel symptoms, gastrointestinal symptom-specific anxiety and quality of life. *Aliment Pharmacol Ther* (2011) 34(3):363–73. doi: 10.1111/j.1365-2036.2011.04731.x

66. Garland EL, Gaylord SA, Palsson O, Faurot K, Douglas Mann J, Whitehead WE. Therapeutic mechanisms of a mindfulness-based treatment for IBS: effects on visceral sensitivity, catastrophizing, and affective processing of pain sensations. *J Behav Med* (2012) 35(6):591–602. doi: 10.1007/s10865-011-9391-z

67. Zernicke KA, Campbell TS, Blustein PK, Fung TS, Johnson JA, Bacon SL, et al. Mindfulness-based stress reduction for the treatment of irritable bowel syndrome symptoms: a randomized wait-list controlled trial. *Int J Behav Med* (2013) 20(3):385–96. doi: 10.1007/s12529-012-9241-6

68. Rokicki LA, Holroyd KA, France CR, Lipchik GL, France JL, Kvaal SA. Change mechanisms associated with combined relaxation/EMG biofeedback training for chronic tension headache. *Appl Psychophysiol Biofeedback* (1997) 22(1):21–41. doi: 10.1023/A:1026285608842

69. Shaw G, Srivastava ED, Sadlier M, Swann P, James JY, Rhodes J. Stress management for irritable bowel syndrome: a controlled trial. *Digestion* (1991) 50(1):36–42. doi: 10.1159/000200738

70. Bennett P, Wilkinson S. A comparison of psychological and medical treatment of the irritable bowel syndrome. *Br J Clin Psychol* (1985) 24(Pt 3):215–6. doi: 10.1111/j.2044-8260.1985.tb01340.x

71. Blanchard EB, Greene B, Scharff L, Schwarz-McMorris SP. Relaxation training as a treatment for irritable bowel syndrome. *Biofeedback Self Regul* (1993) 18 (3):125–32. doi: 10.1007/BF00999789

72. Thakur ER, Holmes HJ, Lockhart NA, Carty JN, Ziadni MS, Doherty HK, et al. Emotional awareness and expression training improves irritable bowel syndrome: A randomized controlled trial. *Neurogastroenterol Motil* (2017) 29 (12). doi: 10.1111/nmo.13143

73. Lynch PM, Zamble E. A controlled behavioral treatment study of irritable bowel syndrome. *Behav Ther* (1989) 20(4):509–23.

74. Keefer L, Blanchard EB. The effects of relaxation response meditation on the symptoms of irritable bowel syndrome: results of a controlled treatment study. *Behav Res Ther* (2001) 39(7):801–11.

75. Kuttner L, Chambers CT, Hardial J, Israel DM, Jacobson K, Evans K. A randomized trial of yoga for adolescents with irritable bowel syndrome. *Pain Res Manage* (2006) 11(4):217–23. doi: 10.1155/2006/731628

76. van der Veek PP, van Rood YR, Masclee AA. Clinical trial: short- and long-term benefit of relaxation training for irritable bowel syndrome. *Aliment Pharmacol Ther* (2007) 26(6):943–52.

77. Shinozaki M, Kanazawa M, Kano M, Endo Y, Nakaya N, Hongo M, et al. Effect of autogenic training on general improvement in patients with irritable bowel syndrome: a randomized controlled trial. *Appl Psychophysiol Biofeedback* (2010) 35(3):189–98. doi: 10.1007/s10484-009-9125-y

78. Boltin D, Sahar N, Gil E, Aizic S, Hod K, Levi-Drummer R, et al. Dickman R. Gut-directed guided affective imagery as an adjunct to dietary modification in irritable bowel syndrome. *J Health Psychol* (2015) 20(6):712–20.

79. Schumann D, Langhorst J, Dobos G, Cramer H. Randomised clinical trial: yoga vs a low-FODMAP diet in patients with irritable bowel syndrome. *Aliment Pharmacol Ther* (2018) 47(2):203–11. doi: 10.1111/apt.14400

80. Hasan SS, Pearson JS, Morris J, Whorwell PJ. Skype Hypnotherapy for irritable bowel syndrome: effectiveness and comparison with face-to-face treatment. *Int J Clin Exp Hypn* (2019) 67(1):69–80. doi: 10.1080/00207144.2019.1553766

6

Therapy of IBS: Is a Low FODMAP Diet the Answer?

Lauren P. Manning[1], C. K. Yao[2] and Jessica R. Biesiekierski[1]*

[1] Department of Rehabilitation, Nutrition and Sport, La Trobe University, Melbourne, VIC, Australia, [2] Department of Gastroenterology, Central Clinical School, Monash University & Alfred Health, Melbourne, VIC, Australia

*Correspondence:
Jessica R. Biesiekierski
j.biesiekierski@latrobe.edu.au

Irritable bowel syndrome (IBS) is the most prevalent functional gastrointestinal disorder with a worldwide prevalence of 11%. It is characterized by abdominal pain and altered bowel habits in the absence of underlying unique pathology. The condition is associated with poor quality of life and high use of healthcare resources required for management. The low FODMAP diet (LFD) is a recognized treatment for symptom management of IBS; however, approximately 30% of patients do not respond. The aim of this review was to understand the effectiveness and application of the LFD compared with other dietary and non-dietary interventions. Ten studies were included, eight of which assessed the LFD against other dietary interventions including traditional dietary advice, modified National Institute for Health and Care Excellence guidelines, a high FODMAP diet, gluten-free diet and Mediterranean diet, generalized dietary advice, probiotics, and a sham diet. Two studies compared a LFD to non-diet interventions of gut directed hypnotherapy or yoga. The findings clearly support the LFD as an effective treatment in IBS, and although it highlights the role for microbiota and current psychosocial state, it remains challenging to identify what combination of treatments may be best to ensure a personalized approach and overall higher response rates to IBS therapy.

Keywords: FODMAP, dietary therapy, symptom management, IBS (irritable bowel syndrome), gut-brain axis

INTRODUCTION

Irritable bowel syndrome (IBS) is a chronic functional gastrointestinal disorder with an estimated worldwide prevalence of 11.2% (1). The condition is characterised by recurrent abdominal pain and altered bowel habits as per the diagnostic Rome IV criteria (1). IBS is associated with decreased quality of life, social productivity, and work performance. Furthermore, IBS not only poses a financial burden to the individual through the cost of seeking medical advice but also impacts the healthcare system by time and resources acquired by patients (2). Nearly 40% of primary care and gastroenterologist visits can be attributed to IBS (3).

Diet, specifically the widely recognized low fermentable, oligosaccharide-, disaccharide-, monosaccharide-, and polyol (FODMAP) diet (LFD), has been a cornerstone therapy for IBS. The LFD involves three phases; a 'FODMAP restriction phase' lasting 4–8 weeks, a 're-introduction and challenge phase' lasting 6–10 weeks, and a 'personalization phase' where tolerated FODMAPs are returned to the diet (4). Several studies have shown the diet to be efficacious in the management of IBS symptoms (5, 6). However, data still suggest that approximately 30% of individuals do not respond to this management option (7). Furthermore, the safety of the LFD has been questioned in regard to its nutritional adequacy, decreased fiber intake, and potential negative impact on the gut microbiome (8).

The major mechanistic pathways *via* which FODMAPs induce symptoms in IBS are *via* osmotic load and colonic gas production in the setting of visceral hypersensitivity and have been reviewed in depth elsewhere (9). In addition, the gut-brain axis has emerged as an important mechanistic pathway directly modulable through various therapies. This axis is a bidirectional interconnection of the vagal and sacral parasympathetic and sympathetic efferent nerves interacting with the enteric nervous system. The higher brain center can receive signals from the enteric intrinsic, external vagal, and spinal afferents. Dysregulation of this pathway can be attributed to depression, anxiety, and psychological stress (10). Signals relayed between the gut and the brain suggest that IBS is responsive to cognitive and emotive triggers such as stress, anxiety, and depression. Given that psychosocial factors are seen in a high proportion of individuals with IBS, it could explain the refractory response to dietary management of IBS in some patients. Abnormalities in the central sensory processing in IBS patients has become the target for non-dietary related therapies. Psychological therapies (including cognitive therapy and gut-directed hypnotherapy) have shown promise in significantly improving IBS symptoms in adults suffering IBS (11).

Despite several treatment options showing good efficacy for IBS management, particularly in the case of the LFD, there is still much to understand about tailoring the right treatment (whether psychotherapy or diet should be employed as a first line therapy, or a combination of both) to the individual patient. Therefore, the aim of this review was to assess the effectiveness of the LFD compared with non-dietary treatments, in reducing symptoms and improving bowel function, as well as safety considerations such as nutritional adequacy and effects on the colonic microbiota. The findings will provide insight into strengths, limitations, and application of the LFD compared with other dietary and non-dietary interventions, thereby addressing gaps in the literature and future directions for the management of IBS.

METHODS

A literature search was conducted using the Medline, Scopus, Cinahl and Embase databases. Search terms included "irritable bowel syndrome," "IBS," "fodmap," "diet," "cognitive behavioral therapy," "complementary and alternative medicine," "hypnotherapy," and "herbal medicine." Intervention studies were included, being either randomized or non-randomized comparative trials that assessed the LFD against another intervention (dietary or otherwise). This inclusion criteria were set so that the LFD could have a clear comparison against another treatment modality. Studies were included if they assessed an adult population, and there was no limitation on year or the therapy the LFD was being compared to. No limitations were placed on IBS subtype. Data reviewed within these studies included diagnostic criteria (Rome III or Rome IV), intervention duration, assessment of symptom measures, changes to gut microbiome, type and overall effectiveness of the intervention implemented (education and resources), gaps in the literature, and future research directions within an IBS population.

RESULTS

Ten studies were included in this review, which assessed the LFD against other treatments (**Table 1**). Six of these studies compared the LFD against other dietary interventions including traditional dietary advice (12), modified National Institute for Health and Care Excellence (NICE) guidelines (13), high FODMAP diet (14), gluten-free diet and Mediterranean diet (15), generalized dietary advice and (8, 16). Two studies compared the LFD to probiotics (17, 18) and two studies compared a LFD to non-diet interventions—gut directed hypnotherapy (19) or yoga (20). One study (17) used a factorial design with participants allocated to either the shame diet/ probiotic, sham diet/placebo, the LFD/probiotics, or the LFD/ placebo; however, no interaction effect for symptoms or microbiota changes were noted, so data for the LFD compared to probiotics was not reported. Therefore, only results for the LFD compared to the sham diet have been included in the current analysis.

This review included studies with a range of comparative study methodologies. All except two studies were randomized controlled trials (RCTs) (8, 15). Of these studies, four were single-blind RCTs (12, 14, 16, 20), one was double-blind (17), with the remainder being open-label (13, 18, 19). Four studies (8, 13, 18, 19) were adequately powered (12, 14–18, 20). Data for IBS subtypes were not available for all studies, but where available (8, 12, 14, 17–19), the evidence has been discussed in relation to its applicability to the specific subtype.

LFD vs. Other Dietary Treatments
Symptom Severity

Five studies (12, 14–17) used the IBS-SSS to compare symptom severity in a LFD compared to other dietary treatment. The IBS-SSS is a five-item questionnaire scored using a VAS. One study (12) found IBS-SSS improved symptoms in each group with no significant difference between groups (p = 0.20). In the remaining studies, the LFD demonstrated superior efficacy in reducing IBS-SSS scores in comparison to traditional dietary advice, a high FODMAP diet (HFD), a gluten-free diet, generalized healthy eating, and a sham diet.

Two studies (8, 13) used scoring systems other than the IBS-SSS to assess changes in symptoms. For both studies, the LFD had a greater reduction in symptoms overall at the end of intervention compared to baseline after a minimum of 4 weeks. One study (8) showed a greater reduction for each individual question and globally with a composite score of the questions on the LFD.

Bristol Stool Form Scale

Five studies assessed bowel habits using the Bristol stool form scale as a measure of stool consistency and frequency (12, 13, 15–17). Overall, there was a trend toward the LFD improving stool consistency (13, 17) and frequency (16). One study reported the LFD having the greatest improvement in IBS-D subtype (15).

None of the remaining interventions produced an effect on stool form or number of bowel motions (12, 15).

IBS Subtype Response to Treatment

The IBS-D subtype showed a positive response to the LFD at 1 week (13) and 6 weeks (16). One study (14) showed that at 4

TABLE 1 | Summary of trials reporting on the assessment of the low FODMAP diet compared with other interventions in the management of IBS.

Author, year, country	Study design	Population, diagnostic criteria, and source of recruitment	Intervention and duration	Gastrointestinal symptom and microbial measures	Effect on symptoms	Practice implications
				LFD vs. other dietary interventions		
Bohn et al. (12) 2015 Sweden	Randomized, multi-center, single blind	n = 67 Adults aged 18–70 years Rome III IBS outpatient clinics	4-week LFD or NICE guidelines (regular meals, reduced fat, fiber, caffeine, and gas reducing foods)	IBS-SSS Bristol stool form scale	Symptoms reduced within both groups (p = <0.00001) but no difference between groups (p =0.2) Mean stool frequency improved significantly within the LFD from baseline to 4 weeks (1.9 ± 0.8) to (1.5 ± 0.7), p = <0.001) as per the Bristol stool form scale. Stool frequency had a non-significant change in the NICE group at baseline) (1.6 ± 0.7) compared to 4 weeks (1.5 ± 0.6), p =0.15). There was a non-significant difference between the groups at 4 weeks (p =0.64)	*Overlap between two diet interventions on reduction in 'gas-forming foods' and other components of FODMAPs suggest efficacy favoring LFD[†] Potential for 'sensible' eating guidelines to have additive effects to LFD*
Eswaran et al. (13) 2016 United States of America	Randomized, single center open label trial	n = 92 Adults aged 18 years and over Rome III (IBS-D subtype) Gastroenterology and primary care clinics	4-week LFD or modified NICE (mNICE) guidelines	11-point likert scale Weekly global symptom assessment Bristol stool form scale	52% LFD vs. 41% mNICE reported adequate relief (p = 0.031) LFD had higher proportion of abdominal pain responders compared with mNICE (51% vs. 23%, p = 0.008) At 4 weeks, stool consistency improved significantly on the LFD compared to the mNICE guidelines (p<0.0001) as per the Bristol stool form scale	*LFD[†] produced a greater improvement in abdominal pain, bloating, stool consistency, stool frequency and urgency at 1-week mNICE guidelines showed no significant improvement in abdominal pain, bloating or stool frequency in any wk Compared to baseline, both diets showed improvement for abdominal pain, bloating, stool consistency, stool frequency and urgency at 4-week*
McIntosh et al. (14) 2017 Canada	Prospective, randomized, single blind parallel study	n = 37 Adults aged 18 years and over Rome III Outpatient clinics	3-week LFD or HFD	IBS-SSS 16s RNA profiling	IBS-SSS reduced in LFD but not in HFD (p = <0.001) No differences in α or β diversity between samples from before or after HFD or LFD across IBS subgroups	*LFD[†] showed greater reduction in abdominal symptoms at 3-week HFD led to increased pain at 3 weeks Subgroup analysis showed IBS-M and IBS-D participants had higher bacterial richness after the LFD at 3 weeks*
Paduano et al. (15) 2019 Italy	Non-randomized cross over clinical trial	n = 92 Adults aged 18–45 years Rome IV GI outpatient clinics	4-week LFD or gluten-free or Mediterranean diet	IBS-SSS VAS for bloating and abdominal pain Bristol stool form scale	All 3 diets reduced symptom severity (<0.01), bloating (p<0.01) and abdominal pain (p<0.01) The LFD improved stool solidarity from a type 6 to a type 4 (p = 0.03) which was further supported by 79% of LFD participants showing a trend to reach type 4 after 4 weeks on the LFD. No statistically significant differences were observed in stool solidarity for the gluten-free and Mediterranean diets at 4 weeks (data not shown)	*Adequate FODMAP distribution over the day was key to preventing overload of FODMAPs in a single meal and inducing symptoms LFD[†] showed superiority for improving overall & individual GI symptoms, including stool consistency*
Staudacher et al. (8) 2011 United Kingdom	Non-randomized clinical control trial	n = 82 Adults aged 18 years and over NICE criteria Dietetic outpatient clinic follow-ups	36-week LFD or standard dietary advice based on NICE guidelines (if a dietitian had already been seen)	16-point VAS scale that included symptoms 7-point Likert scale for symptoms based on IBS global improvement scale	LFD reported greater satisfaction in symptom response (p = 0.38) LFD showed better overall symptom response (p = 0.001), improvement in bloating (p = 0.002), abdominal pain (p = 0.023) and flatulence (p = 0.001)	
Zahedi et al. (16)	Randomized, controlled	n = 110 Adults aged 20–60 years	6-week LFD or British Dietetic	IBS-SSS Bristol stool form scale	LFD decreased IBS-SSS for abdominal pain intensity (p = 0.001) and frequency (0.017), abdominal distention (p = <0.001), dissatisfaction with intestinal	*Both diets reduced symptom severity LFD compared to generalized*

(Continued)

TABLE 1 | Continued

Author, year, country	Study design	Population, diagnostic criteria, and source of recruitment	Intervention and duration	Gastrointestinal symptom and microbial measures	Effect on symptoms	Practice implications
2018 Iran	single blind trial	Rome III (IBS-D) Hospital GI clinic	Association guidelines		transit (p = 0.001) and interference with daily life (p = 0.005) Mean stool consistency significantly improved in the LFD from baseline to week 6 (5.92 ± 0.45 to 4.3 ± 0.5, p = <0.001) and for the generalized dietary advice group from baseline (5.67 ± 0.61) to week 6 (4.61 ± 0.69, p = <0.001) Mean stool frequency significantly improved in the LFD from baseline to week 6 (3.29 ± 0.87 to 1.91 ± 0.56, p = <0.001) and for the generalized dietary advice group from baseline (3.3 ± 0.77) to week 6 (2.6 ± 0.96, p = <0.001)	*dietary advice decreased symptoms for each subset of IBS-SSS and produced relief of symptoms at each timepoint (baseline, 3 weeks, and 6 weeks) Both diets improved stool frequency and consistency at 6 weeks*
Staudacher et al. (17) 2017 United Kingdom	Randomized, Double-blind 2x2 factorial design	n = 104 Adults aged 18–65 years Rome III Tertiary hospitals	4-week LFD or sham diet and placebo or multi-strain probiotic formulation	Gastrointestinal symptom rating system (GSRS) IBS-SSS Bristol stool form scale qPCR and 16sRNA sequencing	A higher proportion of patients on LFD had adequate symptom relief than sham diet (p = 0.042) LFD showed lower IBS-SSS score than sham diet (p = 0.01 but not different between probiotic and placebo (p = 0.721) LFD showed a higher proportion of participants achieved clinically meaningful reduction of >50-point reduction in total IBS-SSS compared to sham diet (73% vs. 42%) There was a significant difference in mean stool consistency at 4 weeks between the sham diet (4.3 ± 1.1) compared to the LFD (3.9 ± 1.0), p = 0.008 as per the Bristol stool form scale. The was no significant difference for the placebo and probiotic group for stool consistency (4.2 ± 1.0 vs. 4.0 ± 1.1), p = 0.544, respectively At 4 weeks here was lower absolute *Bifidobacterium* species abundance in LFD compared to sham diet (8.8 16s rRNA genes/g (SD 0.6) vs. 9.2rRNA genes/g (SD 1.0) mean difference -0.39 rRNA genes/g (95% CI, -0.64 to -0.13, p = 0.008) and greater abundance of *Bifidobacterium* species for probiotic compared to placebo [9.1 rRNA genes/g (SD 0/6) vs. 8.8 rRNA genes/g (SD 1.0) mean difference +0.34 rRNA genes/g (95% CI, 0.05 to 0.61, p = 0.019]	*LFD[†] showed greater efficacy in improving GI specific and overall symptoms compared to sham dietary advice at 4 week LFD-induced effects on microbiota can be modified with adjunct probiotic therapy*
				LFD vs. probiotics		
Pederson et al. (18) 2014 Denmark	Randomized, open label control trial	n = 123 Adults aged 18–74 years Rome III Tertiary hospital	6-week LFD or normal diet (ND) or lactobacillus rhamnoses GG probiotic (LGG)	IBS-SSS	LFD reduced IBS-SSS from baseline to 6 weeks compared to LGG vs. ND (p = <0.01) IBS-SSS scores reduced in LFD and LGG group compared to the normal diet (133 ± 122 vs. 68 ± 107, 133 ± 122 vs. 34 ± 95, p = <0.01) at 6 weeks	*LFD superior over probiotic alone across all IBS subtypes except IBS-C*
				LFD vs. non-dietary interventions		
Peters et al. (19) 2016 Australia	Randomized open-label, parallel study	n = 74 Adult aged 18 years and over Rome III General IBS population	6-week LFD or gut-directed hypnotherapy or a combination of both	100 mm VAS for symptoms (abdominal bloating, wind, abdominal pain, nausea, and satisfaction with stools)	Improvements in all symptoms were observed from baseline to 6 weeks for hypnotherapy, LFD and combination treatment with no difference across groups (p = 0.67)	*While both gut-directed hypnotherapy and LFD were equally efficacious in the short (6 weeks) and longer term (6 months), gut-directed hypnotherapy showed a greater benefit on psychological indices compared to LFD Combining two equally efficacious therapies did not necessarily confer added benefits for IBS patients*

(Continued)

TABLE 1 | Continued

Author, year, country	Study design	Population, diagnostic criteria, and source of recruitment	Intervention and duration	Gastrointestinal symptom and microbial measures	Effect on symptoms	Practice implications
Schumann et al. (20) 2018 Germany	Randomized, single blind study	n = 59 Adults aged 18–75 years Rome III Online and local press, department of internal and integrative medicine	12-week LFD or yoga	IBS-SSS	No significant differences between groups regarding IBS-SSS, except for abdominal distention subscale at 12 weeks (p = 0.040) in favor of LFD IBS subtype analysis showed no significant differences between interventions for effectiveness (data not shown)	LFD[†] showed higher proportion of participants who achieved clinically meaningful reduction in IBS-SSS at 12 weeks Clinical remission was sustained in equal number of patients between both groups at 6-month follow-up

GI, gastrointestinal; GSRS, gastrointestinal symptom rating scale; HFD, high FODMAP diet; IBS-C, irritable bowel syndrome-constipation, IBS-D, irritable bowel syndrome-diarrhea; IBS-M, irritable bowel syndrome-mixed; IBS-SSS, irritable bowel syndrome symptom severity score; NICE, National Institute for Health and Care Excellence; VAS, visual analogue scale; [†]indicates the LFD was superior for treatment response.

weeks, the LFD had the following changes; 14 of 16 IBS-D showed an improvement in bowels, 7 of 10 with IBS-C showed bowel improvement, and of eight with IBS-M, two participants showed improvement, one worsened, and two had no changes. The remaining participants were all IBS-U, undefined at baseline (15). These findings suggest that the LFD benefits each IBS subtype, most consistently for IBS-D.

Delivery of Dietary Intervention

Given the LFD approach is comprehensive due to the elimination, reintroduction, and personalization of the diet, there are potential risks if the diet is not implemented safely. Alterations to gastrointestinal microbiota and nutritional adequacy have been noted after just 4 weeks of a LFD, which is concerning given that the initial restriction phase is usually 6 weeks (4). Personalized dietary advice from a dietitian has been positively associated with compliance and success (21). In all studies evaluating the LFD compared to other dietary intervention, it was promising to see all involved the expertise of a dietitian in delivering the LFD diet (8, 12–16). Additionally, a major factor in determining the success of the LFD was the provision of written resources to facilitate implementing the diet (22). There were varying degrees of contact with the dietitian where some participants received 45 to 90 min on a single occasion or up to four sessions in either an individual or group setting. In some studies, there was limited contact with the dietitian to replicate clinical practice. Commonly noted feedback to study personnel were that participants found the diet relatively easy to follow, but the translation of low FODMAP foods into recipes was difficult. One study, which had the low FODMAP food resource prepared in accordance with Iranian culture, found that adherence was considered difficult; however, it was not reported as a problem in the trial (16). Adherence with the LFD was associated with achieving a clinically important value of a reduction in IBS-SSS ≥50 (12).

For the other dietary interventions, there was insufficient detail provided to ascertain whether participants received the same level of care as those receiving a LFD. Therefore, the quality of dietetic care is less comparable to those who received LFD intervention, and there is insufficient insight what participants were specially instructed to do to elicit symptomatic relief.

Effects on Microbiome
Overall Analysis
Changes in the dietary content of fermentable carbohydrates have previously been shown to have a major influence on the gut microbiota composition. Alpha and beta diversity were not different after the implementation of a HFD or LFD from baseline to end of intervention and the result was consistent across IBS subtypes (14). There were no significant differences in the alpha diversity for the LFD compared to the sham diet (p = 0.401). The LFD compared to the sham diet did not produce a difference in beta diversity either (p = 0.575) (17). At a taxonomic level, the genus *Aldercreutzia*, *Dorea*, and the family Actinomycetaceae were lower after following a HFD (p = 0.02, p = 0.05, and p = 0.04, respectively). However, after just 3 weeks, the LFD produced fecal samples with higher Actinobacteria richness and diversity compared with the HFD group (p = 0.046 and p = 0.02, respectively) (14). Several bacterial groups decreased after following the HFD, with the exception of the Bifidobacteriaceae family and unclassed family within the Lachnospiraceae family, which increased (14). On a species level, the LFD compared with the sham diet produced lower absolute abundance of *Bifidobacterium* (p = 0.08). The LFD did not produce a difference in relative abundance of the *Streptococcus* species or the *Lactobacillus* species compared to the sham diet between baseline and follow-up (17). These findings suggest that the alpha and beta diversity may not be impacted by the implementation of a LFD; however, at a species level, the results are inconsistent.

Subgroup Analysis
When the IBS subtypes IBS-M and IBD-D (both groups having some diarrhoea) were analyzed, there was a greater bacterial richness in those following the LFD compared to the HFD (p = 0.047). Actinobacteria diversity was increased (p = .013), and

Firmicutes, Clostridiales, and Actinobacteria richness was greater (p = 0.029, p = 0.023, and p = 0.029, respectively) (14).

LFD vs. Probiotics
Symptom Severity
Symptom severity was measured using the GSRS (17). The LFD produced a 117-point decrease on the IBS-SSS compared to the probiotic with an 82-point decrease. Probiotics did not produce a statistically significant overall symptom improvement using the GSRS (p = 0.66), but the LFD was significant (p = 0.020) (17).

Bristol Stool Form Scale
Pedersen et al. did not use the Bristol stool form scale.

Delivery of Dietary Intervention
One study compared a LFD to probiotic use whereby participants were seen by either a dietitian or nutritionist (18). Dietary counselling was provided for up to one hour (18) with a complex list of appropriate foods provided by a dietitian (18). Dietary compliance was regularly checked and contact with the dietitian was encouraged (18). Probiotics were administered in capsules (18) whereby participants consumed two capsules each day.

Effects on Microbiome
Data on the LFD and probiotic on microbiome was not reported (18).

IBS Subtype Response to Treatment
The IBS-D subtype showed a positive response to the LFD at 6 weeks (18). In addition, IBS-M subtype showed a positive response to the LFD and LGG probiotic at 6 weeks. The IBS-C subtype did not have a positive response to the LFD, probiotic intervention, or a normal diet (18).

LFD vs. Non-Dietary Treatments
Symptom Severity
For two studies comparing a LFD to non-dietary treatments, there was a significant decrease in symptoms for the LFD from baseline to end of intervention (p < 0.001) (19) and (p < 0.001 and p < 0.001 for yoga and a LFD, respectively) for IBS-SSS scoring (20). For both studies, there were no significant differences between the groups at baseline compared to end of intervention.

Bristol Stool Form Scale
Neither of the studies that assessed non-dietary interventions used the Bristol stool form scale as an outcome.

Delivery of Intervention
The participants receiving gut-directed hypnotherapy were allocated 1 h weekly sessions throughout the 6-week study duration. Each participant received the same script that was also recorded and given to the participants to listen to daily for the duration of the study. The intervention was provided by an experienced clinical hypnotherapist (19).

Participants who received the yoga intervention had twice weekly group sessions, which were 75 min in duration for a 12-week period. The classes were guided by the same certified hatha yoga instructor. Specifically, participants were instructed on customised postures and breathing techniques to improve symptom control (20).

IBS Subtype Response to Treatment
There were no differences in treatment effectiveness between IBS subtypes (19, 20).

DISCUSSION

This review highlights that the LFD is efficacious in the management of IBS. Despite its success, several considerations need to be addressed regarding its use. While there has been greater understanding of the LFD and its mechanism in practice with recent research, there is still a consensus that further understanding of the diet's implications are needed.

Gaps of interest include a deeper understanding on the long-term effects of the LFD on gut microbiota diversity. It should be established whether a change in the microbiota profile can be attributed to a mediated symptom response (8, 14). Although recent reviews indicate that baseline microbiota may not be an accurate predictor of symptom improvement in IBS (23), the volatile organic compound profile may very accurately select responders, suggesting that understanding metabolic function of bacteria is more important for determining response to dietary interventions (24). Modulation of gut microbiota with the use of pre- and probiotics while implementing the LFD should be considered. While prebiotics can infer a symptomatic response in some individuals, it should be ascertained whether a less restrictive LFD mitigates the negative impact on the microbiota.

From a safety perspective, calorie and nutrient inadequacies have been acknowledged when following the LFD. Therefore, excessive restrictions such as the avoidance of complete food groups should be averted (25). The implementation of the LFD is extensive and requires education from a qualified nutrition professional (4). Where the LFD may not be appropriate or possible, other dietary strategies can be considered. Evidence suggests that simple strategies such as a reduction in gut stimulants (caffeine, alcohol, and spicy food) and modulation of meal size and frequency may also be effective. However, it should be noted that the NICE guidelines include recommendations such as reducing polyols, onions, cabbage, and beans and limiting fruit to three portions per day. Despite being considered as generalized dietary advice, these foods contain FODMAPs, which is why a reduction in symptoms may be concurrent if following this advice. Furthermore, dietitians instructed participants in one study who were not randomized to the LFD to limit consumption of foods that contribute to perceived detrimental symptoms (16). While the dietitians did not advise these participants to restrict FODMAPs specifically, it is unknown if any foods restricted did contain FODMAPs, which could have contributed to symptom improvement. From a practical perspective, it appears there is still a need for data on the LFD when followed for a long duration.

Cognitive considerations in IBS also warrant further investigation. The mechanisms in which gut directed hypnotherapy exert an effect on the gut are not fully understood but suggest the control and normalisation of gastrointestinal function can be made to the subconscious mind. Peters et al. found that improved psychological indices were not correlated with symptomatic benefit, although the study was not designed to evaluate mechanisms for efficacy; therefore, further understanding the mechanisms of gut hypnotherapy on symptom improvement is needed (19).

Despite results from Peters et al. that a combination of dietary and psychological interventions showed no additive benefits, areas for further research would be further exploring combining dietary and other non-dietary interventions. Tailored advice based on an individual's current dietary intake and other psychosocial factors should help to inform a management plan. Given that the gut microbiota have an established role in IBS and the gut-brain axis (26), combined dietary and cognitive treatments should be examined to determine the relationship between concurrent changes to the gut microbiota and symptom resolution.

This review highlighted a heterogeneity in LFD study designs and in IBS patient selection, including a lack of inclusion or reporting of specific IBS-subtypes. Regardless, the findings demonstrate consistencies in the evidence that the LFD is efficacious in overall symptom and bowel function improvement for each IBS subtype, allowing practical application across the distribution of IBS patterns.

In conclusion, the LFD is efficacious in reducing symptoms when compared to other dietary and non-dietary treatments, however it remains difficult to understand why some individuals respond to certain treatments while others do not. Future research should focus on identifying which treatment modality specifically or in which combination *via* a multimodal approach is best suited to an individual with IBS, including short- and long-term effects. Current dietary intake and symptom pattern of an individual in conjunction with current psychosocial state regarding depression, anxiety, and stress should be measured to best inform whether dietary or cognitive therapies are likely to be more effective in the management of IBS.

AUTHOR CONTRIBUTIONS

Conceptualization: LM and JB. Writing and draft preparation: LM. Review and editing: CY and JB.

REFERENCES

1. Lacy BE, Mearin F, Chang L, Chey WD, Lembo AJ, Simren M, et al. Bowel Disorders. *Gastroenterology* (2016) 150(6):1393–1407.e5. doi: 10.1053/j.gastro.2016.02.031

2. Canavan C, West J, Card T. Review article: the economic impact of the irritable bowel syndrome. *J Psychosom Res* (2014) 1023–34. doi: 10.1111/apt.12938

3. Kamp KJ, Weaver KR, Sherwin LB, Barney P, Hwang SK, Yang PL, et al. Effects of a comprehensive self-management intervention on extraintestinal symptoms among patients with IBS. *J Psychosom Res* (2019) 126:109821–1. doi: 10.1016/j.jpsychores.2019.109821

4. Whelan K, Martin LD, Staudacher HM, Lomer MC. The low FODMAP diet in the management of irritable bowel syndrome: an evidence-based review of FODMAP restriction, reintroduction and personalisation in clinical practice. *J Hum Nutr Dietetics* (2018) 31(2):239–55. doi: 10.1111/jhn.12530

5. Marsh A, Eslick EM, Eslick GD. Does a diet low in FODMAPs reduce symptoms associated with functional gastrointestinal disorders? A comprehensive systematic review and meta-analysis. *Eur J Nutr* (2016) 55(3):897–906. doi: 10.1007/s00394-015-0922-1

6. Schumann D, Störsrud S, Klose P, Lauche R, Dobos G, Langhorst J, et al. Low fermentable, oligo-, di-, mono-saccharides and polyol diet in the treatment of irritable bowel syndrome: A systematic review and meta-analysis. *Nutrition* (2018) 45:24–31. doi: 10.1016/j.nut.2017.07.004

7. Gibson PR. The evidence base for efficacy of the low FODMAP diet in irritable bowel syndrome: is it ready for prime time as a first-line therapy? *Journal of Gastroenterology* (2017) 32:32–5. doi: 10.1111/jgh.13693

8. Staudacher HM, Whelan K, Irving PM, Lomer MC. Comparison of symptom response following advice for a diet low in fermentable carbohydrates (FODMAPs) versus standard dietary advice in patients with irritable bowel syndrome. *J Hum Nutr Dietetics* (2011) 24(5):487–95. doi: 10.1111/j.1365-277X.2011.01162.x

9. Heidi MS, Staudacher HM, Irving PM, Lomer MC, Whelan K. Mechanisms and efficacy of dietary FODMAP restriction in IBS. *Nat Rev Gastroenterol Hepatol* (2014) 11(4):256. doi: 10.1038/nrgastro.2013.259

10. Chang L, Di Lorenzo C, Farrugia G, Hamilton FA, Mawe GM, Pasricha PJ, et al. Functional Bowel Disorders: A Roadmap to Guide the Next Generation of Research. *Gastroenterology* (2018) 154(3):723–35. doi: 10.1053/j.gastro.2017.12.010

11. Laird KT, Tanner-Smith EE, Russell AC, Hollon SD, Walker LS. Comparative efficacy of psychological therapies for improving mental health and daily functioning in irritable bowel syndrome: A systematic review and meta-analysis. *Clin Psychol Rev* (2017) 51:142–52. doi: 10.1016/j.cpr.2016.11.001

12. Böhn L, Störsrud S, Liljebo T, Collin L, Lindfors P, Törnblom H, et al. Diet Low in FODMAPs Reduces Symptoms of Irritable Bowel Syndrome as Well as Traditional Dietary Advice: A Randomized Controlled Trial. *Gastroenterology* (2015) 149(6):1399–1407.e2. doi: 10.1053/j.gastro.2015.07.054

13. Eswaran SL, Chey WD, Han-Markey T, Ball S, Jackson K. A Randomized Controlled Trial Comparing the Low FODMAP Diet vs. Modified NICE Guidelines in US Adults with IBS-D. *Am J Gastroenterol* (2016) 111(12):1824–32. doi: 10.1038/ajg.2016.434

14. McIntosh K, Reed DE, Schneider T, Dang F, Keshteli AH, De Palma G, et al. FODMAPs alter symptoms and the metabolome of patients with IBS: A randomised controlled trial. *Gut* (2017) 66(7):1241–51. doi: 10.1136/gutjnl-2015-311339

15. Paduano D, Cingolani A, Tanda E, Usai P. Effect of Three Diets (Low-FODMAP, Gluten-free and Balanced) on Irritable Bowel Syndrome Symptoms and Health-Related Quality of Life. *Nutrients* (2019) 11(7):1566. doi: 10.3390/nu11071566

16. Zahedi MJ, Behrouz V, Azimi M. Low fermentable oligo-di-mono-saccharides and polyols diet versus general dietary advice in patients with diarrhea-predominant irritable bowel syndrome: A randomized controlled trial. *J Gastroenterol Hepatol (Aust)* (2018) 33(6):1192–9. doi: 10.1111/jgh.14051

17. Staudacher HM, Lomer MC, Farquharson FM, Louis P, Fava F, Franciosi E, et al. A Diet Low in FODMAPs Reduces Symptoms in Patients With Irritable Bowel Syndrome and A Probiotic Restores Bifidobacterium Species: A Randomized Controlled Trial. *Gastroenterology* (2017) 153(4):936–47. doi: 10.1053/j.gastro.2017.06.010

18. Pedersen N, Andersen NN, Végh Z, Jensen L, Ankersen DV, Felding M, et al. Ehealth: Low FODMAP diet vs Lactobacillus rhamnosus GG in irritable bowel syndrome. *World J Gastroenterol* (2014) 20(43):16215–26. doi: 10.3748/wjg.v20.i43.16215

19. Peters SL, Yao CK, Philpott H, Yelland GW, Muir JG, Gibson PR. Randomised clinical trial: the efficacy of gut-directed hypnotherapy is similar to that of the low FODMAP diet for the treatment of irritable bowel syndrome. *Alimen Pharmacol Ther* (2016) 44(5):447–59. doi: 10.1111/apt.13706

20. Schumann D, Langhorst J, Dobos G, Cramer H. Randomised clinical trial: yoga vs a low-FODMAP diet in patients with irritable bowel syndrome. *Alimen Pharmacol Ther* (2018) 47(2):203–11. doi: 10.1111/apt.14400

21. Tuck CJ, Reed DE, Muir JG, Vanner SJ. Implementation of the low FODMAP diet in functional gastrointestinal symptoms: A real-world experience. *Neurogastroenterol Motil* (2019) 32(1): e13730. doi: 10.1111/nmo.13730

22. Gearry RB, Irving PM, Barrett JS, Nathan DM, Shepherd SJ, Gibson PR. Reduction of dietary poorly absorbed short-chain carbohydrates (FODMAPs) improves abdominal symptoms in patients with inflammatory bowel disease—a pilot study. *J Crohn's Colitis* (2009) 3(1):8–14. doi: 10.1016/j.crohns.2008.09.004

23. Biesiekierski JR, Jalanka J, Staudacher HM. Can Gut Microbiota Composition Predict Response to Dietary Treatments? *Nutrients* (2019) 11(5):1134. doi: 10.3390/nu11051134

24. Rossi M, Aggio R, Staudacher HM, Lomer MC, Lindsay JG, Irving JO, et al. Volatile Organic Compounds in Feces Associate With Response to Dietary Intervention in Patients With Irritable Bowel Syndrome. *Clin Gastroenterol Hepatol* (2018) 16(3):385–391.e1. doi: 10.1016/j.cgh.2017.09.055

25. Staudacher HM, Lomer MC, Anderson JL, Barrett JS, Muir JG, Irving PM, et al. Fermentable carbohydrate restriction reduces luminal bifidobacteria and gastrointestinal symptoms in patients with irritable bowel syndrome. *J Nutr* (2012) 142(8):1510–8. doi: 10.3945/jn.112.159285

26. Bonaz B, Bazin T, Pellissier S. The Vagus Nerve at the Interface of the Microbiota-Gut-Brain Axis. *Front Neurosci* (2018) 12:49. doi: 10.3389/fnins.2018.00049

7

Sex Differences Linking Pain-Related Fear and Interoceptive Hypervigilance: Attentional Biases to Conditioned Threat and Safety Signals in a Visceral Pain Model

Franziska Labrenz, Sopiko Knuf-Rtveliashvili and Sigrid Elsenbruch*

Institute of Medical Psychology & Behavioral Immunobiology, University Hospital Essen, University of Duisburg-Essen, Essen, Germany

Correspondence:
Sigrid Elsenbruch
Sigrid.Elsenbruch@uk-essen.de

Although the broad role of fear and hypervigilance in conditions of the gut-brain axis like irritable bowel syndrome is supported by converging evidence, the underlying mechanisms remain incompletely understood. Even in healthy individuals, it remains unclear how pain-related fear may contribute to pain-related attentional biases for acute visceral pain. Building on our classical fear conditioning work in a clinically relevant model of visceral pain, we herein elucidated pain-related attentional biases shaped by associative learning in healthy women and men, aiming to elucidate possible sex differences and the role of psychological traits. To this end, we compared the impact of differentially conditioned pain-predictive cues on attentional biases in healthy women and men. Sixty-four volunteers accomplished a visual dot-probe task and subsequently underwent pain-related fear conditioning where one visual cue (CS^+) was contingently paired with a painful rectal distention (US) while another cue remained unpaired (CS^-). During the following test phase, the dot-probe task was repeated to investigate changes in attentional biases in response to differentially valenced cues. While pain-related learning was comparable between groups, men revealed more pronounced attentional engagement with the CS^+ and CS^- whereas women demonstrated stronger difficulties to disengage from the CS^+ when presented with a neutral cue. However, when both CS^+ and CS^- were presented together, women revealed stronger difficulties to disengage from the CS^-. Regression analyses revealed an interaction of sex, with negative affect predicting stronger avoidance of the CS^+ and stronger difficulties to disengage attention from the CS^- in men. These results provide first evidence that pain-related fear conditioning may induce attentional biases differentially in healthy women and men. Hence, sex differences may play a role in attentional mechanisms underlying hypervigilance, and may be modulated by psychological vulnerability factors relevant to chronic visceral pain.

Keywords: gut-brain axis, visceral pain, attentional bias, hypervigilance, pain-related fear, anxiety, sex differences

INTRODUCTION

Fear is a potent motivator that drives learning and behavior. It serves to rapidly shift attention toward signals of threat in order to avoid bodily harm, engage in self-protection and seek safety. Although adaptive by nature, fear and ensuing avoidance behaviors can also become maladaptive, with broad implications for the pathophysiology and treatment of chronic pain (1, 2). The fear-avoidance model of pain proposes a vicious cycle of pain-related fear, hypervigilance and avoidance, maintained, and modulated by psychological vulnerability factors like anxiety, catastrophizing, and negative affect (3, 4). Pain-related fear is essentially governed by the principles of classical and instrumental conditioning, engaging attentional resources that are relevant to hypervigilance, and avoidance. As an inherently fear-evoking stimulus, pain attracts strong attentional responses leading to increased sensitivity for negative information and aberrant attentional orienting toward threat (5, 6). These responses involve opposing, yet inextricably linked mechanisms of facilitated engagement toward threat, avoidance and difficulties to disengage with individuals orienting toward or away from threat early during attentional processing and subsequent avoidance at later stages (7, 8). While these processes are broadly established in the context of anxiety and posttraumatic stress (9, 10), evidence in the context of pain-related fear remains scarce and inconsistent (6, 11), especially with regard to interoceptive, visceral pain. Visceral pain is of high clinical relevance, specifically in conditions of the gut-brain axis like irritable bowel syndrome (IBS). Compared to other types of exteroceptive pain, visceral pain is considered to be characterized by a unique biological salience, as supported by greater visceral pain-related fear and enhanced pain-related learning (12, 13), making this a suitable preclinical model to study pain-related attentional biases. While numerous studies addressed attentional biases toward threat only, safety cues signaling the absence of an aversive event were also found to induce attentional biases (14) and are prioritized under threatening conditions (15). Specifically in visceral pain, patients (16, 17) and healthy individuals (18) demonstrated enhanced awareness of safety cues suggesting that attentional biases may also pertain to safety cues.

Building on our conditioning work in a clinically relevant model of visceral pain (19–21), we herein aimed to elucidate attentional biases induced by conditioned pain-related fear and safety signals in healthy volunteers. Inspired by broad knowledge about higher prevalence and incidence of chronic visceral pain in women (22), initial evidence suggesting sex differences in pain-related fear conditioning (23) and attentional coping strategies (24), we a priori committed to elucidating sex differences. Moreover, pain-related attentional biases seem to vary as a function of inter-individual differences in anxiety sensitivity and catastrophizing, but findings are heterogeneous (22, 25–27).

We herein employed a visual dot-probe task to address whether conditioning results in attentional biases related to attentional avoidance, facilitated engagement and/ or difficulties to disengage from pain-related threat and safety cues. We hypothesized that women would demonstrate more pronounced attentional biases toward threat cues, reflected by stronger engagement at short stimulus durations, as well as stronger difficulties to disengage at longer stimulus durations. Moreover, we assumed that women would demonstrate more pronounced biases to safety cues as conditioned inhibitors of fear responses and a clinically relevant phenotype in anxiety-related disorders (28). Finally, we explored the sex-specific role of psychological vulnerability factors as predictors, specifically aiming to assess a greater contribution of anxiety, negative affect as well as coping and catastrophizing to pain-related attentional biases in women.

MATERIALS AND METHODS

Recruitment

The study protocol followed the rules stated in the Declaration of Helsinki and was approved by the local Ethics Committee of the University Hospital Essen, Germany (approval #10-4493). Recruitment and data collection were conducted between August 2016 and December 2017. The recruitment and screening process followed our group's established procedures in place for all visceral pain studies involving rectal distensions, and included a structured telephone screening and personal interview with a medical examination conducted by a physician.

To calculate the required sample size, we performed a power analysis using G*Power (version 3.1.9.2) (29). To detect between-groups effects of sex, we specified two groups, i.e., women and men, and eight measurements, i.e., four conditions of the dot-probe task at baseline and during the test phase presenting CS^+ and CS^- each with a neutral cue, CS^+ and CS^- together and one condition only presenting neutral cues. Based on the meta-analysis by (11) reporting attentional biases toward signals of impending experimental pain in healthy individuals, we assumed a medium effect size of Cohen's $d = 0.676$ (conforming to Cohen's $f = 0.338$). With an actual power of 0.95, the required sample size included 66 participants with a critical F-value of 3.99.

Based on local advertisement, we were initially contacted via telephone or email by a total of $N = 143$ interested individuals. After providing more detailed study information, $N = 102$ individuals agreed to participate in our structured telephone screening. Exclusion criteria were age <18 or >45 years, body mass index (BMI) <18 or >30, any known medical or psychological health condition, chronic medication use except occasional use of over-the-counter allergy or pain medications, and prior participation in any other conditioning study conducted by our group. Moreover, we excluded free-cycling women based on self-report to avoid confounding effects of cyclical fluctuations of sex hormones. During telephone screening, a total of $N = 26$ individuals were excluded. All others ($N = 76$) were then scheduled for a personal interview at the University Hospital Essen. During the interview, participants were screened for current anxiety or depression symptoms using the German version of the Hospital Anxiety and Depression Scale (HADS; Cronbach's alpha $\alpha = 0.80$ for the anxiety subscale and $\alpha = 0.81$ for the depression subscale) (30) and for symptoms suggestive of any functional or organic gastrointestinal condition based on a standardized in-house questionnaire (31). All participants were further evaluated digitally for perianal tissue damage (e.g., painful hemorrhoids). Based on these screening criteria, $N = 5$ individuals were excluded due to HADS scores ≥ 8, $N = 3$ due to increased gastrointestinal symptoms ≥ 13, and $N = 1$ due to anal tissue damage. Further, on the day of the experimental study, two participants missed the appointment and one participant terminated the study during the second run of the dot-probe task. The final sample that we herein report on thus includes 64 healthy volunteers (32 women, 32 men).

Study Design and Procedures

Prior to study participation, all participants were instructed not to eat, drink, or exercise within 2 h before arrival to the laboratory. Participants completed the study protocol within ~2 h between 09:00 and 16:00 h. Upon arrival, participants gave written informed consent and completed the questionnaire battery and then underwent the TMT and Stroop test (see below). For women, pregnancy was routinely excluded by commercially available urinary test upon arrival. All participants were tested in a medically-equipped, sound-shielded, and dimly lit room and were positioned in a hospital bed. The rectal balloon was subsequently placed, sensory thresholds were determined, and distension pressure for implementation during conditioning was individually calibrated based on the rectal pain threshold (for details, see below). All instructions and tasks were presented on a 22-inch widescreen monitor with 60 Hz refresh rate and a display resolution of 1,680 × 1,050 pixels at a viewing distance of ~140 cm. All measurements were performed by the same female tester.

The study design consisted of a mixed-group (women, men) repeated-measures design with three consecutive experimental phases (**Figure 1A**): A visual dot-probe task (baseline, for details on the task see below) was followed by fear conditioning, after which the same visual dot-probe task was repeated during the test phase. For conditioning, explained in detail below, we implemented an established differential delay conditioning paradigm with individually calibrated painful rectal distensions as interoceptive unconditioned stimuli, carried out with a pressure-controlled barostat system, and visual cues as conditioned stimuli (CS). The total duration of the dot-probe task varied between participants with a notional minimum duration of 4.67 min assuming overall reaction times of 200 ms and a maximum duration of 13.07 min assuming the longest possible reaction time of 2,000 ms with an average of 8.87 min. After completion of the first dot-probe task, instructions were given for the conditioning procedure that commenced immediately afterwards. The total duration of the conditioning procedure was 7.77 min. Subsequently, the study investigator informed the participant that a second run of the dot-probe task using the same procedure as during the first run will immediately start. Together, average duration for all three experimental phases was 25.51 min.

Questionnaire Battery and Neuropsychological Testing

On the study day, participants initially completed a questionnaire battery assessing sociodemographic variables as well as several psychological characteristics. Trait anxiety was measured with the State Trait Anxiety Inventory (STAI-T; α between 0.88 and 0.94) (32) as a self-report of stable aspects of anxiety proneness. To assess situation-specific aspects of cognitive coping and catastrophizing with pain, we used the Pain-Related Self Statements Scale (PRSS; $\alpha = 0.92$) (33). In addition, we measured current emotional states and fluctuations using the Positive and Negative Affect Schedule (PANAS; for both subscales $\alpha = 0.86$) (34).

Moreover, the Trail Making Test (TMT) and Stroop Color Word Test were administered as control parameters for possible differences between women and men in attentional and executive functioning. The TMT is a neuropsychological task proposed to measure selective attention and processing speed in version A and set shifting in version B (35, 36), with first evidence suggesting that healthy women perform worse on version B (37). The Stroop test is thought to provide a measure of cognitive inhibition (38, 39). However, evidence regarding sex differences remains scarce and has so far yielded inconclusive results (40, 41).

Visual Dot-Probe Task and Attentional Bias Assessment

The visual dot-probe task employed in the present study was used to assess the phenomenological characteristics of attentional biases that have previously been determined in various empirical investigations (7): attentional avoidance, engagement and disengagement. Most studies on attentional biases in chronic pain so far utilized words or varying categories of pictures or facial expressions that however raised concerns about their ecological validity and that may not be sufficiently intense to induce attentional biases (42). Therefore, it has been proposed that stimuli need to be sufficiently matched to the individual qualities of pain-related fear (26), for instance through instructed fear stimuli (43) or differential conditioning (44, 45). We herein modified the original dot-probe task (46) by utilizing differentially valenced visual stimuli induced through differential, pain-related fear conditioning.

Moreover, many studies utilizing the dot-probe task have encountered methodological and analytical problems due to the absence of baseline measures. Herein, the implementation of neutral stimuli within conditions creates a neutral baseline against which responses toward threat and safety cues can be compared and therefore allows to specifically determine the type of attentional bias observed (47, 48). Likewise, the implementation of a baseline measurement of the dot-probe task before pain-related fear conditioning allows assessing intra-individual changes in attentional biases in response to experimentally induced pain-related fear and safety cues in a within-subject design.

Finally, while common dot-probe tasks often employ static stimulus durations, we furthermore aimed to elucidate the time course of attentional biases by varying the time between stimulus onset and appearance of the probe. According to a two-stage model proposing that initial attentional vigilance is followed by attentional avoidance, some studies yet revealed that the utilization of short and long stimulus durations captures attentional features occurring prior to attentional avoidance (49,

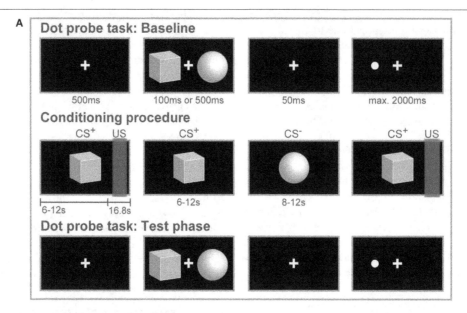

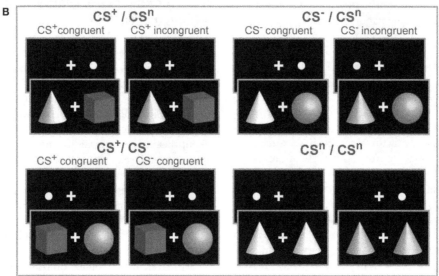

FIGURE 1 | Study design and experimental procedure. Schematic illustration of the experimental procedure **(A)** and conditions during the dot-probe task **(B)**. **(A)** Participants initially accomplished a dot-probe task (baseline) during which three different visual cues were used as stimulus material. Participants were instructed to respond by button press to the dot appearing either on the left or right side of the fixation cross. During the subsequent fear-conditioning procedure, one visual cue (CS+) was repeatedly paired with a rectal distension (US) while a second visual cue (CS−) was presented without US. Only two out of three visual cues were presented during conditioning. Afterwards participants completed a second run of the dot-probe task (test phase) with the same visual stimuli presented during the baseline task. After each phase, visual analog scale (VAS) ratings of CS valence and CS-US contingency (only after fear conditioning) were accomplished. **(B)** In the dot-probe task, counterbalanced and randomized order of the three different visual cues yielded four conditions. The cues are color-coded for visual purposes only to illustrate the different CS valences acquired after conditioning. For the CS+ /CSⁿ and CS− /CSⁿ conditions, trials were considered congruent if the dot-probe appeared at the location previously occupied by the CS+ (shown in red) or CS− (shown in green) and incongruent, if the dot appeared at the location previously occupied by the neutral cue (shown in gray). When CS+ and CS− where presented together, the dot-probe was considered CS+-congruent when it appeared at the location previously occupied by the CS+ and CS−-congruent when the dot appeared at the location previously occupied by the CS−. During the neutral condition, only neutral cues were presented.

50). Moreover, Koster et al. (8) have emphasized the potential interaction of stimulus duration and threat value, indicating that attentional biases may show different phenomenological characteristics which has been corroborated by multiple studies demonstrating stimulus duration to exert a moderating effect

(8, 51, 52). Specifically, stimuli of high biological significance like pain can immediately draw attention to the potential source of threat even before conscious perception and evaluation (53), suggesting that acquired signals of imminent threat as well as safety cues signaling the absence of pain may likewise occupy different phenomenological and temporal characteristics. We herein adopted presentation times from (8) who demonstrated the impact of stimulus duration and threat value on the time course of attentional biases using pictorial stimuli.

Each trial consisted of the following sequence (**Figure 1A**): First, a fixation cross was displayed in the center of the screen for 500 ms. Then, a stimulus pair of geometric symbols was presented with one stimulus presented left and one stimulus presented right from the fixation cross with a variable duration of either 100 or 500 ms. After a blank screen depicting the fixation cross for 50 ms, a dot appeared either on the left or right side from the fixation cross at the same location occupied by one of the stimuli before. Participants were asked to respond as fast as possible to the dot with button press of the corresponding arrow key on a keyboard. If a response was registered, the dot disappeared or if no response was registered, the dot lasted until a maximum response time set at 2,000 ms. Inter-trial intervals (ITI) were 750 ms. Randomizing and counterbalancing stimulus presentation across trials and stimuli across the left and right side of the fixation cross resulted in four conditions (**Figure 1B**), presenting the CS^+ with a neutral cue ($CS^+ + CS^n$; $CS^n + CS^+$), presenting the CS^- with a neutral cue ($CS^- + CS^n$; $CS^n + CS^-$), conditions presenting the CS^+ and CS^- together ($CS^+ + CS^-$; $CS^- + CS^+$) and neutral trials ($CS^n + CS^n$). For each run of the dot-probe task, 280 trials were presented, 80 per each condition presenting a CS^+ and/ or CS^- and 40 trials presenting only neutral cues.

As main outcome, reaction time (RT) was recorded on each trial to assess the speed of response to the location of the dot-probe. Before statistical analyses, premature responses <100 ms, missing and false responses were removed from RT data according to empirical recommendations for analyses of the dot-probe task (50). Mean RT was calculated for each condition, type of congruency (congruent, incongruent) and stimulus duration (100, 500 ms) for the dot-probe task at baseline and during the test phase. Type of congruency was determined using target t and dot-probe d appearing either on the left l or right r side. A trial is considered congruent when the dot appears at the same location as the previously displayed target stimulus, calculating the mean RT as $RT_{congruent} = (RT_{tldl} + RT_{trdr})/2$. On incongruent trials, the dot appears at the location of the neutral stimulus and is calculated as $RT_{incongruent} = (RT_{tldr} + RT_{trdl})/2$. Trials presenting both CS^+ and CS^- represent a special case where trials can be determined as CS^+-congruent if the dot appears at the location of the CS^+, and CS^--congruent if the dot appears at the location of the CS^-. Likewise, mean RT for the neutral condition presenting only neutral CS that were not subjected to fear conditioning were calculated as $RT_{neutral} = (RT_{tldl} + RT_{trdr} + RT_{tldr} + RT_{trdl})/4$. Outlying RT values were then identified based on the interquartile range (IQR) with a lower threshold of $Q1 - 1.5 \times IQR$ and the upper threshold of $Q3 - 1.5 \times IQR$.

Indices of attentional avoidance, engagement and disengagement were calculated for each condition following previous studies (8, 54). Attentional avoidance was calculated as $RT_{incongruent} - RT_{congruent}$ with negative scores indicating stronger attentional avoidance. Attentional engagement was calculated as $RT_{neutral} - RT_{congruent}$ with positive scores indicating enhanced attentional capture and negative scores indicating slower attentional engagement. Attentional disengagement was calculated as $RT_{neutral} - RT_{incongruent}$ with negative scores indicating stronger attentional vigilance with difficulty to divert onto another stimulus and positive scores indicating faster attention away from the cue. For all these indices, a score of zero implies no differences either in attentional avoidance, engagement or disengagement.

Visceral Pain Model and Conditioning

Rectal distensions were carried out with a pressure-controlled barostat system (modified ISOBAR 3 device, G & J Electronics, Toronto, ON, Canada). Sensory and pain thresholds were determined using the ascending method of limits delivering distensions with random pressure increments of 5 mmHg and a maximal distension pressure of 50 mmHg as previously described (31, 55, 56). During conditioning, individually calibrated rectal distensions were implemented as interoceptive painful US. To this end, prior to the baseline dot-probe task, individual US intensity was carefully titrated. Participants rated selected pressures (i.e., starting with pressures just below pain threshold) on a visual analog scale (VAS) ranging from 0 to 100 with endpoints labeled "not painful at all" and "very painful." When participants rated pain intensities between 60 and 70, the corresponding pressure was chosen for US presentation during the conditioning procedure.

During conditioning, one geometric visual symbol (CS^+) was consistently paired with a painful rectal distension (US) while a second visual cue (CS^-) was never followed by the US (differential delay conditioning) (**Figure 1A**). Overall, 32 CS were presented (16 CS^+ and 16 CS^-) in pseudo-randomized order with a 75% reinforcement schedule, i.e., 12 out of 16 CS^+ were followed by a US and 4 CS^+ remained unpaired. Duration of distensions was 16 s and US onset varied randomly between 6 and 12 s after CS^+ onset with both stimuli co-terminating. Please note that reinforced CS^+ were presented longer than non-reinforced CS^+. Inter-trial intervals (ITI) were 20 s. In our previous conditioning studies, this conditioning paradigm revealed successful pain-related learning to threat and safety cues on behavioral and neural measures in healthy individuals (19, 56) and in patients with chronic visceral pain (16, 17).

Behavioral Measures of Emotional Learning and Contingency Awareness

Online visual analog scales (VAS) were used to assess learning-induced changes in CS valence along with expected changes in cognitive aspects that together verify the efficacy of conditioning herein (57). Prior pain-related conditioning studies from our own group [reviewed in (58, 59)] and in the broader fear conditioning literature support the notion that conditioned changes in cue valence constitutes a sensitive and relevant behavioral measure (60, 61). CS valence was assessed at three time points: (1) after the first dot-probe task and prior to conditioning (baseline), (2) after conditioning and (3) following the second dot-probe task. Participants were prompted to indicate how they perceived each of the visual cues by presenting a digitized vertical

200 mm scale with end points labeled "very unpleasant" and "very pleasant," indicating "neutral" in the middle of the scale. These values were then transformed into a scale with end points −100 indicating "very pleasant," 100 indicating "very unpleasant" and "neutral" at 0 as previously accomplished in all of our prior conditioning work with this visceral pain model (13, 19–21). After conditioning, contingency awareness was assessed with ratings on how often each of the visual cues was followed by a rectal distension with corresponding scale end points labeled "never" (0%) and "always" (100%).

Statistical Analyses

Analyses of all data were carried out with the Statistical Package for the Social Sciences (SPSS, IBM Corp. IBM SPSS Statistics for Windows, Version 22.0. Armonk, NY: IBM Corp.). Initially, we analyzed whether women and men were comparable with respect to social demographics, psychological state and trait variables as well as perceptual and pain thresholds. All variables were normally distributed and analyzed by means of two-sample t-tests.

For CS valence ratings, we conducted a repeated measures ANCOVA with within-subject factors CS (CS^+, CS^-, CS^n) and phase (baseline, conditioning, test phase), between-subject factor sex (women, men), and BMI as covariate due to a significant difference between women and men for each condition separately. For CS-US contingency, paired t-tests were calculated with values assessed after conditioning for women and men separately.

For attentional bias indices, we carried out repeated measures ANCOVAs with the within-subject factors phase (baseline, test phase), stimulus duration (100, 500 ms), the between-subject factor sex (women, men), and BMI as covariate. To address the specificity of attentional bias to threat and safety cues, we further compared trials presenting a CS with a neutral cue with trials presenting both CS^+ and CS^- using repeated measures ANCOVAs with within-subject factors condition ($CS + CS^n$, $CS^+ + CS^-$), phase (baseline, test phase), the between-subject factor sex (women, men), and BMI as covariate. Results are reported for significant interactions with Greenhouse-Geisser correction and post-hoc testing was accomplished with Bonferroni correction to adjust for multiple comparisons. To test the effects of response slowing as a potential confound in analyses of attentional biases, we furthermore performed ANCOVAS using reaction time data. For these analyses, conditions presenting the CS^+ with the neutral cue were compared with conditions presenting only neutral cues to test for cue ($CS^+ + CS^n$; $CS^n + CS^n$) × congruency (congruent trials; incongruent trials) interactions.

Finally, we carried out multiple regression analyses to predict changes in indices of attentional avoidance, engagement and disengagement from baseline to test phase for each condition separately. Predictors included sex, psychological vulnerability factors of trait anxiety (STAI-T), positive and negative affect (PANAS-P, PANAS-N), cognitive coping and catastrophizing (PRSS) and CS valence changes. Moreover, interaction terms with sex were calculated by multiplying sex by each predictor. For all regression models, sex was entered into the first block and always maintained. Into the second block, a pair including the main effect and interaction with sex for one predictor was

entered. If the regression model did not yield significance, the interaction term was removed first and the subsequent regression model was set up with sex in the first block and the main effect of the predictor in the second block. If the main effect did not yield significance, it was removed from the model and the subsequent regression model was set up with sex only. Results are reported with F- and p-values, adjusted R^2 and for the coefficients, standardized beta-, t-, and p-values are given. If the main effect and/ or interaction term was found as significant predictor, subsequent regression analyses were carried out with the main effect of the predictor for women and men separately, reporting F- and p-values and adjusted R^2 for the model and for the coefficient the beta- and t-values. Detailed results of the regression analyses are given in the **Supplementary Material**.

All data are given as mean ± standard error of the mean (SEM), unless indicated otherwise.

RESULTS
Sample Characteristics

In total, 64 healthy volunteers (32 women, 32 men) completed the study. Sociodemographic and psychological characteristics were comparable between men and women, except for a lower BMI in women (**Table 1**). Positive and negative affective states (PANAS), trait anxiety (STAI-T) and pain-related cognitions including catastrophizing and active coping (PRSS), all assessed upon arrival to the laboratory on the study day, did not reveal differences between women and men. Likewise, neuropsychological attention tests including the TMT and Stroop task as well as rectal and pain thresholds were comparable between groups (**Table 1**).

CS Valence and CS-US Contingency

For CS valence (**Figure 2**; for single subject data see **Figure S1**), analysis revealed a significant time × CS interaction ($F = 2.79$, $p = .038$, $\eta^2 = .05$), supporting the efficacy of the conditioning procedure without any effect of sex ($F = 0.01$, $p = .943$). While ratings of all CS were expectedly comparable and neutral at baseline (all $p > .598$), after conditioning both women and men perceived the CS^+ as significantly more unpleasant and the CS^- as more pleasant compared to the neutral cue (both $p < .001$). The difference between CS^+ and CS^- was still evident after the test phase ($p < .001$), indicating persisting effects of conditioning. Likewise, both men and women were similarly aware of conditioning contingencies for both CS^+ and CS^-, as supported by changes in CS-US contingency ratings assessed after conditioning with higher perceived contingency for CS^+-US pairings compared to CS^--US pairings in women (CS^+-US contingency M ± SEM: 77.41% ± 2.46; CS^--US contingency: 15.69% ± 3.63; $t = 11.00$, $p < .001$), and men (CS^+-US contingency: 81.63% ± 2.18; CS^--US contingency: 11.41% ± 3.46; $t = 15.42$, $p < .001$).

Sex Differences in Indices of Attentional Bias
Attentional Avoidance

For attentional avoidance indices (**Table 2**; for single subject data see **Figure S2**), analyses yielded no significant interactions

TABLE 1 | Sample characterization.

	Full sample	Women	Men	Statistics
(A) Measured during screening				
Age	28.22 ± 1.00	28.53 ± 1.71	27.91 ± 1.06	$t = 0.31, p = .757$
Body mass index	22.79 ± 0.33	21.92 ± 0.41	23.66 ± 0.47	$t = 2.80, p = .007$
Gastrointestinal symptoms	2.70 ± 0.36	3.13 ± 0.55	2.28 ± 0.46	$t = 1.18, p = .241$
HADS anxiety	3.70 ± 0.32	4.16 ± 0.48	3.25 ± 0.42	$t = 1.44, p = .156$
HADS depression	1.76 ± 0.28	1.29 ± 0.26	2.22 ± 0.48	$t = 1.68, p = .096$
(B) Measured on study day				
STAI Trait	35.67 ± 0.89	36.75 ± 1.35	34.59 ± 1.16	$t = 1.21, p = .230$
PANAS positive	3.25 ± 0.08	3.27 ± 0.12	3.24 ± 0.11	$t = 0.15, p = .885$
PANAS negative	1.39 ± 0.06	1.41 ± 0.09	1.37 ± 0.08	$t = 0.37, p = .715$
PRSS catastrophizing	0.80 ± 0.10	0.77 ± 0.17	0.83 ± 0.12	$t = 0.31, p = .762$
PRSS coping	3.54 ± 0.10	3.57 ± 0.14	3.52 ± 0.15	$t = 0.24, p = .811$
TMT version A	26.30 ± 1.03	26.59 ± 1.60	26.00 ± 1.33	$t = 0.29, p = .776$
TMT version B	53.70 ± 2.36	54.72 ± 2.34	52.69 ± 4.13	$t = 0.43, p = .670$
SCWT word reading	30.65 ± 0.64	30.97 ± 1.09	30.34 ± 0.69	$t = 0.49, p = .628$
SCWT color naming	47.29 ± 1.10	48.32 ± 1.72	46.28 ± 1.39	$t = 0.93, p = .358$
SCWT color-word naming	69.25 ± 1.66	70.61 ± 2.68	67.94 ± 2.00	$t = 0.80, p = .425$
Perception threshold	15.75 ± 0.82	16.33 ± 1.22	15.17 ± 1.11	$t = 0.71, p = .483$
Pain threshold	39.21 ± 1.29	38.04 ± 1.90	40.34 ± 1.75	$t = 0.90, p = .375$

Overview of sociodemographic and psychological variables as well neuropsychological attention test results obtained during screening procedure (A) and on study day (B). Psychological variables were assessed with the Hospital Anxiety and Depression Scale (HADS), State-Trait Anxiety Inventory (STAI) including only the trait subscale, Positive, and Negative Affective Schedule (PANAS) including positive and negative subscales and Pain-Related Self Statements Scale (PRSS) including subscales of pain catastrophizing and coping. Neuropsychological attention tests included the Trail Making Test (TMT) with versions A and B as well as the Stroop color word test (Stroop) with conditions word reading, color naming and the interference condition of color-word naming, all results given in seconds. During the individual rectal distention calibration procedure, perception, and pain thresholds were measured in mmHG. All values are given as mean ± standard error of the mean (M ± SEM). Differences between women and men were calculated by means of independent sample t-tests.

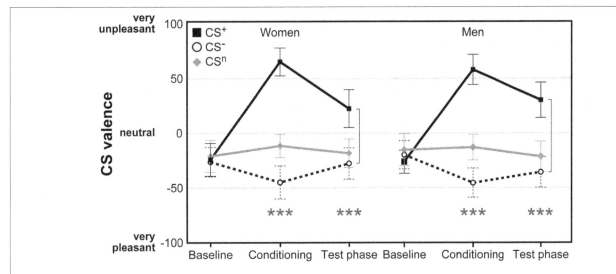

FIGURE 2 | Ratings of CS valence assessed on visual analog scales (VAS) before and after conditioning as well as after the test phase. Both women and men demonstrated significant increases in CS+ aversiveness and increases in CS− pleasantness following acquisition without differences between groups. ***$p < 0.001$.

between phase and sex (all $F < 0.45$, all $p > .507$), and no significant interactions between phase, sex and stimulus duration (all $F < 0.53$, all $p > .470$), indicating no differences in attentional avoidance between women and men.

Attentional Engagement

For attentional engagement indices (**Table 3**, **Figure 3A**; for single subject data see **Figure S3**), analyses revealed significant phase × sex interactions for both conditions presenting the CS+

TABLE 2 | Indices of attentional avoidance.

	Women		Men					
	Baseline	Test phase	Baseline	Test phase	Interaction effect	F	p	η^2
CS^+/CS^n	2.73 ± 2.20	5.55 ± 2.96	3.28 ± 3.67	2.88 ± 2.59	Phase $\times$ sex	0.13	.717	.00
					Phase $\times$ duration $\times$ sex	0.53	.470	.01
CS^-/CS^n	5.99 ± 3.53	1.66 ± 3.51	10.87 ± 2.98	5.96 ± 2.71	Phase $\times$ sex	0.45	.507	.01
					Phase $\times$ duration $\times$ sex	0.16	.691	.00
CS^+/CS^-	-5.89 ± 3.34	-2.78 ± 3.10	-6.72 ± 3.40	-6.17 ± 3.50	Phase $\times$ sex	0.18	.671	.00
					Phase $\times$ duration $\times$ sex	0.38	.542	.01

Descriptive statistics and results from ANCOVAs comparing indices of attentional avoidance across phase (baseline vs. test phase), stimulus duration (100 ms, 500 ms) and sex (women vs. men). Conditions include presentation of CS^+ and CS^- each with a neutral cue and presentation of CS^+ and CS^- together. Descriptive statistics are given as mean values across 100 and 500 ms stimulus duration $\pm$ standard error of the mean (M $\pm$ SEM).

TABLE 3 | Indices of attentional engagement.

	Women		Men					
	Baseline	Test phase	Baseline	Test phase	Interaction effect	F	p	η^2
<u>CS^+</u>/CS^n	5.39 ± 2.62	-1.43 ± 2.19	3.93 ± 3.87	4.90 ± 3.39	Phase $\times$ sex	**9.20**	**.004**	**.16**
					Phase $\times$ duration $\times$ sex	0.12	.731	.00
<u>CS^+</u>/CS^-	3.49 ± 3.30	-3.47 ± 3.09	-6.10 ± 1.81	-2.36 ± 2.29	Phase $\times$ sex	**11.73**	**.001**	**.18**
					Phase $\times$ duration $\times$ sex	0.36	.551	.01
<u>CS^-</u>/CS^n	6.48 ± 4.57	-3.88 ± 2.95	5.40 ± 3.61	5.20 ± 2.43	Phase $\times$ sex	**7.06**	**.011**	**.14**
					Phase $\times$ duration $\times$ sex	0.03	.869	.00
<u>CS^-</u>/CS^+	9.04 ± 4.39	8.89 ± 3.63	0.62 ± 3.51	2.37 ± 3.52	Phase $\times$ sex	2.13	.151	.05
					Phase $\times$ duration $\times$ sex	0.61	.441	.01

Descriptive statistics and results from ANCOVAs comparing indices of attentional engagement across phase (baseline vs. test phase), stimulus duration (100, 500 ms) and sex (women vs. men). Conditions include presentation of CS^+ and CS^- each with a neutral cue and presentation of CS^+ and CS^- together. The underscore indicates the appearance of the dot-probe at the location either of the CS^+ or CS^-. Descriptive statistics are given as mean values across 100 and 500 ms stimulus duration $\pm$ standard error of the mean (M $\pm$ SEM). Significant interactions are given in bold.

and the CS^- with the neutral cue (all $F > 7.06$, all $p < .011$, all $\eta^2 > .14$). However, there was no effect of stimulus duration (all $F < 0.61$, all $p > .441$). *Post-hoc* comparisons revealed during the test phase significantly higher indices for men (all $p < .038$), indicating that men showed higher attentional engagement after fear conditioning compared to women. In contrast, women revealed significant decreases from baseline to test phase in attentional engagement indices across these conditions (all $p < .021$), while revealed a significant increase in response to the CS^+ when presented together with the CS^- ($p = .032$).

To further investigate the specificity of attentional engagement, conditions presenting one CS with the neutral cue were compared with conditions presenting both the CS^+ and CS^-. For the CS^-, analyses revealed an interaction between condition, phase and sex that marginally missed to yield significance ($F = 3.87$, $p = .054$). Exploratory *post-hoc* analyses revealed for women significantly higher attentional engagement with the CS^- when presented with the CS^+ as compared to the concomitant presentation of the neutral cue ($p = .012$) while for men no effects were observed.

Attentional Disengagement

For disengagement indices (**Table 4**, **Figure 3B**; for single subject data see **Figure S4**), analyses revealed significant phase $\times$ sex

interactions for conditions when the CS^+ and CS^- were each presented with the neutral cue as well as for the CS^- when presented with the CS^+ (all $F > 6.44$, all $p < .014$, all $\eta^2 > .11$). Stimulus duration again had no effect (all $F < 0.66$, all $p > .421$). *Post-hoc* comparisons between women and men during the test phase yielded significance only when the CS^+ was presented with the neutral cue ($p = .009$) indicating that women had stronger difficulties to disengage attention from the CS^+. For the remaining conditions, results did not survive Bonferroni correction (CS^-/CS^n $p = .080$; CS^-/CS^+ $p = .062$). Moreover, comparisons between baseline and test phase revealed that women had stronger difficulties to disengage from the CS^+ when presented with the neutral cue ($p = .010$) and from the CS^- when presented with the CS^+ ($p = .023$) while men demonstrated significant increases in these conditions (both $p < .039$). Further analyses on the specificity of attentional disengagement between conditions did not yield significance.

Response Slowing

Previous research on the allocation of visuospatial attention demonstrated a response slowing effect of threat indicating that differences in reaction times between trials containing a threat cue and trials containing a neutral cue might arise from avoidance or freezing of motor responses [e.g.,

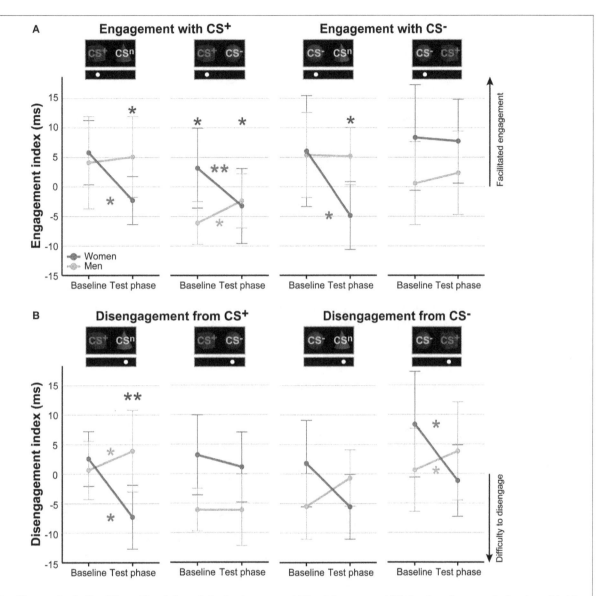

FIGURE 3 | Sex differences in attentional biases. Mean indices of attentional engagement **(A)** and disengagement **(B)** given in ms for women (red) and men (blue) for the dot-probe tasks accomplished at baseline and during the test phase. Please note that mean values depicted in the figure are not corrected for BMI that was used as covariate in statistical analyses. Significant differences between women and men are given with gray asterisks and within-group differences between baseline and test phase are given with the corresponding color code for women and men. Men compared to women showed higher attentional engagement with the CS$^+$ and CS$^-$ when presented with the neutral cue and with the CS$^+$ when presented together with the CS$^-$. Women compared to men demonstrated stronger difficulties to disengage attention from the CS$^+$ when presented with the neutral cue. $^{**}p < .010$; $^{*}p < .050$.

(57, 58)]. We tested for this effect by comparing reaction times from conditions presenting the CS$^+$ with a neutral cue with conditions presenting the neutral cue only for 100 and 500 ms stimulus duration. For 100 ms stimulus duration, the cue x congruency interaction yielded significance ($F = 7.80$, $p = .007$, $\eta^2 = .14$) with *post-hoc* comparisons demonstrating higher reaction times for incongruent compared to congruent CS$^+$ trials ($p = .017$). However, there were no significant differences between the CS$^+$ and the neutral condition for either congruent or incongruent trials (both $p > .102$). For 500 ms stimulus duration, there was no significant cue x congruency

interaction ($F = 1.81$, $p = .184$) indicating no effect of response slowing.

Sex-Specific Associations Between Emotional Learning, Psychological Traits and Attentional Biases

Multiple regression analyses with the main effects of sex, psychological vulnerability factors, and changes in CS valence as well as the interaction terms considering sex were calculated to predict changes in attentional biases from baseline to test phase.

TABLE 4 | Indices of attentional disengagement.

| | Women | | Men | | | | | |
	Baseline	Test phase	Baseline	Test phase	Interaction effect	F	p	η^2
CS+/CS^n	2.47 ± 2.25	−6.98 ± 2.64	0.65 ± 2.47	3.90 ± 3.46	Phase × sex	**10.36**	**.002**	**.18**
					Phase × duration × sex	0.66	.421	.01
CS+/CS−	9.04 ± 4.39	−0.69 ± 2.98	0.62 ± 3.51	3.81 ± 4.16	Phase × sex	1.92	.173	.04
					Phase × duration × sex	0.47	.497	.01
CS−/CS^n	2.21 ± 3.57	−5.54 ± 2.66	−5.48 ± 2.78	−0.67 ± 2.39	Phase × sex	**6.44**	**.014**	**.11**
					Phase × duration × sex	0.05	.831	.00
CS−/CS+	3.49 ± 3.30	1.31 ± 2.88	−6.10 ± 1.81	−6.14 ± 3.03	Phase × sex	**9.73**	**.003**	**.15**
					Phase × duration × sex	0.06	.802	.00

Descriptive statistics and results from ANCOVAs comparing indices of attentional disengagement across phase (baseline vs. test phase), stimulus duration (100, 500 ms) and sex (women vs. men). Conditions include presentation of CS+ and CS− each with a neutral cue and presentation of CS+ and CS− together. The underscore indicates the appearance of the dot-probe at the location either of the CS+ or CS−. Descriptive statistics are given as mean values across 100 and 500 ms stimulus duration ± standard error of the mean (M ± SEM). Significant interactions are given in bold.

For attentional avoidance, the model with the interaction between sex and negative affect as well as the interaction between sex and active coping yielded significance ($F = 4.48$, $p = .007$, adj. $R^2 = .14$). Both, the interaction sex*negative affect ($\beta = 0.48$, $t = 3.04$, $p = .004$) and sex*active coping emerged as significant predictors ($\beta = -0.45$, $t = 2.26$, $p = .028$) while sex alone did not yield significance ($\beta = 0.06$, $t = 0.26$, $p = .797$) (for more details, see **Table S1**). Subsequent analyses revealed a larger slope for men ($F = 9.03$, $p = .005$, adj. $R^2 = .23$, $\beta = 0.48$, $t = 3.01$) compared to women ($F = 0.02$, $p = .879$, adj. $R^2 = -.03$, $\beta = 0.03$, $t = 0.15$), indicating that only in men higher negative affect was associated with stronger avoidance of the CS+ when presented with the CS−. However, for active coping neither regression model yielded significance although the slope observed for men ($F = 2.76$, $p = .107$, adj. $R^2 = .06$, $\beta = -0.29$, $t = 1.67$) was higher compared to women ($F = 2.76$, $p = .107$, adj. $R^2 = .06$, $\beta = -0.29$, $t = 1.67$).

For attentional engagement, sex was found as a significant predictor ($F = 4.27$, $p = .043$, adj. $R^2 = .05$, $\beta = 0.25$, $t = 2.07$) for the condition presenting the CS+ together with the CS− while regression models including psychological vulnerability factors and changes in CS valence failed to reach significance ($F = 3.77$, $p = .057$, adj. $R^2 = .04$) (**Table S2**).

For attentional disengagement, sex emerged as a significant predictor for conditions presenting the CS+ with the neutral cue ($F = 4.95$, $p = .030$, adj. $R^2 = .06$, $\beta = 0.27$, $t = 2.22$) and the CS− with the neutral cue ($F = 5.14$, $p = .027$, adj. $R^2 = .06$, $\beta = 0.28$, $t = 2.27$) (**Tables S3, S4**). Moreover, for the condition presenting the CS− together with the CS+, the model including sex, negative affect and sex*negative affect yielded significance ($F = 4.93$, $p = .004$, adj. $R^2 = .16$) (**Table S5**). Herein, sex ($\beta = 1.13$, $t = 3.18$, $p = .002$), negative affect ($\beta = 0.84$, $t = 2.36$, $p = .022$) and the interaction between sex and negative affect ($\beta = 1.54$, $t = 3.19$, $p = .002$) were found as significant predictors. Subsequent regression analyses for the interaction effect revealed a larger slope for men ($F = 16.99$, $p < .001$, adj. $R^2 = .34$, $\beta = -0.60$, $t = 4.12$) compared to women ($F = 0.36$, $p = .555$, adj. $R^2 = -.02$, $\beta = 0.11$, $t = 0.60$), indicating that only in men higher

negative affect was related to stronger difficulties to disengage from the CS−.

DISCUSSION

Although the broad role of fear and hypervigilance in the transition from acute to chronic pain is widely acknowledged, pain-related attentional biases as putative neurocognitive mechanism remain incompletely understood. In addition, sex differences as they are considered highly relevant to both acute and chronic pain are rarely systematically studied, especially in the context of visceral pain (62). The aim of this study was to elucidate attentional biases induced by pain-related conditioning in healthy women and men. To this end, we implemented a visual dot-probe task before and after differential fear conditioning with visceral pain as highly salient and clinically relevant interoceptive US (12, 13, 63). Conditioning successfully induced emotional pain-related learning to threat and safety cues, as evidenced by differential changes in cue valence. Consistent with behavioral and neural findings in our earlier conditioning studies (12, 19, 21), visual cues that were contingently paired with visceral pain became highly unpleasant predictors of threat, likely reflecting conditioned pain-related fear in anticipation of visceral pain. In contrast, cues that predicted the absence of impending pain acquired positive emotional valence, consistent with their role as conditioned safety signals. There was no evidence of sex differences in emotional pain-related learning, confirming earlier behavioral results in a different, smaller sample of healthy volunteers (23). Similarly, men and women did not differ in contingency awareness of cue-pain relationships, which was fairly accurate in both sexes. Interestingly, comparing men and women with respect to attentional avoidance, facilitated engagement, and difficulties to disengage from visceral pain-related threat and safety cues revealed novel evidence supporting sex differences in attentional biases. Specifically, men showed more facilitated attentional engagement with both threat and safety cues. Women, on the other hand, demonstrated more pronounced difficulties to disengage from threat in the presence of a neutral cue. However, when both threat and safety cues were presented, women showed stronger difficulties to disengage from the safety cue. While these findings do not support our hypothesis of facilitated threat engagement in women, they are consistent with a proposed bias toward safety cues. While the role of conditioned safety signals remains incompletely understood and arguably underappreciated, we previously reported distinctly altered neural processes during safety learning in healthy women (18) as well as in women with IBS (17). Specifically, IBS patients demonstrated a more pronounced positive valence increase to conditioned safety cues, higher awareness of safety cue contingencies, as well as greater neural responses involving regions relevant to reward processing (17) and conditioned autonomic, somatomotor and cognitive fear responses (16). Distinct neural networks engaged during the acquisition and extinction of conditioned threat vs. safety cues have not only been reported in our model, but also more broadly in the fear conditioning literature (64). Together, our findings support that visceral pain-related fear conditioning induces attentional biases differently in healthy women and men, supporting a role of sex or gender in attentional mechanisms underlying hypervigilance.

Attentional biases to signals predicting experimental pain have previously been shown, albeit outside of interoceptive, visceral pain, as summarized in recent meta-analyses (11, 65). Our results complement results gathered in different conditioning paradigms (47, 48, 66–69), and extend knowledge regarding the role of pain-related fear as a putative mediator. Moreover, several psychological state and trait factors demonstrably contribute to inter-individual differences in the modulation of pain (22, 70, 71), which have thus far rarely been considered in experimental studies on pain-related attentional biases. Therefore, we explored sex differences in relationships between attentional biases and positive and negative affect, trait anxiety, pain-related coping and catastrophizing using regression analyses. Our results revealed an influence of sex on negative affect in predicting attentional threat avoidance and difficulties to disengage from the safety cue. This finding is well in line with the fear avoidance model of chronic pain, emphasizing that a higher propensity toward experiencing negative emotions impacts upon pain control and increases pain-related fear, thereby promoting avoidance behaviors (72). Interestingly, these effects were observed in men while no relationships between psychological vulnerability factors and attentional biases were observed in women. While this is at odds with our hypothesis, we cannot with certainty exclude a self-selection bias for participation due to the research setting at a university hospital and the nature of the study, specifically concerning the application of painful stimuli (73). This may have resulted in an overall sample of healthy individuals presenting with rather low anxiety and negative affect and may have specifically discouraged healthy women with higher experience of gastrointestinal symptoms. Therefore, the translation to the general population or patient populations is limited. Moreover, it has previously been suggested that individuals with high fear of pain exhibit a selective attention bias toward pain-related information, supporting that biased attentional processes mediate increased susceptibility to negative pain experience (74, 75). Our conditioning model experimentally induces fear

as a state, rather than a trait assessed by questionnaire. This calls attention to the fact that fear of pain and by inference pain-related attentional biases are likely shaped by more permanent, trait-like factors, as well as more state-like learning processes regarding threat and reward. Hence, inter-individual differences in pain-related attentional biases could be explained by pre-existing differences in fear of pain, as previously shown in our visceral pain model (12), as well as by sex differences, as suggested herein.

Herein, men and women were comparable with respect to pain thresholds and pain ratings, and the intensity of pain stimuli implemented during conditioning was individually calibrated, supporting that sex differences in attentional biases were not attributable to differences in the response to pain or in the strength of emotional learning to either threat or safety cues. Further strengths of this study include the ecological validity and translational qualities of the visceral pain model, as rectal distension-induced pain is highly salient even in healthy individuals (12) and closely resembles clinical pain and related symptoms such as urgency (73) in functional gastrointestinal disorders like IBS (76). In the context of attentional bias research, the utilization of semantic and pictorial threat stimuli has raised concerns about their ecological validity and generalizability (26), resulting in calls for research with paradigms that closely resemble real-life situations (77) or consider motivational context (69). In line with these efforts, our model offers research perspectives in patient populations, especially those with somatic symptom disorder or chronic visceral pain such as in IBS. Utilizing modified Stroop and exogenous cueing tasks, IBS patients revealed alterations in attentional processing for pain and symptom-related words (78, 79) as well as situational threat words (80). This attentional bias was moreover associated with symptom severity, illness behaviors and anxiety (49, 80, 81). Hence, increased attention to interoceptive, visceral sensations may lead to the exacerbation of symptoms and distress (82) in line with the fear avoidance model, which has yet to be more fully tested in the context of chronic visceral pain and the gut-brain axis. Neuroimaging studies support this assumption by demonstrating increased functional connectivity in the salience network in IBS patients during resting state (83), rectal stimulation (84) and contextual threat situations (85). Initial support that the behavioral modification of attentional bias may improve attentional functioning and regulation of brain mechanisms related to anxiety and attention in IBS patients (86, 87), provides a treatment perspective to complement more basic mechanistic research.

Lastly, our findings are relevant toward further elucidating the neurocognitive and emotional mechanisms of associative learning and memory processes in the context of visceral pain. Brain imaging studies revealed conditioning-induced changes in the brain emotional arousal and salience networks, supporting that conditioning processes contribute to hypervigilance, possibly by engaging nocebo mechanisms (58). It has also been proposed that pain-related conditioning may impair perceptual discrimination acuity (88), enhance fear generalization (89) or interfere with normal habituation processes (90). Although our attempts to show hyperalgesia as a result of conditioning provided negative results (21, 63), data from other groups do support sensitization (91, 92) and lowered pain thresholds (93). Regardless of these inconsistencies and a clear need for further study, it is important to emphasize that different yet intricately intertwined mechanisms engaged during associative learning are clearly not mutually exclusive. They may indeed play distinct roles in modulating responses to acute pain, shaping the transition from acute to chronic pain and the maintenance of pain. Importantly, attentional biases arguably play a role in many if not all of these proposed processes, and could thus be viewed as a fundamental neurocognitive mechanism that is shaped by pain-related learning and memory processes (48, 94). This is supported by first evidence that attentional bias to threat signals is still present after extinction (47) and re-emerges during reinstatement (48), consistent with our brain imaging work on the reactivation of previously extinguished responses to conditioned pain and safety cues induced by reinstatement (20, 56) or renewal (19).

ETHICS STATEMENT

The studies involving human participants were reviewed and approved by the Ethics Committee of the University Hospital Essen, Germany. The patients/participants provided their written informed consent to participate in this study.

AUTHOR CONTRIBUTIONS

FL and SE planned the study, contributed to data analysis and interpretation and wrote the manuscript. FL and SK-R were involved in conducting the study. All authors: revision of the manuscript for critical intellectual content and approval of the final draft submitted. All authors contributed to manuscript revision, read and approved the submitted version.

ACKNOWLEDGMENTS

The authors thank Christoph Ritter and Ann-Kathrin Stock for excellent technical support and Madeleine Hetkamp and Simone Kotulla for excellent support in conducting this project.

REFERENCES

1. Flor H. New developments in the understanding and management of persistent pain. *Curr Opin Psychiatry.* (2012) 25:109–13. doi: 10.1097/YCO.0b013e3283503510
2. Harvie DS, Moseley GL, Hillier SL, Meulders A. Classical conditioning differences associated with chronic pain: a systematic review. *J Pain.* (2017) 18:889–98. doi: 10.1016/j.jpain.2017.02.430
3. Crombez G, Eccleston C, Van Damme S, Vlaeyen JWS, Karoly P. Fear-Avoidance model of chronic pain. *Clin J Pain.* (2012) 28:475–83. doi: 10.1097/AJP.0b013e3182385392
4. Hollander M den, de Jong JR, Volders S, Goossens ME, Smeets RJ, Vlaeyen JW. Fear reduction in patients with chronic pain: a learning theory perspective. *Expert Rev Neurother.* (2010) 10:1733–45. doi: 10.1586/ern.10.115
5. Van Ryckeghem DML, Crombez G, Goubert L, De Houwer J, Onraedt T, Van Damme S. The predictive value of attentional bias towards pain-related information in chronic pain patients: a diary study. *Pain.* (2013) 154:468–75. doi: 10.1016/j.pain.2012.12.008
6. Schoth DE, Nunes VD, Liossi C. Attentional bias towards pain-related information in chronic pain; a meta-analysis of visual-probe investigations. *Clin Psychol Rev.* (2012) 32:13–25. doi: 10.1016/j.cpr.2011.09.004
7. Cisler JM, Bacon AK, Williams NL. Phenomenological characteristics of attentional biases towards threat: a critical review. *Cognit Ther Res.* (2009) 33:221–34. doi: 10.1007/s10608-007-9161-y
8. Koster EHW, Crombez G, Verschuere B, Van Damme S, Wiersema JR. Components of attentional bias to threat in high trait anxiety: facilitated engagement, impaired disengagement, and attentional avoidance. *Behav Res Ther.* (2006) 44:1757–71. doi: 10.1016/j.brat.2005.12.011
9. Mogg K, Bradley BP. Anxiety and attention to threat: cognitive mechanisms and treatment with attention bias modification. *Behav Res Ther.* (2016) 87:76–108. doi: 10.1016/j.brat.2016.08.001
10. Schoorl M, Putman P, Van Der Werff S, Van Der Does AJW. Attentional bias and attentional control in posttraumatic stress disorder. *J Anxiety Disord.* (2014) 28:203–10. doi: 10.1016/j.janxdis.2013.10.001
11. Crombez G, Van Ryckeghem DML, Eccleston C, Van Damme S. Attentional bias to pain-related information: a meta-analysis. *Pain.* (2013) 154:497–510. doi: 10.1016/j.pain.2012.11.013
12. Koenen LR, Icenhour A, Forkmann K, Pasler A, Theysohn N, Forsting M, et al. Greater fear of visceral pain contributes to differences between visceral and somatic pain in healthy women. *Pain.* (2017) 158:1599–608. doi: 10.1097/j.pain.0000000000000924
13. Koenen LR, Icenhour A, Forkmann K, Theysohn N, Forsting M, Bingel U, et al. From anticipation to the experience of pain: the importance of visceral versus somatic pain modality in neural and behavioral responses to pain-predictive cues. *Psychosom Med.* (2018) 80:826–35. doi: 10.1097/PSY.0000000000000612
14. Schmidt LJ, Belopolsky AV, Theeuwes J. The time course of attentional bias to cues of threat and safety. *Cogn Emot.* (2017) 31:845–57. doi: 10.1080/02699931.2016.1169998
15. Vogt J, Koster EHW, De Houwer J. Safety first: instrumentality for reaching safety determines attention allocation under threat. *Emotion.* (2017) 17:528–37. doi: 10.1037/emo0000251
16. Claassen J, Labrenz F, Ernst TM, Icenhour A, Langhorst J, Forsting M, et al. Altered cerebellar activity in visceral pain-related fear conditioning in irritable bowel syndrome. *Cerebellum.* (2017) 16:508–17. doi: 10.1007/s12311-016-0832-7
17. Icenhour A, Langhorst J, Benson S, Schlamann M, Hampel S, Engler H, et al. Neural circuitry of abdominal pain-related fear learning and reinstatement in irritable bowel syndrome. *Neurogastroenterol Motil.* (2015) 27:114–27. doi: 10.1111/nmo.12489
18. Labrenz F, Icenhour A, Thürling M, Schlamann M, Forsting M, Timmann D, et al. Sex differences in cerebellar mechanisms involved in pain-related safety learning. *Neurobiol Learn Mem.* (2015) 123:92–9. doi: 10.1016/j.nlm.2015.05.006
19. Icenhour A, Kattoor J, Benson S, Boekstegers A, Schlamann M, Merz CJ, et al. Neural circuitry underlying effects of context on human pain-related fear extinction in a renewal paradigm. *Hum Brain Mapp.* (2015) 36:3179–93. doi: 10.1002/hbm.22837

20. Kattoor J, Gizewski ER, Kotsis V, Benson S, Gramsch C, Theysohn N, et al. Fear conditioning in an abdominal pain model: neural responses during associative learning and extinction in healthy subjects. *PLoS ONE*. (2013) 8:e51149. doi: 10.1371/journal.pone.0051149

21. Labrenz F, Icenhour A, Schlamann M, Forsting M, Bingel U, Elsenbruch S. From Pavlov to pain: how predictability affects the anticipation and processing of visceral pain in a fear conditioning paradigm. *Neuroimage*. (2016) 130:104–14. doi: 10.1016/j.neuroimage.2016.01.064

22. Fillingim RB, King CD, Ribeiro-Dasilva MC, Rahim-Williams B, Riley JL. Sex, gender, and pain: a review of recent clinical and experimental findings. *J Pain*. (2009) 10:447–85. doi: 10.1016/j.jpain.2008.12.001

23. Benson S, Kattoor J, Kullmann JS, Hofmann S, Engler H, Forsting M, et al. Towards understanding sex differences in visceral pain: enhanced reactivation of classically-conditioned fear in healthy women. *Neurobiol Learn Mem*. (2014) 109:113–21. doi: 10.1016/j.nlm.2013.12.014

24. Keogh E, Hatton K, Ellery D. Avoidance versus focused attention and the perception of pain: differential effects for men and women. *Pain*. (2000) 85:225–30. doi: 10.1016/S0304-3959(99)00270-5

25. Brookes M, Sharpe L, Kozlowska K. Attentional and interpretational biases toward pain-related stimuli in children and adolescents: asystematic review of the evidence. *J Pain*. (2018) 19:1091–101. doi: 10.1016/j.jpain.2018.04.010

26. Dear BF, Sharpe L, Nicholas MK, Refshauge K. Pain-related attentional biases: the importance of the personal relevance and ecological validity of stimuli. *J Pain*. (2011) 12:625–32. doi: 10.1016/j.jpain.2010.11.010

27. MacLeod C, Grafton B. Anxiety-linked attentional bias and its modification: illustrating the importance of distinguishing processes and procedures in experimental psychopathology research. *Behav Res Ther*. (2016) 86:68–86. doi: 10.1016/j.brat.2016.07.005

28. Christianson JP, Fernando ABP, Kazama AM, Jovanovic T, Ostroff LE, Sangha S. Inhibition of fear by learned safety signals: a mini-symposium review. *J Neurosci*. (2012) 32:14118–24. doi: 10.1523/JNEUROSCI.3340-12.2012

29. Erdfelder E, Faul F, Buchner A, Lang AG. Statistical power analyses using G*Power 3.1: tests for correlation and regression analyses. *Behav Res Methods*. (2009) 41:1149–60. doi: 10.3758/BRM.41.4.1149

30. Herrmann-Lingen C, Buss U, Snaith R. *Hospital Anxiety and Depression Scale - Deutsche Version. Second*. Bern: Hans Huber (2005).

31. Lacourt TE, Houtveen JH, Doornen LJP, Benson S, Grigoleit JS, Cesko E, et al. Biological and psychological predictors of visceral pain sensitivity in healthy premenopausal women. *Eur J Pain*. (2014) 18:567–74. doi: 10.1002/j.1532-2149.2013.00397.x

32. Laux L, Glanzmann P, Schaffner P, Spielberger C. *Das State-Trait-Angstinventar. Theoretische Grundlagen und Handanweisung*. Weinheim: Beltz (1981).

33. Flor H, Behle DJ, Birbaumer N. Assessment of pain-related cognitions in chronic pain patients. *Behav Res Ther*. (1993) 31:63–73. doi: 10.1016/0005-7967(93)90044-U

34. Watson D, Clark LA, Tellegen A. Development and validation of brief measures of positive and negative affect: the PANAS scales. *J Pers Soc Psychol*. (1988) 54:1063–70. doi: 10.1037/0022-3514.54.6.1063

35. Partington J, Leiter R. Partington's pathway test. *Psychol Serv Cent J*. (1949) 1:9–20.

36. Tombaugh TN. Trail making test a and b: normative data stratified by age and education. *Arch Clin Neuropsychol*. (2004) 19:203–14. doi: 10.1016/S0887-6177(03)00039-8

37. Foroozandeh E. Gender differences in trail making test performance in a nonclinical sample of adults. *Int J Clin Exp Neurol*. (2014) 2:1–3. doi: 10.12691/ijcen-2-1-1

38. Macleod CM. The stroop task: the "gold standard" of attentional measures. *J Exp Psychol Gen*. (1992) 121:12–4. doi: 10.1037/0096-3445.121.1.12

39. Stroop JR. Studies of interference. *J Exp Psychol*. (1935) 18:643–62. doi: 10.1037/h0054651

40. MacLeod Colin M. Half a century of research on the stroop effect: an integrative review. *Psychol Bull*. (1991) 109:163–203. doi: 10.1037/0033-2909.109.2.163

41. Mekarski JE, Cutmore TRH, Suboski W. Gender differences during processing of the stroop task. *Percept Mot Skills*. (1996) 83:563–8. doi: 10.2466/pms.1996.83.2.563

42. Frewen PA, Dozois DJA, Joanisse MF, Neufeld RWJ. Selective attention to threat versus reward: meta-analysis and neural-network modeling of the dot-probe task. *Clin Psychol Rev*. (2008) 28:307–37. doi: 10.1016/j.cpr.2007.05.006

43. Deltomme B, Mertens G, Tibboel H, Braem S. Instructed fear stimuli bias visual attention. *Acta Psychol (Amst)*. (2018) 184:31–8. doi: 10.1016/j.actpsy.2017.08.010

44. Koenig S, Uengoer M, Lachnit H. Attentional bias for uncertain cues of shock in human fear conditioning: evidence for attentional learning theory. *Front Hum Neurosci*. (2017) 11:1–13. doi: 10.3389/fnhum.2017.00266

45. Schrooten MGS, Van Damme S, Crombez G, Peters ML, Vogt J, Vlaeyen JWS. Nonpain goal pursuit inhibits attentional bias to pain. *Pain*. (2012) 153:1180–6. doi: 10.1016/j.pain.2012.01.025

46. MacLeod C, Mathews A, Tata P. Attentional bias in emotional disorders. *J Abnorm Psychol*. (1986) 95:15–20. doi: 10.1037/0021-843X.95.1.15

47. Van Damme S, Crombez G, Eccleston C, Koster EHW. Hypervigilance to learned pain signals: a componential analysis. *J Pain*. (2006) 7:346–57. doi: 10.1016/j.jpain.2005.12.006

48. Van Damme S, Crombez G, Hermans D, Koster EHW, Eccleston C. The role of extinction and reinstatement in attentional bias to threat: a conditioning approach. *Behav Res Ther*. (2006) 44:1555–63. doi: 10.1016/j.brat.2005.11.008

49. Boyer MC, Compas BE, Stanger C, Colletti RB, Konik BS, Morrow SB, et al. Attentional biases to pain and social threat in children with recurrent abdominal pain. *J Pediatr Psychol*. (2006) 31:209–20. doi: 10.1093/jpepsy/jsj015

50. Price RB, Kuckertz JM, Siegle GJ, Ladouceur CD, Silk JS, Ryan ND, et al. Empirical recommendations for improving the stability of the dot-probe task in clinical research. *Psychol Assess*. (2015) 27:365–76. doi: 10.1037/pas0000036

51. Koster EHW, Verschuere B, Crombez G, Van Damme S. Time-course of attention for threatening pictures in high and low trait anxiety. *Behav Res Ther*. (2005) 43:1087–98. doi: 10.1016/j.brat.2004.08.004

52. Mogg K, Bradley BP, Miles F, Dixon R. Time course of attentional bias for threat scenes: testing the vigilance-avoidance hypothesis. *Cogn Emot*. (2004) 18:689–700. doi: 10.1080/02699930341000158

53. Bar-Haim Y, Lamy D, Pergamin L, Bakermans-Kranenburg MJ, Van Ijzendoorn MH. Threat-related attentional bias in anxious and nonanxious individuals: a meta-analytic study. *Psychol Bull*. (2007) 133:1–24. doi: 10.1037/0033-2909.133.1.1

54. Koster EHW, Crombez G, Verschuere B, De Houwer J. Selective attention to threat in the dot probe paradigm: differentiating vigilance and difficulty to disengage. *Behav Res Ther*. (2004) 42:1183–92. doi: 10.1016/j.brat.2003.08.001

55. Elsenbruch S, Rosenberger C, Enck P, Forsting M, Schedlowski M, Gizewski ER. Affective disturbances modulate the neural processing of visceral pain stimuli in irritable bowel syndrome: an fMRI study. *Gut*. (2010) 59:489–95. doi: 10.1136/gut.2008.175908

56. Gramsch C, Kattoor J, Icenhour A, Forsting M, Schedlowski M, Gizewski ER, et al. Learning pain-related fear: neural mechanisms mediating rapid differential conditioning, extinction and reinstatement processes in human visceral pain. *Neurobiol Learn Mem*. (2014) 116:36–45. doi: 10.1016/j.nlm.2014.08.003

57. Lonsdorf TB, Menz MM, Andreatta M, Fullana MA, Golkar A, Haaker J, et al. Don't fear 'fear conditioning': methodological considerations for the design and analysis of studies on human fear acquisition, extinction, and return of fear. *Neurosci Biobehav Rev*. (2017) 77:247–85. doi: 10.1016/j.neubiorev.2017.02.026

58. Elsenbruch S, Labrenz F. Nocebo effects and experimental models in visceral pain. *Int Rev Neurobiol*. (2018) 138:285–306. doi: 10.1016/bs.irn.2018.01.010

59. Enck P, Chae Y, Elsenbruch S. Novel designs and paradigms to study the placebo response in gastroenterology. *Curr Opin Pharmacol*. (2017) 37:72–9. doi: 10.1016/j.coph.2017.10.003

60. Dirikx T, Hermans D, Vansteenwegen D, Baeyens F, Eelen P. Reinstatement of extinguished conditioned responses and negative stimulus valence as a pathway to return of fear in humans. *Learn Mem*. (2004) 11:549–54. doi: 10.1101/lm.78004

61. Dour HJ, Brown LA, Craske MG. Positive valence reduces susceptibility to return of fear and enhances approach behavior. *J Behav Ther Exp Psychiatry*. (2016) 50:277–82. doi: 10.1016/j.jbtep.2015.09.010

62. Icenhour A, Labrenz F, Roderigo T, Siebert C, Elsenbruch S, Benson S. Are there sex differences in visceral sensitivity in young healthy men and women? *Neurogastroenterol Motil*. (2019) 31:e13664. doi: 10.1111/nmo.13664

63. Icenhour A, Labrenz F, Ritter C, Theysohn N, Forsting M, Bingel U, et al. Learning by experience? visceral pain-related neural and behavioral responses in a classical conditioning paradigm. *Neurogastroenterol Motil.* (2017) 29:e13026. doi: 10.1111/nmo.13026

64. Fullana MA, Harrison BJ, Soriano-Mas C, Vervliet B, Cardoner N, Àvila-Parcet A, et al. Neural signatures of human fear conditioning: an updated and extended meta-analysis of fMRI studies. *Mol Psychiatry.* (2016) 21:500-8. doi: 10.1038/mp.2015.88

65. Todd J, van Ryckeghem DML, Sharpe L, Crombez G. Attentional bias to pain-related information: a meta-analysis of dot-probe studies. *Health Psychol Rev.* (2018) 12:419-36. doi: 10.1080/17437199.2018.1521729

66. Van Damme S, Lorenz J, Eccleston C, Koster EH, De Clercq A, Crombez G. Fear-conditioned cues of impending pain facilitate attentional engagement. *Neurophysiol Clin.* (2004) 34:33-9. doi: 10.1016/j.neucli.2003.11.001

67. Van Damme S, Crombez G, Eccleston C, Goubert L. Impaired disengagement from threatening cues of impending pain in a crossmodal cueing paradigm. *Eur J Pain.* (2004) 8:227-36. doi: 10.1016/j.ejpain.2003.08.005

68. Van Damme S, Crombez G, Eccleston C. The anticipation of pain modulates spatial attention: evidence for pain-specificity in high-pain catastrophizers. *Pain.* (2004) 111:392-9. doi: 10.1016/j.pain.2004.07.022

69. Schrooten MGS, Van Damme S, Crombez G, Kindermans H, Vlaeyen JWS. Winning or not losing? The impact of non-pain goal focus on attentional bias to learned pain signals. *Scand J pain.* (2018) 18:675-86. doi: 10.1515/sjpain-2018-0055

70. Quartana PJ, Campbell CM, Edwards RR. Pain catastrophizing: a critical review. *Expert Rev Neurother.* (2009) 9:745-58. doi: 10.1586/ern.09.34

71. Wiech K, Tracey I. The influence of negative emotions on pain: behavioral effects and neural mechanisms. *Neuroimage.* (2009) 47:987-94. doi: 10.1016/j.neuroimage.2009.05.059

72. Vlaeyen JWS, Crombez G, Linton SJ. The fear-avoidance model of pain. *Pain.* (2016) 157:1588-9. doi: 10.1097/j.pain.0000000000000574

73. Roderigo T, Benson S, Schöls M, Hetkamp M, Schedlowski M, Enck P, et al. Effects of acute psychological stress on placebo and nocebo responses in a clinically relevant model of visceroception. *Pain.* (2017) 158:1489-98. doi: 10.1097/j.pain.0000000000000940

74. Keogh E, Ellery D, Hunt C, Hannent I. Selective attentional bias for pain-related stimuli amongst pain fearful individuals. *Pain.* (2001) 91:91-100. doi: 10.1016/S0304-3959(00)00422-X

75. Todd J, Sharpe L, Colagiuri B. Attentional bias modification and pain: the role of sensory and affective stimuli. *Behav Res Ther.* (2016) 83:53-61. doi: 10.1016/j.brat.2016.06.002

76. Keszthelyi D, Troost FJ, Masclee AA. Irritable bowel syndrome: methods, mechanisms, and pathophysiology. Methods to assess visceral hypersensitivity in irritable bowel syndrome. *AJP Gastrointest Liver Physiol.* (2012) 303:G141-54. doi: 10.1152/ajpgi.00060.2012

77. Schoth DE, Ma Y, Liossi C. Exploring attentional bias for real-world, pain-related information in chronic musculoskeletal pain using a novel change detection paradigm. *Clin J Pain.* (2015) 31:680-8. doi: 10.1097/AJP.0000000000000149

78. Afzal M, Potokar JP, Probert CSJ, Munafò MR. Selective processing of gastrointestinal symptom-related stimuli in irritable bowel syndrome. *Psychosom Med.* (2006) 68:758-61. doi: 10.1097/01.psy.0000232270.78071.28

79. Phillips K, Wright BJ, Kent S. Irritable bowel syndrome and symptom severity: evidence of negative attention bias, diminished vigour, and autonomic dysregulation. *J Psychosom Res.* (2014) 77:13-9. doi: 10.1016/j.jpsychores.2014.04.009

80. Tkalcic M, Domijan D, Pletikosic S, Setic M, Hauser G. Attentional biases in irritable bowel syndrome patients. *Clin Res Hepatol Gastroenterol.* (2014) 38:621-8. doi: 10.1016/j.clinre.2014.02.002

81. Chapman S, Martin M. Attention to pain words in irritable bowel syndrome: increased orienting and speeded engagement. *Br J Heal Psychol.* (2011) 16:47-60. doi: 10.1348/135910710X505887

82. Hauser G, Pletikosic S, Tkalcic M. Cognitive behavioral approach to understanding irritable bowel syndrome. *World J Gastroenterol.* (2014) 20:6744-58. doi: 10.3748/wjg.v20.i22.6744

83. Icenhour A, Witt ST, Elsenbruch S, Lowén M, Engström M, Tillisch K, et al. Brain functional connectivity is associated with visceral sensitivity in women with irritable bowel syndrome. *NeuroImage Clin.* (2017) 15:449-57. doi: 10.1016/j.nicl.2017.06.001

84. Liu X, Silverman A, Kern M, Ward BD, Li SJ, Shaker R, et al. Excessive coupling of the salience network with intrinsic neurocognitive brain networks during rectal distension in adolescents with irritable bowel syndrome: a preliminary report. *Neurogastroenterol Motil.* (2016) 28:43-53. doi: 10.1111/nmo.12695

85. Hong JY, Naliboff B, Labus JS, Gupta A, Kilpatrick LA, Ashe-Mcnalley C, et al. Altered brain responses in subjects with irritable bowel syndrome during cued and uncued pain expectation. *Neurogastroenterol Motil.* (2016) 28:127-38. doi: 10.1111/nmo.12710

86. Tayama J, Saigo T, Ogawa S, Takeoka A, Hamaguchi T, Hayashida M, et al. Effect of attention bias modification on brain function and anxiety in patients with irritable bowel syndrome: a preliminary electroencephalogram and psycho-behavioral study. *Neurogastroenterol Motil.* (2017) 29:e13131. doi: 10.1111/nmo.13131

87. Tayama J, Saigo T, Ogawa S, Takeoka A, Hamaguchi T, Inoue K, et al. Effect of attention bias modification on event-related potentials in patients with irritable bowel syndrome: a preliminary brain function and psycho-behavioral study. *Neurogastroenterol Motil.* (2018) 29:e13402. doi: 10.1111/nmo.13402

88. Zaman J, Vlaeyen JWS, Van Oudenhove L, Wiech K, Van Diest I. Associative fear learning and perceptual discrimination: a perceptual pathway in the development of chronic pain. *Neurosci Biobehav Rev.* (2015) 51:118-25. doi: 10.1016/j.neubiorev.2015.01.009

89. Meulders A, Jans A, Vlaeyen JWS. Differences in pain-related fear acquisition and generalization. *Pain.* (2015) 156:108-22. doi: 10.1016/j.pain.0000000000000016

90. Lowén MBO, Mayer E, Tillisch K, Labus J, Naliboff B, Lundberg P, et al. Deficient habituation to repeated rectal distensions in irritable bowel syndrome patients with visceral hypersensitivity. *Neurogastroenterol Motil.* (2015) 27:646-55. doi: 10.1111/nmo.12537

91. Jensen K, Kirsch I, Odmalm S, Kaptchuk T, Ingvar M. Classical conditioning of analgesic and hyperalgesic pain responses without conscious awareness. *Proc Natl Acad Sci USA.* (2015) 112:7863-7. doi: 10.1073/pnas.1504567112

92. Bruce Overmier J. Sensitization, conditioning, and learning: can they help us understand somatization and disability? *Scand J Psychol.* (2002) 43:105-12. doi: 10.1111/1467-9450.00275

93. Williams AE, Rhudy JL. The influence of conditioned fear on human pain thresholds: does preparedness play a role? *J Pain.* (2007) 8:598-606. doi: 10.1016/j.jpain.2007.03.004

94. Vlaeyen JWS, Morley S, Crombez G. The experimental analysis of the interruptive, interfering, and identity-distorting effects of chronic pain. *Behav Res Ther.* (2016) 86:23-34. doi: 10.1016/j.brat.2016.08.016

8

Placebo Responses and Placebo Effects in Functional Gastrointestinal Disorders

Paul Enck* and Sibylle Klosterhalfen

Department of Internal Medicine VI: Psychosomatic Medicine and Psychotherapy, University Hospital Tübingen, Tübingen, Germany

*Correspondence:
Paul Enck
paul.enck@uni-tuebingen.de

Much has been written about the placebo effects in functional gastrointestinal disorders (FGD), especially in irritable bowel syndrome (IBS), driven by the early hypothesis that in randomized controlled trials (RCTs) of IBS, the placebo effect might be specifically high and thus, corrupts the efficacy of novel drugs developed for this condition. This narrative review is based on a specific search method, a database (www.jips.online) developed since 2004 containing more than 4,500 papers (data papers, meta-analyses, systematic reviews, reviews) pertinent to the topic placebo effects/placebo response. Three central questions—deducted from the body of current literature—are addressed to explore the evidence behind this hypothesis: What is the size placebo effect in FGD, especially in IBS, and is it different from the placebo effect seen in other gastrointestinal disorders? Is the placebo effect in FGD different from other functional, non-intestinal disorders, *e.g.* in other pain syndromes? Is the placebo effect in FGD related to placebo effects seen in psychiatry, *e.g.* in depression, anxiety disorders, and alike? Following this discussion, a fourth question is raised as the result of the three: What are the consequences of this for future drug trials in FGD? In summary it is concluded that, contrary to common belief and discussion, the placebo effect seen in RCT in FGD is not specifically high and extraordinary as compared to other comparable (*i.e.* functional) disorders. It shares less than expected commonalities with the placebo effect in psychiatry, and very few predictors have yet been identified that determine its effect size, especially some that are driven by design features of the studies. Current practice of RCT in IBS seems to limit and control the placebo effect quite well, and future trial practice, *e.g.* head-to-head trial, still offers options to maintain this control, even in the absence of placebos used.

Keywords: irritable bowel syndrome, clinical trial, functional dyspepsia, placebo, nocebo

INTRODUCTION

Much has been written—by us (1–4) and by others (5–7)—about the placebo effects in functional gastrointestinal disorders (FGD), especially in irritable bowel syndrome (IBS), driven by the early hypothesis that in randomized controlled trials (RCTs) of IBS, the placebo effect might be specifically high (8) and thus, corrupts the efficacy of novel drugs developed for this condition

(9). This has been a popular statement over the next two decades and is still around among many gastroenterologists when explaining the difficulties of IBS RCT and the lack of effective treatment. Previous reviews have attempted to contradict this common belief, but until very recently, a comparison between placebo response rates in IBS, in other functional bowel disorders, in non-functional gastrointestinal disorders and in associated disorders in psychiatry was lacking. While systematic reviews and meta-analyses to estimate the effect size of placebos in comparison to those of drugs were published, a direct comparison of the determinants of the placebo response, *e.g.* in psychiatry, was and is not available.

METHODS

The specific approach taken to assess the relevant papers for the topic of this review is described in more detail elsewhere (10). In an attempt to comprehensively screen the entire medical literature published for papers reporting the placebo effect/placebo response, a PubMed search using the single search term "placebo" was conducted in early 2004. This resulted in more than 100,000 papers at that time. The title and abstracts of these papers were screened retrospectively (at a frequency of maximally 1,000 per day, 7 days a week for about one year), to identify the approximately 1% of all papers relevant for placebo research. These papers were stored in an *Endnote*-like database, respective PDFs were collected, and made available to the local working group in Tübingen. A few years later, a similar search using the term "nocebo" was added. Papers found occasionally and incidentally in book chapters and papers not available *via* PUBMED were added manually to the database, as were papers suggested by colleagues and other researchers.

At the same time (2003), a *prospective* PUBMED search was started that resulted in weekly reports of newly published papers with either of the two terms (on average 200 per week altogether) and again screened for relevance for placebo research. The 1% outcome has increased to about 2% over the years. Overall, this resulted in a database of approximately 4,500 papers (data papers, meta-analyses, systematic reviews, reviews, commentaries, and a limited number of letters) as of mid 2020. These references and monthly updates thereof were made available to the scientific community *via* a newsletter that can be subscribed at <www.jips. online> and has currently a few hundred subscribers. For the purpose of this review and other papers published in the last few years by us and others, this database is screen for new papers relevant to specific topics, such as placebo effects in functional bowel disorders.

So, why another review of the topic, especially in times when drug testing tends to move away from placebo-controlled trials and towards "real life" studies, studies that mimic daily medical routine rather than promote (self-)selection of patients willing to take part in a placebo-controlled test, while others, and presumably the more severely affected patients, prefer open-label treatment, even with novel compounds. Such "observational studies" are experiencing rediscovery and support not only by patients and patient organizations but also by approval authorities. However, eliminating placebos in drug testing does not eliminate the placebo response that is inherent to all medical (and psychological) interventions, even when provided by computerized algorithms—the digital placebo response (11). It has recently been proposed that even with open-label observational studies, proper control of some of the mediators of the placebo response is feasible (12) and thereby insists on a scientific rather than a pragmatic approach.

RESULTS

In the following, an answer to three major questions that are posed by the continuing discussion is attempted:

A: How large is placebo effect in FGD, especially in IBS, and is it different from the placebo effect seen in other gastrointestinal disorders, such as in IBD?

B: Is the placebo effect in FGD different from other functional, non-intestinal disorders, *e.g.* in other pain syndromes?

C: Is the placebo effect in FGD related to placebo effects seen in psychiatry, *e.g.* in depression, anxiety disorders, and alike?

Following this discussion, a fourth question is raised as a consequence of the three:

D: What are the consequences of this for future drug trials in FGD?

While most of the current knowledge about the placebo effect and the placebo response can be easily accessed *via* the web-platform that was established (www.jips.online) and that currently (end of 2019) contains nearly 4,500 papers (data paper, reviews, meta-analyses) genuinely discussing the placebo effects in medicine (10), final answers are far from being readily available. It may just be that this is *our* final contribution to the discussion.

In the following, the terms placebo effect and placebo response are used more or less interchangeably, but this is in light of the fact that this is a deviation from common practice and definitions [*e.g.* (13)]; for the purpose of this paper it may, however, be acceptable to simplify explanations and ease understanding.

A: Is The Placebo Effect in FGD (IBS) Different From Other Gastrointestinal Disorders?

The first step to answer this question is to check how large the placebo effect in IBS is, overall and not only in a few but in all studies. According to some meta-analyses the overall size of the placebo effect in IBS is in the range of 40%, be it in conventional drug trials (14), in complementary and alternative medicine interventions (7), or in nutritional interventions (15), with the latter challenged by larger difficulties to maintain some of the standards of good scientific practice, *e.g.* appropriate double-blinding, compliance control, and other features (16).

While attributing 40% of improvement to placebo effects in RCT in IBS seems a lot, this has much to do with the chosen primary endpoints of these studies: Clinical experts and/or approval authorities may have agreed on meaningful degrees of improvement (*e.g.* at least 30% change in average pain rating for one week on a visual analog scale (VAS) between 0 = no pain and 10 = highest imagined—or experienced—pain); the subsequent division of patients into responders meeting these criteria and non-responders simplifies decision making for the benefit of the approval process, but not for clinical routine: are the patients responding with a 29% improvement *only* really non-responders in comparison to the ones with a 30% improvement, and is the patient with the 90% improvement really the same type of responder than the one just meeting the 30% threshold? Dichotomizations of this kind may ignore potentially clinically meaningful differences by reducing data variance, but they ease power calculations, efficacy statistics, and publishing attempts, as well as marketing strategies of the drug. However, for the meta-analyses that have found the 40% to be the average size of the placebo effect, the dichotomization effect may be less pronounced, as long as the same entry criteria into the studies were used. Whether or not this was the case is not as much a consequence of the patient definitions at times (Rom to Rome IV) (17) but rather of the recruitment strategies at the level of the single centers.

The hypothesis that IBS studies yield a higher-than-usual placebo response stems from the times before the Rome definitions of IBS and was first mentioned in a review by Klein (8) as early as 1988. It was Spillers (9) 1999 prediction that the placebo effect would decline to an average rate of 20% once longer studies than the usual 4-week trials were conducted (**Figure 1**). However, as was shown (19), the high placebo response rates in earlier studies were not as much a function of the trial duration but rather a function of the number of patients included (**Figure 2**). Small sample sizes carried the risk of higher

variability of the placebo effect across studies, and it was the trials with the highest response rates that drove the impression and stuck in peoples mind; on average, the placebo response was always around 40%. Another fact that may have driven higher placebo response rates in individual RCTs was the fact that most of these studies were single center trials, while multi-centric studies became only the rule after 2000 (**Figure 3**). In monocentric studies, a single empathic doctor can eliminate the entire drug effect by raising the placebo response, especially with small samples, while nowadays block-randomization prevents or at least minimizes a disbalance in efficacy between centers.

Much less is published about the placebo effects in RCT with FGD other than IBS, *e.g.* in functional dyspepsia (FD), but a systematic review from 2001 (20) yielded an overall placebo response rate of 230/619 (37.2%) patients with functional ("non-ulcer") dyspepsia in 19 studies with gastroprokinetics, and it was 350/754 (46.4%) in 10 studies with acid blocking agents, resulting in an overall placebo response of 42.2%. The placebo effect varied between 6 and 73% (**Figure 4**) and therefore, was quite similar to the IBS studies at the time (3 to 83%) (22). This was noted by others as well (23) but has not (yet) led to an updated meta-analysis of the response rate across all (or many) trials. A 2018 systematic review and meta-analysis of 43 prokinetic RCT in functional dyspepsia (24) noted a 60% risk to be not symptom-free after prokinetic treatment compared to a 74% risk after placebo, with a rather high risk of bias in many studies. Thus, in FD the placebo response seems to be of similar size to that in IBS RCT. However, predictor analyses of the placebo response in FGD other than IBS have never been performed.

A 2015 systematic review of placebo response rates across many medical conditions (25) listed other gastrointestinal diseases, such as gastric and duodenal ulcers, reflux disease, and inflammatory bowel diseases that were meta-analyzed—a few additional meta-analyses have been published ever since (see **Table 1**). As can be seen, compared to IBS, the placebo response rates in IBD, both ulcerative colitis (UC) and Crohn´s Disease (CD), are somewhat lower and in the range of 15 to 30%, depending on whether the endpoints were clinical benefit (improvement) or remission (based on standardized, *e.g.* endoscopic or histological criteria) and whether the studies were to initiate or to maintain remission.

However, it is evident from these data that in chronic, recurrent diseases as IBD the placebo response also includes cases of spontaneous remission of the disease and are not easily separated from these—for this, "no treatment control groups" would be needed and that definitively is not possible in severe and life-threatening diseases such as UC and CD, while it would be possible (but never has been done) in IBS. Since spontaneous waxing and waning of symptoms is also a characteristic on FGD, care has to be taken not to overinterpret the placebo response rates in IBS by ignoring spontaneous symptom variation and others, *e.g.* methodological contributions to the placebo effect in RCT. Across many mild or minor diseases, this has been done by some authors (37–39), and they estimated these contributions to explain 50% of the placebo effect.

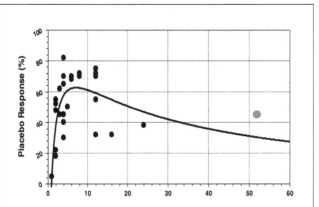

FIGURE 1 | Association between placebo response rates and the duration of treatment in 26 IBS studies from a review (9), supplemented by the first 1-year study (18) (blue dot). The non-linear (rational) regression function is highly significant, but note there are only two studies that lasted longer than 12 weeks at that time. Evidently (what we know now) with longer treatment duration the placebo response rate will be substantially higher (40%) than the 25% in the initial prediction. (Reproduced with permission from Elsevier).

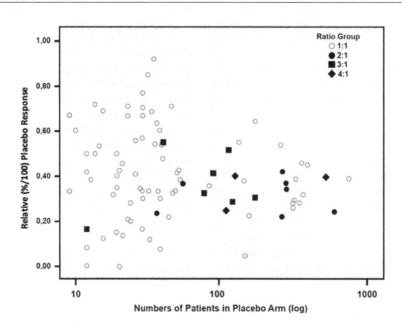

FIGURE 2 | Scatterplot between relative placebo response rates (n/N) and number of patients (log transformed) in the placebo arm of 102 randomized, double-blinded placebo-controlled irritable bowel syndrome studies. It is evident that with sample sizes of more than 100 patients the placebo response tends toward 40%. Open circles indicate studies powered 1:1, and dark marks indicate studies with different unbalanced randomization ratios. (Reproduced from Weimer & Enck (19), with permission from Springer).

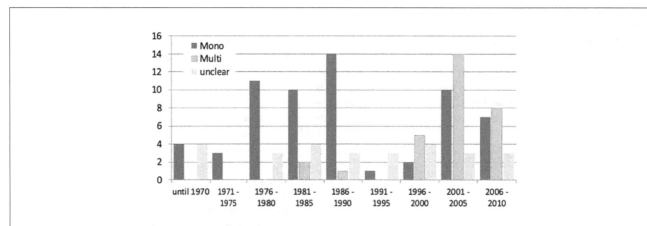

FIGURE 3 | Number of IBS studies published between 1975 and 2010 (data according to Klein (8), Spiller (9), and own data compilations) according to their mono-centric or multicentric nature. Note that monocentric studies dominated until 1990, while multi-center trials became more prevalent thereafter and were the rule after 2010.

Not surprisingly, some meta-analyses in IBD have used the placebo response rates in drug RCT to rather calculate the relative risk of <u>disease recurrence</u> and relapse in maintenance studies with IBD and found an increased risk compared to drug in the range of 23.7% in CD patients after surgery (40), while others (41) found the relapse rate in gastric ulcer studies to be 3.29% higher with placebo as compared to the (acid suppressing) drug. This is not to mix up the so-called nocebo effects (42, 43) with the reports of adverse events (AE) while on placebo during a double-blinded RCT, although this as well is difficult to separate without adequate control groups, *e.g.* register studies that include a "monitoring only" arm (12) (see below).

B: Is the Placebo Effect in FGD Different From Other Functional Non-GI Disorders?

The question specifically addresses pain syndromes, as (visceral) pain is the central characteristic of most FGD, although it is admitted that among the very many functional syndromes the Rome Committee has identified—altogether 38 in the Rome III

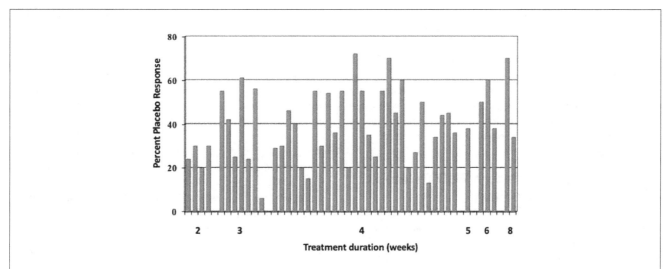

FIGURE 4 | Placebo response rates (in %) in 29 functional dyspepsia studies [data according to Mearin et al. (21) and Allescher et al. (20)], sorted according to length of study (in weeks). Each bar represents one study. The mean placebo response across all 45 trials is 40%. (Reproduced from Enck & Klosterhalfen (1), with permission from Wiley).

TABLE 1 | Systematic Reviews and meta-analyses of placebo response rates in different functional and non-functional gastrointestinal diseases.

Author, Year	Ref No	Clinical Condition	Number of studies/patients	Pooled Placebo Response (%)
Pitz et al., 2005	(5)	IBS	53/6326	36 (global improvement)
Pitz et al., 2005	(5)	IBS	39/5445	28 (abdominal pain)
Patel et al., 2005	(6)	IBS	45/3352	40.2
Dorn 2010	(26)	IBS	19/658	42.6 (CAM treatment)
Ford et al., 2010	(14)	IBS	73/8364	37.5
Allescher et al., 2001	(19)	NUD	29/1373	37.2/46.6[###]
Ilnyckyj et al., 1997	(27)	IBD-UC*	16/11/8	26.7/30.3/25.2
Su et al., 2004	(28)	IBD-CD**	21/327	18
Jairath et al., 2017	(29)	IBD-UC[+]	57/4062	19/22–10/33
Jairath et al., 2017	(30)	IBD-CD[++]	100/7638	32/26–18/28
Estevinho et al., 2018	(31)	IBD (UC,CD)[#]	26/2842	17.7/27.5–13.2/27.6
Ma et al., 2018	(32)	IBD-UC[##]	64/5282	14/20–23/35
Macluso et al., 2018	(33)	IBD-UC	31/2702	9/34/26°
Duijvestein et al., 2019	(34)	IBD-CD	5/188	16.2/5.2°°
de Craen et al., 1999	(35)	DU	79/1350	44.2/36.2°°°
Cremonini et al., 2010	(36)	GERD	24/3041	18.9

IBS, irritable bowel syndrome; NUD, non-ulcer dyspepsia; IBD, Inflammatory Bowel Disease; UC, Ulcerative colitis; CD, Crohn's Disease; CAM, Complementary and alternative medicine; DU, Duodenal Ulcers; GERD, Gastroesophageal reflux disease.
*data for % clinical benefit, not for % remission, with clinical, endoscopic, or histological endpoints, respectively. For % remission the respective values are 9.1, 13.5, and 8.6%.
**CDAI as endpoint, % received remission (CDAI score decrease varied from >50 to >100).
[+]data for maintenance trials (N = 9) and for induction trials (N = 48); endpoint remission and clinical response rates for maintenance and induction, respectively, are listed.
[++]data for maintenance trials (N = 40) and for induction trials (N = 67); endpoint remission and clinical response rates for maintenance and for induction, respectively, are listed.
[#]Quality of life improvement (IBDQ, SF36); data for IBDQ, separated for induction and maintenance in UC and CD, respectively.
[##]data for maintenance trials (N = 8) and for induction trials (N = 56); endpoint remission and clinical response rates for maintenance and induction, respectively, are listed.
[###]Response rates for prokinetics vs acid-suppressing treatments are given.
°induction rates for remission, response, and mucosal healing, respectively, are given; for maintenance, the respective data are 14, 23, and 19%.
°°placebo response for endoscopic improvement and remission, respectively.
°°°placebo response data for 4/day versus 2/day regiments are given.

edition—some are not associated with pain but rather with disturbed bowel function (motility) only. However, pain is a prerequisite to receive the diagnosis of IBS, and only data on placebo effects and responses in IBS are in the focus and have been studied extensively.

The already mentioned systematic reviews and meta-analyses (25) listed quite a number of functional syndromes outside the gastrointestinal tract in which the placebo effect has

been studied. **Table 2** summarized these data but restricted the studies to those meta-analyses of trials in painful clinical conditions. Three not pain-associated diseases (overactive bladder syndrome, OAB; premenstrual syndrome, PMS; chronic fatigue syndrome, CFS) are single examples listed for comparison.

As can be seen, painful non-GI clinical conditions are all associated with placebo response rates of 20% and higher, and up to 40% as is regularly the case in FGD, especially when visceral tissue is involved (pouchitis, pancreatitis); effect sizes are moderate to strong. A similarly strong placebo effect seems to dominate in pains associated with vascular mechanisms (migraine). Whether this moderate increase of visceral placebo analgesia over somatic placebo analgesia is a consequence of the rather diffuse nature of visceral pain, its specific characteristic as being deep, dark, and poorly locatable, or specifics of the "personality" of the patients affected cannot be answered from such meta-analyses.

C: Is the Placebo Effect in FGD Related to Effects Seen in Psychiatry?

The area in which placebo effects and their determinants are best investigated is psychiatry, and it was psychiatry in which increased placebo response rates in RCT were first noted—in fact, drug development has occasionally been hindered by too strong placebo effects rather than by weak drugs (60, 61). It was psychiatry as well where the first evidence of increasing placebo effects over time were noted. It is, therefore not surprising that increased placebo response rates in non-psychiatric, e.g. gastrointestinal conditions were attributed to psychiatric comorbidity in otherwise somatically affected patients. This is specifically true for FGD of IBS-type, as the overall placebo response rate in IBS is 40% (as discussed above), and the overall

response rates in depression trials match these 40% quite well (62).

A similar systematic review of meta-analyses than the one introduced above for all medical conditions (25) summarized the placebo effect in RCT in psychiatric disorders recently (63). Here it is discussed whether the various predictors of the placebo response especially in depression trials match findings from prediction analysis in IBS and FD. These predictors are classified into three groups: Disease characteristics, patient characteristics, and study design characteristics. To the best of our knowledge, only one regression analysis has been performed with data from the placebo arm of a trial with 599 patients with constipation-predominant IBS (64) to identify predictors of the placebo response, as well as predictors of a non-response to placebo in the same trial,

Disease Characteristics

The overwhelming finding from most such prediction analyses is that patients with a lower symptom severity at study start will show stronger placebo effects than patients with more severe symptoms (25). This may reflect the tendency of drug companies to recruit a mildly-to-moderately affected patient population for their studies, but it may as well reflect the fact that patients with milder symptoms may be more willing to participate in a placebo-controlled therapy trial. The downside of this tendency is that

TABLE 2 | Placebo response rates in different clinical pain conditions.

Author, Year	Ref No	Clinical Condition	Number of studies/patients	Pooled Placebo Response: % or ES or SMD
Diener et al., 1999	(44)	migraine	15/1345	25.9 (44/13)*
Macedo et al., 2008	(45)	migraine	98/11793	9/18/28/32**
Macedo et al., 2006	(46)	migraine	32/1416	21
Ho et al., 2009	(47)	migraine	8/1322	36.2/38.1–9.5/10.5***
Meissner et al., 2013	(48)	migraine	79/2828	22/26/23/38/24+
Quessy et al., 2008	(49)	NP	35/3265	26.5–15.5++
Zhang et al., 2008	(50)	osteoarthritis	193/16364	ES: 0.51/0.77+++
Häuser et al., 2011	(51)	fibromyalgia/DNP	72	SDM: 0.42/0.72 (45/62)#
Capurso et al., 2012	(52)	pain/pancreatitis	7/202	19.9
Chen et al., 2017	(53)	osteoarthritis	124/15633	ES: 0.52
Athayde et al., 2018	(54)	pouchitis	12/229	47/24°°°
Huang et al., 2019	(55)	osteoarthritis	21	SMD: −0.16–0.34/−0.31°°
Porporatti et al., 2019	(56)	TMD	42/1657	29/19/26°
Freeman et al., 1999	(57)	PMS	2/247	33
Cho et al., 2005	(58)	CFS	29/985	19.6 (14/16.5/24)###
Lee et al., 2009	(59)	OAB	36/5735	PE: −1.15/−1.27/12.4##

NP, Neuropathic pain; DPN, diabetic polyneuropathy; TMD, temporomandibular disorders; PMS, premenstrual syndrome; CFS, chronic fatigue syndrome; OAB, overactive bladder; ES, effect size; SMD, standardized mean difference.

*overall, headache response and pain-free response are listed.

**responses for 30 min, 1, 2, and >2 h after intake.

***for pain relief and pain free in females/males.

+for oral pharmacologic, CAM, injection therapies, sham acupuncture/surgery and sham CBT/electromagnetic stimulation therapies, respectively.

++for NP in DPN and post-herpes neuropathy, respectively.

+++ES estimate: Clinically, an ES of 0.2 suggests a small effect, 0.5 means a moderate effect, and 0.8 and over indicates a large effect. ES are given for all trials and for three trials comparing treatment with a no-treatment control, respectively.

#SDM for DNP and fibromyalgia, respectively, are given; percentage relates to the improvement in the active group that can be attributed to placebo.

##Point estimated (PE) from meta-analysis for incontinence episodes, micturition frequency, and voiding volume, respectively, are given (all highly significant).

###Overall response and response in low, medium, and high expectation groups, respectively.

°response for laser therapy, drugs, and other therapies.

°°SMD for patient-reported outcome (PRO) for pain, muscle strength, and range of motion.

°°°for induction and maintenance trials, respectively.

RCT may not represent the medical reality in terms of patients tested, and this may corroborate the representativeness of the study results. It has been noted that drugs such as serotoninergic antidepressants are by far less effective in daily routine than had been reported in RCT (65). However, this may as well be due to overinterpretation of the RCT data. A lower symptom severity is often associated with a shorter disease history that was found to predict higher placebo responses, while previously untreated patients were sometimes found to generate higher responses but in other cases, lower responses. Rather than previous treatment *per se*, treatment success or failure may determine the response to subsequent trials. Another of the concerns related to the representativeness of antidepressant trials is that patients recruited may have been taken off their regular medicines and may have experienced symptom worsening before being included into a RCT, and thereby the gap between drug and placebo arms may have been artificially widened.

The only meta-analysis that has studied the prediction in IBS (14) did not find disease severity to affect placebo responses, mainly because patient definition for recruitment was based on the IBS diagnostic criteria (Rome) that regularly do not include assessments of symptom severity, *e.g.* by the IBS-SSS score (66). The different Rome criteria used over time did not result in differences of the placebo effect (14). The re-analysis of the data from a single IBS-C RCT (64), confirmed that placebo responders had lower baseline pain severity than non-responders, and that a pain response as early as week two of the trial was associated with a higher placebo response with respect to the primary endpoints, a >30% pain relief and "adequate pain relief"; the latter response was also associated with a placebo response for spontaneous bowel movements. A higher number of baseline spontaneous bowel movements were associated with lower placebo response.

For functional dyspepsia, two re-analyses of individualized data from RCT can be used to answer this question: in one (67), a lower symptom burden at baseline and a symptom increase during run-in were associated with higher placebo responses, while in the other (68) this could not be confirmed; instead, an unstable symptom pattern was predictive of higher placebo responses as was a higher Body Mass Index (BMI). The BMI data are probably accidental findings in this specific cohort as was the smoking status in the other one (67), or it may represent a more general feature (69) yet to be explored.

Patient Characteristics

At least in some conditions, especially in psychiatric diseases, younger patient age was usually associated with higher placebo response rates (25) and has led to speculation about reasons for this (70) that are not conclusive overall; however, conflicting evidence exists as well. On the contrary, the widely believed idea that women may generate higher placebo response rates in RCTs was not supported by our analysis of clinical trials (25), while experimental placebo studies tend to confirm sex difference, albeit in both directions: Men seem more prone to show placebo responses in expectancy-based designs, while women responded stronger in learning (conditioning) experiments—the reasons for this difference are discussed elsewhere (71).

Age and sex were not reported to drive the placebo effect in the largest meta-analysis (14), while at least one (5) noted younger age to be associated with higher placebo effects in IBS. Data from FD studies (67, 68) did not find evidence for the influence of age and sex. Other patient characteristics, especially personality variables, are usually not assessed in RCT outside psychiatry because of the risk of limiting the indication of the drug under investigation. And pieces of evidence from experimental trials (72) have never been confirmed in clinical studies.

Study Design Characteristics

Probably the most consistent and surprising finding in psychiatric and neurological trials is the fact that the so-called "unbalanced randomization" determines the placebo effect: with a higher chance to receive active treatment in enrichment trials, trials with more than one drug arm, different dosages, comparator trials or trials which attempt to motivate more patients in general, the placebo effect rises [*e.g.* (44, 73), for a discussion see (63)]. It is of utmost importance to note that this feature has not been replicated in IBS studies at all (3). However, in IBS such studies were usually multi-center trials with large patient populations conducted by the pharmaceutical industry (see **Figure 2**), while in psychiatry, many such trials were small scale with an *a priori* risk of high placebo effects.

Another feature that has steered the placebo discussion, especially in depression, is an increase of the placebo effect over time, noted as early as 2002 (74). This is counter-intuitive towards the fact that more recent studies tend to be longer, and that shorter trial duration usually was found to be prone to higher placebo response rates (63). In depression, this trend was at least questioned (75–77), and it was not confirmed in IBS trials either (3) Neither was it found in IBS studies that trials between the US and Europe differed in the placebo effect (with higher responses in the US in depression), and with industry-initiated studies producing higher placebo effect than investigator-initiated studies, as was the case in some psychiatric trials (63).

One characteristic that was similar between psychiatric trials and FGD trials is the number of planned study visits during a trial: the more visits are planned the higher is the placebo response, a feature that was not only found in IBS (5, 6)—though with conflicting trends, see (78) —but also in IBD trials (27).

A very specific drug design feature in FGD (IBS), requested by the European Medical Agency (EMA) and matched by neither the Federal Drug Administration (FDA) rules in the US nor the EMA/FDA rules in any other class of diseases, is to either conduct long-term (*e.g.* six months) trials or to conduct a short-term (week) trial and repeat the treatment after re-randomization for another short-term to verify the drug is still effective. To the best of our knowledge, only one IBS RTC has been conducted with the second option (79) and showed the placebo effect in the second treatment period to be of similar size than in the first treatment phase. However, most of the assessment tools for outcome measures used have not been validated for such test strategy, but this also holds true for other endpoints, *e.g.* the "global assessment of improvement" (GAI) for 6-month trials in IBS.

In summary of this part of the review therefore, none of the study characteristics (disease, patient, and design) driving the placebo response in psychiatry seem to contribute to the placebo effects seen in FGD, and except for the number of study visits and the effects of symptom severity at baseline, seem to be of relevance in IBS. Hence, the prediction capability of placebo meta-analyses remains to be rather poor in FGD in gastroenterology.

D: What Are the Consequences of These Findings for Future Drug Trials in FGD?

A number of immediate conclusions can be drawn from the above discussed data:

- For one, the placebo effect in RCT in FGD, especially in IBS, may be slightly higher than in other functional and organic diseases, but with around 40% it is not extraordinarily high as long as the sample size is sufficiently high (say: more than 100 patients per study arm). Studies with lower sample sizes should be avoided.
- Patient reported outcomes usually produce higher placebo response rates than biomarker readouts as is evident e.g. from differences between symptomatic readouts and endoscopic/histological endpoints. It would therefore be advisable to add one or more biomarkers to IBS studies, currently relying on symptom reports in diaries mainly.
- Because time trend observed in psychiatric and neurological disorders (increased placebo response rates in more recent RCT) has not been confirmed in FGD, this underlines the importance to maintain current patient definition and endpoint selection in IBS trials as manifested in the Rome criteria.
- Since unbalanced randomization appears not to be a factor influencing the size of the placebo response, such strategies, e.g. adding comparator drugs to a trial, should be encouraged in gastroenterology, especially in FGD where they are literally non-existing. On the other hand, enrichment trials to enhance the drug effects and to limit placebo effects, as they become popular in psychiatry, seem not to be needed in FGD in gastroenterology.
- A trial length of 12 weeks seems to be reasonable, as longer trials do not eliminate the placebo effect, as was previously hoped, but shorter trials definitively carry the risk to increase placebo response rates.
- Unbalancing the sex ratio in RCT with IBS and FD patient may be a risk factor for sex-related drug effects, but is obviously not affecting the placebo effects. There is, however, evidence for different placebo responses in relation to age that should be kept in mind when planning a RCT.

Eliminating placebo-controlled studies and replacing them with comparator trials (also called head-to-head trials) do not eliminate the placebo effect but make it more difficult to identify and quantify it—placebo effects are immanent to all medical and psychological therapeutic interventions and may also affect diagnostic procedures (43, 80, 81). It has been shown (e.g. in psychiatry) that in fact the 100% chance to receive active treatment may drive the placebo effect to another height (62). On the other hand, as has been argued above, a substantial fraction of what appears to be the placebo effect in RCT is in fact a contribution of spontaneous symptom variation and—in chronic recurrent diseases—remission and relapse. To control both, the placebo effect without placebo provision and the contribution of the spontaneous course of the disease, in "real world studies" (studies under realistic conditions in daily medical routine), other measures may be needed that are discussed in more detail elsewhere (12, 19):

- From a methodological standpoint, even comparator trials comparing two or more drugs, the novel one and the one already on the market, should always include a placebo arm as well, to allow testing the non-inferiority of the novel compound against the established one as well as its superiority against placebo.
- To include a "no treatment" control arm into conventional placebo-controlled trials, studies should make use of the "cohort multiple randomized controlled trial" (CMRCT) (82), also called "Zelen design" (83): The "monitoring only" study is separated from the interventional study recruitment, e.g. by using large cohorts in disease registries. Patients recruited to participate in disease monitoring are subsequently asked to volunteer for the interventional part, and those not agreeing remain in the monitoring arm for control purposes.
- With open-label observational studies and no apparent randomization, monitoring spontaneous symptom variation can also be achieved by utilizing the same strategy, called "controlled open-label trial" (COLT) discussed in a recent paper (12).
- Finally, open label placebo treatment (84) can be added to a conventional placebo-controlled trial, either with full double-blinded randomization (85) or allowing patient preferences for either arm, what has been called preference design (19).

SUMMARY AND CONCLUSION

Contrary to common belief and discussion, the placebo effect seen in RCT in FGD is not specifically high and extraordinary as compared to other comparable (i.e. functional) disorders. It shares less than expected commonalities with the placebo effect in psychiatry, and very few predictors have yet been identified that determine its effect size, especially very few that are driven by design features of the studies. Current practice of RCT in IBS seems to limit and control the placebo effect quite well, and future trial practice, e.g. head-to-head trial still offers options to maintain this control even in the absence of placebos used.

AUTHOR CONTRIBUTIONS

SK and PE conceptualized the paper. PE wrote the paper. SK corrected and approved the manuscript.

REFERENCES

1. Enck P, Klosterhalfen S. The placebo response in functional bowel disorders: perspectives and putative mechanisms. *Neurogastroenterol Motil* (2005) 17 (3):325–31. doi: 10.1111/j.1365-2982.2005.00676.x

2. Musial F, Klosterhalfen S, Enck P. Placebo responses in patients with gastrointestinal disorders. *World J Gastroenterol* (2007) 13(25):3425–9. doi: 10.3748/wjg.v13.i25.3425

3. Elsenbruch S, Enck P. Placebo effects and their determinants in gastrointestinal disorders. *Nat Rev Gastroenterol Hepatol* (2015) 12(8):472–85. doi: 10.1038/nrgastro.2015.117

4. Enck P, Chae Y, Elsenbruch S. Novel designs and paradigms to study the placebo response in gastroenterology. *Curr Opin Pharmacol* (2017) 37:72–9. doi: 10.1016/j.coph.2017.10.003

5. Pitz M, Cheang M, Bernstein CN. Defining the predictors of the placebo response in irritable bowel syndrome. *Clin Gastroenterol Hepatol* (2005) 3 (3):237–47. doi: 10.1016/S1542-3565(04)00626-3

6. Patel SM, Stason WB, Legedza A, Ock SM, Kaptchuk TJ, Conboy L, et al. The placebo effect in irritable bowel syndrome trials: a meta-analysis. *Neurogastroenterol Motil* (2005) 17(3):332–40. doi: 10.1111/j.1365-2982.2005.00650.x

7. Dorn SD, Kaptchuk TJ, Park JB, Nguyen LT, Canenguez K, Nam BH, et al. A meta-analysis of the placebo response in complementary and alternative medicine trials of irritable bowel syndrome. *Neurogastroenterol Motil* (2007) 19(8):630–7. doi: 10.1111/j.1365-2982.2007.00937.x

8. Klein KB. Controlled treatment trials in the irritable bowel syndrome: a critique. *Gastroenterology* (1988) 95(1):232–41. doi: 10.1016/0016-5085(88) 90319-8

9. Spiller RC. Problems and challenges in the design of irritable bowel syndrome clinical trials: experience from published trials. *Am J Med* (1999) 107(5a):91s–7s. doi: 10.1016/S0002-9343(99)00086-8

10. Enck P, Horing B, Broelz E, Weimer K. Knowledge Gaps in Placebo Research: With Special Reference to Neurobiology. *Int Rev Neurobiol* (2018) 139:85–106. doi: 10.1016/bs.irn.2018.07.018

11. Torous J, Firth J. The digital placebo effect: mobile mental health meets clinical psychiatry. *Lancet Psychiatry* (2016) 3(2):100–2. doi: 10.1016/S2215-0366(15) 00565-9

12. Enck P, Klosterhalfen S. Placebos and the Placebo Effect in Drug Trials. *Handb Exp Pharmacol* (2019) 260:399–431. doi: 10.1007/164_2019_269

13. Evers AWM, Colloca L, Blease C, Annoni M, Atlas LY, Benedetti F, et al. Implications of Placebo and Nocebo Effects for Clinical Practice: Expert Consensus. *Psychother Psychosom* (2018) 87(4):204–10.

14. Ford AC, Moayyedi P. Meta-analysis: factors affecting placebo response rate in the irritable bowel syndrome. *Aliment Pharmacol Ther* (2010) 32(2):144–58. doi: 10.1111/j.1365-2036.2010.04328.x

15. Masi A, Lampit A, Glozier N, Hickie IB, Guastella AJ. Predictors of placebo response in pharmacological and dietary supplement treatment trials in pediatric autism spectrum disorder: a meta-analysis. *Transl Psychiatry* (2015) 5:e640. doi: 10.1038/tp.2015.143

16. Staudacher HM, Irving PM, Lomer MCE, Whelans K. The challenges of control groups, placebos and blinding in clinical trials of dietary interventions. *Proc Nutr Soc* (2017) 76(3):203–12. doi: 10.1017/S0029665117002816

17. Thompson WG. The road to rome. *Gastroenterology* (2006) 130(5):1552–6. doi: 10.1053/j.gastro.2006.03.011

18. Chey WD, Chey WY, Heath AT, Dukes GE, Carter EG, Northcutt A, et al. Long-term safety and efficacy of alosetron in women with severe diarrhea-predominant irritable bowel syndrome. *Am J Gastroenterol* (2004) 99 (11):2195–203. doi: 10.1111/j.1572-0241.2004.30509.x

19. Weimer K, Enck P. Traditional and innovative experimental and clinical trial designs and their advantages and pitfalls. *Handb Exp Pharmacol* (2014) 225:237–72. doi: 10.1007/978-3-662-44519-8_14

20. Allescher HD, Bockenhoff A, Knapp G, Wienbeck M, Hartung J. Treatment of non-ulcer dyspepsia: a meta-analysis of placebo-controlled prospective studies. *Scand J Gastroenterol* (2001) 36(9):934–41. doi: 10.1080/003655201750305440

21. Mearin F, Balboa A, Zárate N, Cucala M, Malagelada JR. Placebo in functional dyspepsia: symptomatic, gastrointestinal motor, and gastric sensorial responses. *Am J Gastroenterol* (1999) 94(1):116–25. doi: 10.1111/j.1572-0241.1999.00781.x

22. Enck P, Horing B, Weimer K, Klosterhalfen S. Placebo responses and placebo effects in functional bowel disorders. *Eur J Gastroenterol Hepatol* (2012) 24 (1):1–8. doi: 10.1097/MEG.0b013e32834bb951

23. Savarino E, De Cassan C, Bodini G, Furnari M, de Bortoli N, Savarino V. The placebo effect is a relevant factor in evaluating effectiveness of therapies in functional gastrointestinal disorders. *J Gastroenterol* (2014) 49(9):1362–3. doi: 10.1007/s00535-014-0974-7

24. Pittayanon R, Yuan Y, Bollegala NP, Khanna R, Lacy BE, Andrews CN, et al. Prokinetics for Functional Dyspepsia: A Systematic Review and Meta-analysis of Randomized Control Trials. *Am J Gastroenterol* (2019) 114(2):233–43. doi: 10.1038/s41395-018-0258-6

25. Weimer K, Colloca L, Enck P. Age and sex as moderators of the placebo response - an evaluation of systematic reviews and meta-analyses across medicine. *Gerontology* (2015) 61(2):97–108. doi: 10.1159/000365248

26. Dorn SD. Systematic review: self-management support interventions for irritable bowel syndrome. *Aliment Pharmacol Ther* (2010) 32(4):513–21. doi: 10.1111/j.1365-2036.2010.04374.x

27. Ilnyckyj A, Shanahan F, Anton PA, Cheang M, Bernstein CN. Quantification of the placebo response in ulcerative colitis. *Gastroenterology* (1997) 112 (6):1854–8. doi: 10.1053/gast.1997.v112.pm9178676

28. Su C, Lichtenstein GR, Krok K, Brensinger CM, Lewis JD. A meta-analysis of the placebo rates of remission and response in clinical trials of active crohn's disease. *Gastroenterology* (2004) 126(5):1257–69. doi: 10.1053/j.gastro.2004.01.024

29. Jairath V, Zou G, Parker CE, Macdonald JK, Mosli MH, Khanna R, et al. Systematic Review and Meta-analysis: Placebo Rates in Induction and Maintenance Trials of Ulcerative Colitis. *J Crohns Colitis* (2016) 10(5):607–18. doi: 10.1093/ecco-jcc/jjw004

30. Jairath V, Zou G, Parker CE, MacDonald JK, Mosli MH, AlAmeel T, et al. Systematic review with meta-analysis: placebo rates in induction and maintenance trials of Crohn's disease. *Aliment Pharmacol Ther* (2017) 45 (8):1021–42. doi: 10.1111/apt.13973

31. Estevinho MM, Afonso J, Rosa I, Lago P, Trindade E, Correia L, et al. Placebo effect on the health-related quality of life of inflammatory bowel disease patients: a systematic review with meta-analysis. *J Crohns Colitis* (2018) 12 (10):1232–44. doi: 10.1093/ecco-jcc/jjy100

32. Ma C, Guizzetti L, Panaccione R, Fedorak RN, Pai RK, Parker CE, et al. Systematic review with meta-analysis: endoscopic and histologic placebo rates in induction and maintenance trials of ulcerative colitis. *Aliment Pharmacol Ther* (2018) 47(12):1578–96. doi: 10.1111/apt.14672

33. Macaluso FS, Maida M, Ventimiglia M, Renna S, Cottone M, Orlando A. Factors Affecting Clinical and Endoscopic Outcomes of Placebo Arm in Trials of Biologics and Small Molecule Drugs in Ulcerative Colitis: A Meta-Analysis. *Inflamm Bowel Dis* (2018) 25(6):987–97. doi: 10.1093/ibd/izy365

34. Duijvestein M, Jeyarajah J, Guizzetti L, Zou G, Parker CE, van Viegen T, et al. Response to Placebo, Measured by Endoscopic Evaluation of Crohn's Disease Activity, in a Pooled Analysis of Data from 5 Randomized Controlled Induction Trials. *Clin Gastroenterol Hepatol* (2020) 18(5):1121–32. doi: 10.1016/j.cgh.2019.08.025

35. de Craen AJ, Moerman DE, Heisterkamp SH, Tytgat GN, Tijssen JG, Kleijnen J. Placebo effect in the treatment of duodenal ulcer. *Br J Clin Pharmacol* (1999) 48 (6):853–60. doi: 10.1046/j.1365-2125.1999.00094.x

36. Cremonini F, Ziogas DC, Chang HY, Kokkotou E, Kelley JM, Conboy L, et al. Meta-analysis: the effects of placebo treatment on gastro-oesophageal reflux disease. *Aliment Pharmacol Ther* (2010) 32(1):29–42. doi: 10.1111/j.1365-2036.2010.04315.x

37. Krogsboll LT, Hrobjartsson A, Gotzsche PC. Spontaneous improvement in randomised clinical trials: meta-analysis of three-armed trials comparing no treatment, placebo and active intervention. *BMC Med Res Methodol* (2009) 9:1. doi: 10.1186/1471-2288-9-1

38. Rutherford BR, Mori S, Sneed JR, Pimontel MA, Roose SP. Contribution of spontaneous improvement to placebo response in depression: a meta-analytic review. *J Psychiatr Res* (2012) 46(6):697–702. doi: 10.1016/j.jpsychires.2012.02.008

39. Hengartner MP. Is there a genuine placebo effect in acute depression treatments? A reassessment of regression to the mean and spontaneous

remission. *BMJ Evid Based Med* (2020) 25(2):46–8. doi: 10.1136/bmjebm-2019-111161

40. Renna S, Camma C, Modesto I, Cabibbo G, Scimeca D, Civitavecchia G, et al. Meta-analysis of the placebo rates of clinical relapse and severe endoscopic recurrence in postoperative Crohn's disease. *Gastroenterology* (2008) 135 (5):1500–9. doi: 10.1053/j.gastro.2008.07.066

41. Yuan YH, Wang C, Yuan Y, Hunt RH. Meta-analysis: incidence of endoscopic gastric and duodenal ulcers in placebo arms of randomized placebo-controlled NSAID trials. *Aliment Pharmacol Ther* (2009) 30(3):197–209. doi: 10.1111/j.1365-2036.2009.04038.x

42. Bingel U. Placebo Competence Team,. Avoiding nocebo effects to optimize treatment outcome. *JAMA* (2014) 312(7):693–4. doi: 10.1001/jama.2014.8342

43. Schedlowski M, Enck P, Rief W, Bingel U. Neuro-Bio-Behavioral Mechanisms of Placebo and Nocebo Responses: Implications for Clinical Trials and Clinical Practice. *Pharmacol Rev* (2015) 67(3):697–730. doi: 10.1124/pr.114.009423

44. Diener HC, Dowson AJ, Ferrari M, Nappi G, Tfelt-Hansen P. Unbalanced randomization influences placebo response: scientific versus ethical issues around the use of placebo in migraine trials. *Cephalalgia* (1999) 19(8):699–700. doi: 10.1046/j.1468-2982.1999.019008699.x

45. Macedo A, Banos JE, Farre M. Placebo response in the prophylaxis of migraine: a meta-analysis. *Eur J Pain* (2008) 12(1):68–75. doi: 10.1016/j.ejpain.2007.03.002

46. Macedo A, Farre M, Banos JE. A meta-analysis of the placebo response in acute migraine and how this response may be influenced by some of the characteristics of clinical trials. *Eur J Clin Pharmacol* (2006) 62(3):161–72. doi: 10.1007/s00228-005-0088-5

47. Ho TW, Fan X, Rodgers A, Lines CR, Winner P, Shapiro RE. Age effects on placebo response rates in clinical trials of acute agents for migraine: pooled analysis of rizatriptan trials in adults. *Cephalalgia* (2009) 29(7):711–8. doi: 10.1111/j.1468-2982.2008.01788.x

48. Meissner K, Fassler M, Rucker G, Kleijnen J, Hrobjartsson A, Schneider A, et al. Differential effectiveness of placebo treatments: a systematic review of migraine prophylaxis. *JAMA Intern Med* (2013) 173(21):1941–51. doi: 10.1001/jamainternmed.2013.10391

49. Quessy SN, Rowbotham MC. Placebo response in neuropathic pain trials. *Pain* (2008) 138(3):479–83. doi: 10.1016/j.pain.2008.06.024

50. Zhang W, Robertson J, Jones AC, Dieppe PA, Doherty M. The placebo effect and its determinants in osteoarthritis: meta-analysis of randomised controlled trials. *Ann Rheum Dis* (2008) 67(12):1716–23. doi: 10.1136/ard.2008.092015

51. Hauser W, Bartram-Wunn E, Bartram C, Reinecke H, Tolle T. Systematic review: Placebo response in drug trials of fibromyalgia syndrome and painful peripheral diabetic neuropathy-magnitude and patient-related predictors. *Pain* (2011) 152(8):1709–17. doi: 10.1016/j.pain.2011.01.050

52. Capurso G, Cocomello L, Benedetto U, Camma C, Delle Fave G. Meta-analysis: the placebo rate of abdominal pain remission in clinical trials of chronic pancreatitis. *Pancreas* (2012) 41(7):1125–31. doi: 10.1097/MPA.0b013e318249ce93

53. Chen X, Zou K, Abdullah N, Whiteside N, Sarmanova A, Doherty M, et al. The placebo effect and its determinants in fibromyalgia: meta-analysis of randomised controlled trials. *Clin Rheumatol* (2017) 36(7):1623–30. doi: 10.1007/s10067-017-3595-8

54. Athayde J, Davies SC, Parker CE, Guizzetti L, Ma C, Khanna R, et al. Placebo Rates in Randomized Controlled Trials of Pouchitis Therapy. *Dig Dis Sci* (2018) 63(10):2519–28. doi: 10.1007/s10620-018-5199-9

55. Huang Z, Chen J, Hu QS, Huang Q, Ma J, Pei FX, et al. Meta-analysis of pain and function placebo responses in pharmacological osteoarthritis trials. *Arthritis Res Ther* (2019) 21(1):173. doi: 10.1186/s13075-019-1951-6

56. Porporatti AL, Costa YM, Reus JC, Stuginski-Barbosa J, Conti PCR, Velly AM, et al. Placebo and nocebo response magnitude on temporomandibular disorders related-pain: a systematic review and meta-analysis. *J Oral Rehabil* (2019) 46(9):862–82. doi: 10.1111/joor.12827

57. Freeman EW, Rickels K. Characteristics of placebo responses in medical treatment of premenstrual syndrome. *Am J Psychiatry* (1999) 156(9):1403–8. doi: 10.1176/ajp.156.9.1403

58. Cho HJ, Hotopf M, Wessely S. The placebo response in the treatment of chronic fatigue syndrome: a systematic review and meta-analysis. *Psychosom Med* (2005) 67(2):301–13. doi: 10.1097/01.psy.0000156969.76986.e0

59. Lee S, Malhotra B, Creanga D, Carlsson M, Glue P. A meta-analysis of the placebo response in antimuscarinic drug trials for overactive bladder. *BMC Med Res Methodol* (2009) 9:55. doi: 10.1186/1471-2288-9-55

60. Greist JH, Mundt JC, Kobak K. Factors contributing to failed trials of new agents: can technology prevent some problems? *J Clin Psychiatry* (2002) 63 (Suppl 2):8–13.

61. Kobak KA, Kane JM, Thase ME, Nierenberg AA. Why do clinical trials fail? The problem of measurement error in clinical trials: time to test new paradigms? *J Clin Psychopharmacol* (2007) 27(1):1–5. doi: 10.1097/JCP.0b013e31802eb4b7

62. Rutherford BR, Sneed JR, Roose SP. Does study design influence outcome? The effects of placebo control and treatment duration in antidepressant trials. *Psychother Psychosom* (2009) 78(3):172–81. doi: 10.1159/000209348

63. Weimer K, Colloca L, Enck P. Placebo effects in psychiatry: mediators and moderators. *Lancet Psychiatry* (2015) 2(3):246–57. doi: 10.1016/S2215-0366(14)00092-3

64. Ballou S, Beath A, Kaptchuk TJ, Hirsch W, Sommers T, Nee J, et al. Factors associated with response to placebo in patients with irritable bowel syndrome and constipation. *Clin Gastroenterol Hepatol.* (2018) 16(11):1738–44e1. doi: 10.1016/j.cgh.2018.04.009

65. Kirsch I. Placebo Effect in the Treatment of Depression and Anxiety. *Front Psychiatry* (2019) 10:407. doi: 10.3389/fpsyt.2019.00407

66. Drossman DA, Chang L, Bellamy N, Gallo-Torres HE, Lembo A, Mearin F, et al. Severity in irritable bowel syndrome: a Rome Foundation Working Team report. *Am J Gastroenterol* (2011) 106(10):1749–59. doi: 10.1038/ajg.2011.201

67. Enck P, Vinson B, Malfertheiner P, Zipfel S, Klosterhalfen S. The placebo response in functional dyspepsia–reanalysis of trial data. *Neurogastroenterol Motil* (2009) 21(4):370–7. doi: 10.1111/j.1365-2982.2008.01241.x

68. Talley NJ, Locke GR, Lahr BD, Zinsmeister AR, Cohard-Radice M, D'Elia TV, et al. Predictors of the placebo response in functional dyspepsia. *Aliment Pharmacol Ther* (2006) 23(7):923–36. doi: 10.1111/j.1365-2036.2006.02845.x

69. Enck P, Weimer K, Klosterhalfen S. Are all placebo respondents non-smokers? *Med Hypotheses* (2014) 83(3):355–8. doi: 10.1016/j.mehy.2014.06.012

70. Weimer K, Gulewitsch MD, Schlarb AA, Schwille-Kiuntke J, Klosterhalfen S, Enck P. Placebo effects in children: a review. *Pediatr Res* (2013) 74(1):96–102. doi: 10.1038/pr.2013.66

71. Enck P, Klosterhalfen S. Does Sex/Gender Play a Role in Placebo and Nocebo Effects? Conflicting Evidence From Clinical Trials and Experimental Studies. *Front Neurosci* (2019) 13:130. doi: 10.3389/fnins.2019.00160

72. Horing B, Weimer K, Muth ER, Enck P. Prediction of placebo responses: a systematic review of the literature. *Front Psychol* (2014) 5:1079. doi: 10.3389/fpsyg.2014.01079

73. Rutherford BR, Sneed JR, Tandler JM, Rindskopf D, Peterson BS, Roose SP. Deconstructing pediatric depression trials: an analysis of the effects of expectancy and therapeutic contact. *J Am Acad Child Adolesc Psychiatry* (2011) 50(8):782–95. doi: 10.1016/j.jaac.2011.04.004

74. Walsh BT, Seidman SN, Sysko R, Gould M. Placebo response in studies of major depression: variable, substantial, and growing. *JAMA* (2002) 287 (14):1840–7. doi: 10.1001/jama.287.14.1840

75. Enck P. Placebo response in depression: is it rising? *Lancet Psychiatry* (2016) 3 (11):1005–6. doi: 10.1016/S2215-0366(16)30308-X

76. Khan A, Fahl Mar K, Faucett J, Khan Schilling S, Brown WA. Has the rising placebo response impacted antidepressant clinical trial outcome? Data from the US Food and Drug Administration 1987-2013. *World Psychiatry* (2017) 16 (2):181–92. doi: 10.1002/wps.20421

77. Furukawa TA, Cipriani A, Leucht S, Atkinson LZ, Ogawa Y, Takeshima N, et al. Is placebo response in antidepressant trials rising or not? A reanalysis of datasets to conclude this long-lasting controversy. *Evid Based Ment Health* (2018) 21(1):1–3. doi: 10.1136/eb-2017-102827

78. Enck P, Klosterhalfen S, Kruis W. Factors affecting therapeutic placebo response rates in patients with irritable bowel syndrome. *Nat Clin Pract Gastroenterol Hepatol* (2005) 2(8):354–5. doi: 10.1038/ncpgas thep0237

79. Rao S, Lembo AJ, Shiff SJ, Lavins BJ, Currie MG, Jia XD, et al. A 12-week, randomized, controlled trial with a 4-week randomized withdrawal period to evaluate the efficacy and safety of linaclotide in irritable bowel syndrome with

constipation. *Am J Gastroenterol* (2012) 107(11):1714–24. doi: 10.1038/ajg.2012.255

80. Enck P, Bingel U, Schedlowski M, Rief W. The placebo response in medicine: minimize, maximize or personalize? *Nat Rev Drug Discov* (2013) 12(3):191–204. doi: 10.1038/nrd3923

81. Rief W, Bingel U, Schedlowski M, Enck P. Mechanisms involved in placebo and nocebo responses and implications for drug trials. *Clin Pharmacol Ther* (2011) 90(5):722–6. doi: 10.1038/clpt.2011.204

82. Relton C, Torgerson D, O'Cathain A, Nicholl J. Rethinking pragmatic randomised controlled trials: introducing the "cohort multiple randomised controlled trial" design. *BMJ* (2010) 340:c1066. doi: 10.1136/bmj.c1066

83. Zelen M. A new design for randomized clinical trials. *N Engl J Med* (1979) 300 (22):1242–5. doi: 10.1056/NEJM197905313002203

84. Kaptchuk TJ. Open-Label Placebo: Reflections on a Research Agenda. *Perspect Biol Med* (2018) 61(3):311–34. doi: 10.1353/pbm.2018.0045

85. Schaefer M, Enck P. Effects of a probiotic treatment (Enterococcus faecalis) and open-label placebo on symptoms of allergic rhinitis: study protocol for a randomised controlled trial. *BMJ Open* (2019) 9(10):e031339. doi: 10.1136/bmjopen-2019-031339

9

The Role of GI Peptides in Functional Dyspepsia and Gastroparesis

Karen Van den Houte, Emidio Scarpellini, Wout Verbeure, Hideki Mori, Jolien Schol, Imke Masuy, Florencia Carbone and Jan Tack*

Translational Research Center for Gastrointestinal Diseases, University of Leuven, Leuven, Belgium

*Correspondence:
Jan Tack
jan.tack@kuleuven.be

Functional dyspepsia (FD) and gastroparesis (GP) are common disorders of the upper gastrointestinal tract. The pathophysiology of these conditions is likely to be heterogenous, and factors such as altered motility, sensitivity and response to nutrition have been identified as putative underlying mechanisms. Motility, sensitivity as well as responses to nutrition can be influenced or mediated by peptide hormones and serotonin released from the gastrointestinal mucosa. This review summarizes the role of GI peptides in functional dyspepsia and gastroparesis. In most studies, the levels of somatostatin, ghrelin, and motilin did not differ between healthy volunteers and FD or GP patients, but higher symptom burden was often correlated with higher peptide levels. Ghrelin and motilin receptor agonists showed promising results in improvement of the gastric emptying, but the link with improvement of symptoms is less predictable. Serotonin agonists have a potential to improve symptoms in both FD and idiopathic gastroparesis. Drugs acting on the GLP-1 and on the PYY receptors deserve further investigation. There is a need for systematic large scale studies.

Keywords: functional dyspepsia, gastroparesis, gastrointestinal peptides, cholecystokinin, glucagonlike peptide 1, peptide YY, motilin, ghrelin

INTRODUCTION

Functional Dyspepsia

Functional dyspepsia (FD), defined as "epigastric symptoms affecting daily life, such as postprandial fullness, early satiation, epigastric pain and burning, in the absence of underlying organic abnormalities" (1), is an extremely common functional gastrointestinal disorder. In the general population, the prevalence of FD is found to be up to 21% (2, 3). Although only a minority of *H. pylori* infected patients remain asymptomatic after successful eradication therapy, patients reporting *helicobacter pylori*-associated dyspeptic symptoms are now being recognized as a separate entity referred to as *H. pylori* associated dyspepsia (1, 4, 5).

To facilitate the management of FD, the Rome Consensus subdivided FD into two subtypes: Postprandial Distress Syndrome (PDS) (60%) characterized by meal-related symptoms, such as postprandial fullness, early satiation, postprandial epigastric pain and other symptoms triggered by food ingestion, and Epigastric Pain Syndrome (EPS) (20%) characterized by epigastric pain and burning (4, 6). Approximately 20% of FD patients overlaps between PDS and EPS.

FD is extremely common, with estimates of 10–30% prevalence in the general population, and is associated with substantial medical care costs and a considerable health economic impact (7–9). A proportion of 20–25% of the patients with severe and refractory GI symptoms also have psychosocial co-morbidities such as anxiety, depression or somatization and severely impaired daily functioning (about 10% of these patients have work disability). Somatization, namely multiple stress-related symptoms of unknown origin resulted to be the most important risk factor for impaired QOL in patients with severe functional dyspepsia (10). This FD subgroup is often referred to advanced care, which may be associated with even higher health economic costs (11).

Finally, FD patients also show an important degree of overlap with gastro-esophageal reflux disease (GERD) (12, 13) and irritable bowel syndrome (IBS), and are, thus, often misclassified.

Gastroparesis

Gastroparesis is characterized by delayed gastric emptying and by upper gastrointestinal symptoms (nausea, vomiting, abdominal pain, early satiety, bloating) in the absence of mechanical obstruction (14). Two of the most common types of gastropareses are idiopathic gastroparesis and diabetic gastroparesis (15). Gastroparesis can also be a complication of upper gastrointestinal surgery, neurological disease, collagen vascular disorders, viral infections, or drugs use (16). It is associated with a major impact on the patients' quality of life and substantial social and health economic costs (17).

Gastrointestinal Peptides

In the classical pathophysiological model, functional gastrointestinal disorders (FGIDs) are considered heterogeneous conditions, and symptoms are attributed to a combination of motility disturbances, visceral hypersensitivity, low grade mucosal immune activation, and altered processing of gut-brain signals (18). This is based on the presence of impaired gastric storage and emptying function in FD and gastroparesis, as well as findings of visceral hypersensitivity and increased levels of depression, somatization and anxiety, which are considered markers of altered gut-brain interaction (19–21).

Recent research has focused on visceral hypersensitivity as a common mechanism determining symptom severity and impact across several functional gastrointestinal disorders (19). To date, the focus of research has mainly been on hypersensitivity to mechanical stimuli, studied by balloon distention (22). However, there is increasing evidence for a role for visceral hypersensitivity to specific nutrients as well, suggested amongst other by the observation that FODMAPs induce symptoms and the observation that specific nutrients induce local immune activation in irritable bowel syndrome (IBS) patients but not in health (23, 24).

The gastrointestinal mucosa expresses a wide range of chemosensing receptors, which detect the presence and nature of nutrients in the lumen (25, 26). Nutrients are mainly sensed in the duodenum and jejunum, and initiate an avalanche-effect by releasing gut peptides from entero-endocrine cells into the blood stream. The brain receives these signals through activation of the vagus nerve or directly via the fenestrated blood brain region, the area postrema (25, 26).

There is recent evidence of nutrient-specific enhanced release of gut peptide hormones [motilin, ghrelin, peptide YY (PYY), cholecystokinin (CCK), and glucagon-like peptide 1 (GLP-1)]

in FD, which was correlated to intensities of the provoked symptoms. However, most studies are somewhat artificial as they used intraduodenal tube administration of selected nutrients, rather than ingestion of a true meal (27).

The aim of this review was to describe the current evidence on the role of gastrointestinal (GI) peptides in FGID, especially in FD and gastroparesis. We will also address implications for future applications or modulations of gastrointestinal peptides for FD and idiopathic and diabetic gastroparesis treatment.

METHODS

We conducted a Pubmed and Medline search for papers, reviews, metanalyses, case series, and RCTs using the following keywords and their associations: functional dyspepsia, gastroparesis, gastrointestinal peptides, CCK, GLP-1, PYY, motilin, ghrelin, and dipeptidyl peptidase (**Figure 1**). We included also included preliminary evidence from abstracts belonging to main national and international gastroenterological meetings (e.g., United European Gastroenterology Week, Digestive Disease Week, Neurogastroenterology and Motility meetings, and the Belgian Gastroenterology week).

RESULTS
Preliminary Consideration

Both in FD-PDS and in gastroparesis, symptoms are triggered by ingestion of a meal (28, 29). The release of gut peptides in response to nutrient intake is expected to be triggered sequentially, driven by the location of the entero-endocrine cells that are expressing them. Thus, nutrient arrival in the stomach is thought to affect the release of gastrin, ghrelin and potentially somatostatin, while duodenal exposure to nutrients may impact on the release of CCK, motilin, PYY, and GLP-1, among others (25–27). In addition, serotonin release is expected to occur when nutrients enter the duodenum (25) (**Figure 2**). The association between peptide levels and symptoms in FD and gastroparesis is summarized in **Table 1**.

Gastrin

Gastrin is released by G-cells in the stomach and is a major stimulus for gastric acid secretion (25). As a group, FD patients do not seem to have altered gastrin levels according to a study of Jonsson et al. (30). However, in a study by He et al., FD patients with delayed gastric emptying had significantly higher gastrin levels (31). A recent study from Poland confirmed these findings, with elevated gastrin levels in both PDS and EPS (32). Use of acid suppressive therapy, often applied in FD as first-line therapy, may increase gastrin levels and it remains unclear to which extent the studies could rigorously exclude such confounder. In a relatively small study from Japan, gastrin serum level did not predict the response to H2 blocker therapy in FD (33).

Somatostatin

Somatostatin is released in the stomach but also in the small bowel, and has a strong inhibitory effect on gastrointestinal motility and secretion (25). In the study by He et al., plasma

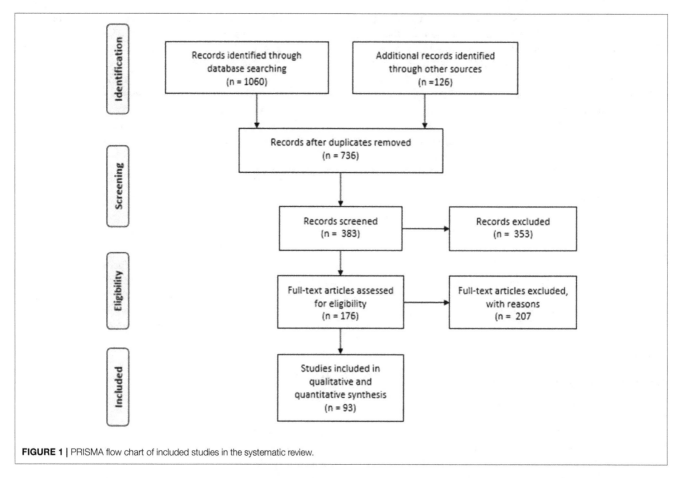

FIGURE 1 | PRISMA flow chart of included studies in the systematic review.

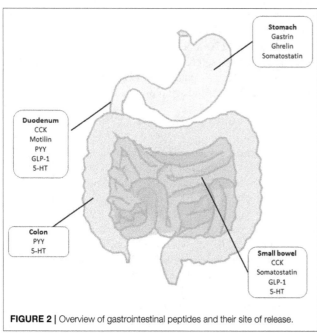

FIGURE 2 | Overview of gastrointestinal peptides and their site of release.

somatostatin levels and mucosal expression of somatostatin in the antrum and the duodenum did not differ between health and FD, with normal or delayed emptying (31). The same

was found in FD patients as a group in the study by Jonsson et al., but higher symptom burden was associated with higher fasting somatostatin levels in FD, and somatostatin levels were also correlated with heartburn severity scores (30). FD patients displayed a rapid, transient, somatostatin peak during a stress interview compared to matched controls (30). In a study by Russo et al., comparing gut peptide levels between 42 PDS and 12 EPS patients, somatostatin levels tended to be lower in PDS compared to EPS but this did not reach statistical significance (34). Itopride, a prokinetic agent with mixed dopamine-2 receptor and cholinesterase inhibitory actions, was reported to acutely increase somatostatin plasma levels (35). The somatostatin analog octreotide was reported to slow gastric emptying, enhance fasting gastric volumes and suppress meal-induced volume increments in healthy subjects (36). Clinical reports with somatostatin analogs in FD patients are lacking.

Ghrelin

Ghrelin is produced by endocrine P/D1 cells in the stomach, with plasma levels that increase during fasting and decrease after food intake (25, 88). Ghrelin a 28 amino acid peptide which needs to have an octanoyl group attached to its third serine residue to be biologically active (25). Ghrelin levels are inversely related to body weight (89, 90) and decrease with increasing extent of gastric mucosal atrophy (91, 92). Several studies have investigated ghrelin release in FD and gastroparesis,

TABLE 1 | Summary findings on the link between gut peptides, functional dyspepsia, and gastroparesis.

References	Peptide	Method	Subjects	Major findings
Jonnson et al. (30)	Gastrin	Gastrin dosage	FD patients	No altered gastrin levels.
He et al. (31)	Gastrin	Gastrin dosage	FD patients with delayed gastric emptying and HV	Higher gastrin levels
Walecka-Kapica et al. (32)	Gastrin	Gastrin dosage	PDS and EPS patients and HV	Higher gastrin levels
Yoshikawa et al. (33)	Gastrin	Gastrin dosage	FD patients on H2-blockers	Gastrin levels do not predict H2-blockers response
He et al. (29)	Somatostatin	Plasma somatostatin dosage and mucosal expression	FD with normal/delayed gastric emptying and HV	No differences between FD and HV
Jonnson et al. (30)	Somatostatin	Plasma somatostatin dosage	FD with normal/delayed gastric emptying and HV	Higher somatostatin levels associated with higher symptoms' burden and higher heartburn severity scores; rapid, transient, somatostatin peak during a stress interview
Russo et al. (34)	Somatostatin	Plasma somatostatin dosage	42 PDS and 12 EPS patients	Somatostatin levels tendency to be lower in PDS vs. EPS, without reaching statistical significance
Katagiri et al. (35)	Somatostatin	Plasma somatostatin dosage	HV administered with Itopride	Acute increase of somatostatin levels
Foxx-Orenstein et al. (36)	Somatostatin	Somatostatin analog Octreotide administration	HV	Slowed gastric emptying, enhanced fasting gastric volumes and suppressed meal-induced volume increments
Yagi et al. (37)	Ghrelin	Ghrelin dosage	Gastroparesis and HV (multiple studies)	No significant difference between patients and HV
Kim et al. (38)	Ghrelin	Ghrelin dosage	PDS and EPS patients vs. HV	Significant correlation between ghrelin levels and symptom severity, namely epigastric pain in EPS, early satiation in PDS patients
Shindo et al. (39)	Ghrelin	Ghrelin dosage	PDS and EPS patients with NERD	Negative correlation between plasma ghrelin levels and gastric emptying rate in PDS but not with EPS patients
Takamori et al. (40)	Ghrelin	Ghrelin dosage	Dismotility-like dyspepsia patients (Rome II criteria) vs. HV	Lower Ghrelin levels vs. HV
Nishizawa et al. (41)	Ghrelin	Ghrelin dosage	FD patients vs. HV	Higher Ghrelin levels vs. HV
Pilichiewicz et al. (42)	Ghrelin	Ghrelin dosage	FD patients vs. HV with high-fat meal ingestion	Ingestion of the meal did not affect plasma ghrelin levels in FD vs. HV
Akamizu et al. (43)	Ghrelin	Ghrelin i.v. administration b.i.d. for 2 weeks	FD patients with loss of appetite	Significantly increased appetite and tendency to increased daily food intake in FD patients with loss of appetite
Arai et al. (44)	Ghrelin	Rikkunshito administration	FD patients	Improved upper gastrointestinal symptoms, correlating with increased plasm ghrelin levels
Suzuki et al. (45)	Ghrelin	Rikkunshito administration	*Helicobacter pylori*-infected participants with increased plasma ghrelin levels	Improved upper gastrointestinal symptoms
Gaddipati et al. (46)	Ghrelin	Ghrelin dosage	Idiopathic, diabetic and post-surgical Gastroparesis patients vs. HV gastroparesis	Increased ghrelin levels after sham feeding in HV and IG patients vs. diabetic and postsurgical gastroparesis
Tack et al. (47)	Ghrelin	Gastric emptying and meal-related symptoms evaluation	IG patients	Increased gastric emptying and improved symptoms
Murray et al. (48)	Ghrelin	Gastric emptying and meal-related symptoms evaluation	Diabetic gastroparesis patients	Increased gastric emptying
Binn et al. (49)	Ghrelin	Gastric emptying evaluation	Neurogenic Gastroparesis patients	Increased gastric emptying
Ejskjaer et al. (50)	Ghrelin	Ulimorelin (ghrelin agonist) i.v. administration	Diabetic gastroparesis patients	Increased gastric emptying

(Continued)

TABLE 1 | Continued

References	Peptide	Method	Subjects	Major findings
Heyland et al. (51)	Ghrelin	Ulimorelin (ghrelin agonist) i.v. administration vs. Metoclopramide	Critical ill patients with enteral feeding intolerance	Increased gastric emptying for both treatments, impossible differentiation
Ejskjaer et al. (52)	Ghrelin	TZP-102 (ghrelin agonist) Phase 2a study, 12 weeks study	Diabetic gastroparesis patients	Increased gastric emptying
Mc Callum et al. (53)	Ghrelin	TZP-102 ghrelin agonist) Phase 2b study, 12 weeks study	Diabetic gastroparesis patients	Failed to confirm Increased gastric emptying
Lembo et al. (54)	Ghrelin	Relamorelin injections	Diabetic gastroparesis patients	Reduced vomiting frequency/severity; accelerated gastric emptying
Camilleri et al. (55)	Ghrelin	Relamorelin injections	Diabetic gastroparesis patients	Accelerated gastric emptying
Russo et al. (34)	Motilin	Motilin dosage	PDS and EPS patients	Higher motilin levels in EPS vs. PDS patients
Labo et al. (56)	Motilin	Motilin dosage	FD patients with delayed gastric emptying	Absence of motilin levels fluctuations during the interdigestive state; gastric phase III contractions absence
Achem-Karam et al. (57)	Motilin	Motilin dosage	Diabetic gaastroparesis patients	Elevated and fluctuating motilin plasma levels during the interdigestive state; antral phase III activity is absent
Talley et al. (58)	Motilin	ABT-229 administration	FD patients with and without delayed gastric emptying	No significant symptoms improvement
Talley et al. (59)	Motilin	ABT-229 administration	Type 1 diabetes mellitus patients	No significant symptoms improvement
McCallum et al. (60)	Motilin	Mitemcinal	Patients with idiopathic and diabetic gastroparesis	Accelerates gastric empying
Mccallum et al. (61)	Motilin	Mitemcinal	Diabetic patients with gastroparesis symptoms	Symptoms relief vs. placebo
Cuomo et al. (62)	Motilin	Motilin dosage	HV	Contraction of proximal stomach, increases satiety
Deloose et al. (63)	Motilin	Camicinal	HV	Stimulates MMC and gastric emptying
Hellstrom et al. (64)	Motilin	Camicinal single dose administration (25, 50, or 125 mg)	Type 1 Diabetic patients with gastroparesis symptoms	significantly accelerated gastric emptying of solids by 125 mg dose
Barton et al. (65)	Motilin	Camicinal	Diabetic patients with gastroparesis symptoms	Significantly accelerated gastric emptying
Chapman et al. (66)	Motilin	Camicinal	Critical ill patients with enteral feeding intolerance	Camicinal single dose (50 mg) acceleratedgastric emptying and increased glucose absorption
Chiloiro et al. (67)	CCK	Standard solid-liquid meal (gastric emptying)	H. pylori associated dyspepsia patients	Significantly lower basal values compared to H. pylori negative patients
Bharucha et al. (27)	CCK	Intraduodenal dextrose and lipid adminstration	FD patients vs. HV	Correlation between plasma concentrations of CCK and provoked symptoms Early increase of CCK plasma levels
Barbera et al. (68)	CCK	Intraduodenal administration of lipids	FD patients	Increases sensitivity to gastric distention
Feinle et al. (69)	CCK	Duodenal lipid infusion + CCK-A antagonist dexloxiglumide	FD patients	Lipid increased plasma CCK levels Dexloxiglumide reduced gastric compliance Gastric distention relieved by dexloxiglumide
van Boxel et al. (70)	CCK	Duodenal perfusion	FD patients vs. HV	Mean mucosal CCK concentration was lower in FD patients
Feinle-Bisset et al. (71)	CCK	High (HF) and low (LF) fat yogurt	FD patients	Plasma CCK was higher after HF compared to LF
Rotondo et al. (72)	GLP-1	Dipeptidyl peptidase-4 inhibitor (vildagliptin)	HV	Inhibition of gastric accommodation and increased GLP-1 plasma levels

(Continued)

TABLE 1 | Continued

References	Peptide	Method	Subjects	Major findings
Mano et al. (73)	GLP-1	Hot water and broth (with rice)	HV	Rise in GLP-1 after ingestion of synthesized broth
Witte et al. (74)	GLP-1	Liquid meal	FD patients (EPS)	Similar GLP-1 levels to HV, correlation with nausea
Pilichiewicz et al. (42)	PYY	PYY dosage	FD patients vs. HV with high-fat meal ingestion	Lower postprandial PYY levels compared to HV
Witte et al. (74)	PYY	Liquid meal	FD patients (EPS)	PYY3-36 is correlated with the sensation of fullness
Tack et al. (75)	5-HT	Cisapride (5-HT4 agonist)	HV	Enhances gastric distension and accommodation
Kessing et al. (76)	5-HT	Prucalopride (5-HT4 agonist)	HV after a standardized meal	Accelerates gastric emptying in male volunteers
Carbone et al. (77)	5-HT	Prucalopride (5-HT4 agonist)	Patients with gastroparesis	Enhances gastric emptying
Netzer et al. (78)	5-HT	Ondansetron (5-HT3 antagonist)	HV	No effect on gastric emptying
Janssen et al. (79)	5-HT	Ondansetron (5-HT3 antagonist)	HV	No effect on gastric compliance, gastric tone
Van Oudenhove et al. (80)	5-HT	Busprione (5-HT1A agonist)	HV	Relaxation of the proximal stomach + decreases gastric emptying
Tack et al. (81)	5-HT	Busprione (5-HT1A agonist)	FD patients	Decreased symptoms + increased gastric accommodation
Geeraerts et al. (82)	5-HT	Acute tryptophan depletion	HV	Reduction in 5-HT levels in duodenum
Tack et al. (83)	5-HT	Paroxetine	HV	Enhances gastric accommodation
Janssen et al. (84)	5-HT	Citalopram (5-HT reuptake inhibitor)	HV	Preprandial gastric relaxation, lower postprandial volume increase + enhances liquid emptying
Jannsen et al. (85)	5-HT	Citalopram (5-HT reuptake inhibitor)	HV	Suppresses gastric phase 2 Stimulates intestinal phase 3
Wilmer et al. (86)	5-HT	Ondansetron (5-HT3 antagonist)	HV	Suppresses gastric component of phase 3
Chueng et al. (87)	5-HT	5-HT postprandial levels	FD patients	Decreased levels of 5-HT

and the findings are conflicting (38). Most studies found no difference in fasting ghrelin levels in FD compared to health (37, 39–41, 93, 94). However, in a small group of EPS and PDS patients compared to health, correlations were reported between ghrelin levels and symptom severity, in particular epigastric pain in EPS and early satiation in PDS (38). Shindo et al. found a negative correlation between plasma acylated ghrelin levels and gastric emptying rate in patients with PDS but not with EPS (39). Takamori et al. reported lower levels of des-acyl ghrelin (the inactive form after hydrolysis of the octanoyl group), in dysmotility-like dyspepsia according to the Rome II criteria (40) while Nishizawa et al. reported higher ghrelin levels in FD patients as a group (41). The ingestion of a high fat meal in FD patients did not differently affect the plasma ghrelin levels in FD compared to healthy subjects (42). Intravenous administration of ghrelin, twice daily for 2 weeks, significantly increased appetite and tended to increase daily food intake in FD patients with loss of appetite (43). Furthermore, Arai et al. observed a clear improvement in upper gastrointestinal symptoms in FD patients after administration of the Japanese Kampo medicine Rikkunshito, which increased plasma ghrelin levels (44). Suzuki et al. also showed Rikkunshito was effective

among H. pylori-infected participants with increased plasma ghrelin levels (45).

Plasma ghrelin levels increased with sham feeding in healthy controls and patients with idiopathic gastroparesis but not in patients with diabetic or postsurgical gastroparesis, indicative of a role for intact vagal signaling in the control of ghrelin release (46). In pilot studies, acute intravenous administration of ghrelin enhanced gastric emptying rate in idiopathic and diabetic gastroparesis (47–49). In idiopathic gastroparesis patients, symptoms were also improved.

Subsequently, several ghrelin agonists have been studied, with a major focus on diabetic gastroparesis. The intravenously administered macrocylic peptidomimetic molecule ulimorelin, enhanced gastric emptying, and was subsequently mainly studied in critical care patients, with lack of differentiation from metoclopramide (50, 51). The orally administered TZP-102 showed promising results in phase 2a, but this was not confirmed in phase 2b (52, 53). Relamorelin, an injectable ghrelin receptor agonist, showed efficacy in diabetic gastroparesis patients with active vomiting symptoms in two placebo-controlled phase 2 studies and is being evaluated in phase 3 studies (54, 55).

Motilin

Motilin is released from M-cells situated in the proximal duodenum during the fasted state, is a stimulus for strong antral contractions and has a hunger signaling function (25, 95). Several studies evaluated plasma motilin levels in FD and gastroparesis (34, 56, 96–98). FD patients as a group have comparable fasting plasma levels to those in health (95). Russo et al. reported higher fasting motilin plasma levels in EPS compared to PDS (34). In the same study, elevated CRF levels were also reported in PDS. The relevance of this finding is unclear. It is well-known that motilin plasma levels fluctuate with interdigestive motility and are maximal during gastric phase III (95). The study by Russo et al. did not correct for migrating motor complex (MMC) cycle, which could be a major confounder, as it is conceivable that PDS patients have less occurrence of gastric phase III (96).

In patients with FD and delayed gastric emptying, motilin plasma levels did not display the normal fluctuations during the interdigestive state and gastric phase III contractions were absent (56). In patients with diabetic gastroparesis, motilin plasma levels were elevated but still fluctuating during the interdigestive state, although antral phase III activity was absent (57, 98). In FD patients with unexplained loss of appetite, gastric phase III contractions are suppressed, suggesting low plasma levels, but these were not measured in this study (99).

Several macrolide antibiotics such as erythromycin and azithromycin have motilin receptor agonistic effects, and have a stimulatory effect on gastric emptying rate (100–102). The impact on symptoms, however, was often disappointing (101). A number of macrolides without antibiotics but with motilin receptor agonistic properties were developed for the treatment of FD and diabetic gastroparesis (103). However, invariably, they failed to provide significant symptomatic benefit in phase 2 studies and no agent progressed into phase 3 studies (58–61, 104). The main reasons that have been put forward to explain the lack of success in trials with motilin agonist drugs for gastroparesis have been the use of too high doses, which impact on gastric accommodation, and the use of long-acting agents which are prone to desensitization (62, 103).

Camicinal is a novel small molecule motilin receptor agonist with short half-life, which was shown to induce gastric phase III contractions during the fasting state and dose-dependently enhance gastric emptying rate (63, 64). In a phase 2 study, the lowest dose of camicinal significantly improved symptoms, confirming the therapeutic potential of this class of agents, whereas only the highest dose studied enhanced gastric emptying. Indicating that enhanced emptying rate does not underlie the symptom improvement (65). Camicinal was also studied in critical care patients, but the drug has not advanced to phase 3 in any indication (66).

Cholecystokinin (CCK)

CCK is a brain-gut peptide released from I-cells in the upper small intestine upon food intake, especially after meals containing high fat or protein amounts (25). In *H. pylori* associated dyspepsia patients, significantly lower CCK basal values were demonstrated in comparison to *H. pylori* negative patients (67). Hyper responsiveness to CCK can be one of the

pathophysiological pathways for the occurrence of symptoms in FD patients (105). A recent study showed a correlation between the release of gut peptide hormones as CCK and provoked symptoms after infusion of nutrients into the duodenum (27). However, in this study, intraduodenal tube administration of selected nutrients was used, rather than ingestion of a true meal. An early increase of CCK plasma levels was found, followed later by a rise of other peptides such as GLP-1 and PYY. Previously, it has also been shown that the intraduodenal infusion of fat may trigger symptoms as fullness and discomfort and to sensitize the stomach to gastric distension (68, 105). Duodenal lipids induce higher CCK levels in patients with FD compared to health, and the CCK-A receptor antagonist dexloxiglumide, was able to reduced sensitivity to gastric distension after lipid administration (69, 70, 106). However, ingestion of a low fat meal when patients perceived intake of a high fat meal (cognitive factors) did not significantly change the CCK level but was associated with higher symptom scores (71).

In addition, a CCK antagonist accelerated the gastric emptying rate which could lead to a benefit in both functional dyspepsia as gastroparesis patients (107). The improvement in gastric emptying probably involves an effect of CCK on capsaicin-sensitive vagal pathways (107). Infusion of CCK in healthy volunteers resulted in an increase in gastric compliance, but this was not confirmed in a study with FD patients (108). Unfortunately, in spite of a number of positive mechanistic observations, CCK-receptor antagonists were not further developed for the treatment of FD.

Glucagon-Like Peptide 1 (GLP-1)

GLP-1, secreted by intestinal endocrine L-cells upon food intake, slows the gastric emptying in diabetes with a decrease in glycemia (108). In healthy controls, elevated GLP-1 plasma levels after administration of the Dipeptidyl peptidase-4 inhibitor vildagliptin, were associated with impaired gastric accommodation (72). In Japan, gastric emptying was measured in healthy subjects and increased significantly after ingestion of a broth with rice, which was accompanied by a significantly more rapid rise in plasma GLP-1 and glucose levels compared to rice with water (73). In an earlier study, it was shown that GLP-1 was correlated with nausea in a single meal experiment in FD patients subtype EPS as well as in healthy volunteers (74). This would be an interesting fact for the use of medication acting on the GLP-1 receptor for the treatment of gastroparesis patients with nausea as one of their main symptoms.

Peptide YY (PYY)

PYY is a gut hormone secreted from endocrine L-cells in the gut mucosa, most prominently present in the ileum and the colon, and released into the circulation after ingestion of food (25, 109). As mentioned above, the intake of lipids is often a trigger for symptoms in FD. In FD patients, ingestion of a high fat meal was associated with lower postprandial PYY levels compared to healthy volunteers (42). In addition, PYY was found to be correlated with symptoms such as a sensation of fullness in EPS patients after a single drink test and a satiety test (74). However, based on the literature, little is known about the effect of PYY in FD patients.

Serotonin (5-HT)

5-HT is also released by entero-endocrine cells in the gastrointestinal tract, in response to mechanical stimulation or the presence of nutrients or toxins (25, 110, 111). It has its effect via 14 known serotonin receptors, but we will focus on the most relevant ligands in this review. The role of 5-HT in upper gastrointestinal physiology remains unclear, due to a lack of suitable agonists and antagonists for human application (110). While 5-HT4 agonists enhance gastric accommodation and gastric emptying, 5-HT3 antagonists had no significant effect on these functions, and 5-HT_{1A} agonists enhance gastric accommodation and tend to slow gastric emptying (75–81). Alternative approaches to unravel a role for 5-HT in gastric sensorimotor function has been the use of tryptophan depletion (82) and the administration of selective serotonin reuptake inhibitors (SSRIs) (83, 84). Acute tryptophan depletion enhanced gastric accommodation, which was also observed with short-term SSRI use, while acute intravenous SSRI administration inhibited accommodation, suggesting that endogenous serotonin release serves to limit gastric accommodation (82–84). In terms of interdigestive gastric motility, acute intravenous SSRI administration suppresses gastric phase 3 while stimulating intestinal phase 3, and ondansetron also inhibited the occurrence of gastric phase 3 (85, 86).

Studies focusing on IBS have shown that circulating 5-HT levels rise after a meal, and that this rise is exaggerated in IBS with diarrhea and suppressed in IBS with constipation (112, 113). These studies used platelet-depleted plasma to measure circulating plasma levels of gastrointestinal origin, thereby eliminating the confounding effect of storage in thrombocytes. Similar studies in FD are lacking. One study measured plasma 5-HT in FD and found decreased basal and postprandial plasma compared to health (87). This is in agreement with a recent study reporting a decreased number of duodenal serotonin containing endocrine cells in FD patients (74).

Several 5-HT receptor agonists/antagonists, such as cisapride (5-HT4 agonist, 5-HT2, and 5-HT3 antagonist), tegaserod (5-HT4 and 5-HT1 agonist, 5-HT2a/b antagonist), mosapride (5-HT4 agonist, 5-HT3 antagonist) and revexepride (5-HT4 agonist) have been evaluated for the treatment of dyspepsia and gastroparesis, although not all studies show efficacy (114–116). A recent metanalysis showed that FD patients treated with serotonin receptor agonists have a significantly better symptom response compared to placebo (117) and the most recently published evidence indicates efficacy for prucalopride in idiopathic gastroparesis and emerging efficacy for velusetrag in gastroparesis (118, 119). Case series suggest potential benefit of the 5-HT_3 antagonists granisetron or ondansetron for symptoms of nausea and vomiting in gastroparesis, but formal studies are lacking (120, 121).

SUMMARY AND CONCLUSIONS

FD and gastroparesis, two of the most common FGIDs, are both characterized by upper GI symptoms. FD patients are subdivided in PDS and EPS patients, defined by symptoms as postprandial fullness, early satiety, epigastric pain, and epigastric burning. Patients with gastroparesis are characterized by nausea with or without vomiting, and often also similar symptoms as in FD, with a significantly delayed gastric emptying in the absence of mechanical obstruction. The most common subgroups are idiopathic and diabetic gastroparesis. The pathophysiology of both FGIDs is based on a combination of motility disturbances, visceral hypersensitivity, low grade mucosal immune activation, and altered processing of gut-brain-signals. Recent observations support a new pathophysiological model in at least subsets of patients with FD and gastroparesis, which involves visceral hypersensitivity to nutrients. Nutrient sensing occurs in the stomach and duodenum and is signaled to the brain through neural pathways, but especially through the release of gut peptides, which was shown in some studies to be correlated with symptoms in FD and gastroparesis.

In this review, the effect of peptides as gastrin, somatostatin, and ghrelin, all released by endocrine cells in the stomach, and of motilin, CCK, GLP-1, PYY and 5-HT, secreted in the duodenum, was summarized. Previous studies showed contradictory results regarding an increase in peptide levels in FD patients compared to health, but the impact of confounders, as the use of acid suppressive therapy for gastrin, the impact of MMC cycle for motilin, and the accumulation of 5-HT in thrombocytes, was not taken into account (28–30, 50). In most studies, the levels of somatostatin, ghrelin, and motilin did not differ between healthy volunteers and FD patients, however higher symptom burden was often correlated with higher peptide levels (28, 29, 36, 48). Nevertheless, most of these studies are limited by small sample sizes. Furthermore, a study by Russo et al. showed a trend toward higher somatostatin and motilin levels in EPS patients compared to PDS patients (32). However, the effect of gut peptides was mainly analyzed in FD patients as a group compared to healthy controls and only rarely in terms of EPS vs. PDS subgroups. In addition, little is known about the relation of gut peptides in FD patients fulfilling Rome IV criteria. *H. pylori* associated dyspepsia patients were shown to have lower CCK levels compared to *H.pylori* negative patients (67).

In patients with FD and gastroparesis, the correlation of gut peptides and gastric emptying was studied. Previously, a negative correlation was found between acylated ghrelin and gastric emptying (39). Intravenous administration of ghrelin increased the appetite in FD and enhanced gastric emptying and symptoms in idiopathic gastroparesis (43, 47–49). In addition, intraduodenal administration lipid administration provoked FD symptoms whose severity was correlated with CCK levels (27). Nevertheless, studies in which gut peptides are examined after eating a standard meal with an analysis on symptoms and motility disturbances, are lacking.

Based on the literature, low grade inflammation with increased mast cell and eosinophil count would underlie in the pathophysiological mechanisms of FGIDs and lead to an impaired barrier function. Duodenal factors, such as nutrients, may play a role in the activation of those eosinophils and mast cells. Therefore, it would be interesting to further investigate the effect of nutrients or diets on the release of GI peptides and evaluate this as a potential treatment option for FD or gastroparesis. Drugs acting on peptide receptors have already been tested in both groups, but is the scope of the available data is limited. Ghrelin agonists such as ulimorelin, relamorelin, and TZP-102, as well as 5-HT4 agonists and CCK antagonists all showed promising results in terms of improvement of the gastric emptying (50, 52–55, 66, 117–119). In addition, the use of motilin receptor agonists (macrolide antibiotics and camicinal) enhanced the gastric emptying, but there the link with improvement of symptoms is less predictable (66, 101). Serotonin agonists have a potential to improve symptoms in both FD and idiopathic

gastroparesis (114, 117 119). Drugs acting on the GLP-1 and on the PYY receptors deserve further investigation, because of the link between GLP-1 release and nausea, and the link between PYY release and postprandial fullness (74).

In summary, there is a clear need for in-depth evaluation of release of GI peptides after a standard meal in larger sample sizes of Rome IV PDS and EPS and gastroparesis patients. This should be complemented with detailed studies of drugs altering the level of GI peptides or their effect on their receptors.

AUTHOR CONTRIBUTIONS

KV, ES, and JT drafted the manuscript. All authors made edits and corrections and reviewed and approved the final version of the test.

REFERENCES

1. Stanghellini V, Chan FK, Hasler WL, Malagelada JR, Suzuki H, Tack J, et al. Gastroduodenal disorders. *Gastroenterology*. (2016) 150:1380–92. doi: 10.1053/j.gastro.2016.02.011
2. Mahadeva S, Goh KL. Epidemiology of functional dyspepsia: a global perspective. *World J Gastroenterol*. (2006) 12:2661–6. doi: 10.3748/wjg.v12.i17.2661
3. Piessevaux H, De Winter B, Louis E, Muls V, De Looze D, Pelckmans P, et al. Dyspeptic symptoms in the general population: a factor and cluster analysis of symptom groupings. *Neurogastroenterol Motil*. (2009) 21:378–88. doi: 10.1111/j.1365-2982.2009.01262.x
4. Sugano K, Tack J, Kuipers EJ, Graham DY, El-Omar EM, Miura S, et al. Kyoto global consensus report on Helicobacter pylori gastritis. *Gut*. (2015) 64:1353–67. doi: 10.1136/gutjnl-2015-309252
5. Ford AC, Moayyedi P, Jarbol DE, Logan RF, Delaney BC. Meta-analysis: *Helicobacter pylori* 'test and treat' compared with empirical acid suppression for managing dyspepsia. *Aliment Pharmacol Ther*. (2008) 28:534–44. doi: 10.1111/j.1365-2036.2008.03784.x
6. Tack J, Talley NJ. Functional dyspepsia–symptoms, definitions and validity of the Rome III criteria. *Nat Rev Gastroenterol Hepatol*. (2013) 10:134–41. doi: 10.1038/nrgastro.2013.14
7. Lacy BE, Weiser KT, Kennedy AT, Crowell MD, Talley NJ. Functional dyspepsia: the economic impact to patients. *Aliment Pharmacol Ther*. (2013) 38:170–7. doi: 10.1111/apt.12355
8. Aro P, Talley NJ, Agréus L, Johansson SE, Bolling-Sternevald E, Storskrubb T, et al. Functional dyspepsia impairs quality of life in the adult population. *Aliment Pharmacol Ther*. (2011) 33:1215–24. doi: 10.1111/j.1365-2036.2011.04640.x
9. El-Serag HB, Talley NJ. Health-related quality of life in functional dyspepsia. *Aliment Pharmacol Ther*. (2003) 18:387–93. doi: 10.1046/j.1365-2036.2003.01706.x
10. Van Oudenhove L, Vandenberghe J, Vos R, Fischler B, Demyttenaere K, Tack J. Abuse history, depression, and somatization are associated with gastric sensitivity and gastric emptying in functional dyspepsia. *Psychosom Med*. (2011) 73:648–55. doi: 10.1097/PSY.0b013e31822f32bf
11. Drossman DA. Functional gastrointestinal disorders: history, pathophysiology, clinical features and Rome IV. *Gastroenterology*. (2016) 150:1262–79. doi: 10.1053/j.gastro.2016.02.032
12. Quigley EM, Lacy BE. Overlap of functional dyspepsia and GERD–diagnostic

and treatment implications. *Nat Rev Gastroenterol Hepatol*. (2013) 10:175–86. doi: 10.1038/nrgastro.2012.253
13. Pleyer C, Bittner H, Locke GR, Choung RS, Zinsmeister AR, Schleck CD, et al. Overdiagnosis of gastro-esophageal reflux disease and underdiagnosis of functional dyspepsia in a USA community. *Neurogastroenterol Motil*. (2014) 26:1163–71. doi: 10.1111/nmo.12377
14. Tack J, Camilleri M. New developments in the treatment of gastroparesis and functional dyspepsia. *Curr Opin Pharmacol*. (2018) 43:111–7. doi: 10.1016/j.coph.2018.08.015
15. Stanghellini V Tack J. Gastroparesis: separate entity or just a part of dyspepsia? *Gut*. (2014) 63:1972–8. doi: 10.1136/gutjnl-2013-306084
16. Hasler WL. Gastroparesis: pathogenesis, diagnosis and management. *Nat Rev Gastroenterol Hepatol*. (2011) 8:438–53. doi: 10.1038/nrgastro.2011.116
17. Hirsch W, Nee J, Ballou S, Petersen T, Friedlander D, Lee HN, et al. Emergency Department Burden of Gastroparesis in the United States, 2006 to 2013. *J Clin Gastroenterol*. (2019) 53:109–13. doi: 10.1097/MCG.0000000000000972
18. Drossman DA, Hasler WL. Rome IV-functional GI disorders: disorders of gut-brain interaction. *Gastroenterology*. (2016) 150:1257–61. doi: 10.1053/j.gastro.2016.03.035
19. Simrén M, Törnblom H, Palsson OS, van Tilburg MAL, Van Oudenhove L, Tack J, et al. Visceral hypersensitivity is associated with GI symptom severity in functional GI disorders: consistent findings from five different patient cohorts. *Gut*. (2018) 67:255–62. doi: 10.1136/gutjnl-2016-312361
20. Jones MP, Tack J, Van Oudenhove L, Walker MM, Holtmann G, Koloski NA, et al. Mood and anxiety disorders precede development of functional gastrointestinal disorders in patients but not in the population. *Clin Gastroenterol Hepatol*. (2017) 15:1014–20.e4. doi: 10.1016/j.cgh.2016.12.032
21. Van Den Houte K, Carbone F, Tack J. Postprandial distress syndrome: stratification and management. *Expert Rev Gastroenterol Hepatol*. (2019) 13:37–46. doi: 10.1080/17474124.2019.1543586
22. Farré R, Vanheel H, Vanuytsel T, Masaoka T, Törnblom H, Simrén M, et al. In functional dyspepsia, hypersensitivity to postprandial distention correlates with meal-related symptom severity. *Gastroenterology*. (2013) 145:566–73. doi: 10.1053/j.gastro.2013.05.018
23. Halmos EP, Power VA, Shepherd SJ, Gibson PR, Muir JG. A diet low in FODMAPs reduces symptoms of irritable bowel syndrome. *Gastroenterology*. (2014) 146:67–75.e5. doi: 10.1053/j.gastro.2013.09.046
24. Fritscher-Ravens A, Pflaum T, Mösinger M, Ruchay Z, Röcken C, Milla PJ, et al. Many patients with irritable bowel syndrome have atypical food allergies not associated with immunoglobulin E. *Gastroenterology*. (2019) 157:109–18.e5. doi: 10.1053/j.gastro.2019.03.046

25. Farré R, Tack J. Food and symptom generation in functional gastrointestinal disorders: physiological aspects. *Am J Gastroenterol.* (2013) 108:698–706. doi: 10.1038/ajg.2013.24

26. Depoortere I. Taste receptors of the gut: emerging roles in health and disease. *Gut.* (2014) 63:179–90. doi: 10.1136/gutjnl-2013-305112

27. Bharucha AE, Camilleri M, Burton DD, Thieke SL, Feuerhak KJ, Basu A, et al. Increased nutrient sensitivity and plasma concentrations of enteral hormones during duodenal nutrient infusion in functional dyspepsia. *Am J Gastroenterol.* (2014) 109:1910–20; quiz 09:21. doi: 10.1038/ajg.2014.330

28. Bisschops R, Karamanolis G, Arts J, Caenepeel P, Verbeke K, Janssens J, et al. Relationship between symptoms and ingestion of a meal in functional dyspepsia. *Gut.* (2008) 57:1495–503. doi: 10.1136/gut.2007.137125

29. Karamanolis G, Caenepeel P, Arts J, Tack J. Determinants of symptom pattern in idiopathic severely delayed gastric emptying: gastric emptying rate or proximal stomach dysfunction? *Gut.* (2007) 56:29–36. doi: 10.1136/gut.2005.089508

30. Jonsson BH, Uvnäs-Moberg K, Theorell T, Gotthard R. Gastrin, cholecystokinin, and somatostatin in a laboratory experiment of patients with functional dyspepsia. *Psychosom Med.* (1998) 60:331–7. doi: 10.1097/00006842-199805000-00020

31. He MR, Song YG, Zhi FC. Gastrointestinal hormone abnormalities and G and D cells in functional dyspepsia patients with gastric dysmotility. *World J Gastroenterol.* (2005) 11:443–6. doi: 10.3748/wjg.v11.i3.443

32. Walecka-Kapica E, Klupinska G, Stec-Michalska K, Olszowiec K, Pawłowicz M, Chojnacki C. [Gastrin secretion in patients with functional dyspepsia]. *Pol Merkur Lekarski.* (2009) 26:362–5.

33. Yoshikawa I, Murata I, Kume K, Kanagawa K, Hirohata Y, Nakamura H, et al. Serum pepsinogen can predict response to H2-receptor antagonist in patients with functional dyspepsia. *Aliment Pharmacol Ther.* (2002) 16:1805–9. doi: 10.1046/j.1365-2036.2002.01352.x

34. Russo F, Chimienti G, Clemente C, Riezzo G, D'Attoma B, Martulli M. Gastric activity and gut peptides in patients with functional dyspepsia: postprandial distress syndrome versus epigastric pain syndrome. *J Clin Gastroenterol.* (2017) 51:136–44. doi: 10.1097/MCG.0000000000000531

35. Katagiri F, Shiga T, Inoue S, Sato Y, Itoh H, Takeyama M. Effects of itopride hydrochloride on plasma gut-regulatory peptide and stress-related hormone levels in healthy human subjects. *Pharmacology.* (2006) 77:115–21. doi: 10.1159/000093485

36. Foxx-Orenstein A, Camilleri M, Stephens D, Burton D. Effect of a somatostatin analogue on gastric motor and sensory functions in healthy humans. *Gut.* (2003) 52:1555–61. doi: 10.1136/gut.52.11.1555

37. Yagi T, Asakawa A, Ueda H, Miyawaki S, Inui A. The role of ghrelin in patients with functional dyspepsia and its potential clinical relevance (Review). *Int J Mol Med.* (2013) 32:523–31. doi: 10.3892/ijmm.2013.1418

38. Kim YS, Lee JS, Lee TH, Cho JY, Kim JO, Kim WJ, et al. Plasma levels of acylated ghrelin in patients with functional dyspepsia. *World J Gastroenterol.* (2012) 18:2231–7. doi: 10.3748/wjg.v18.i18.2231

39. Shindo T, Futagami S, Hiratsuka T, Horie A, Hamamoto T, Ueki N, et al. Comparison of gastric emptying and plasma ghrelin levels in patients with functional dyspepsia and non-erosive reflux disease. *Digestion.* (2009) 79:65–72. doi: 10.1159/000205740

40. Takamori K, Mizuta Y, Takeshima F, Akazawa Y, Isomoto H, Ohnita K, et al. Relation among plasma ghrelin level, gastric emptying, and psychologic condition in patients with functional dyspepsia. *J Clin Gastroenterol.* (2007) 41:477–83. doi: 10.1097/01.mcg.0000225614.94470.47

41. Nishizawa T, Suzuki H, Nomoto Y, Masaokas T, Hosoda H, Mori M, et al. Enhanced plasma ghrelin levels in patients with functional dyspepsia. *Aliment Pharmacol Ther.* (2006) 24(Suppl. 4):S104–10. doi: 10.1111/j.1365-2036.2006.00032.x

42. Pilichiewicz AN, Feltrin KL, Horowitz M, Holtmann G, Wishart JM, Jones KL, et al. Functional dyspepsia is associated with a greater symptomatic response to fat but not carbohydrate, increased fasting and postprandial CCK, and diminished PYY. *Am J Gastroenterol.* (2008) 103:2613–23. doi: 10.1111/j.1572-0241.2008.02041.x

43. Akamizu T, Iwakura H, Ariyasu H, Hosoda H, Murayama T, Yokode M, et al. Repeated administration of ghrelin to patients with functional dyspepsia: its effects on food intake and appetite. *Eur J Endocrinol.* (2008) 158:491–8. doi: 10.1530/EJE-07-0768

44. Arai M, Matsumura T, Tsuchiya N, Sadakane C, Inami R, Suzuki T, et al. Rikkunshito improves the symptoms in patients with functional dyspepsia, accompanied by an increase in the level of plasma ghrelin. *Hepatogastroenterology.* (2012) 59:62–6. doi: 10.5754/hge11246

45. Suzuki H, Matsuzaki J, Fukushima Y, Suzaki F, Kasugai K, Nishizawa T, et al. Randomized clinical trial: rikkunshito in the treatment of functional dyspepsia–a multicenter, double-blind, randomized, placebo-controlled study. *Neurogastroenterol Motil.* (2014) 26:950–61. doi: 10.1111/nmo.12348

46. Gaddipati KV, Simonian HP, Kresge KM, Boden GH, Parkman HP. Abnormal ghrelin and pancreatic polypeptide responses in gastroparesis. *Dig Dis Sci.* (2006) 51:1339–46. doi: 10.1007/s10620-005-9022-z

47. Tack J, Depoortere I, Bisschops R, Verbeke K, Janssens J, Peeters T. Influence of ghrelin on gastric emptying and meal-related symptoms in idiopathic gastroparesis. *Aliment Pharmacol Ther.* (2005) 22:847–53. doi: 10.1111/j.1365-2036.2005.02658.x

48. Murray CD, Martin NM, Patterson M, Taylor SA, Ghatei MA, Kamm MA, et al. Ghrelin enhances gastric emptying in diabetic gastroparesis: a double blind, placebo controlled, crossover study. *Gut.* (2005) 54:1693–8. doi: 10.1136/gut.2005.069088

49. Binn M, Albert C, Gougeon A, Maerki H, Coulie B, Lemoyne M, et al. Ghrelin gastrokinetic action in patients with neurogenic gastroparesis. *Peptides.* (2006) 27:1603–6. doi: 10.1016/j.peptides.2005.12.008

50. Ejskjaer N, Vestergaard ET, Hellström PM, Gormsen LC, Madsbad S, Madsen JL, et al. Ghrelin receptor agonist (TZP-101) accelerates gastric emptying in adults with diabetes and symptomatic gastroparesis. *Aliment Pharmacol Ther.* (2009) 29:1179–87. doi: 10.1111/j.1365-2036.2009.03986.x

51. Heyland DK, van Zanten ARH, Grau-Carmona T, Evans D, Beishuizen A, Schouten J, et al. A multicenter, randomized, double-blind study of ulimorelin and metoclopramide in the treatment of critically ill patients with enteral feeding intolerance: PROMOTE trial. *Intensive Care Med.* (2019) 45:647–56. doi: 10.1007/s00134-019-05593-2

52. Ejskjaer N, Wo JM, Esfandyari T, Mazen Jamal M, Dimcevski G, Tarnow L, et al. A phase 2a, randomized, double-blind 28-day study of TZP-102 a ghrelin receptor agonist for diabetic gastroparesis. *Neurogastroenterol Motil.* (2013) 25:e140–50. doi: 10.1111/nmo.12064

53. McCallum RW, Lembo A, Esfandyari T, Bhandari BR, Ejskjaer N, Cosentino C, et al. Phase 2b, randomized, double-blind 12-week studies of TZP-102, a ghrelin receptor agonist for diabetic gastroparesis. *Neurogastroenterol Motil.* (2013) 25:e705–17. doi: 10.1111/nmo.12184

54. Lembo A, Camilleri M, McCallum R, Sastre R, Breton C, Spence S, et al. Relamorelin reduces vomiting frequency and severity and accelerates gastric emptying in adults with diabetic gastroparesis. *Gastroenterology.* (2016) 151:87–96.e6. doi: 10.1053/j.gastro.2016.03.038

55. Camilleri M, McCallum RW, Tack J, Spence SC, Gottesdiener K, Fiedorek FT. Efficacy and safety of relamorelin in diabetics with symptoms of gastroparesis: a randomized, Placebo-Controlled Study. *Gastroenterology.* (2017) 153:1240–50.e2. doi: 10.1053/j.gastro.2017.07.035

56. Labo G, Bortolotti M, Vezzadini P, Bonora G, Bersani G. Interdigestive gastroduodenal motility and serum motilin levels in patients with idiopathic delay in gastric emptying. *Gastroenterology.* (1986) 90:20–6. doi: 10.1016/0016-5085(86)90069-7

57. Achem-Karam SR, Funakoshi A, Vinik AI, Owyang C. Plasma motilin concentration and interdigestive migrating motor complex in diabetic gastroparesis: effect of metoclopramide. *Gastroenterology.* (1985) 88:492–9. doi: 10.1016/0016-5085(85) 90512-8

58. Talley NJ, Verlinden M, Snape W, Beker JA, Ducrotte P, Dettmer A, et al. Failure of a motilin receptor agonist (ABT-229) to relieve the symptoms of functional dyspepsia in patients with and without delayed gastric emptying: a randomized double-blind placebo-controlled trial. *Aliment Pharmacol Ther.* (2000) 14:1653–61. doi: 10.1046/j.1365-2036.2000.00868.x

59. Talley NJ, Verlinden M, Geenen DJ, Hogan RB, Riff D, McCallum RW, et al. Effects of a motilin receptor agonist (ABT-229) on upper gastrointestinal symptoms in type 1 diabetes mellitus: a randomised, double blind, placebo controlled trial. *Gut.* (2001) 49:395–401. doi: 10.1136/gut.49.3.395

60. McCallum RW, Cynshi O, Investigative Team. Clinical trial: effect of mitemcinal (a motilin agonist) on gastric emptying in patients with gastroparesis - a randomized, multicentre, placebo-controlled study. *Aliment*

Pharmacol Ther. (2007) 26:1121–30. doi: 10.1111/j.1365-2036.2007.03461.x

61. McCallum RW, Cynshi O, US investigative team. Efficacy of mitemcinal, a motilin agonist, on gastrointestinal symptoms in patients with symptoms suggesting diabetic gastropathy: a randomized, multi-center, placebo-controlled trial. *Aliment Pharmacol Ther.* (2007) 26:107–16. doi: 10.1111/j.1365-2036.2007.03346.x

62. Cuomo R, Vandaele P, Coulie B, Peeters T, Depoortere I, Janssens J, et al. Influence of motilin on gastric fundus tone and on meal-induced satiety in man: role of cholinergic pathways. *Am J Gastroenterol.* (2006) 101:804–11. doi: 10.1111/j.1572-0241.2005.00339.x

63. Deloose E, Depoortere I, de Hoon J, Van Hecken A, Dewit OE, Vasist Johnson LS, et al. Manometric evaluation of the motilin receptor agonist camicinal (GSK962040) in humans. *Neurogastroenterol Motil.* (2018) 30:e13173. doi: 10.1111/nmo.13173

64. Hellström P, Tack J, Johnson L, Hacqouil K, Barton M, Richards D, et al. The pharmacodynamics, safety, and pharmacokinetics of single doses of the motilin agonist, camicinal, in type 1 diabetes mellitus with slow gastric emptying. *Br J Pharmacol.* (2016) 173:1768–77. doi: 10.1111/bph.13475

65. Barton ME, Otiker T, Johnson LV, Robertson DC, Dobbins RL, Parkman HP, et al. A randomized, double-blind, placebo-controlled phase II study (MOT114479) to evaluate the safety and efficacy and dose response of 28 days of orally administered camicinal, a motilin receptor agonist, in diabetics with gastroparesis. *Gastroenterology.* (2014) 146:S20. doi: 10.1016/S0016-5085(14)60070-6

66. Chapman MJ, Deane AM, O'Connor SL, Nguyen NQ, Fraser RJ, Richards DB, et al. The effect of camicinal (GSK962040), a motilin agonist, on gastric emptying and glucose absorption in feed-intolerant critically ill patients: a randomized, blinded, placebo-controlled, clinical trial. *Crit Care.* (2016) 20:232. doi: 10.1186/s13054-016-1420-4

67. Chiloiro M, Russo F, Riezzo G, Leoci C, Clemente C, Messa C, et al. Effect of Helicobacter pylori infection on gastric emptying and gastrointestinal hormones in dyspeptic and healthy subjects. *Dig Dis Sci.* (2001) 46:46–53. doi: 10.1023/A:1005601623363

68. Barbera R, Feinle C, Read NW. Abnormal sensitivity to duodenal lipid infusion in patients with functional dyspepsia. *Eur J Gastroenterol Hepatol.* (1995) 7:1051–7. doi: 10.1097/00042737-199511000-00007

69. Feinle C, Meier O, Otto B, D'Amato M, Fried M. Role of duodenal lipid and cholecystokinin A receptors in the pathophysiology of functional dyspepsia. *Gut.* (2001) 48:347–55. doi: 10.1136/gut.48.3.347

70. van Boxel OS, ter Linde JJ, Oors J, Otto B, Weusten BL, Feinle-Bisset C, et al. Functional dyspepsia patients have lower mucosal cholecystokinin concentrations in response to duodenal lipid. *Eur J Gastroenterol Hepatol.* (2014) 26:205–12. doi: 10.1097/MEG.0000000000000001

71. Feinle-Bisset C, Meier B, Fried M, Beglinger C. Role of cognitive factors in symptom induction following high and low fat meals in patients with functional dyspepsia. *Gut.* (2003) 52:1414–8. doi: 10.1136/gut.52.10.1414

72. Rotondo A, Masuy I, Verbeure W, Biesiekierski JR, Deloose E, Tack J. Randomised clinical trial: the DPP-4 inhibitor, vildagliptin, inhibits gastric accommodation and increases glucagon-like peptide-1 plasma levels in healthy volunteers. *Ent Pharmacol Ther.* (2019) 49:997–1004. doi: 10.1111/apt.15195

73. Mano F, Ikeda K, Joo E, Yamane S, Harada N, Inagaki N. Effects of three major amino acids found in Japanese broth on glucose metabolism and gastric emptying. *Nutrition.* (2018) 46:153–8.e1. doi: 10.1016/j.nut.2017.08.007

74. Witte AB, Hilsted L, Holst JJ, Schmidt PT. Peptide YY3-36 and glucagon-like peptide-1 in functional dyspepsia. Secretion and role in symptom generation. *Scand J Gastroenterol.* (2016) 51:400–9. doi: 10.3109/00365521.2015.1101780

75. Tack J, Broeckaert D, Coulie B, Janssens J. Influence of cisapride on gastric tone and on the perception of gastric distension. *Alim Pharmacol Ther.* (1998) 12:761–6. doi: 10.1046/j.1365-2036.1998.00366.x

76. Kessing BF, Smout AJ, Bennink RJ, Kraaijpoel N, Oors JM, Bredenoord AJ. Prucalopride decreases esophageal acid exposure and accelerates gastric emptying in healthy subjects. *Neurogastroenterol Motil.* (2014) 26:1079–86. doi: 10.1111/nmo.12359

77. Carbone F, Tack J. The effect of prucalopride on gastric accommodation in healthy volunteers. *Neurogastroenterol Motil.* (2014) 26(Suppl. 1):3–4. doi: 10.1111/nmo.12411

78. Netzer P, Gaia C, Lourens ST, Reber P, Wildi S, Noelpp U, et al. Does intravenous ondansetron affect gastric emptying of a solid meal, gastric electrical activity or blood hormone levels in healthy volunteers? *Aliment Pharmacol Ther.* (2002) 16:119–27. doi: 10.1046/j.1365-2036.2002.01152.x

79. Janssen P, Vos R, Van Oudenhove L, Tack J. Influence of the 5-HT(3) receptor antagonist ondansetron on gastric sensorimotor function and nutrient tolerance in healthy volunteers. *Neurogastroenterol Motil.* (2011) 23:444–9.e175. doi: 10.1111/j.1365-2982.2010.01655.x

80. Van Oudenhove L, Kindt S, Vos R, Coulie B, Tack J. Influence of buspirone on gastric sensorimotor function in man. *Aliment Pharmacol Ther.* (2008) 28:1326–33. doi: 10.1111/j.1365-2036.2008.03849.x

81. Tack J, Janssen P, Masaoka T, Farré R, Van Oudenhove L. Efficacy of buspirone, a fundus-relaxing drug, in patients with functional dyspepsia. *Clin Gastroenterol Hepatol.* (2012) 10:1239–45. doi: 10.1016/j.cgh.2012.06.036

82. Geeraerts B, Van Oudenhove L, Boesmans W, Vos R, Vanden Berghe P, Tack J. Influence of acute tryptophan depletion on gastric sensorimotor function in humans. *Am J Physiol Gastrointest Liver Physiol.* (2011) 300:G228–35. doi: 10.1152/ajpgi.00020.2010

83. Tack J, Broekaert D, Coulie B, Fischler B, Janssens J. Influence of the selective serotonin reuptake inhibitor paroxetine on gastric sensorimotor function in man. *Alim Pharmacol Ther.* (2003) 17:603–8. doi: 10.1046/j.1365-2036.2003.01469.x

84. Janssen P, Van Oudenhove L, Casteels C, Vos R, Verbeke K, Tack J. The effects of acute citalopram dosing on gastric motor function and nutrient tolerance in healthy volunteers. *Aliment Pharmacol Ther.* (2011) 33:395–402. doi: 10.1111/j.1365-2036.2010.04522.x

85. Janssen P, Vos R, Tack J. The influence of citalopram on interdigestive gastrointestinal motility in man. *Aliment Pharmacol Ther.* (2010) 32:289–95. doi: 10.1111/j.1365-2036.2010.04351.x

86. Wilmer A, Tack J, Coremans G, Janssens J, Peeters T, Vantrappen G. 5-Hydroxytryptamine3 receptors are involved in the initiation of gastric phase 3 motor activity in man. *Gastroenterology.* (1993) 105:773–80. doi: 10.1016/0016-5085(93)90895-J

87. Cheung CK, Lee YY, Chan Y, Cheong PK, Law WT, Lee SF, et al. Decreased Basal and postprandial plasma serotonin levels in patients with functional dyspepsia. *Clin Gastroenterol Hepatol.* (2013) 11:1125–9. doi: 10.1016/j.cgh.2013.03.026

88. Cummings DE, Purnell JQ, Frayo RS, Schmidova K, Wisse BE, Weigle DS. A preprandial rise in plasma ghrelin levels suggests a role in meal initiation in humans. *Diabetes.* (2001) 50:1714–9. doi: 10.2337/diabetes.50.8.1714

89. Shiiya T, Nakazato M, Mizuta M, Date Y, Mondal MS, Tanaka M, et al. Plasma ghrelin levels in lean and obese humans and the effect of glucose on ghrelin secretion. *J Clin Endocrinol Metab.* (2002) 87:240–4. doi: 10.1210/jcem.87.1.8129

90. Tschöp M, Weyer C, Tataranni PA, Devanarayan V, Ravussin E, Heiman ML. Circulating ghrelin levels are decreased in human obesity. *Diabetes.* (2001) 50:707–9. doi: 10.2337/diabetes.50.4.707

91. Suzuki H, Masaoka T, Hosoda H, Nomura S, Ohara T, Kangawa K, et al. Plasma ghrelin concentration correlates with the levels of serum pepsinogen I and pepsinogen I/II ratio–a possible novel and non-invasive marker for gastric atrophy. *Hepatogastroenterology.* (2004) 51:1249–54.

92. Kawashima J, Ohno S, Sakurada T, Takabayashi H, Kudo M, Ro S, et al. Circulating acylated ghrelin level decreases in accordance with the extent of atrophic gastritis. *J Gastroenterol.* (2009) 44:1046–54. doi: 10.1007/s00535-009-0120-0

93. Lee KJ, Cha DY, Cheon SJ, Yeo M, Cho SW. Plasma ghrelin levels and their relationship with gastric emptying in patients with dysmotility-like functional dyspepsia. *Digestion.* (2009) 80:58–63. doi: 10.1159/000215389

94. Shinomiya T, Fukunaga M, Akamizu T, Irako T, Yokode M, Kangawa K, et al. Plasma acylated ghrelin levels correlate with subjective symptoms of functional dyspepsia in female patients. *Scand J Gastroenterol.* (2005) 40:648–53. doi: 10.1080/00365520510015403

95. Deloose E, Janssen P, Depoortere I, Tack J. The migrating motor complex: control mechanisms and its role in health and disease. *Nat Rev Gastroenterol Hepatol.* (2012) 9:271–85. doi: 10.1038/nrgastro.2012.57

96. Wilmer A, Van Cutsem E, Andrioli A, Tack J, Coremans G, Janssens

J. Prolonged ambulatory gastrojejunal manometry in severe motility-like dyspepsia: lack of correlation between dysmotility, symptoms and gastric emptying. *Gut.* (1998) 42:235–42. doi: 10.1136/gut.42.2.235

97. Kamerling IM, Van Haarst AD, Burggraaf J, Schoemaker RC, Biemond I, Heinzerling H, et al. Motilin effects on the proximal stomach in patients with functional dyspepsia and healthy volunteers. *Am J Physiol Gastrointest Liver Physiol.* 284:G776–81. doi: 10.1152/ajpgi.00456.2002

98. Imura H, Seino Y, Mori K, Itoh Z, Yanaihara N. Plasma motilin levels in normal subjects and patients with diabetes mellitus and certain other diseases. Fasting levels and responses to food and glucose. *Endocrinol Jpn.* (1980) 27(Suppl. 1):151–5. doi: 10.1507/endocrj1954.27.Supplement_151

99. Tack J, Deloose E, Ang D, Scarpellini E, Vanuytsel T, Van Oudenhove L, et al. Motilin-induced gastric contractions signal hunger in man. *Gut.* (2016) 65:214–24. doi: 10.1136/gutjnl-2014-308472

100. Janssens J, Peeters TL, Vantrappen G, Tack J, Urbain JL, De Roo M, et al. Improvement of gastric emptying in diabetic gastroparesis by erythromycin. Preliminary studies. *N Engl J Med.* (1990) 322:1028–31. doi: 10.1056/NEJM199004123221502

101. Arts J, Caenepeel P, Verbeke K, Tack J. Influence of erythromycin on gastric emptying and meal related symptoms in functional dyspepsia with delayed gastric emptying. *Gut.* (2005) 54:455–60. doi: 10.1136/gut.2003.035279

102. Larson JM, Tavakkoli A, Drane WE, Toskes PP, Moshiree B. Advantages of azithromycin over erythromycin in improving the gastric emptying half-time in adult patients with gastroparesis. *J Neurogastroenterol Motil.* (2010) 16:407–13. doi: 10.5056/jnm.2010.16.4.407

103. Tack J, Peeters TL. What comes after macrolides and other motilin stimulants? *Gut.* (2001) 49:317–8. doi: 10.1136/gut.49.3.317

104. Russo A, Stevens JE, Giles N, Krause G, O'Donovan DG, Horowitz M, et al. Effect of the motilin agonist KC 11458 on gastric emptying in diabetic gastroparesis. *Aliment Pharmacol Ther.* (2004) 20:333–8. doi: 10.1111/j.1365-2036.2004.02066.x

105. Chua AS, Keeling PW, Dinan TG. Role of cholecystokinin and central serotonergic receptors in functional dyspepsia. *World J Gastroenterol.* (2006) 12:1329–35. doi: 10.3748/wjg.v12.i9.1329

106. Fried M, Feinle C. The role of fat and cholecystokinin in functional dyspepsia. *Gut.* (2002) 51(Suppl. 1):i54–7. doi: 10.1136/gut.51.suppl_1.i54

107. Scarpignato C, Varga G, Corradi C. Effect of CCK and its antagonists on gastric emptying. *J Physiol.* (1993) 87:291–300. doi: 10.1016/0928-4257(93)90035-R

108. Chua AS, Keeling PW. Cholecystokinin hyperresponsiveness in functional dyspepsia. *World J Gastroenterol.* (2006) 12:2688–93. doi: 10.3748/wjg.v12.i17.2688

109. Adrian TE, Ferri GL, Bacarese-Hamilton AJ, Fuessl HS, Polak JM, Bloom SR. Human distribution and release of a putative new gut hormone, peptide YY. *Gastroenterology.* (1985) 89:1070–7. doi: 10.1016/0016-5085(85)90211-2

110. Gershon MD, Tack J. The serotonin signalling system: from basic understanding to drug development for functional GI disorders. *Gastroenterology.* (2007) 219:172–80. doi: 10.1053/j.gastro.2006.11.002

111. Kidd M, Modlin IM, Gustafsson BI, Drozdov I, Hauso O, Pfragner R. Luminal regulation of normal and neoplastic human EC cell serotonin release is mediated by bile salts, amines, tastants, and olfactants. *Am J Physiol Gastrointest Liver Physiol.* (2008) 295:G260–72. doi: 10.1152/ajpgi.00056.2008

112. Atkinson W, Lockhart S, Whorwell PJ, Keevil B, Houghton LA. Altered 5-hydroxytryptamine signaling in patients with constipation- and diarrhea-predominant irritable bowel syndrome. *Gastroenterology.* (2006) 130:34–43. doi: 10.1053/j.gastro.2005.09.031

113. Dunlop SP, Coleman NS, Blackshaw E, Perkins AC, Singh G, Marsden CA, et al. Abnormalities of 5-hydroxytryptamine metabolism in irritable bowel syndrome. *Clin Gastroenterol Hepatol.* (2005) 3:349–57. doi: 10.1016/S1542-3565(04)00726-8

114. Tack J, Van den Houte K, Carbone F. The unfulfilled promise of prokinetics for functional dyspepsia/postprandial distress syndrome. *Am J Gastroenterol.* (2019) 114:204–6. doi: 10.14309/ajg.0000000000000072

115. Hallerback BI, Bommelaer G, Bredberg E, Campbell M, Hellblom M, Lauritsen K, et al. Dose finding study of mosapride in functional dyspepsia: a placebo-controlled, randomized study. *Aliment Pharmacol Ther.* (2002) 16:959–67. doi: 10.1046/j.1365-2036.2002.01236.x

116. Tack J, Rotondo A, Meulemans A, Thielemans L, Cools M. Randomized clinical trial: a controlled pilot trial of the 5-HT4 receptor agonist revexepride in patients with symptoms suggestive of gastroparesis. *Neurogastroenterol Motil.* (2016) 28:487–97. doi: 10.1111/nmo.12736

117. Jin M, Mo Y, Ye K, Chen M, Liu Y, He C. Efficacy of serotonin receptor agonists in the treatment of functional dyspepsia: a meta-analysis. *Arch Med Sci.* (2019) 15:23–32. doi: 10.5114/aoms.2017.69234

118. Carbone F, Van den Houte K, Clevers E, Andrews CN, Papathanasopoulos A, Holvoet L, et al. Prucalopride in gastroparesis: a randomized placebo-controlled crossover study. *Am J Gastroenterol.* (2019) 114:1265–74. doi: 10.14309/ajg.0000000000000304

119. Abell T, Kuo B, Esfandyari T, Canafax D, Camerini R, Grimaldi M, et al. Velusetrag improves gastroparesis both in symptoms and gastric emptying in patients with diabetic or idiopathic gastroparesis in a 12-week global phase 2B study. *Gastroenterology.* (2019) 156:S164. doi: 10.1016/S0016-5085(19)37201-4

120. Midani D, Parkman HP. Granisetron transdermal system for treatment of symptoms of gastroparesis: a prescription registry study. *J Neurogastroenterol Motil.* (2016) 22:650–5. doi: 10.5056/jnm15203

121. Simmons K, Parkman HP. Granisetron transdermal system improves refractory nausea and vomiting in gastroparesis. *Dig Dis Sci.* (2014) 59:1231–4. doi: 10.1007/s10620-014-3097-3

10

Epigenetic Mechanisms in Irritable Bowel Syndrome

*Swapna Mahurkar-Joshi and Lin Chang**

G. Oppenheimer Center for Neurobiology of Stress and Resilience, Division of Digestive Diseases, Department of Medicine at UCLA, Los Angeles, CA, United States

*Correspondence:
Lin Chang
linchang@mednet.ucla.edu

Irritable bowel syndrome (IBS) is a brain-gut axis disorder characterized by abdominal pain and altered bowel habits. IBS is a multifactorial, stress-sensitive disorder with evidence for familial clustering attributed to genetic or shared environmental factors. However, there are weak genetic associations reported with IBS and a lack of evidence to suggest that major genetic factor(s) contribute to IBS pathophysiology. Studies on animal models of stress, including early life stress, suggest a role for environmental factors, specifically, stress associated with dysregulation of corticotropin releasing factor and hypothalamus-pituitary-adrenal (HPA) axis pathways in the pathophysiology of IBS. Recent evidence suggests that epigenetic mechanisms, which constitute molecular changes not driven by a change in gene sequence, can mediate environmental effects on central and peripheral function. Epigenetic alterations including DNA methylation changes, histone modifications, and differential expression of non-coding RNAs (microRNA [miRNA] and long non-coding RNA) have been associated with several diseases. The objective of this review is to elucidate the molecular factors in the pathophysiology of IBS with an emphasis on epigenetic mechanisms. Emerging evidence for epigenetic changes in IBS includes changes in DNA methylation in animal models of IBS and patients with IBS, and various miRNAs that have been associated with IBS and endophenotypes, such as increased visceral sensitivity and intestinal permeability. DNA methylation, in particular, is an emerging field in the realm of complex diseases and a promising mechanism which can provide important insights into IBS pathogenesis and identify potential targets for treatment.

Keywords: irritable bowel syndrome, IBS, epigenetics, visceral hypersensitivity, DNA methylation, microRNA, histone modifications, long non-coding RNA

INTRODUCTION

Irritable bowel syndrome (IBS) is a complex condition characterized by alterations of bidirectional brain-gut interactions affecting gastrointestinal (GI) function. It is a widely prevalent disorder affecting about 5% to 11% of general population and occurs in children and adults and in men and women although it is considered a female-predominant condition. Hallmark symptoms include the presence of chronic or recurrent abdominal pain associated with altered bowel habits without underlying structural abnormalities (1–4). IBS has been subdivided on the basis of predominant bowel habits into diarrhea-predominant (IBS-D), constipation-predominant (IBS-C), or a mix of diarrhea and constipation (IBS-M) subtypes (3). IBS can coexist with other GI disorders including gastroesophageal reflux disease and functional dyspepsia, as well as somatic syndromes including fibromyalgia, interstitial cystitis, migraine headaches, and psychologic disorders (5). Due to its high prevalence, recurrent nature of symptoms and a negative impact on health-related quality of life (6), IBS is associated with substantial cost to patients, the health care system, and society (7).

IBS is considered to be a multi-factorial disorder, however, its pathophysiology is not completely understood. IBS and other functional GI disorders have more recently been redefined by experts as "disorders of gut-brain interactions (DGBI) classified by GI symptoms related to any combination of the following: motility disturbance, visceral hypersensitivity, altered mucosal and immune function, altered gut microbiota, and altered central nervous system (CNS) processing" (4). The presence of emotional and psychological factors and food intolerance contribute to the clinical presentation and can exacerbate IBS symptoms (8, 9).

Studies have shown that genetic factors have a modest effect in IBS (10). In addition, there is increasing evidence of a strong influence of environmental factors such as stress in its pathogenesis. A number of studies have found that IBS patients have a higher prevalence of stressful events including early adverse life events (EALs), or traumatic experiences during childhood, as well as current stressful life events in adulthood (11–13). The mechanisms underlying long-term effects of stress and EALs may result from epigenetic programing (14). Epigenetic changes refer to molecular alterations that potentially lead to altered gene expression resulting in a change in phenotype in absence of alteration in the underlying gene sequence.

In this review, we summarize the genetic factors associated with IBS and describe the role of epigenetic factors including DNA methylation and histone modifications as links between genes and environmental factors (e.g., stress) in the etiopathology of IBS. We review the current knowledge of epigenetic modifications associated with IBS in patients as well as in early life stress animal models of IBS, and those associated with IBS endophenotypes (defined as intermediate phenotypes of subclinical traits) including stress and hypothalamic–pituitary–adrenal (HPA) axis function, visceral hypersensitivity and abdominal pain, and GI motility. Further, we briefly outline the role of other epigenetic factors including non-coding RNAs (long non-coding RNAs [lncRNAs] and microRNAs [miRNAs]) in IBS. Finally, we will present a schematic model of our current understanding of factors associated with IBS pathogenesis. A better understanding of the epigenetic mechanisms in IBS can open new avenues for the identification of novel therapeutic targets.

GENETIC CHANGES ASSOCIATED WITH IBS

Familial Aggregation and Twin Studies in IBS

IBS is often associated with familial clustering in which patients report a family history of IBS (15–17). However, the strength of the genetic association varies between studies. One study reported familial aggregation in IBS but found no evidence of association in spouses, suggesting either a possible genetic etiology or an exposure to a shared household environmental factor early in life as an underlying cause of IBS (18). Additional evidence in favor of both a genetic and environmental etiology of IBS comes from twin studies. Twin studies by Morris-Yates et al. (19) and Svedberg et al. (20) provided evidence for genetic basis of IBS in Australian and Swedish populations. In two large studies on 281 twin pairs in the United States (21) and 3334 twin pairs in Norway (22), Levy et al. and Bengtson et al. showed a higher concordance rate among monozygotic twins than in dizygotic twins for IBS. However, one study by Mohammed et al. (23), failed to replicate the differences in the concordance rates between the monozygotic and dizygotic twin groups. Interestingly, Levy et al. also reported that the presence of IBS in the mother was a strong predictor of having IBS. The proportion of twins who had mothers with IBS was 15.2% which was significantly higher than the 6.7% of twins with IBS who had a co-twin with IBS. Since dizygotic twins share about the same number of genes with each other as each twin shares with their mother, this study suggested that in addition to heredity, social learning, and behavior may contribute to the development of IBS (24).

Candidate Gene Studies in IBS

IBS has been associated with genetic variants in a number of candidate genes. Genes associated with IBS in various studies are listed in **Table 1**. These include single nucleotide polymorphisms (SNPs) in genes related to signaling systems important in the control of gut motility or sensation in IBS, which includes serotoninergic (5-HT) system including tryptophan hydroxylase (TPH), serotonin reuptake transporter (SERT), a, cholecystokinin (CCK), voltage-gated sodium channels (Nav), Catechol-O-methyltransferase (COMT), cannabinoids, and ion channels, such as transient receptor potential (TRP) channels (TRPV1). Immune related SNPs have been of particular interest in IBS based on accumulating evidence showing immune activation in IBS (25). However, findings have been variable across studies and association of genes such as tumor necrosis factor (TNFα) and IL-10 have not been consistent (26). A recent meta-analysis, which included 12 published case-control studies found no significant association with IBS with polymorphisms in genes such as IL-4, IL-6, IL-8, IL-10, TNFA, IL-1R1, and IL-23R. However, SNP rs4263839 which encodes for TNFSF15 was only moderately associated with IBS, in particular with IBS-C (25). Candidate gene association studies in IBS have been comprehensively reviewed by Cheung et al. (27), Camilleri (28), and Gazouli et al. (29).

Despite these genetic associations, it is not entirely unexpected that the effects of an individual polymorphism on the overall phenotype are modest because IBS is a complex, multifactorial condition. Moreover, the development of disease likely involves more than the presence of just a moderately associated common variant. While SNPs of these genes alone may not be sufficient to cause IBS or other complex chronic pain conditions, they may interact with other genes and

TABLE 1 | Genetic changes associated with irritable bowel syndrome (IBS).

Function	Gene	Polymorphism	Endophenotype	PMID
Neurotransmission				
Serotonin biosynthesis	Tryptophan hydroxylase (*TPH1* and *TPH2* isoforms)	rs4537731, rs211105, rs4570625	IBS-D, IBS-C	21073637, 24060757
Serotonin reuptake; Seretonin receptors	Serotonin reuptake transporter (*SERT* or *SLC6A4*); 5-HT receptor 3A (*HTR3A*)	5-HT transporter linked promoter region (5-HTT LPR) deletion; rs25531; rs1062613	IBS-C, IBS; IBS-D, symptom severity and anxiety	12135035, 15361494, 17040410, 17564628, 17074108, 17241856, 18511740, 19426812, 19125330; 19125330, 24069428, 24512255, 21420406.
Adrenergic receptors, Catecholamine metabolism	Adrenergic receptors alpha (*ADR2A*, *ADR2C*, *ADRA1D*), Catechol-o-methyl transferase (*COMT*)	alpha(2C) Del 322–325; alpha(2A) –1291; rs1556832, val158met	IBS-C, severity, alterations in brain regions, IBS	19833115, 26288143
Neuropeptide receptors	Neuropeptide S receptor1 (*NPSR1*)	rs2609234, rs6972158, rs1379928, rs1379928	colonic transit, pain and gas	21437260
Cannabinoid mechanisms	Cannabinoid receptor1, (*CNR1/CB1*), Fatty acid amide hydrolase (*FAAH*), Corticotropin-releasing hormone binding protein (*CRHBP*)	AAT repeat frequency, rs806378 C385A, rs10474485	IBS, abdominal pain, IBS-D, colonic motility, transit time, emotional abnormalities	19732772
Barrier function, Immune and Inflammatory Mediators				
Barrier function, adhesion	Toll-like receptor 9 (*TLR9*), Cadherein 1 (*CDH1*)	rs5743836	PI-IBS, epithelial cell barrier function	20044998
Cytokines	Interleukin (*IL*)-6, *IL-10*, Tumor necrosis factor-alpha (*TNFα*), *IL-8*, *TNFSF15*	rs1800870, rs1800872, rs6478108, rs6478109, rs7848647, rs4263839	PI-IBS, IBS, IBS-D, innate immune response	20044998; 22837345
Ion Channels and Bile acids				
	Voltage-gated sodium channel NaV 1.5 (*SCN5A*), G protein-coupled bile acid receptor 1 (*GPBAR1*), Klotho Beta (*KLB*)	rs11554825, rs17618244	IBS, colonic transit, fecal bile acid	20044998, 21752155, 16279907, 23595519, 12477767, 15765388, 20337945, 22158028, 24409078, 22684480, 21636646, 25824902

Table 1 shows genetic changes associated with IBS and IBS endophenotypes. PMID, PubMed ID; IBS-D, IBS diarrhea subtype; IBS-C, IBS constipation subtype.

environmental factors including EALs and contribute to the disease etiology. Therefore, an alternative approach has been to evaluate an association of gene variants with specific IBS subtypes (IBS-D, IBS-C, and IBS-M) as well as endophenotypes. For example, we found that the SNP rs1556832 in the catecholaminergic gene, adrenoceptor alpha 1D (ADRA1D), was associated with IBS symptom severity and morphological changes in brain regions that modulate sensory processing (30). In another study, we demonstrated that the presence of IBS was significantly associated with SNPs in corticotropin releasing hormone receptor 1 (CRH-R1) gene. These SNPs were associated with increased GI symptom-related anxiety and acoustic startle response to threat in IBS patients, suggesting that that CRH-R1 is involved in altered stress responsiveness in IBS (30).

Genome Wide Association Studies (GWAS) in IBS

Considering the challenges of identifying individual risk alleles in case-control studies and the difficulty of defining significant gene association with IBS, a GWAS using large samples has been proposed as an alternative approach in an attempt to increase sample size and homogeneity. Ek et al. reported a GWAS study in IBS comprising of 534 IBS patients and 4,932 healthy controls, followed by six independent clinical case-control replication studies from different countries (31) where they identified variants in KDLER2 and GRIP2IP (chromosome 7p22.1) genes to be associated with IBS. KDLER2 codes for a family of integral membrane protein with seven transmembrane domains involved in intracellular signaling of bacterial toxins

(32), potentially relevant to the role of microbiota in IBS. The GRID2IP gene encodes for a protein (delphilin) expressed on fiber-Purkinje cell synapses in the brain involved in glutamatergic neurotransmission, potentially relevant to pain signaling (31, 33). Another GWAS with a smaller sample size (172 IBS cases and 1,398 controls) conducted in an Australian cohort found an association of protocadherin 15 (PCDH15) gene, encoding an integral membrane protein that mediates calcium-dependent cell–cell adhesion (P~9 × 10−9).

GWAS studies have also evaluated other SNP associations in IBS. TNFSF15 was found to be only nominally significant in the GWAS study, contrasting with prior reports as mentioned previously. Similar nominal associations were detected for other genes such as Cell Division Cycle 42 (CDC42), Neurexophilin 1 (NXPH1) (34), 5-HT Receptor 3E (HTR3E) (35), Klothoβ (KLB) (36) and Sodium Voltage-Gated Channel Alpha Subunit 5 (SCN5A). Interestingly, SCN5A encodes the α-subunit of the voltage-gated sodium channel NaV1.5. About 2% of patients with IBS were found to carry mutations in SCN5A, most of which were loss-of-function mutations that disrupted NaV1.5 channel function (37). Additionally, in a GWAS study on self-reported IBS patients and controls, Bonfiglio et al. identified variants at 9q31.2 locus that were associated with IBS in women suggesting a role for sex hormones in IBS (38). However, most genes associated with IBS thus far represent non-validated findings and therefore their role in IBS needs to be cautiously interpreted. Moreover, such discrepancies are believed to arise from multifactorial nature of the disease, phenotype heterogeneity (including variability in endophenotypes) and/or sample sizes, among others.

Additionally, the mechanisms involved in pain sensitization and altered motility are likely multifactorial as demonstrated in multiple clinical and animal studies in the past decades (39). These functional alterations are mediated through cellular and molecular changes mediated by genetic and epigenetic alterations (40) detailed in the following sections. At the CNS level, proposed mechanisms include plasticity of the endogenous pain modulation system and structural changes in the brain (41, 42). An important step towards understanding the complex pathogenesis of IBS lies in the ability to discover the interface between genetic pathways and epigenetic regulation mediated by gene-environment interaction at peripheral (gut) and central (CNS) levels.

STRESS: AN ENVIRONMENTAL TRIGGER FOR IBS

IBS is associated with various environmental factors including chronic stress in early life and/or adulthood, diet (43–45), and gastrointestinal infections (46, 47). Chronic stress can increase an individual's vulnerability to developing IBS and/or can trigger or exacerbate the symptoms of IBS (48, 49). Stress is the body's reaction to a physical or psychological stimulus that disturbs the homeostasis of an organism. Stress has wide-spread effects on gut physiology, including changes in intestinal motility, mucosal transport, and gut barrier function leading to changes in permeability, and visceral perception. The biological effects of stress are mediated by the sympathetic nervous system and corticotropin releasing factor (CRF)/HPA axis pathways. Glucocorticoids, which are major effector molecules of the HPA axis, bind to their intracellular receptors and regulate the physiological adaptations to stress (50, 51). Glucocorticoids including cortisol/corticosterone initiates negative feedback control *via* binding to glucocorticoid receptors (GR) and mineralocorticoid receptors (MR) in brain regions including hippocampus, paraventricular nucleus (PVN), and anterior pituitary gland (52). However, in response to chronic and uncontrollable stressors, maladaptive changes can be elicited resulting in malfunctioning of stress systems affecting the brain structure and function (53, 54).

Stress-Induced Visceral Hypersensitivity and Motility Abnormalities in IBS

Many studies support an important role for stress in the IBS pathophysiology and symptoms (8). The stress-induced activation or augmentation of the CRF and HPA axis systems has been associated with visceral hypersensitivity, an important feature of IBS, in animal models (55–58). IBS patients have a greater reactivity to stress compared to healthy subjects, as manifested by a dysregulated HPA axis response, enhanced visceral perception and gut motility, among other findings (59–61). IBS has been associated with increased prevalence of EALs and a growing body of evidence from both animal and human studies supports the hypothesis that chronic stress, including EALs, represent an important mechanism leading to changes in glucocorticoid receptor (GR) expression, thereby increasing

responsiveness of the HPA axis (62). The HPA axis response is regulated by a negative feedback though binding of cortisol to GRs at multiple levels including the hypothalamus and hippocampus. Impairment of this negative feedback mechanism can lead to a dysregulation of the HPA axis, specifically an enhanced HPA axis response due to reduced negative feedback from reduced expression of GRs. The importance of an early life and adulthood stress on this IBS phenotype was demonstrated in the maternal separation (MS) animal model, where pups that were maternally separated in early life and later subjected to psychologic stress as an adult displayed post-stress visceral hypersensitivity, increased corticosterone levels, and reduced expression of GRs in the hippocampus (63, 64). Additionally, stress-induced visceral hyperalgesia has been investigated in repeated water avoidance stress (WAS), a validated rat model of psychological stress that demonstrates many human IBS-like traits. A knockdown of GRs has also been shown to increase visceromotor response to colonic distention in animal models (65). Additionally, a neonatal inflammation rat model suggested a role for inflammatory insult in early life, which upregulates vasoactive intestinal peptide (Vip) in the colon muscularis externa contributing to altered motility and diarrhea-like symptoms as seen in IBS-D patients (66–68).

We found that GR expression was decreased in peripheral blood mononuclear cells (PBMCs) in IBS patients in comparison to healthy controls and that GR expression levels negatively correlated with pituitary responsiveness (ACTH levels) to CRF stimulation (69). That is, reduced GR expression was associated with an enhanced HPA axis response. HPA axis function was assessed in PBMCs because they are accessible and feasible to study. Although GRs regulate HPA axis *via* negative feedback in the CNS, changes in GRs on PBMCs have been reported in psychiatric diseases, including changes in the number and sensitivity of GRs (70, 71) and GR promoter methylation status and mRNA expression (69, 72–74). Furthermore, the transcriptome of peripheral blood has been shown to share >80% homology with genes expressed in the brain, heart, liver, spleen, colon, kidney, prostate, and stomach, and that there is a broad movement of leukocyte subsets to and from the gut at steady state, suggesting that PBMCs can reflect the molecular events at the central and peripheral locations (75).

Stress, Intestinal Epithelial Barrier Function and Immune System

Various animal models representing different stress paradigms (e.g. restraint stress, WAS, neonatal MS, etc.) as well as studies in human subjects have demonstrated an impairment in mucosal barrier function, the enteric nervous system (ENS), and immune system (76–78). These stress-induced changes result in alterations in GI functions including increased intestinal permeability, altered ion transport and hypersecretion, and mucus secretion and are mediated by neuro-immune mechanisms including the CRF system, which consists of CRF, urocortins 1–3 (Ucn) and their receptors CRF-1R and CRF-2R (79, 80). Barrier dysfunction may also occur early in IBS and is hypothesized to contribute to low-grade intestinal immune activation and increased visceral perception (81), specifically in

IBS-D patients (82, 83) and post-infection IBS (PI-IBS) (84). Additionally, an increase in paracellular permeability has been correlated with the magnitude of visceral pain in IBS-D patients (83). Furthermore, an exaggerated response to CRH infusion in IBS patients was associated with an increase in cytokine levels suggesting a correlation between stress and increased cytokine levels (85). This is hypothesized to be mediated by glucocorticoid-related epigenetic changes leading to inadequate suppression of proinflammatory cytokines (40). It conceivable that this contributes, at least in part, to the higher plasma levels of cytokines reported in some IBS patients (86, 87).

Both local (intestinal) and systemic factors contribute to the altered epithelial barrier function. Recent data indicate that soluble mediators from fecal supernatants and mucosal homogenates of IBS patients affect the epithelial integrity, thereby increasing colonic permeability (88, 89). These studies showed that the impairment of barrier integrity may be mediated *via* the release of various mediators such as serine proteases or histamine. Additionally, molecular alterations such as expression of genes involved in barrier function (90) can mediate permeability changes, which can in turn lead to permeation of bacteria and their products.

EPIGENETIC MODIFICATIONS: A BRIDGE BETWEEN ENVIRONMENT AND GENES IN IBS

Epigenetic mechanisms alter gene expression without alterations of underlying DNA sequence (91) and are key to the normal development, cellular function, and differentiation into specific lineages (92). These mechanisms broadly include DNA methylation, histone modification, and non-coding RNA mediated gene regulation as shown in **Figure 1**. Epigenetic mechanisms play a role in synaptic plasticity, learning, and memory (93), as well as in various neuropsychiatric conditions including depression and pain (94). Long-lasting epigenetic changes have been linked to early stress, childhood trauma or abuse. Epigenetic changes are amenable to exogenous influences and involve complex and dynamic interaction between the DNA sequence, DNA and histone modifications and environmental factors, all of which combine to produce the phenotype, thus providing an important link between environment and phenotype (95).

DNA Methylation in Animal Models of IBS and IBS Patients

In vertebrates, DNA methylation occurs mostly in the context of CpG dinucleotides by a covalent attachment of a methyl group to the C5 position of cytosine (91). CpG islands (CGIs) are short interspersed DNA sequences (usually 1000 base-pairs) with a high concentration of CpG residues, which are normally non-methylated in contrast to the rest of the genome, which is globally methylated. CGIs typically occur at or near the transcription start site of genes (96) and when a CGI in the promoter region of a gene is methylated, expression of the gene is

repressed. The exact mechanism of DNA methylation mediated repression of gene expression has begun to be elucidated in recent years. DNA methylation results in binding of methyl-binding-domain (MBD) proteins, which are associated with large protein complexes that contain histone deacetylases (HDACs) and recruit histone methyl transferases (HMTs) leading to chromatin remodeling (97). Both DNA methylation and the proteins associated with MDBs are being investigated as promising therapeutic targets (98). Additionally, recent studies have demonstrated that methylation of CpG sites in the gene body are positively correlated with gene expression and is a potential therapeutic target in cancer (99). The quantification of DNA methylation in diseased or environmentally impacted cells could provide useful information for detection and treatment of the disease.

DNA methylation changes, in particular, have been studied in various chronic conditions including cancer (100), chronic pain (101), and psychiatric diseases (102). Stress and other environmental factors including EALs, diet and gut microbial metabolites can potentially trigger epigenetic alterations (103, 104). For example, studies have demonstrated that maternal care influences HPA axis function through epigenetic programming of GR (coded by Nuclear Receptor Subfamily 3 Group C Member 1, or *NR3C1*) expression and that environment-induced remodeling of the epigenome, or during chronic stress, can result in long-term changes in gene expression (105–107). **Table 2A** lists the epigenetic modifications reported in association with IBS or animal models of IBS. The role of central epigenetic regulatory mechanisms in stress-induced visceral hypersensitivity has been demonstrated in MS and WAS rat models. While MS animal models mimic the early life stress, WAS simulates both acute and chronic effects of a psychological stressor on colonic sensitivity, which have been extensively reviewed by Greenwood-Van Meerveld et al. (108). Stress-induced visceral hypersensitivity has been associated with an increase in DNA methylation in the GR gene promoter and a decreased expression of the GR gene in the amygdala of WAS rats (109, 110). Additionally, the study identified a decrease in DNA methylation and increased expression of the CRF gene associate with visceral hypersensitivity in the amygdala of the stressed rats. Hong et al. demonstrated that chronic stress increased methylation of genes that regulate visceral pain sensation in the peripheral nervous system of rats. They reported that chronic stress resulted in increased promoter methylation and reduced expression of the *NR3C1* (or GR) gene in L6-S2 dorsal root ganglia (111). In human subjects, DNA methylation in brains of suicide victims with a history of childhood abuse was associated with increased methylation and decreased expression of GR gene compared to suicide victims with no history of childhood maltreatment (106). However, no clear consensus exists regarding DNA methylation of the GR gene in IBS patients.

In a genome-wide methylation scan followed by targeted sequencing, we previously demonstrated an association of DNA methylation of several CpG sites in PBMCs in IBS patients compared to healthy controls (112). We reported an

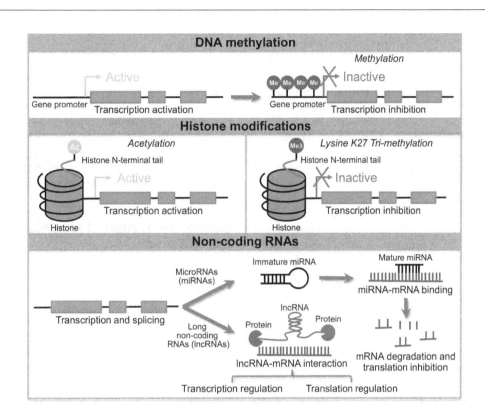

FIGURE 1 | Major epigenetic changes studied in the context of irritable bowel syndrome (IBS). Shows a conceptual model of major epigenetic changes studied in the context of IBS. Lines with blue boxes represent genes with promoter regions. Blue boxes represent exons, lines before exon 1 represents promoter region and the lines between exons represent introns. The top panel shows active transcription in the unmethylated state of the gene, which when methylated (Me) at the promoter region leads to transcription inactivation. Middle panel shows two representative histone modifications, histone acetylation at the N-terminal tail, which is usually associated with activation of transcription and histone methylation, specifically, addition of a tri-methyl group (Me3) at 27th lysine (K) on the N-terminal tail, which is associated with transcription repression. The bottom panel shows mechanism of transcription regulation by non-coding RNAs. MicroRNA genes are transcribed to immature precursor miRNAs that are processed to form mature miRNAs, which bind to miRNAs either leading to mRNA degradation or inhibition of translation. Long non-coding RNAs regulate transcription and translation, and function at the level of chromatin *via* interaction with RNA binding proteins.

increase in DNA methylation in genes including sub-commissural organ (SCO)-Spondin (*SSPO*), glutathione-S-transferases mu 5 (*GSTM5*) and tubulin polymerization promoting protein (*TPPP*) in IBS patients compared to healthy controls. SSPO is associated with neuronal function (113) and has been suggested to play a role in depression and evidence suggests that SCO secretory activity is regulated by the serotonin system, which plays an important role in stress-related pathways and in IBS (114). Additionally, an increased methylation of *GSTM5*, a gene that codes an enzyme that plays an important role in antioxidant defense was associated with decreased gene expression compared to controls. Although a role for oxidative stress and the significance of epigenetic silencing of *GSTM5* in IBS is not known, DNA methylation mediated repression of *GSTM5* gene expression has been shown in other conditions (115). Although larger independent studies may be required to confirm the functional role of the associated genes, these studies highlight the importance of epigenetic changes in IBS. DNA methylation changes in blood cells can provide insights into

systemic changes associated with IBS and can serve as important diagnostic and prognostic biomarkers (116).

Epigenetic changes in the gut mucosa can provide important insights into the peripheral mechanisms of IBS. A recent study investigated the genome-wide methylation predominantly in promoter regions of genes, and gene expression in the colon of rat WAS model and suggested an association of Notch signaling and focal adhesion pathways with psychological stress (117). In a recent study that included a relatively large cohort of IBS subjects and healthy controls (n=102 and 36, respectively), we found several DNA methylation changes in PBMCs as well as colonic mucosa that were associated with IBS. There was increased methylation of stress-related genes such as *NR3C1*, *CRHR1*, brain-derived neurotrophic factor (BDNF) in PBMCs and/or colon (118). In the colonic mucosa of IBS patients, we identified distinct clusters of DNA methylation patterns highlighting the heterogeneity in the epigenetic profiles of colonic mucosa of IBS patients. A hyper-methylated cluster was associated with higher symptom severity and abdominal pain compared to clusters with lower methylation levels and included genes such as protocadherins (PCDHs), cadherins (CDHs), VIP, TRPV4, and Guanylate Cyclase 1, Soluble, Beta 3 (GUCY1B3) which were significant after correcting for multiple comparisons. Thus, these studies suggest that DNA methylation changes are important pathophysiologic mechanisms in IBS and should be further evaluated.

Histone Modifications in Animal Models of IBS

In eukaryotic cells, genes complex with histone and other chromosomal proteins to form a chromatin scaffold. Histone modifications play an important role in regulation of gene expression. The histone tails undergo a variety of covalent modifications, that include lysine acetylation, methylation, ubiquitination, and sumoylation, among others (119) (**Figure 1**). Acetylation and methylation are some of the most studied histone modifications so far. In general, acetylation of core histone tails leads to open chromatin structure to allow transcription and the histone deacetylases (HDACs) oppose the effects of histone acetylases and are predominantly transcriptional repressors (120). Histone methylation is more complex and can occur on a specific lysine or arginine residue. Depending on the residues being methylated and the number of methylation molecules added (each methylated lysine residue can exist in a mono-, di-, or tri-methylated state), histone methylation may be associated with either an active or a silent state of chromatin. For example, H3K27me3 is associated with transcription repression whereas, H3K4me3 is generally associated with active transcription.

Recent studies have highlighted antinociceptive effects of histone acetylation and lysine tri-methylation in inflammatory and neuropathic pain models (121, 122). In the partial sciatic nerve ligation model of neuropathic pain, an increase in the expression levels of monocyte chemotactic protein-3 (MCP3), a pro-inflammatory cytokine was associated with reduced levels of repressive histone methylation, H3K27me3 (123). A role for histone acetylation has been suggested in the pathophysiology of visceral hypersensitivity induced by early-life stress in the MS animal model of IBS (124). Moloney et al. showed that HDAC inhibitor, suberoylanilide hydroxamic acid (SAHA), reversed visceral hypersensitivity, and the effects of stress on fecal pellet output in animal models of early life stress highlighting the importance of histone acetylation in stress-related conditions (125). Hong et al. demonstrated an increased expression of histone acetyltransferase EP300, which induced acetylation of histone H3 of promoter of nociceptive endovanilloid TRPV1 gene in the chronic WAS model of IBS. Moreover, they demonstrated that siRNA mediated knockdown of EP300 prevented visceral hyperalgesia (126).

Animal models suggest that neonatal inflammation may contribute to altered gut motility *via* histone modification. In rats subjected to neonatal inflammation, Vip levels increased, which reduced the interaction of histone deacetylase 3 (HDAC3) with α1C-subunit of Cav1.2b channel (Cacna1c or α1C1b). This resulted in increased acetylation of histone H3 lysine 9 (H3K9) in the promoter region inducing the transcription of α1C1b which may result in gut dysmotility and diarrhea (67). Similarly, neonatal immune challenge led to an upregulation of tyrosine hydroxylase in the locus coeruleus, mediated by epigenetic programming (127). The study showed a cascade of events involving upregulation of norepinephrine, activation of adrenergic receptors, and involvement of enhanced pCREB binding to the cAMP response element, which resulted in recruitment of histone acetylene transferase (HAT) to the brain derived neurotrophic factor (BDNF) gene. This led to an enhanced expression of the BDNF and aggravated visceromotor response to colorectal distension.

MicroRNA in Animal Models of IBS and IBS Patients

MiRNAs are endogenous noncoding RNAs of small size (18–25 nucleotides) that have been characterized as important gene expression regulators *via* binding through complementary sequence homology to the 3′-untranslated region (UTR) of target mRNAs thereby causing repression of translation or mRNA degradation (128) (**Figure 1**). Involvement of miRNA in cancer is well established and emerging research indicates a role of miRNA in the regulation of genes that play a role in nociceptive circuits (129). It has been suggested that miRNAs interacting with nervous and immune systems may act as "master switches" regulating a network of genes orchestrating the pain response and may be targeted for therapeutic purposes contrasting with the current strategy focusing on single targets (129). This approach is highly relevant to the GI tract where neuroimmune interactions are key contributors to the control of GI functions.

Recent translational studies in IBS have identified several miRNAs (**Table 2B**) that appear to be important in regulating the expression of genes involved in visceral pain response or intestinal permeability. In a study conducted in two independent cohorts of IBS-D women in in the UK and Germany, there was an association between the c.*76G>A variant in the 3′UTR of the serotonin receptor 3 subunit gene (*HTR3E*), leading to increased expression of the 5HT3E subunit, and (131). Using luciferase assays, this variation was located in the binding element sequence of miR-510 suggesting a functional implication of the *HTR3E* variation in the ability of miR-510 to regulate its gene expression.

Fourie et al. investigated whether circulating miRNAs are differentially expressed in a small number of IBS patients compared to healthy controls (132). This study found an upregulation of miR-150 and miR-342-3p, which are involved in inflammatory (133) and pain pathways, in IBS patients compared to healthy controls (134). Subsequent studies from Zhou et al, using a miRNA microarray approach, revealed increased expression of miR-29a in blood microvesicles, small bowel and colonic biopsies from IBS-D patients compared to healthy controls, and it was associated with increased intestinal permeability (135). Glutamine synthetase was confirmed as a

TABLE 2A | Epigenetic changes associated with irritable bowel syndrome (IBS).

Functional category	Gene	Sample	IBS vs controls	Phenotype	PMID
DNA methylation					
Oxidative stress	Glutathione-S-transferases mu 5 (*GSTM5*)	PBMCs	Hyper-methylated	IBS-D	26670691
Neuronal genes	SCO-Spondin (*SSPO*)	PBMCs	Hyper-methylated	IBS; HAD[#] depression	26670691
	Tubulin polymerization promoting protein (*TPPP*)	PBMCs	Hyper-methylated	IBS-C	26670691
	SSX family member 2 interacting protein (*Ssx2ip*)	Colon of WAS[$]	Hyper-methylated	Visceral hypersensitivity	30106160
	Par-3 family cell polarity regulator (*Pard3*)	Colon of WAS[$]	Hyper-methylated	Visceral hypersensitivity	30106160
	Vinculin (*Vcl*)	Colon of WAS[$]	Hyper-methylated	Visceral hypersensitivity	30106160
	Glucocorticoid receptor (*Nr3c1*)	MS Amygdala/DRG[%] neurons in WAS[$]	Hyper-methylated	Visceral hypersensitivity	25263804; 23084728
	Corticotropin-releasing factor (*Crf*)	Amygdala/DRG neurons in WAS[$]	Hypo-methylated	Visceral hypersensitivity	23084728
	Cannabinoid receptor 1(*Cnr1*)	DRG[%] neurons in WAS[$]	Hyper-methylated	Visceral hypersensitivity	25263804
Histone modifications					
Neuronal genes	Transient receptor potential cation channel subfamily V member 1 (*Trpv1*)	DRG[%] neurons in WAS[$]	Increased histone (H3) acetylation	Visceral hypersensitivity	25263804
	Brain derived neurotrophic factor (*Bdnf*)	Neonatal inflammation	histone acetylene transferase (HAT)	Visceral sensitivity	28439935
Calcium channels	*Cacna1c*	Neonatal inflammation	Reduced interaction with histone deacetylase 3 (HDAC3)	Altered motility and diarrhea	23886858

Table 2A shows epigenetic changes, including DNA methylation and histone modifications associated with IBS or IBS models. [#]HAD, hospital anxiety depression scale; PMID, PubMed ID; [$]WAS, water avoidance stress; [%]DRG, dorsal root ganglia; IBS-D, IBS diarrhea subtype; IBS-C, IBS constipation subtype; Hyper-methylation, increased methylation; Hypo-methylation, decreased methylation.

target of miR-29A and was significantly reduced in the small bowel mucosa in IBS patients suggesting a relationship between miR-29a, glutamine dependent signaling pathways and intestinal permeability in IBS patients. In a randomized placebo-controlled trial, glutamate was shown to safely and effectively reduce IBS symptoms in post-infection IBS-D patients with increased intestinal permeability (136). Subsequently, Zhou et al. showed increased levels of mir-29A/B and reduced expression of NFKB Repressing Factor (*NKRF*) and Claudin 1 (*CLDN1*) genes in intestinal tissue from IBS-D patients as well as TNBS colitis and WAS rat models of IBS (137). Additionally, they showed that miR-199a was significantly decreased in IBS-D patients compared to controls and an upregulation in animal models decreased visceral pain *via* inhibition of TRPV1 signaling.

Subsequently, the role of other miRNAs has been identified in IBS. CGN and CLDN2, associated with barrier function were shown to be the targets of hsa-miR-125b-5p and hsa-miR-16, which were downregulated in jejunal mucosal samples of IBS-D (138). Similarly, occludin (OCLN) and zonula occludens 1 (ZO1/ TJP1), which are associated with intestinal permeability, were identified as direct targets of miR-144 in the colon of IBS-D rat models (139). In addition, the role of miRNAs in visceral hyperalgesia has been suggested by altered levels of miRNAs, including miR-200a which targets cannabinoid receptor 1 (CNR1) and serotonin transporter (SERT) (140), miR-214 which targets SERT (141), and miR-16 and miR-103 which target HTR4 (142) in a rat model of IBS-D and human IBS-D colonic epithelial cells.

These studies have led to an increased understanding of the molecular mechanisms underlying some of the endophenotypes of IBS. Thus, they may be explored as diagnostic tools and have potential to form a basis for the therapeutic interventions being proposed in IBS (135). However, further studies examining their exact mechanisms in IBS and that can reproduce previous findings in a larger population are needed. These translational discoveries have prompted growing interest in miRNA-based therapy for IBS, although delivering drugs targeting miRNA to the intestinal tissue currently stands as a major obstacle and is being actively investigated (143).

Long Non-Coding RNAs in IBS

LncRNAs are transcripts that measure more than 200 nucleotides in length and are processed similar to protein-coding mRNAs (144). Although the functional mechanisms of most lncRNAs are not fully understood, they are known to exhibit diverse functional roles, including the gene regulation by chromatin remodeling, modulation of gene expression, localization, and stability (145) (**Figure 1**). Recently, Videlock et al. investigated the entire colonic mucosal transcriptome and found that a lncRNA, GREHLOS, which regulates the expression of motilin involved in smooth muscle contraction, was downregulated in IBS patients compared to healthy controls (130). Recently, increased expression of a lncRNA, X inactivate-specific transcript (XIST) was associated with decrease SERT transcription and increased visceral hypersensitivity in mouse

TABLE 2B | Non-coding RNAs associated with irritable bowel syndrome (IBS).

	Targets	Endophenotype	Sample	miRNA regulation in IBS/model	PMID
MicroRNAs					
miR-510	5-hydroxytryptamine receptor 3E(HTR3E), PRDX1	IBS-D	Colonic mucosa, and cells	Downregulated	18614545 26787495 31934286
miR-150 and miR-342-3p	Exploratory	Inflammatory and pain pathways	Whole blood	Upregulated	24768587
miR-199a	Transient receptor potential cation channel subfamily V member 1(TRPV1)	IBS-D, visceral pain	Colonic biopsies	Downregulated	25681400
miR-29a	Glutamate-ammonia ligase (GLUL), Aquaporin (AQP) 1, AQP3 and AQP8	Intestinal permeability	Colon and duodenum of IBS; colonic epithelial cells of IBS-D rat models	Upregulated	19951903 29156760
miR-16	HTR4 CLDN2	Intestinal sensitivity and motility; permeability	Colon of IBS-D; Jejunum of IBS-D	Downregulated	29089619 28082316
miR-103	5-hydroxytryptamine receptor 4 (HTR4)	Intestinal sensitivity and motility	Colon of IBS-D	Downregulated	29089619
miR-125b	Cingulin (CGN)	Permeability	Jejunum of IBS-D	Downregulated	28082316
miR-144	Occluding (OCLN), Zona Occludens1 (ZO1)	Intestinal permeability	Colon of BS-D rat model	Upregulated	29258088
miR-200a	Cannabinoid receptor 1(CNR1), Serotonin transporter (SERT)	Visceral hypersensitivity	Colon of IBS-D rat model	Upregulated	30347941
miR-24	SERT	Pain and nociception	Epithelial cells of colon and mouse model of IBS	Upgregulated	26631964
LncRNAs					
GHRLOS	Motilin	Smooth muscle contraction	Colonic mucosa of IBS	Downregulated	Videlock et al. (130)
XIST	SERT	Visceral hypersenitivity	Colon of mouse model of IBS	Upregulated	32446903

Table 2B shows epigenetic changes including miRNA and long non-coding RNA expression changes associated with IBS or IBS models. IBS-D, IBS diarrhea subtype.

model of IBS-D. The study suggested a role for XIST in recruiting DNA methyl transferases, DNMT1, DNMT3A, and DNMT3B to reduce SERT transcription *via* promoter methylation.

Microbiome and Diet as Environmental Factors Mediating Epigenetic Changes in IBS

Recent studies are starting to investigate an interaction of microbiome, diet, and epigenetics defined as "microbiota-nutrient metabolism-epigenetics axis" in complex diseases (146). Evidence suggests that epigenetic events are dynamic and responsive to changing nutrient availability and microbiome (104, 146, 147). Although the role of microbes and their metabolites on epigenetic machinery in the manifestation of IBS symptoms has not been investigated, there is indirect evidence for the role of microbial products involved in epigenetic modifications in eliciting visceral hypersensitivity (148). These interactions may be mediated by metabolites synthesized by commensal bacteria including neurotransmitters or short-chain fatty acids (SCFAs) (149). SCFAs, including butyrate, propionate, and acetate produced by the fermentation of host dietary polysaccharides, have neuroactive properties (150) and may play an important role in the brain-gut microbiome axis in IBS (151). SFCAs have been shown to regulate post-translational modifications of histones by inhibiting histone deacetylases, promoting active chromatin state and thereby promoting transcription (152, 153).

Nutrigenomics, the study of interaction of diet and genomic factors is an emerging topic in the context of IBS (154, 155). The majority of patients with IBS report meal-related symptoms and dietary modifications is an increasing treatment intervention used in IBS. For example, a low FODMAP (fermentable oligo-, di-, and mono-saccharides and polyols) diet has been associated with alleviation of IBS symptoms (156–157). Additionally, nutrition or diet can affect the epigenomic state. The role of diet in regulating epigenetic pathways is highlighted by a recent study, which showed that calorie restriction changes gene expression and DNA methylation profile of subcutaneous adipose tissue (147). It is suggested that diet and microbial metabolites influence the epigenome by impacting the pool of compounds or enzymes involved in epigenetic pathways (102). In particular, dietary components, co-factors, and vitamins including, S-adenosyl methionine (SAM), folate, vitamin B12, vitamin B6, acetyl-CoA have been shown to play a role in regulating histone modifications or DNA methylation levels (146). Therefore, investigating interactions between diet, microbiome and epigenetic factors may be important in understanding the etiology of IBS and developing personalized therapy for IBS.

MODEL FOR ETIOPATHOGENESIS OF IBS

Genetic, epigenetic, and other factors associated with IBS have been summarized in a schematic figure (**Figure 2**). IBS is a

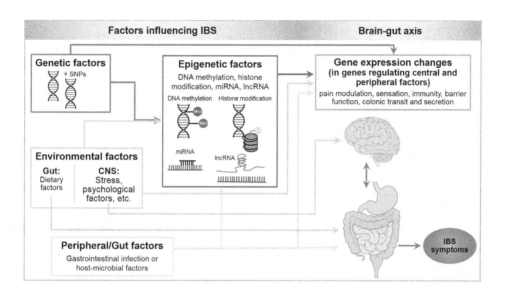

FIGURE 2 | Genetic, epigenetic, environmental and peripheral factors in irritable bowel syndrome. Shows a schematic model of genetic and epigenetic factors influencing IBS. Pink arrows illustrate that genetic factors including SNPs can influence the gene expression either directly or mediated by epigenetic factors including DNA methylation, histone modifications, miRNA and lncRNA expression (purple arrow). Environmental factors including stress and psychological factors at CNS level and dietary factors at gastrointestinal level can induce changes in gene expression mediated by epigenetic or non-genetic/epigenetic factors, and can have a direct influence on CNS and gut function (blue arrows). Peripheral or gut factors including GI infection or other host or microbial factors, can potentially modify the function of genes mediated by epigenetic or non-epigenetic factors, and influence the CNS and gut function (green arrows) such as, pain modulation, sensation, immunity, barrier function, colonic transit and secretion to manifest the symptoms of IBS (orange-red arrow).

multifactorial disorder of gut-brain interactions. In addition to stress, diet, and other environmental factors, changes at molecular level including genetic and epigenetic factors may contribute to pain modulation at the CNS level and/or periphery, and affect immune function, oxidative stress, mucosal barrier function, and GI motor and secretory function at the peripheral level in IBS. Moreover, gut microbiota and their metabolites likely contribute to this integrated system and play a major role in the pathogenesis of IBS. Given that IBS is a complex, multifactorial disorder, we propose that epigenomic mechanisms imprint dynamic environmental effects on the fixed genome resulting in alterations in phenotype leading to a disease state. These changes are potentially reversible and can be powerful diagnostic and prognostic markers and therapeutic targets (158).

CONCLUSION

Understanding the role of neuroimmune, genetic, epigenetic, and microbial underpinnings in IBS is crucial to understanding the pathophysiology of IBS. The mechanisms of visceral pain and

neuro-motor dysfunction, resulting in the symptoms of IBS are influenced by several factors including stress, genetic, epigenetic as well as microbiota. An in-depth investigation of these factors independently, as well as integratively, in a sufficiently large, well-characterized patient and control populations is crucial in understanding the etio-pathology of IBS and in identifying reliable and validated diagnostic biomarkers and therapeutic targets in IBS.

AUTHOR CONTRIBUTIONS

SM-J reviewed the literature and wrote the manuscript. LC reviewed the literature, wrote and edited the manuscript and provided the resources.

ACKNOWLEDGMENTS

We would like to thank Cathy Liu for her assistance in the creation of the figures.

REFERENCES

1. Lovell RM, Ford AC. Global prevalence of and risk factors for irritable bowel syndrome: a meta-analysis. *Clin Gastroenterol Hepatol.* (2012) 10:712–721.e4. doi: 10.1016/j.cgh.2012.02.029

2. Heitkemper M, Jarrett M, Bond EF, Chang L. Impact of sex and gender on irritable bowel syndrome. *Biol Res Nurs* (2003) 5:56–65. doi: 10.1177/1099800403005001006

3. Longstreth GF, Thompson WG, Chey WD, Houghton LA, Mearin F, Spiller RC. Functional bowel disorders. *Gastroenterology* (2006) 130:1480–91. doi: 10.1053/j.gastro.2005.11.061

4. Drossman DA, Hasler WL. Rome IV-Functional GI Disorders: Disorders of Gut-Brain Interaction. *Gastroenterology* (2016) 150:1257–61. doi: 10.1053/j.gastro.2016.03.035

5. Kim SE, Chang L. Overlap between functional GI disorders and other functional syndromes: what are the underlying mechanisms? *Neurogastroenterol. Motil* (2012) 24:895–913. doi: 10.1111/j.1365-2982.2012.01993.x

6. Gralnek IM, Hays RD, Kilbourne A, Naliboff B, Mayer EA. The impact of irritable bowel syndrome on health-related quality of life. *Gastroenterology* (2000) 119:654–60. doi: 10.1053/gast.2000.16484

7. Canavan C, West J, Card T. Review article: the economic impact of the irritable bowel syndrome. *Aliment. Pharmacol Ther* (2014) 40:1023–34. doi: 10.1111/apt.12938

8. Chang L. The role of stress on physiologic responses and clinical symptoms in irritable bowel syndrome. *Gastroenterology* (2011) 140:761–5. doi: 10.1053/j.gastro.2011.01.032

9. Monsbakken KW, Vandvik PO, Farup PG. Perceived food intolerance in subjects with irritable bowel syndrome- etiology, prevalence and consequences. *Eur J Clin Nutr* (2006) 60:667–72. doi: 10.1038/sj.ejcn.1602367

10. Saito YA, Mitra N, Mayer EA. Genetic approaches to functional gastrointestinal disorders. *Gastroenterology* (2010) 138:1276–85. doi: 10.1053/j.gastro.2010.02.037

11. Bradford K, Shih W, Videlock EJ, Presson AP, Naliboff BD, Mayer EA, et al. Association between early adverse life events and irritable bowel syndrome. *Clin Gastroenterol Hepatol.* (2012) 10:385–390.e1–3. doi: 10.1016/j.cgh.2011.12.018

12. Park SH, Videlock EJ, Shih W, Presson AP, Mayer EA, Chang L. Adverse childhood experiences are associated with irritable bowel syndrome and gastrointestinal symptom severity. *Neurogastroenterol. Motil* (2016) 28:1252–60. doi: 10.1111/nmo.12826

13. Parker CH, Naliboff BD, Shih W, Presson AP, Videlock EJ, Mayer EA, et al. Negative Events During Adulthood Are Associated With Symptom Severity and Altered Stress Response in Patients With Irritable Bowel Syndrome. *Clin Gastroenterol Hepatol.* (2019) 17:2245–52. doi: 10.1016/j.cgh.2018.12.029

14. Meaney MJ, Szyf M. Environmental programming of stress responses through DNA methylation: life at the interface between a dynamic environment and a fixed genome. *Dialogues Clin Neurosci* (2005) 7:103–23.

15. Whorwell PJ, McCallum M, Creed FH, Roberts CT. Non-colonic features of irritable bowel syndrome. *Gut* (1986) 27:37–40. doi: 10.1136/gut.27.1.37

16. Levy RL, Whitehead WE, Von Korff MR, Feld AD. Intergenerational transmission of gastrointestinal illness behavior. *Am J Gastroenterol* (2000) 95:451–6. doi: 10.1111/j.1572-0241.2000.01766.x

17. Locke GR, Zinsmeister AR, Talley NJ, Fett SL, Melton LJ. Familial association in adults with functional gastrointestinal disorders. *Mayo Clin Proc* (2000) 75:907–12. doi: 10.4065/75.9.907

18. Saito YA, Petersen GM, Larson JJ, Atkinson EJ, Fridley BL, de Andrade M, et al. Familial Aggregation of Irritable Bowel Syndrome: A Family Case-Control Study. *Am J Gastroenterol* (2010) 105:833–41. doi: 10.1038/ajg.2010.116

19. Morris-Yates A, Talley NJ, Boyce PM, Nandurkar S, Andrews G. Evidence of a genetic contribution to functional bowel disorder. *Am J Gastroenterol* (1998) 93:1311–7. doi: 10.1111/j.1572-0241.1998.440_j.x

20. Svedberg P, Johansson S, Wallander M-A, Hamelin B, Pedersen NL. Extra-intestinal manifestations associated with irritable bowel syndrome: a twin study. *Aliment. Pharmacol Ther* (2002) 16:975–83. doi: 10.1046/j.1365-2036.2002.01254.x

21. Levy RL, Jones KR, Whitehead WE, Feld SI, Talley NJ, Corey LA. Irritable bowel syndrome in twins: heredity and social learning both contribute to etiology. *Gastroenterology* (2001) 121:799–804. doi: 10.1053/gast.2001.27995

22. Bengtson M-B, Rønning T, Vatn MH, Harris JR. Irritable bowel syndrome in twins: genes and environment. *Gut* (2006) 55:1754–9. doi: 10.1136/gut.2006.097287

23. Mohammed I, Cherkas LF, Riley SA, Spector TD, Trudgill NJ. Genetic influences in irritable bowel syndrome: a twin study. *Am J Gastroenterol* (2005) 100:1340–4. doi: 10.1111/j.1572-0241.2005.41700.x

24. Levy RL, Jones KR, Whitehead WE, Feld SI, Talley NJ, Corey LA. Irritable bowel syndrome in twins: heredity and social learning both contribute to etiology. *Gastroenterology* (2001) 121:799–804. doi: 10.1053/gast.2001.27995

25. Czogalla B, Schmitteckert S, Houghton LA, Sayuk GS, Camilleri M, Olivo-Diaz A, et al. A meta-analysis of immunogenetic Case-Control Association Studies in irritable bowel syndrome. *Neurogastroenterol. Motil* (2015) 27:717–27. doi: 10.1111/nmo.12548

26. Bashashati M, Rezaei N, Shafieyoun A, McKernan DP, Chang L, Öhman L, et al. Cytokine imbalance in irritable bowel syndrome: a systematic review and meta-analysis. *Neurogastroenterol. Motil* (2014) 26:1036–48. doi: 10.1111/nmo.12358

27. Cheung CKY, Wu JCY. Genetic polymorphism in pathogenesis of irritable bowel syndrome. *World J Gastroenterol* (2014) 20:17693–8. doi: 10.3748/wjg.v20.i47.17693

28. Camilleri M. Genetics of Human Gastrointestinal Sensation. *Neurogastroenterol. Motil* (2013) 25:458–66. doi: 10.1111/nmo.12132

29. Gazouli M, Wouters MM, Kapur-Pojskić L, Bengtson M-B, Friedman E, Nikčević G, et al. Lessons learned — resolving the enigma of genetic factors in IBS. *Nat Rev Gastroenterol. Hepatol.* (2016) 13:77–87. doi: 10.1038/nrgastro.2015.206

30. Orand A, Gupta A, Shih W, Presson AP, Hammer C, Niesler B, et al. Catecholaminergic Gene Polymorphisms Are Associated with GI Symptoms and Morphological Brain Changes in Irritable Bowel Syndrome. *PLoS One* (2015) 10:e0135910. doi: 10.1371/journal.pone.0135910

31. Ek WE, Reznichenko A, Ripke S, Niesler B, Zucchelli M, Rivera NV, et al. Exploring the genetics of irritable bowel syndrome: a GWA study in the general population and replication in multinational case-control cohorts. *Gut* (2015) 64:1774–82. doi: 10.1136/gutjnl-2014-307997

32. Kreitman RJ, Pastan I. Importance of the glutamate residue of KDEL in increasing the cytotoxicity of Pseudomonas exotoxin derivatives and for increased binding to the KDEL receptor. *Biochem J* (1995) 307(Pt 1):29–37. doi: 10.1042/bj3070029

33. Miyagi Y, Yamashita T, Fukaya M, Sonoda T, Okuno T, Yamada K, et al. Delphilin: a novel PDZ and formin homology domain-containing protein that synaptically colocalizes and interacts with glutamate receptor delta 2 subunit. *J Neurosci* (2002) 22:803–14. doi: 10.1523/JNEUROSCI.22-03-00803.2002

34. Wouters MM, Lambrechts D, Knapp M, Cleynen I, Whorwell P, Agréus L, et al. Genetic variants in CDC42 and NXPH1 as susceptibility factors for constipation and diarrhoea predominant irritable bowel syndrome. *Gut* (2014) 63:1103–11. doi: 10.1136/gutjnl-2013-304570

35. Gu Q-Y, Zhang J, Feng Y-C, Dai G-R, Du W-P. Association of genetic polymorphisms in HTR3A and HTR3E with diarrhea predominant irritable bowel syndrome. *Int J Clin Exp Med* (2015) 8:4581–5.

36. Wong BS, Camilleri M, Carlson PJ, Guicciardi ME, Burton D, McKinzie S, et al. Gores GJ. A Klothoβ variant mediates protein stability and associates with colon transit in irritable bowel syndrome with diarrhea. *Gastroenterology* (2011) 140:1934–42. doi: 10.1053/j.gastro.2011.02.063

37. Beyder A, Mazzone A, Strege PR, Tester DJ, Saito YA, Bernard CE, et al. Loss-of-function of the voltage-gated sodium channel NaV1.5 (channelopathies) in patients with irritable bowel syndrome. *Gastroenterology* (2014) 146:1659–68. doi: 10.1053/j.gastro.2014.02.054

38. Bonfiglio F, Zheng T, Garcia-Etxebarria K, Hadizadeh F, Bujanda L, Bresso F, et al. Female-Specific Association Between Variants on Chromosome 9 and Self-Reported Diagnosis of Irritable Bowel Syndrome. *Gastroenterology* (2018) 155:168–79. doi: 10.1053/j.gastro.2018.03.064

39. Lee YJ, Park KS. Irritable bowel syndrome: emerging paradigm in pathophysiology. *World J Gastroenterol* (2014) 20:2456–69. doi: 10.3748/wjg.v20.i10.2456

40. Dinan TG, Cryan J, Shanahan F, Keeling PWN, Quigley EMM. IBS: An epigenetic perspective. *Nat Rev Gastroenterol Hepatol.* (2010) 7:465–71. doi: 10.1038/nrgastro.2010.99

41. Mayer EA, Tillisch K. The brain-gut axis in abdominal pain syndromes. *Annu Rev Med* (2011) 62:381–96. doi: 10.1146/annurev-med-012309-103958

42. Seminowicz DA, Labus JS, Bueller JA, Tillisch K, Naliboff BD, Bushnell MC, et al. Regional gray matter density changes in brains of patients with irritable bowel syndrome. *Gastroenterology* (2010) 139:48–57.e2. doi: 10.1053/j.gastro.2010.03.049

43. Singh R, Salem A, Nanavati J, Mullin GE. The Role of Diet in the Treatment of Irritable Bowel Syndrome: A Systematic Review. *Gastroenterol Clin North Am* (2018) 47:107–37. doi: 10.1016/j.gtc.2017.10.003

44. Hayes PA, Fraher MH, Quigley EMM. Irritable bowel syndrome: the role of food in pathogenesis and management. *Gastroenterol Hepatol. (N. Y.)* (2014) 10:164–74.

45. Dimidi E, Rossi M, Whelan K. Irritable bowel syndrome and diet: where are we in 2018? *Curr Opin Clin Nutr Metab Care* (2017) 20:456–63. doi: 10.1097/MCO.0000000000000416

46. Koloski NA, Jones M, Weltman M, Kalantar J, Bone C, Gowryshankar A, et al. Identification of early environmental risk factors for irritable bowel syndrome and dyspepsia. *Neurogastroenterol. Motil* (2015) 27:1317–25. doi: 10.1111/nmo.12626

47. Barbara G, Grover M, Bercik P, Corsetti M, Ghoshal UC, Ohman L, et al. Rome Foundation Working Team Report on Post-Infection Irritable Bowel Syndrome. *Gastroenterology* (2019) 156:46–58.e7. doi: 10.1053/j.gastro.2018.07.011

48. Lackner JM, Brasel AM, Quigley BM, Keefer L, Krasner SS, Powell C, et al. The ties that bind: perceived social support, stress, and IBS in severely affected patients. *Neurogastroenterol. Motil* (2010) 22:893–900. doi: 10.1111/j.1365-2982.2010.01516.x

49. Bennett EJ, Tennant CC, Piesse C, Badcock CA, Kellow JE. Level of chronic life stress predicts clinical outcome in irritable bowel syndrome. *Gut* (1998) 43:256–61. doi: 10.1136/gut.43.2.256

50. Munck A, Guyre PM, Holbrook NJ. Physiological functions of glucocorticoids in stress and their relation to pharmacological actions. *Endocr Rev* (1984) 5:25–44. doi: 10.1210/edrv-5-1-25

51. Bamberger CM, Schulte HM, Chrousos GP. Molecular determinants of glucocorticoid receptor function and tissue sensitivity to glucocorticoids. *Endocr Rev* (1996) 17:245–61. doi: 10.1210/edrv-17-3-245

52. Herman JP, Cullinan WE. Neurocircuitry of stress: central control of the hypothalamo-pituitary-adrenocortical axis. *Trends Neurosci* (1997) 20:78–84. doi: 10.1016/s0166-2236(96)10069-2

53. Nutt DJ, Malizia AL. Structural and functional brain changes in posttraumatic stress disorder. *J Clin Psychiatry* (2004) 65 Suppl 1:11–7.

54. Lupien SJ, McEwen BS, Gunnar MR, Heim C. Effects of stress throughout the lifespan on the brain, behaviour and cognition. *Nat Rev Neurosci* (2009) 10:434–45. doi: 10.1038/nrn2639

55. Venkova K, Johnson AC, Myers B, Greenwood-Van Meerveld B. Exposure of the amygdala to elevated levels of corticosterone alters colonic motility in response to acute psychological stress. *Neuropharmacology* (2010) 58:1161–7. doi: 10.1016/j.neuropharm.2010.02.012

56. Greenwood-Van Meerveld B, Moloney RD, Johnson AC, Vicario M. Mechanisms of Stress-Induced Visceral Pain: Implications in Irritable Bowel Syndrome. *J Neuroendocrinol.* (2016) 28. doi: 10.1111/jne.12361

57. Taché Y, Million M. Role of Corticotropin-releasing Factor Signaling in Stress-related Alterations of Colonic Motility and Hyperalgesia. *J Neurogastroenterol. Motil* (2015) 21:8–24. doi: 10.5056/jnm14162

58. Larauche M, Moussaoui N, Biraud M, Bae WK, Duboc H, Million M, et al. Brain corticotropin-releasing factor signaling: Involvement in acute stress-induced visceral analgesia in male rats. *Neurogastroenterol. Motil* (2019) 31: e13489. doi: 10.1111/nmo.13489

59. Welgan P, Meshkinpour H, Beeler M. Effect of anger on colon motor and myoelectric activity in irritable bowel syndrome. *Gastroenterology* (1988) 94:1150–6. doi: 10.1016/0016-5085(88)90006-6

60. Posserud I, Agerforz P, Ekman R, Björnsson ES, Abrahamsson H, Simrén M. Altered visceral perceptual and neuroendocrine response in patients with irritable bowel syndrome during mental stress. *Gut* (2004) 53:1102–8. doi: 10.1136/gut.2003.017962

61. Dickhaus B, Mayer EA, Firooz N, Stains J, Conde F, Olivas TI, et al. Irritable bowel syndrome patients show enhanced modulation of visceral perception by auditory stress. *Am J Gastroenterol* (2003) 98:135–43. doi: 10.1111/j.1572-0241.2003.07156.x

62. Videlock EJ, Adeyemo M, Licudine A, Hirano M, Ohning G, Mayer M, et al. Childhood trauma is associated with hypothalamic-pituitary-adrenal axis responsiveness in irritable bowel syndrome. *Gastroenterology* (2009) 137:1954–62. doi: 10.1053/j.gastro.2009.08.058

63. Coutinho SV, Plotsky PM, Sablad M, Miller JC, Zhou H, Bayati AI, et al. Neonatal maternal separation alters stress-induced responses to viscerosomatic nociceptive stimuli in rat. *Am J Physiol Gastrointest. Liver Physiol* (2002) 282:G307–316. doi: 10.1152/ajpgi.00240.2001

64. Welting O, Van Den Wijngaard RM, De Jonge WJ, Holman R, Boeckxstaens GE. Assessment of visceral sensitivity using radio telemetry in a rat model of maternal separation. *Neurogastroenterol. Motil* (2005) 17:838–45. doi: 10.1111/j.1365-2982.2005.00677.x

65. Winston JH, Xu G-Y, Sarna SK. Adrenergic stimulation mediates visceral hypersensitivity to colorectal distension following heterotypic chronic stress. *Gastroenterology* (2010) 138:294–304.e3. doi: 10.1053/j.gastro.2009.09.054

66. Sarna SK. *Colonic Motility: From Bench Side to Bedside* (2010). San Rafael (CA: Morgan & Claypool Life Sciences. Available at: http://www.ncbi.nlm.nih.gov/books/NBK53477/ (Accessed July 13, 2020).

67. Li Q, Winston JH, Sarna SK. Developmental origins of colon smooth muscle dysfunction in IBS-like rats. *Am J Physiol Gastrointest. Liver Physiol* (2013) 305:G503–512. doi: 10.1152/ajpgi.00160.2013

68. Choudhury BK, Shi X-Z, Sarna SK. Gene plasticity in colonic circular smooth muscle cells underlies motility dysfunction in a model of postinfective IBS. *Am J Physiol Gastrointest. Liver Physiol* (2009) 296: G632–642. doi: 10.1152/ajpgi.90673.2008

69. Videlock EJ, Shih W, Adeyemo M, Mahurkar-Joshi S, Presson AP, Polytarchou C, et al. The effect of sex and irritable bowel syndrome on HPA axis response and peripheral glucocorticoid receptor expression. *Psychoneuroendocrinology* (2016) 69:67–76. doi: 10.1016/j.psyneuen.2016.03.016

70. de Kloet CS, Vermetten E, Bikker A, Meulman E, Geuze E, Kavelaars A, et al. Leukocyte glucocorticoid receptor expression and immunoregulation in veterans with and without post-traumatic stress disorder. *Mol Psychiatry* (2007) 12:443–53. doi: 10.1038/sj.mp.4001934

71. Yehuda R, Golier JA, Yang R-K, Tischler L. Enhanced sensitivity to glucocorticoids in peripheral mononuclear leukocytes in posttraumatic stress disorder. *Biol Psychiatry* (2004) 55:1110–6. doi: 10.1016/j.biopsych.2004.02.010

72. Yehuda R, Flory JD, Bierer LM, Henn-Haase C, Lehrner A, Desarnaud F, et al. Lower methylation of glucocorticoid receptor gene promoter 1F in peripheral blood of veterans with posttraumatic stress disorder. *Biol Psychiatry* (2015) 77:356–64. doi: 10.1016/j.biopsych.2014.02.006

73. Gola H, Engler A, Morath J, Adenauer H, Elbert T, Kolassa I-T, et al. Reduced peripheral expression of the glucocorticoid receptor α isoform in individuals with posttraumatic stress disorder: a cumulative effect of trauma burden. *PLoS One* (2014) 9:e86333. doi: 10.1371/journal.pone.0086333

74. Hepgul N, Cattaneo A, Zunszain PA, Pariante CM. Depression pathogenesis and treatment: what can we learn from blood mRNA expression? *BMC Med* (2013) 11:28. doi: 10.1186/1741-7015-11-28

75. Liew C-C, Ma J, Tang H-C, Zheng R, Dempsey AA. The peripheral blood transcriptome dynamically reflects system wide biology: a potential diagnostic tool. *J Lab Clin Med* (2006) 147:126–32. doi: 10.1016/j.lab.2005.10.005

76. Lennon EM, Maharshak N, Elloumi H, Borst L, Plevy SE, Moeser AJ. Early life stress triggers persistent colonic barrier dysfunction and exacerbates colitis in adult IL-10-/- mice. *Inflammation Bowel Dis* (2013) 19:712–9. doi: 10.1097/MIB.0b013e3182802a4e

77. Santos J, Benjamin M, Yang PC, Prior T, Perdue MH. Chronic stress impairs rat growth and jejunal epithelial barrier function: role of mast cells. *Am J Physiol Gastrointest. Liver Physiol* (2000) 278:G847–854. doi: 10.1152/ajpgi.2000.278.6.G847

78. Castagliuolo I, Lamont JT, Qiu B, Fleming SM, Bhaskar KR, Nikulasson ST, et al. Acute stress causes mucin release from rat colon: role of corticotropin releasing factor and mast cells. *Am J Physiol* (1996) 271:G884–892. doi: 10.1152/ajpgi.1996.271.5.G884

79. Hoffman JM, Baritaki S, Ruiz JJ, Sideri A, Pothoulakis C. Corticotropin-Releasing Hormone Receptor 2 Signaling Promotes Mucosal Repair Responses after Colitis. *Am J Pathol* (2016) 186:134–44. doi: 10.1016/j.ajpath.2015.09.013

80. Moss AC, Anton P, Savidge T, Newman P, Cheifetz AS, Gay J, et al. Urocortin II mediates pro-inflammatory effects in human colonocytes *via* corticotropin-releasing hormone receptor 2alpha. *Gut* (2007) 56:1210–7. doi: 10.1136/gut.2006.110668

81. Bertiaux-Vandaële N, Youmba SB, Belmonte L, Lecleire S, Antonietti M, Gourcerol G, et al. The expression and the cellular distribution of the tight junction proteins are altered in irritable bowel syndrome patients with differences according to the disease subtype. *Am J Gastroenterol* (2011) 106:2165–73. doi: 10.1038/ajg.2011.257

82. Dunlop SP, Hebden J, Campbell E, Naesdal J, Olbe L, Perkins AC, et al. Abnormal intestinal permeability in subgroups of diarrhea-predominant irritable bowel syndromes. *Am J Gastroenterol* (2006) 101:1288–94. doi: 10.1111/j.1572-0241.2006.00672.x

83. Zhou Q, Zhang B, Verne GN. Intestinal membrane permeability and hypersensitivity in the irritable bowel syndrome. *Pain* (2009) 146:41–6. doi: 10.1016/j.pain.2009.06.017

84. Marshall JK, Thabane M, Garg AX, Clark W, Meddings J, Collins SM, et al. Intestinal permeability in patients with irritable bowel syndrome after a waterborne outbreak of acute gastroenteritis in Walkerton, Ontario. *Aliment. Pharmacol Ther* (2004) 20:1317–22. doi: 10.1111/j.1365-2036.2004.02284.x

85. O'Mahony L, McCarthy J, Kelly P, Hurley G, Luo F, Chen K, et al. Lactobacillus and bifidobacterium in irritable bowel syndrome: symptom responses and relationship to cytokine profiles. *Gastroenterology* (2005) 128:541–51. doi: 10.1053/j.gastro.2004.11.050

86. Dinan TG, Quigley EMM, Ahmed SMM, Scully P, O'Brien S, O'Mahony L, et al. Hypothalamic-Pituitary-Gut Axis Dysregulation in Irritable Bowel Syndrome: Plasma Cytokines as a Potential Biomarker? *Gastroenterology* (2006) 130:304–11. doi: 10.1053/j.gastro.2005.11.033

87. Clarke G, Quigley EMM, Cryan JF, Dinan TG. Irritable bowel syndrome: towards biomarker identification. *Trends Mol Med* (2009) 15:478–89. doi: 10.1016/j.molmed.2009.08.001

88. Gecse K, Róka R, Ferrier L, Leveque M, Eutamene H, Cartier C, et al. Increased faecal serine protease activity in diarrhoeic IBS patients: a colonic lumenal factor impairing colonic permeability and sensitivity. *Gut* (2008) 57:591–9. doi: 10.1136/gut.2007.140210

89. Barbara G, Wang B, Stanghellini V, de Giorgio R, Cremon C, Di Nardo G, et al. Mast cell-dependent excitation of visceral-nociceptive sensory neurons in irritable bowel syndrome. *Gastroenterology* (2007) 132:26–37. doi: 10.1053/j.gastro.2006.11.039

90. Piche T, Barbara G, Aubert P, Bruley des Varannes S, Dainese R, Nano JL, et al. Impaired intestinal barrier integrity in the colon of patients with irritable bowel syndrome: involvement of soluble mediators. *Gut* (2009) 58:196–201. doi: 10.1136/gut.2007.140806

91. Bird A. DNA methylation patterns and epigenetic memory. *Genes Dev* (2002) 16:6–21. doi: 10.1101/gad.947102

92. Kiefer JC. Epigenetics in development. *Dev Dyn.* (2007) 236:1144–56. doi: 10.1002/dvdy.21094

93. Géranton SM, Fratto V, Tochiki KK, Hunt SP. Descending serotonergic controls regulate inflammation-induced mechanical sensitivity and methyl-CpG-binding protein 2 phosphorylation in the rat superficial dorsal horn. *Mol Pain* (2008) 4:35. doi: 10.1186/1744-8069-4-35

94. Géranton SM, Morenilla-Palao C, Hunt SP. A role for transcriptional repressor methyl-CpG-binding protein 2 and plasticity-related gene serum- and glucocorticoid-inducible kinase 1 in the induction of inflammatory pain states. *J Neurosci* (2007) 27:6163–73. doi: 10.1523/JNEUROSCI.1306-07.2007

95. McGowan PO, Sasaki A, D'Alessio AC, Dymov S, Labonté B, Szyf M, et al. Epigenetic regulation of the glucocorticoid receptor in human brain associates with childhood abuse. *Nat Neurosci* (2009) 12:342–8. doi: 10.1038/nn.2270

96. Deaton AM, Bird A. CpG islands and the regulation of transcription. *Genes Dev* (2011) 25:1010–22. doi: 10.1101/gad.2037511

97. Teodoridis JM, Strathdee G, Brown R. Epigenetic silencing mediated by CpG island methylation: potential as a therapeutic target and as a biomarker. *Drug Resist Update* (2004) 7:267–78. doi: 10.1016/j.drup.2004.06.005

98. Patnaik S. Anupriya null. Drugs Targeting Epigenetic Modifications and Plausible Therapeutic Strategies Against Colorectal Cancer. *Front Pharmacol* (2019) 10:588. doi: 10.3389/fphar.2019.00588

99. Yang X, Han H, De Carvalho DD, Lay FD, Jones PA, Liang G. Gene body methylation can alter gene expression and is a therapeutic target in cancer. *Cancer Cell* (2014) 26:577–90. doi: 10.1016/j.ccr.2014.07.028

100. Esteller M. Epigenetics in cancer. *N. Engl J Med* (2008) 358:1148–59. doi: 10.1056/NEJMra072067

101. Denk F, McMahon SB. Chronic pain: emerging evidence for the involvement of epigenetics. *Neuron* (2012) 73:435–44. doi: 10.1016/j.neuron.2012.01.012

102. Radley JJ, Kabbaj M, Jacobson L, Heydendael W, Yehuda R, Herman JP. Stress risk factors and stress-related pathology: neuroplasticity, epigenetics and endophenotypes. *Stress* (2011) 14:481–97. doi: 10.3109/10253890.2011.604751

103. Vaiserman AM. Epigenetic programming by early-life stress: Evidence from human populations. *Dev Dyn.* (2015) 244:254–65. doi: 10.1002/dvdy.24211

104. Hullar MAJ, Fu BC. Diet, the gut microbiome, and epigenetics. *Cancer J* (2014) 20:170–5. doi: 10.1097/PPO.0000000000000053

105. Weaver ICG, Cervoni N, Champagne FA, D'Alessio AC, Sharma S, Seckl JR, et al. Epigenetic programming by maternal behavior. *Nat Neurosci* (2004) 7:847–54. doi: 10.1038/nn1276

106. Labonte B, Yerko V, Gross J, Mechawar N, Meaney MJ, Szyf M, et al. Differential glucocorticoid receptor exon 1(B), 1(C), and 1(H) expression and methylation in suicide completers with a history of childhood abuse. *Biol Psychiatry* (2012) 72:41–8. doi: 10.1016/j.biopsych.2012.01.034

107. Watkeys OJ, Kremerskothen K, Quidé Y, Fullerton JM, Green MJ. Glucocorticoid receptor gene (NR3C1) DNA methylation in association with trauma, psychopathology, transcript expression, or genotypic variation: A systematic review. *Neurosci Biobehav Rev* (2018) 95:85–122. doi: 10.1016/j.neubiorev.2018.08.017

108. Greenwood-Van Meerveld B, Johnson AC. Stress-Induced Chronic Visceral Pain of Gastrointestinal Origin. *Front Syst Neurosci* (2017) 11:86. doi: 10.3389/fnsys.2017.00086

109. Perroud N, Paoloni-Giacobino A, Prada P, Olié E, Salzmann A, Nicastro R, et al. Increased methylation of glucocorticoid receptor gene (NR3C1) in adults with a history of childhood maltreatment: a link with the severity and type of trauma. *Transl Psychiatry* (2011) 1:e59. doi: 10.1038/tp.2011.60

110. Tran L, Chaloner A, Sawalha AH, Greenwood Van-Meerveld B. Importance of epigenetic mechanisms in visceral pain induced by chronic water avoidance stress. *Psychoneuroendocrinology* (2013) 38:898–906. doi: 10.1016/j.psyneuen.2012.09.016

111. Hong S, Zheng G, Wiley JW. Epigenetic regulation of genes that modulate chronic stress-induced visceral pain in the peripheral nervous system. *Gastroenterology* (2015) 148:148–157.e7. doi: 10.1053/j.gastro.2014.09.032

112. Mahurkar S, Polytarchou C, Iliopoulos D, Pothoulakis C, Mayer EA, Chang L. Genome-wide DNA methylation profiling of peripheral blood mononuclear cells in irritable bowel syndrome. *Neurogastroenterol. Motil* (2016) 28:410–22. doi: 10.1111/nmo.12741

113. Grondona JM, Hoyo-Becerra C, Visser R, Fernández-Llebrez P, López-Ávalos MD. The subcommissural organ and the development of the posterior commissure. *Int Rev Cell Mol Biol* (2012) 296:63–137. doi: 10.1016/B978-0-12-394307-1.00002-3

114. Richter HG, Tomé MM, Yulis CR, Vío KJ, Jiménez AJ, Pérez-Fígares JM, et al. Transcription of SCO-spondin in the subcommissural organ: evidence for down-regulation mediated by serotonin. *Brain Res Mol Brain Res* (2004) 129:151–62. doi: 10.1016/j.molbrainres.2004.07.003

115. Hunter A, Spechler PA, Cwanger A, Song Y, Zhang Z, Ying G, et al. DNA Methylation Is Associated with Altered Gene Expression in AMD. *Invest Ophthalmol Vis Sci* (2012) 53:2089–105. doi: 10.1167/iovs.11-8449

116. Leygo C, Williams M, Jin HC, Chan MWY, Chu WK, Grusch M, et al. DNA Methylation as a Noninvasive Epigenetic Biomarker for the

Detection of Cancer. *Dis Markers* (2017) 2017:3726595. doi: 10.1155/2017/3726595

117. Zhu S, Min L, Guo Q, Li H, Yu Y, Zong Y, et al. Transcriptome and methylome profiling in a rat model of irritable bowel syndrome induced by stress. *Int J Mol Med* (2018) 42:2641–9. doi: 10.3892/ijmm.2018.3823

118. Mahurkar-Joshi S, Videlock EJ, Iliopoulos D, Pothoulakis C, Mayer EA, Chang L. Epigenetic Changes in Blood Cells and Colonic Mucosa are Associated with Irritable Bowel Syndrome (IBS). *Gastroenterology* (2018) 154:S–214. doi: 10.1016/S0016-5085(18)31105-3

119. Hake SB, Xiao A, Allis CD. Linking the epigenetic "language" of covalent histone modifications to cancer. *Br J Cancer* (2004) 90:761–9. doi: 10.1038/sj.bjc.6601575

120. Bannister AJ, Kouzarides T. Regulation of chromatin by histone modifications. *Cell Res* (2011) 21:381–95. doi: 10.1038/cr.2011.22

121. Bai G, Wei D, Zou S, Ren K, Dubner R. Inhibition of class II histone deacetylases in the spinal cord attenuates inflammatory hyperalgesia. *Mol Pain* (2010) 6:51. doi: 10.1186/1744-8069-6-51

122. Imai S, Ikegami D, Yamashita A, Shimizu T, Narita M, Niikura K, et al. Epigenetic transcriptional activation of monocyte chemotactic protein 3 contributes to long-lasting neuropathic pain. *Brain* (2013) 136:828–43. doi: 10.1093/brain/aws330

123. Imai S, Ikegami D, Yamashita A, Shimizu T, Narita M, Niikura K, et al. Epigenetic transcriptional activation of monocyte chemotactic protein 3 contributes to long-lasting neuropathic pain. *Brain* (2013) 136:828–43. doi: 10.1093/brain/aws330

124. Moloney RD, Stilling RM, Dinan TG, Cryan JF. Early-life stress-induced visceral hypersensitivity and anxiety behavior is reversed by histone deacetylase inhibition. *Neurogastroenterol. Motil* (2015) 27:1831–6. doi: 10.1111/nmo.12675

125. Moloney RD, Johnson AC, O'Mahony SM, Dinan TG, Greenwood-Van Meerveld B, Cryan JF. Stress and the Microbiota-Gut-Brain Axis in Visceral Pain: Relevance to Irritable Bowel Syndrome. *CNS Neurosci Ther* (2016) 22:102–17. doi: 10.1111/cns.12490

126. Hong S, Zheng G, Wiley JW. Epigenetic regulation of genes that modulate chronic stress-induced visceral pain in the peripheral nervous system. *Gastroenterology* (2015) 148:148–157.e7. doi: 10.1053/j.gastro.2014.09.032

127. Aguirre JE, Winston JH, Sarna SK. Neonatal immune challenge followed by adult immune challenge induces epigenetic-susceptibility to aggravated visceral hypersensitivity. *Neurogastroenterol. Motil* (2017) 29:125. doi: 10.1111/nmo.13081

128. Filipowicz W, Bhattacharyya SN, Sonenberg N. Mechanisms of post-transcriptional regulation by microRNAs: are the answers in sight? *Nat Rev Genet* (2008) 9:102–14. doi: 10.1038/nrg2290

129. Kress M, Hüttenhofer A, Landry M, Kuner R, Favereaux A, Greenberg D, et al. microRNAs in nociceptive circuits as predictors of future clinical applications. *Front Mol Neurosci* (2013) 6:33. doi: 10.3389/fnmol.2013.00033

130. Videlock EJ, Mahurkar-Joshi S, Iliopoulos D, Pothoulakis C, Meyer EA, Chang L. Dysregulation of the long-noncoding RNA, GHRLOS, in irritable bowel syndrome. *Gastroenterology* (2017) 152:S722. doi: 10.1016/S0016-5085(17)32511-8

131. Kapeller J, Houghton LA, Mönnikes H, Walstab J, Möller D, Bönisch H, et al. First evidence for an association of a functional variant in the microRNA-510 target site of the serotonin receptor-type 3E gene with diarrhea predominant irritable bowel syndrome. *Hum Mol Genet* (2008) 17:2967–77. doi: 10.1093/hmg/ddn195

132. Fourie NH, Peace RM, Abey SK, Sherwin LB, Rahim-Williams B, Smyser PA, et al. Elevated circulating miR-150 and miR-342-3p in patients with irritable bowel syndrome. *Exp Mol Pathol* (2014) 96:422–5. doi: 10.1016/j.yexmp.2014.04.009

133. Gheinani AH, Burkhard FC, Monastyrskaya K. Deciphering microRNA code in pain and inflammation: lessons from bladder pain syndrome. *Cell Mol Life Sci* (2013) 70:3773–89. doi: 10.1007/s00018-013-1275-7

134. Pekow JR, Kwon JH. MicroRNAs in inflammatory bowel disease. *Inflammation Bowel Dis* (2012) 18:187–93. doi: 10.1002/ibd.21691

135. Zhou Q, Souba WW, Croce CM, Verne GN. MicroRNA-29a regulates intestinal membrane permeability in patients with irritable bowel syndrome. *Gut* (2010) 59:775–84. doi: 10.1136/gut.2009.181834

136. Randomised placebo-controlled trial of dietary glutamine supplements for postinfectious irritable bowel syndrome. *Gut*. Available at: https://gut.bmj.com/content/68/6/996 (Accessed December 20, 2019).

137. Zhou Q, Costinean S, Croce CM, Brasier AR, Merwat S, Larson SA, et al. MicroRNA 29 targets nuclear factor-κB-repressing factor and Claudin 1 to increase intestinal permeability. *Gastroenterology* (2015) 148:158–169.e8. doi: 10.1053/j.gastro.2014.09.037

138. Martinez C, Rodino-Janeiro BK, Lobo B, Stanifer ML, Klaus B, Granzow M, et al. miR-16 and miR-125b are involved in barrier function dysregulation through the modulation of claudin-2 and cingulin expression in the jejunum in IBS with diarrhoea. *Gut* (2017) 66:1537–8. doi: 10.1136/gutjnl-2016-311477

139. Hou Q, Huang Y, Zhu S, Li P, Chen X, Hou Z, et al. MiR-144 Increases Intestinal Permeability in IBS-D Rats by Targeting OCLN and ZO1. *Cell Physiol Biochem* (2017) 44:2256–68. doi: 10.1159/000486059

140. Hou Q, Huang Y, Zhang C, Zhu S, Li P, Chen X, et al. MicroRNA-200a Targets Cannabinoid Receptor 1 and Serotonin Transporter to Increase Visceral Hyperalgesia in Diarrhea-predominant Irritable Bowel Syndrome Rats. *J Neurogastroenterol. Motil* (2018) 24:656–68. doi: 10.5056/jnm18037

141. Liao X-J, Mao W-M, Wang Q, Yang G-G, Wu W-J, Shao S-X. MicroRNA-24 inhibits serotonin reuptake transporter expression and aggravates irritable bowel syndrome. *Biochem Biophys Res Commun* (2016) 469:288–93. doi: 10.1016/j.bbrc.2015.11.102

142. Wohlfarth C, Schmitteckert S, Härtle JD, Houghton LA, Dweep H, Fortea M, et al. miR-16 and miR-103 impact 5-HT 4 receptor signalling and correlate with symptom profile in irritable bowel syndrome. *Sci Rep* (2017) 7:1–14. doi: 10.1038/s41598-017-13982-0

143. Merhautova J, Demlova R, Slaby O. MicroRNA-Based Therapy in Animal Models of Selected Gastrointestinal Cancers. *Front Pharmacol* (2016) 7:329. doi: 10.3389/fphar.2016.00329

144. Chen L-L. Linking Long Noncoding RNA Localization and Function. *Trends Biochem Sci* (2016) 41:761–72. doi: 10.1016/j.tibs.2016.07.003

145. Yarani R, Mirza AH, Kaur S, Pociot F. The emerging role of lncRNAs in inflammatory bowel disease. *Exp Mol Med* (2018) 50. doi: 10.1038/s12276-018-0188-9

146. Miro-Blanch J, Yanes O. Epigenetic Regulation at the Interplay Between Gut Microbiota and Host Metabolism. *Front Genet* (2019) 10:638. doi: 10.3389/fgene.2019.00638

147. Bouchard L, Rabasa-Lhoret R, Faraj M, Lavoie M-E, Mill J, Pérusse L, et al. Differential epigenomic and transcriptomic responses in subcutaneous adipose tissue between low and high responders to caloric restriction. *Am J Clin Nutr* (2010) 91:309–20. doi: 10.3945/ajcn.2009.28085

148. Rea K, O'Mahony SM, Dinan TG, Cryan JF. The Role of the Gastrointestinal Microbiota in Visceral Pain. In: Greenwood-Van Meerveld B, editor. *Gastrointestinal Pharmacology Handbook of Experimental Pharmacology*. Cham: Springer International Publishing (2017). p. 269–87. doi: 10.1007/164_2016_115

149. Stilling RM, Dinan TG, Cryan JF. Microbial genes, brain & behaviour – epigenetic regulation of the gut–brain axis. *Genes Brain Behav* (2014) 13:69–86. doi: 10.1111/gbb.12109

150. Russell WR, Hoyles L, Flint HJ, Dumas M-E. Colonic bacterial metabolites and human health. *Curr Opin Microbiol.* (2013) 16:246–54. doi: 10.1016/j.mib.2013.07.002

151. Martin CR, Osadchiy V, Kalani A, Mayer EA. The Brain-Gut-Microbiome Axis. *Cell Mol Gastroenterol. Hepatol.* (2018) 6:133–48. doi: 10.1016/j.jcmgh.2018.04.003

152. Maslowski KM, Mackay CR. Diet, gut microbiota and immune responses. *Nat Immunol* (2011) 12:5–9. doi: 10.1038/ni0111-5

153. Krautkramer KA, Rey FE, Denu JM. Chemical signaling between gut microbiota and host chromatin: What is your gut really saying? *J Biol Chem* (2017) 292:8582–93. doi: 10.1074/jbc.R116.761577

154. Vaiopoulou A, Karamanolis G, Psaltopoulou T, Karatzias G, Gazouli M. Molecular basis of the irritable bowel syndrome. *World J Gastroenterol* (2014) 20:376–83. doi: 10.3748/wjg.v20.i2.376

155. DeBusk RM, Fogarty CP, Ordovas JM, Kornman KS. Nutritional genomics in practice: where do we begin? *J Am Diet Assoc* (2005) 105:589–98. doi: 10.1016/j.jada.2005.01.002

156. de Roest RH, Dobbs BR, Chapman BA, Batman B, O'Brien LA, Leeper JA, et al. The low FODMAP diet improves gastrointestinal symptoms in patients with irritable bowel syndrome: a prospective study. *Int J Clin Pract* (2013) 67:895–903. doi: 10.1111/ijcp.12128

157. Halmos EP, Power VA, Shepherd SJ, Gibson PR, Muir JG. A diet low in FODMAPs reduces symptoms of irritable bowel syndrome. *Gastroenterology* (2014) 146:67–75.e5. doi: 10.1053/j.gastro.2013.09.046

158. Kelly TK, De Carvalho DD, Jones PA. Epigenetic Modifications as Therapeutic Targets. *Nat Biotechnol* (2010) 28:1069–78. doi: 10.1038/nbt.1678

11

The Role of Chronic Stress in Normal Visceroception: Insights from an Experimental Visceral Pain Study in Healthy Volunteers

Adriane Icenhour*, Franziska Labrenz, Till Roderigo, Sven Benson[†] and Sigrid Elsenbruch[†]

Institute of Medical Psychology and Behavioral Immunobiology, University Hospital Essen, University of Duisburg-Essen, Essen, Germany

*Correspondence:
Adriane Icenhour
adriane.icenhour@uk-essen.de

[†]These authors have contributed equally to this work

Visceroception is a complex phenomenon comprising the sensation, interpretation, and integration of sensations along the gut-brain axis, including pain or defecatory urgency. Stress is considered a crucial risk factor for the development and maintenance of disorders of gut-brain signaling, which are characterized by altered visceroception. Although the broad role of stress and stress mediators in disturbed visceroception is widely acknowledged, the putative contribution of chronic stress to variations in normal visceroception remains incompletely understood. We aimed to elucidate the role of chronic stress in shaping different facets of visceroception. From a well-characterized, large sample of healthy men and women (N = 180, 50% female), volunteers presenting with low (n = 57) and elevated (n = 61) perceived chronic stress were identified based on the validated Trier Inventory for Chronic Stress (TICS). Visceral sensitivity together with perceived and recalled intensity and defecatory urgency induced by repeated rectal distensions was experimentally assessed, and compared between low and elevated stress groups. Subgroups were compared regarding state anxiety and salivary cortisol concentrations across experimental phases and with respect to psychological measures. Finally, in the full sample and in chronic stress subgroups, a recall bias in terms of a discrepancy between the perception of experimentally-induced symptoms and their recall was tested. Participants with elevated chronic stress presented with increased state anxiety and higher cortisol concentrations throughout the experimental phases compared to the group with low chronic stress. Group differences in visceral sensitivity were not evident. The elevated stress group perceived significantly higher urgency during the stimulation phase, and recalled substantially higher feelings of urgency induced by rectal distensions, while perceived and recalled intensity were comparable between groups. Volunteers with elevated stress exhibited a recall bias in terms of a higher recall relative to mean perception of urgency, whereas no such bias was observed for the intensity of experimental visceral stimulation. Our findings in healthy men and women provide first evidence that the troublesome symptom of urgency might be particularly modifiable by chronic stress and support the relevance of memory biases in visceroception. These results may help to disentangle the impact of chronic stress on altered visceroception in disturbances of gut-brain communication.

Keywords: chronic stress, visceroception, gut-brain axis, visceral pain, urgency, recall bias, memory

INTRODUCTION

Visceroception is defined as the perception and processing of interoceptive signals arising from visceral organs (1, 2). Importantly, visceroception is not fully captured by visceral sensitivity alone, which primarily reflects sensory-discriminative aspects of perception. It is rather conceptualized more broadly as a specific facet of interoception, involving the sensation, interpretation, and integration of visceral signals (2) along the gut-brain axis. The complex affective-motivational and cognitive dimensions of visceroception shape gastrointestinal (GI) symptom perception, including visceral pain and defecatory urgency, in healthy individuals as well as in patients with chronic GI symptoms (3). The clinical relevance of disturbed visceroception is particularly evident in the context of disorders of disturbed gut-brain interactions, like irritable bowel syndrome (IBS) and functional dyspepsia. Altered GI symptoms perception, involving visceral hyperalgesia and hypervigilance, plays a pivotal role in their pathophysiology and treatment. However, the complex mechanisms underlying altered visceroception remain incompletely understood, especially with respect to psychological modulation.

As a crucial psychological factor, stress plays a broad role in disorders of disturbed gut-brain interactions (4–6). This has most clearly been underscored by evidence that acute stress or stress mediators of the hypothalamus-pituitary-adrenal (HPA) axis increase visceral sensitivity and neural processing of visceral stimuli in patients (7) but also in healthy volunteers (8). Chronic stress burden has been identified as an important risk factor for disease onset (9), and for the exacerbation of GI symptoms, particularly of visceral pain in patients with IBS (10, 11). Importantly, symptom burden in patients is often not limited to pain, but also involves defecatory urgency as a highly troublesome symptom in a broad range of GI conditions (12–14). Psychological modulation of defecatory urgency has previously been proposed (15), and our own recent data suggested that acute stress amplified nocebo effects especially for the symptom of distension-induced urgency more so then the symptom of pain in healthy volunteers (16). While together these findings clearly support a role of acute as well as chronic stress in different dimensions of visceroception, experimental work particularly on effects of chronic stress remains scarce.

Building on our earlier work on the modulation of visceroception by acute stress and stress mediators (7, 8, 16), we herein aimed to elucidate the putative role of chronic stress in different clinically-relevant facets of normal visceroception.

From a large sample of well-characterized healthy men and women that underwent rectal sensitivity testing and repeated painful rectal distensions as part of a larger study (16, 17), we compared individuals with elevated and low perceived chronic stress with respect to sensory and pain thresholds and rectal distension-induced symptom reports of pain and urgency. We hypothesized that individuals with elevated levels of stress would reveal increased sensitivity, as reflected by lower thresholds for graded distensions of the rectum as well as higher pain and urgency ratings in response to individually-calibrated repeated distensions. In addition to analyses of symptom reports based on individual distensions, we also elucidated overall symptom recall based on a retrospective symptom rating. This was accomplished given evidence that retrospective overall symptom ratings may be more susceptible to psychological modulation, especially in patients with IBS (18). Given our interest in visceral pain-related memory effects (8, 19–22), together with evidence supporting the role of reporting bias in IBS (23), we introduced a new "memory bias" measure. This measure was based on the difference between perceptual ratings of individual distensions and retrospective overall ratings, the former being presumably more reflective of sensory-discriminative facts of visceroception, the latter possibly more prone to psychological modulation, both with relevance to collective symptom reporting in experimental and clinical trials as well as clinical practice.

METHODS

Participants

From a well-characterized large sample of young healthy men and women (N = 180; 90 women), tertiles based on the validated Trier Inventory for Chronic Stress (TICS) were identified. The top and bottom tertile were chosen to define participants with low and elevated perceived chronic stress, as detailed below, and included in the current analysis. Participants had been recruited through local advertisements for the primary study on the modulation of placebo and nocebo effects by acute experimental stress (16) or relaxation (17) in visceral pain. They had been informed that the aim of the study would be to investigate psychological mechanisms underlying effects of different drugs on experimentally-induced visceral symptoms. Of note, all measures included in the current analyses were assessed prior to randomization of participants for subsequent experimental manipulations. They served as baseline measures in the primary studies, and observations reported herein were therefore independent of subsequent manipulations. Participants were excluded according to the following criteria: age < 18 or > 65 years, body mass index (BMI) < 18 or > 30, a history of or acute medical and psychiatric conditions and current medication use except for hormonal contraceptives, thyroid medication, and occasional use of over-the-counter pain or allergy medication. Moreover, subclinical gastrointestinal (GI) symptoms experienced during a 3 month period preceding study participation were measured using a standardized in-house questionnaire (24). As in our prior studies (19, 21, 24) a cut-off score of 11 was used as an indicator of a putative undiagnosed gastrointestinal condition, which led to exclusion from study participation. Only women using hormonal contraception were included and pregnancy was ruled out on the study day with a commercially available urinary test. All participants underwent a physical examination to exclude perianal tissue damage (e.g., fissures or painful hemorrhoids), which might interfere with the experimental procedure. Participants gave written informed consent and received 200€ for their participation. The study protocol was approved by the local ethics committee (protocol number 13-5565-BO) and followed the provisions of the Declaration of Helsinki.

Experimental Design and Study Procedures

An overview over the experimental design and the study procedures relevant to the current analyses is given in **Figure 1**. All experimental procedures were conducted between 12:00 and 18:00 h to account for effects of the circadian rhythm. Initially, an inflatable balloon attached to a pressure-controlled barostat system (modified ISOBAR 3 device; G & J Electronics, ON, Toronto, Canada) was placed 5 cm from the anal verge, for the application of rectal distensions. Rectal sensory and pain thresholds were determined using a double-random staircase distension protocol with random pressure increments between 2 and 6 mmHg and a maximal distension pressure of 55 mmHg. Participants rated each sensation on a Likert-type scale labeled

1 = no perception, 2 = doubtful perception, 3 = sure perception, 4 = little discomfort, 5 = severe discomfort, and 6 = pain, not tolerable distension. The sensory threshold was defined as a pressure when ratings changed from 2 to 3 and the pain threshold was determined at the change from 5 to 6. The individual pain threshold was used as an anchor for a subsequent pressure calibration to identify a moderately painful intensity for the repeated application of rectal distensions. Specifically, a pressure corresponding to a pain intensity rating not higher than 80 on a visual analog scale (VAS) with endpoints labeled 0 = none at all and 100 = very much was identified, as previously described (16). This intensity was used for the subsequent stimulation phase, during which six rectal distensions with a duration of 30 s and a rest interval of 30 s following each stimulus were applied. Salivary cortisol concentrations and state anxiety as measures of acute stress and arousal were collected at different time points across the experimental phases and ratings of stimulus intensity and urgency perception and recall as different facets of visceroception were assessed, as detailed below.

Measures of Visceroception

In addition to sensory and pain thresholds, mean scores of trial-by-trial VAS ratings of stimulus intensity and urgency perception and ratings of overall recalled intensity and urgency induced by the experienced rectal distensions during the stimulation phase were assessed as measures of visceroception. Specifically, during the stimulation phase, participants were prompted to rate the intensity of each distension and the urgency it induces on separate VAS with endpoints labeled "none" (0) and "very much" (100) for intensity and "none (0) and "very high" (100) for urgency. Following the stimulation phase, participants were asked to recall the overall intensity of and urgency induced by the experienced distensions using separate VAS. In order to elucidate a potential memory bias in visceroception in terms of a deviation of recalled from mean perceived visceral sensations, delta values between perceived and

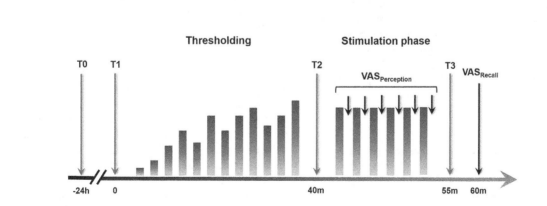

FIGURE 1 | Study design and experimental procedures. Twenty-four hours prior to study participation (T0), a salivary cortisol sample was collected as a baseline measure unaffected by the experimental procedure. On the study day, salivary cortisol and state anxiety were assessed upon arrival (T1), before (T2), and after (T3) the stimulation phase. Visual analog scale (VAS) ratings of intensity and urgency perception were acquired during the stimulation phase. At the conclusion of the experimental phase, VAS ratings assessing intensity and urgency recall were accomplished.

recalled intensity and urgency were calculated, respectively, to test for recall biases in measures of visceroception.

Assessment of State Anxiety and Salivary Cortisol

Twenty-four hours prior to the study appointment (time point T0), a baseline salivary cortisol sample was collected by participants in their home environment, using Salivettes (Sarstedt, Nürnbrecht, Germany), and stored at 4°C until transport to the laboratory on the study day. On the study day, salivary cortisol as a marker of acute stress and HPA axis activation was collected upon arrival (T1), following the thresholding procedure before the stimulation phase (T2), and after the stimulation phase (T3). As a self-report measure of acute arousal, state anxiety was assessed at time points T1–T3 along with cortisol sample collection, using the state version of the validated State Trait Anxiety Inventory (STAI-S) (25, 26). Saliva samples were centrifuged (2,000 rpm, 2 min, 4°C) and stored at −20°C until analysis. Cortisol concentrations were measured using an enzyme-linked immunosorbent assay (ELISA; IBL International, Hamburg, Germany) in accordance with the manufacturer's protocol with a detection limit at 0.138 nmol/L.

Assessment of Chronic Stress and Identification of Stress Subgroups

Following informed consent, participants completed the validated Trier Inventory for Chronic Stress (TICS) screening scale (27). The self-assessment instrument allows an evaluation of individual experiences with chronic stressors in everyday life, providing a reliable global measure of perceived stress during the previous 3 months with a Cronbach's α of .91 (28). Each of the 12 items is scored on a five-point Likert-scale as "never" (0), "rarely" (1), "sometimes" (2), "often" (3), and "very often" (4 points). The total score ranges from 0 to 48 points, expressing the subjectively perceived presence and frequency of chronic stressors. Norm values from healthy volunteers are available (22), with a mean TICS score of 13 corresponding to T = 50. TICS sum scores were used herein to evaluate overall perceived chronic stress and to allocate participants to a subgroup with low or elevated chronic stress. This was accomplished by subdividing participants into tertile subgroups based on TICS scores. Participants in the top tertile were defined as an elevated stress subgroup, the bottom tertile as a group with low chronic stress.

Questionnaires

In addition to TICS for the assessment of chronic stress, participants completed the following comprehensive questionnaire battery for a characterization with respect to psychological factors of putative relevance to both, stress, and visceroception: The trait version of the State Trait Anxiety Inventory (STAI-T) (25, 26) for the assessment of trait anxiety (sum scores between 20 and 80), the Pain-Related Self

Statements Scale (PRSS) (29) to measure pain-related cognitions in terms of maladaptive pain catastrophizing and adaptive pain coping (sum scores ranging from 0 to 45, respectively), and the Generalized Self-efficacy (GSE) Scale (30) to assess optimistic self-beliefs to cope with life demands (total scores 10–40) as a marker of resilience to stressors.

Statistical Analyses

All statistical analyses were performed using IBM SPSS version 25 (IBM Corporation, Armonk, NY, USA). As described above, participants were stratified based on the level of perceived chronic stress, allowing to define and compare groups with low and elevated perceived chronic stress. Notably, due to this stratification strategy, the investigated samples displayed non-normal distribution in some of the relevant outcome measures, as evidenced by significant Kolmogorov-Smirnov tests. However, no outliers were detected in either sample. Given sufficient sample sizes and the robustness of parametric statistical approaches under these circumstances, parametric tests were performed. Accordingly, stress subgroups were compared with respect to sociodemographic and psychological characteristics using two sample t-tests or chi square test where appropriate. Group comparisons of sensory and pain thresholds as measures of visceral sensitivity, as well as baseline cortisol (T0) were accomplished using two sample t-tests. Repeated measures ANOVA with the within-group factor *time* and the between-group factor *stress subgroup* were applied to analyze state anxiety and salivary cortisol concentrations on the study day (T1–T3). Independent sample t-tests were further conducted for group comparisons of mean perceived and recalled measures of visceroception, as assessed with VAS. In addition, bias scores based on the difference between perceptual and retrospective ratings were entered into one sample t-tests for effects in the full sample and into two sample t-tests for stress subgroup comparisons. To account for a possible impact of acute stress and arousal on effects of chronic stress on visceroception, analyses of covariance (ANCOVA) with mean cortisol concentrations and mean state anxiety scores as covariates were additionally conducted for measures of visceroception. Further, to address possibly divergent effects of chronic stress on measures of visceroception in men and women, interactions between the factors *sex* and *stress subgroup* were explored using ANOVA. Finally, to confirm the specificity of findings to chronic stress, stepwise multiple regression analyses (probability to enter ≤.05, probability to remove ≥.10) were performed in the full sample, entering TICS scores as a measure of perceived chronic stress together with closely related psychological traits, such as trait anxiety, pain coping, and self-efficacy, as predictors of variance in visceroceptive markers. Results from ANOVA and ANCOVA are reported with Greenhouse-Geisser correction to account for a possible violation of the sphericity assumption and results from *post hoc* t-tests were Bonferroni corrected for multiple comparisons where appropriate. Alpha level was set at $p < .05$, exact two-tailed p values are reported and η_p^2, Cohen's d, or

Cramer's V are provided as indicators of effect size, respectively. All descriptive statistics are reported as mean ± standard error of the mean (SEM), unless indicated otherwise.

RESULTS

Sample Characterization

A characterization of the full sample and comparisons of stress subgroups with respect to sociodemographic and psychological measures are summarized in **Table 1**. TICS scores in the full sample indicated an average level of perceived chronic stress according to available norm values (28). The mean score in the low stress group corresponded to an average level of chronic stress within a lower range in a healthy population. The elevated stress group presented with mean TICS scores above average, confirming the stratification strategy and the identification of healthy volunteers with low and elevated levels of perceived chronic stress. Accordingly, chronic stress scores were substantially higher in the elevated chronic stress group. Subgroups were comparable regarding age, BMI, and distribution of men and women. Participants with elevated stress presented with increased trait anxiety, lower self-efficacy, and reported more catastrophizing cognitions when coping with pain, whereas groups did not differ regarding the use of active pain coping.

Salivary Cortisol and State Anxiety

Baseline cortisol concentrations 24 h prior to the study appointment (T0) were significantly increased in the group with elevated chronic stress (13.29 ± 1.24 nmol/l) relative to individuals with low perceived chronic stress (10.09 ± 0.72 nmol/l; $t = 2.24$; $p = .027$; $d = .042$). Analysis of cortisol concentrations on the study day (T1–T3) revealed a significant effect of *stress subgroup* ($F = 6.60$; $p = .011$; $\eta_p^2 = .054$), which was attributable to higher cortisol levels across the experimental phases in participants with elevated perceived chronic stress (**Figure 2A**). No effect of *time* was evident ($p = .372$). Analysis of state anxiety also demonstrated a significant effect of *stress subgroup* ($F = 19.76$; $p < .001$; $\eta_p^2 = .146$), with higher state anxiety in the elevated stress compared to the low stress group (**Figure 2B**). No effect of *time* was observed ($p = .257$).

Visceroception in Subgroups With Low and Elevated Chronic Stress
Sensory and Pain Thresholds

Analyses of sensory and pain thresholds in individuals with elevated and low perceived chronic stress revealed comparable thresholds for both, first sensation ($p = .789$; **Figures 3A, C**) and pain ($p = .794$; **Figures 3B, D**). Controlling for state anxiety and salivary cortisol concentrations did not affect these results (data not shown).

TABLE 1 | Characterization of the full sample and chronic stress groups with respect to sociodemographic and psychological variables.

	Full sample N = 180	Low stress n = 57	Elevated stress n = 61	t/χ²	p	d/V
Female (n, %)	90 (50%)	29 (50.9%)	29 (47.5%)	0.13	.717	.033
Age	26.38 ± 0.45	27.23 ± 0.92	26.43 ± 0.82	0.65	.516	.012
BMI	23.29 ± 0.21	23.40 ± 0.36	23.67 ± 0.41	0.49	.623	.009
Chronic stress (T)	17.58 ± 0.65 (55)	7.93 ± 0.49 (44)	26.98 ± 0.64 (63)	23.68	**<.001**	.434
Trait anxiety	36.03 ± 0.64	29.81 ± 0.67	43.03 ± 1.14	9.98	**<.001**	.182
Pain catastrophizing	1.88 ± 0.06	1.45 ± 0.09	2.45 ± 0.11	6.96	**<.001**	.128
Active pain coping	3.41 ± 0.06	3.46 ± 0.11	3.36 ± 0.10	0.74	.460	.014
Self-efficacy	30.25 ± 0.30	32.14 ± 0.44	28.00 ± 0.53	6.01	**<.001**	.111

Data are given as mean ± SEM, unless indicated otherwise and significant group differences are indicated in bold. BMI, body mass index; T, T-score for TICS screening scale.

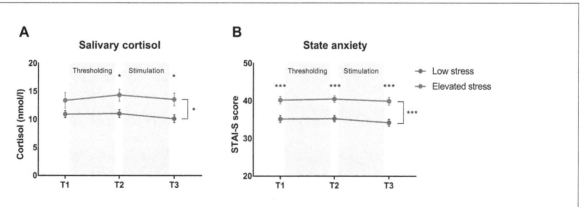

FIGURE 2 | Group comparisons of **(A)** salivary cortisol concentrations and **(B)** state anxiety across the experimental phases (T1–T3) in subjects with elevated (n = 61) *versus* those with low chronic stress (n = 57). Data are given as mean ± SEM. *p < .05 ***p < .001.

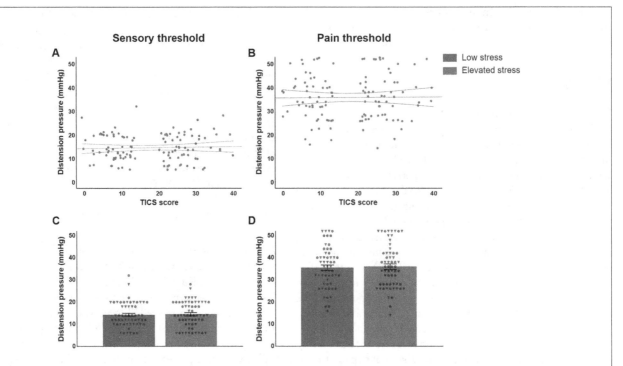

FIGURE 3 | Jittered scatterplots with regression curves and 95% confidence intervals of individual **(A)** sensory and **(B)** pain thresholds in participants with low (n = 57, blue) and elevated chronic stress (n = 61, red) and group comparisons regarding mean thresholds **(C, D)**, provided ± SEM and depicted with individual data points for women (indicated as circles) and men (shown as triangles).

Perception and Recall of Visceroceptive Stimulation

Subgroup comparisons of mean perceived urgency based on trial-by-trial ratings following each visceral sensation during the stimulation phase revealed significantly higher urgency in the group with elevated stress (t = 2.04; p = .043; d = 0.37; **Figure 4A**), whereas groups did not differ regarding mean perceived intensity (p = .507; **Figure 4C**). Similarly, participants with elevated perceived chronic stress recalled significantly higher overall urgency experienced during the stimulation phase (t = 3.57; p = .001; d = 0.66; **Figure 4B**), but no group difference in recalled intensity was observed (p = .517; **Figure 4D**). In covariance analyses, group differences in mean perceived urgency failed statistical significance (p = .095) when including mean state anxiety and mean cortisol concentrations, while differences in urgency recall remained widely unaffected (F = 9.44; p = .003; η_p^2 = .076) and no changes were evident regarding perceived or recalled intensity (data not shown).

Recall Bias

To elucidate a putative exaggeration of intensity or urgency recall, the full sample and stress subgroups were tested for a recall bias in visceroception, operationalized as the differences between mean reported perception during the stimulation phase and overall recall, respectively. One sample t-tests revealed significant effects for both, intensity (t = 2.48; p = .014; d = 0.18) and, more pronounced, for urgency (t = 8.38; p < .001; d = 0.62), indicating higher recall relative to mean perception in the full sample. Individuals with elevated chronic

stress exhibited a significant bias for recalled defecatory urgency, i.e., recalled more intense feelings of urgency relative to their mean perception (t = 2.96; p = .004; d = 0.55; **Figure 5A**). The recall bias for intensity was comparable between stress subgroups (p = .132; **Figure 5B**). ANCOVA including mean state anxiety and cortisol did not affect these finding (urgency recall bias: F = 6.68; p = .011; η_p^2 = .055; intensity recall bias: p = .305).

Interactions Between Chronic Stress and Sex

Possible sex differences in the effects of perceived chronic stress on visceroception were addressed in exploratory analyses. For thresholds, results revealed no interaction between stress level and sex for either first sensation (p = .950; **Figure 3C**) or pain (p = .451; **Figure 3D**). No evidence of sex-specific effects of chronic stress emerged for perceived (p = .503; **Figure 4A**) and recalled urgency (p = .824; **Figure 4B**) or intensity (perceived: p = .143; **Figure 4C**; recalled: p = .222; **Figure 4D**). Finally, neither urgency (p = .352; **Figure 5A**) nor intensity recall bias (p = .793; **Figure 5B**) indicated sex-specific effects of perceived chronic stress.

Specificity to Chronic Stress

Stepwise multiple regression analyses were performed in the full sample of N = 180 participants to evaluate whether the observed effects were specific to chronic stress or could also be attributed to effects of other psychological traits, including trait anxiety, pain coping strategies, and self-efficacy. This exploratory approach focused on significant findings from subgroup

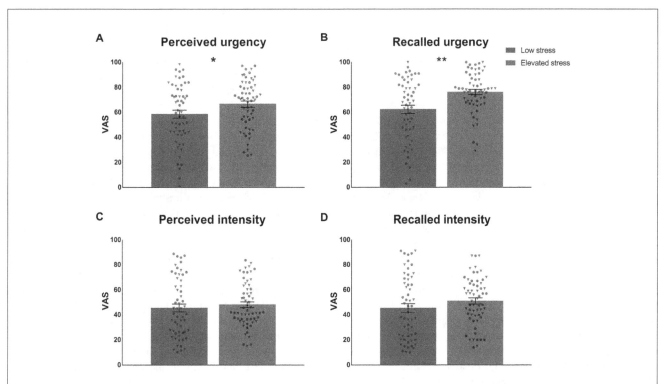

FIGURE 4 | Group comparisons of **(A)** mean perception and **(B)** recall of urgency and **(C, D)** intensity of repeated rectal distensions during the stimulation phase in participants with low (n = 57) and elevated (n = 61) chronic stress. Data are given as mean ± SEM and individual data points for women (circles) and men (triangles) are provided. *$p < .05$; **$p < .01$.

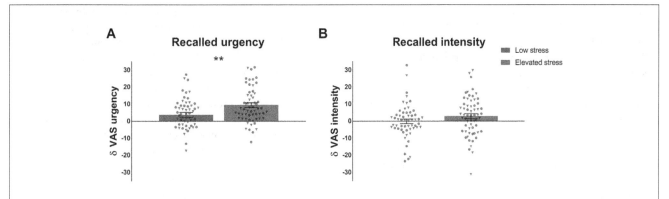

FIGURE 5 | Group comparisons in recall bias of **(A)** defecatory urgency and **(B)** intensity of rectal distensions during the stimulation phase, operationalized as the difference between mean perceived and recalled symptoms. Data from individuals with low (n = 57) and elevated chronic stress levels (n = 61) are given as mean ± SEM and individual data points are illustrated as circles for women and as triangles for men. **$p < .01$.

analyses, and was therefore conducted on perceived and recalled urgency as well as the urgency recall bias. These analyses confirmed chronic stress to be the main predictor of visceroception. Specifically, TICS scores were a single significant predictor of mean perceived ($F = 4.49$; $p = 0.035$; adj. $R^2 = 0.018$; $\beta = 0.157$) and, more pronounced, recalled urgency ($F = 12.84$; $p < .001$; adj. $R^2 = 0.062$; $\beta = 0.259$). Further, perceived chronic stress was identified as a single predictor of variance in the urgency recall bias ($F = 8.59$; $p = .004$; adj. $R^2 = 0.041$; $\beta = 0.215$). Trait anxiety, pain coping, and self-efficacy did

not contribute additionally to explaining variance in visceroception.

DISCUSSION

The relevance of interoception for both health and disease is increasingly acknowledged (1, 2, 31), especially in the context of visceral hypersensitivity in disorders of gut-brain interactions. Although the broad role of stress and stress mediators in disturbed visceroception is widely appreciated (32–34), the putative contribution of chronic stress to variations in normal visceroception remains incompletely understood. To fill this research gap, we herein assessed the impact of chronic stress on different dimensions of visceroception induced by rectal distensions by comparing stress subgroups classified based on a validated chronic stress questionnaire. While individuals with elevated *versus* low levels of perceived chronic stress did not differ in rectal sensory or pain thresholds, both the perception as well as the recall of rectal urgency were significantly enhanced in individuals with elevated chronic stress. Furthermore, a recall bias for previously experienced distension-induced urgency was more pronounced in the group with elevated stress. Together, these findings support that the sensation of urgency might be particularly modifiable by chronic stress in healthy young men and women, with implications for the pathophysiology of chronic GI symptoms.

A link between chronic stress and the perception and recall of urgency complements our previous result that the symptom of urgency was demonstrably highly modifiable by acute psychosocial stress in a placebo/nocebo paradigm (16). Psychological modulation of urgency is interesting from a clinical perspective for a broad range of conditions characterized by chronic gastrointestinal symptoms, which are often not limited to the experience of visceral pain. For example, defecatory urgency is a symptom frequently reported by patients with IBS (12), which has recently been identified as the most troublesome symptom in diarrhea-predominant IBS (13). Urgency has also emerged as an independent predictor of quality of life not only in IBS and other disturbances of gut-brain communication (35, 36), but also in the general population (37).

In light of the fact that symptom reports guide diagnosis and treatment in many conditions involving the gut-brain axis, our findings suggesting a putative role of chronic stress in GI symptom recall are noteworthy and deserve more attention. The recall of defecatory urgency induced by previously experienced visceral sensations was enhanced in participants with elevated chronic stress. Further, individuals who reported more chronic stress also demonstrated a more pronounced recall bias for urgency, herein quantified as the difference between the individual distension ratings and the overall urgency recall. The role of reporting bias and its possible contribution to findings of visceral hypersensitivity in IBS has previously been elegantly demonstrated (23). Our results expand on these data using a somewhat simpler yet clinically-relevant method, following a line of research on memory processes in visceroception (8, 19–22), with a particular focus on interoceptive hypervigilance. It is indeed intriguing to speculate that chronic stress may contribute to interoceptive hypervigilance, either indirectly involving a reporting bias or more directly by biasing specific memory processes, including immediate recall, toward more "negative" memories of symptoms. Future studies should therefore test the hypothesis that altered visceroceptive recall may constitute a nocebo mechanism in the pathophysiology of altered gut-brain

interactions. Support for this assumption is provided by experimental findings from the field of associative visceral pain-related conditioning (19, 21, 22), with documented alterations in pain-related learning and memory processes in patients with IBS (20, 38). Stress and stress mediators might play a key role in these alterations, as evidenced by findings that antagonizing corticotropin releasing factor, one of the main signaling peptides of the HPA axis released in response to stress, normalized aberrant neural and psychophysiological correlates of abdominal pain-related learning and memory in women with IBS (38). In healthy individuals, we recently observed pharmacologically increased cortisol levels to induce a reduction in visceral pain thresholds and to affect the formation of pain-related emotional memories (8). Importantly, these effects appeared to be specific to the visceral domain and were not observed for somatic stimuli of identical intensities, in line with prior research on distinct mechanisms underlying the processing of visceral and somatic pain (39–42), and suggesting that visceroception might be particularly vulnerable to stress and stress mediators. Our findings expand this evidence to the dimension of chronic stress, with putative clinical implications for vulnerability and resilience in health and in disorders of gut-brain communication.

On a critical note, some of the mechanisms underlying our findings remain difficult to discern. We observed significantly elevated state anxiety and cortisol concentrations in our cohort of individuals with higher perceived chronic stress across experimental time points. Hence, higher perceived chronic stress was clearly associated with differences in "state" measures, which reportedly modulate visceral pain processing (43), but also with psychological traits, such as increased trait anxiety, maladaptive pain coping, and lower self-efficacy. While our explorative covariance and regression analyses widely supported the observed effects to be distinctly attributable to chronic stress, our study design and the present results do not allow conclusive answers. Clearly, there exists a large overlap between chronic stress and trait anxiety, including its underlying neurobiology (44) and maladaptive coping is likely to further increase not only acute stress responsivity but also the burden arising from physical or psychological stressors (45). These psychological factors might therefore further increase detrimental effects of chronic stress in patients with disorders of gut-brain interactions. Future studies may consider including patients with disturbed visceroception with and without a comorbidity with anxiety. This could shed more light on additive or interactive relations between stress and anxiety in visceroception, which cannot be fully captured in our sample of young, healthy individuals with overall low anxiety symptom burden and adaptive coping skills. Likewise, although we identified a group of healthy individuals in our sample reporting levels of chronic stress above average, the stress burden was not substantially increased to clinically-relevant levels (20, 46). While posing a limitation regarding the generalizability of our findings to the impact of severe chronic stress in patients with disturbed visceroception, our data support that even subtle increases in perceived chronic stress might modulate visceroception. Finally, we addressed our research questions regarding the role of chronic stress in visceroception in a mixed sample of men and women. A recent analysis conducted in a large pooled sample including the current study cohort confirmed no differences between healthy male and female participants with respect to visceral sensitivity, yet did not test other aspects of visceroception (47). Stress subgroups in the current sample did not differ in the relation between male and female participants, suggesting that men and women suffered from elevated chronic stress to comparable extents. Further, exploratory analyses indicated no sex- or gender-specific effects of perceived chronic stress on the tested dimensions of visceroception, suggesting that, at least in young healthy men and women, chronic stress and sex/gender do not interact in altering visceroception. On the other hand, pharmacologically increased cortisol was recently shown to affect visceral sensitivity distinctly in women (8), in support of a role of sex/gender in the impact of the stress mediator on visceroception. Importantly, such putative sex-dependent effects of stress or stress markers might be mediated by interactions with gonadal hormone status, which in women is subject to substantial variations across the menstrual cycle, reportedly impacts visceroception (48), and appears to affect the vulnerability and responsivity to stressors (49, 50). To control for confounding effects of menstrual cycle phase, all women in the sample under investigation were on hormonal contraception. However, this selection does not allow a generalization to women with a natural menstrual cycle, calling for future research including female participants in different mentrual cycle phases.

Taken together, our findings support that elevated perceived chronic stress affects visceroception in healthy individuals, particularly the perception and recall of defecatory urgency as a highly disturbing and clinically-relevant marker in patients with disturbances of gut-brain interactions (35, 36). As two major pathways in the communication along the gut-brain axis, the descending stress system and the ascending visceroceptive system are tightly interacting (32) and their dysfunction may have profound detrimental effects on the communication pathways connecting the brain and the gut. Therefore, investigating chronic stress also in otherwise healthy individuals may aid to gain further insights into mechanisms contributing to long-lasting disturbances along the gut-brain

axis. Importantly, the relevance of a dysfunctional gut-brain interaction is increasingly acknowledged beyond disorders primarily characterized by GI symptoms. These developments are not least owed to a growing appreciation of the crucial role of gut microbiota in health and disease (51–53). Particularly, tremendous advances have been made in understanding the impact of pre- and postnatal microbial composition on responsivity to stress later in life (54). These transdisciplinary findings strongly suggest a key role of the microbiota-gut-brain axis and its neural, humoral, endocrine, and immunological communication pathways in stress-related disturbances. This has implications for both the pathophysiology, and also the therapy of diseases affecting visceroception (6, 55), as well as highly comorbid stress-related central nervous system (CNS) disorders (56), such as anxiety (57), depression (58), and posttraumatic stress disorder (PTSD) (59). Interdisciplinary research on the complex communication pathways along the gut-brain axis bridging neurogastroenterology, psychiatry, and the neurosciences therefore promises important new insights into pathophysiological processes and may inspire new treatments of diseases characterized by altered stress responsivity, including those with visceroceptive malfunction.

ETHICS STATEMENT

The studies involving human participants were reviewed and approved by the Institutional Ethics Review Board of the Medical Faculty of the University of Duisburg-Essen. The patients/participants provided their written informed consent to participate in this study.

AUTHOR CONTRIBUTIONS

SE and SB designed the research study. TR performed the research. AI and FL analyzed the data. AI, SB, and SE wrote the paper. All authors revised the manuscript for critical intellectual content and approved the final version of the manuscript.

REFERENCES

1. Ceunen E, Vlaeyen JWSS, Van Diest I. On the origin of interoception. *Front Psychol* (2016) 7:743. doi: 10.3389/fpsyg.2016.00743

2. Khalsa SS, Adolphs R, Cameron OG, Critchley HD, Davenport PW, Feinstein JS, et al. Interoception and Mental Health: A Roadmap. *Biol Psychiatry Cogn Neurosci Neuroimaging* (2018) 3:501–13. doi: 10.1016/j.bpsc.2017.12.004

3. Elsenbruch S. Abdominal pain in irritable bowel syndrome: a review of putative psychological, neural and neuro-immune mechanisms. *Brain Behav Immun* (2011) 25:386–94. doi: 10.1016/j.bbi.2010.11.010

4. Meerveld BG-V, Johnson AC. Mechanisms of Stress-induced Visceral Pain. *J Neurogastroenterol Motil* (2018) 24:7–18. doi: 10.5056/jnm17137

5. Moloney RD, O'Mahony SM, Dinan TG, Cryan JF. Stress-induced visceral pain: Toward animal models of irritable-bowel syndrome and associated comorbidities. *Front Psychiatry* (2015) 6:15. doi: 10.3389/fpsyt.2015.00015

6. Moloney RD, Johnson AC, O'Mahony SM, Dinan TG, Greenwood-Van Meerveld B, Cryan JF. Stress and the microbiota–gut–brain axis in visceral pain: relevance to irritable bowel syndrome. *CNS Neurosci Ther* (2016) 22:102–17. doi: 10.1111/cns.12490

7. Elsenbruch S, Rosenberger C, Bingel U, Forsting M, Schedlowski M, Gizewski ER. Patients with irritable bowel syndrome have altered emotional modulation of neural responses to visceral stimuli. *Gastroenterology* (2010) 139:1310–9. doi: 10.1053/j.gastro.2010.06.054

8. Benson S, Siebert C, Koenen LR, Engler H, Kleine-Borgmann J, Bingel U, et al. Cortisol affects pain sensitivity and pain-related emotional learning in experimental visceral but not somatic pain: a randomized-controlled study in healthy men and women. *Pain* (2019) 160:1719–28. doi: 10.1097/j.pain.0000000000001579

9. Creed F. Review article: the incidence and risk factors for irritable bowel syndrome in population-based studies. *Aliment Pharmacol Ther* (2019) 50:507–16. doi: 10.1111/apt.15396

10. Fukudo S. Stress and visceral pain: focusing on irritable bowel syndrome. *Pain* (2013) 154 Suppl1:S63–S70. doi: 10.1016/j.pain.2013.09.008

11. Boeckxstaens GE, Wouters MM. Neuroimmune factors in functional gastrointestinal disorders: a focus on irritable bowel syndrome. *Neurogastroenterol Motil* (2017) 29:e13007. doi: 10.1111/nmo.13007

12. Polster A, Van Oudenhove L, Jones M, Ohman L, Tornblom H, Simren M. Mixture model analysis identifies irritable bowel syndrome subgroups characterised by specific profiles of gastrointestinal, extraintestinal somatic and psychological symptoms. *Aliment Pharmacol Ther* (2017) 46:529–39. doi: 10.1111/apt.14207

13. Tornblom H, Goosey R, Wiseman G, Baker S, Emmanuel A. Understanding symptom burden and attitudes to irritable bowel syndrome with diarrhoea: Results from patient and healthcare professional surveys. *U Eur Gastroenterol J* (2018) 6:1417–27. doi: 10.1177/2050640618787648

14. Spiegel BMR, Khanna D, Bolus R, Agarwal N, Khanna P, Chang L. Understanding gastrointestinal distress: a framework for clinical practice. *Am J Gastroenterol* (2011) 106:380–5. doi: 10.1038/ajg.2010.383

15. Posserud I, Agerforz P, Ekman R, Bjornsson ES, Abrahamsson H, Simren M. Altered visceral perceptual and neuroendocrine response in patients with irritable bowel syndrome during mental stress. *Gut* (2004) 53:1102–8. doi: 10.1136/gut.2003.017962

16. Roderigo T, Benson S, Schöls M, Hetkamp M, Schedlowski M, Enck P, et al. Effects of acute psychological stress on placebo and nocebo responses in a clinically relevant model of visceroception. *Pain* (2017) 158:1489–98. doi: 10.1097/j.pain.0000000000000940

17. Elsenbruch S, Roderigo T, Enck P, Benson S. Can a brief relaxation exercise modulate placebo or nocebo effects in a visceral pain model? *Front Psychiatry* (2019) 10:144. doi: 10.3389/fpsyt.2019.00144

18. Elsenbruch S, Rosenberger C, Enck P, Forsting M, Schedlowski M, Gizewski ER. Affective disturbances modulate the neural processing of visceral pain stimuli in irritable bowel syndrome: an fMRI study. *Gut* (2010) 59:489–95. doi: 10.1136/gut.2008.175000

19. Icenhour A, Labrenz F, Ritter C, Theysohn N, Forsting M, Bingel U, et al. Learning by experience? Visceral pain-related neural and behavioral responses in a classical conditioning paradigm. *Neurogastroenterol Motil* (2017) 29: e13026–n/a. doi: 10.1111/nmo.13026

20. Icenhour A, Langhorst J, Benson S, Schlamann M, Hampel S, Engler H, et al. Neural circuitry of abdominal pain-related fear learning and reinstatement in irritable bowel syndrome. *Neurogastroenterol Motil* (2015) 27:114–27. doi: 10.1111/nmo.12489

21. Icenhour A, Kattoor J, Benson S, Boekstegers A, Schlamann M, Merz CJ, et al. Neural circuitry underlying effects of context on human pain-related fear extinction in a renewal paradigm. *Hum Brain Mapp* (2015) 36:3179–93. doi: 10.1002/hbm.22837

22. Labrenz F, Icenhour A, Schlamann M, Forsting M, Bingel U, Elsenbruch S. From Pavlov to pain: How predictability affects the anticipation and processing of visceral pain in a fear conditioning paradigm. *Neuroimage* (2016) 130:104–14. doi: 10.1016/j.neuroimage.2016.01.064

23. Dorn SD, Palsson OS, Thiwan SIM, Kanazawa M, Clark WC, van Tilburg MAL, et al. Increased colonic pain sensitivity in irritable bowel syndrome is the result of an increased tendency to report pain rather than increased neurosensory sensitivity. *Gut* (2007) 56:1202–9. doi: 10.1136/gut.2006.117390

24. Lacourt TE, Houtveen JH, Doornen LJP, Benson S, Grigoleit J-S, Cesko E, et al. Biological and psychological predictors of visceral pain sensitivity in healthy premenopausal women. *Eur J Pain* (2014) 18:567–74. doi: 10.1002/j.1532-2149.2013.00397.x

25. Laux L, Glanzmann P, Schaffner P, Spielberger C. *Das State-Trait-Angstinventar. Theoretische Grundlagen und Handanweisung.* Weinheim: Beltz (1981).

26. Spielberger C. *State-Trait Anxiety Inventory: Bibliography.* 2nd ed. Palo Alto, CA: Consulting Psychologists Press (1989).

27. Petrowski K, Paul S, Albani C, Brähler E. Factor structure and psychometric properties of the trier inventory for chronic stress (TICS) in a representative German sample. *BMC Med Res Methodol* (2012) 12:42. doi: 10.1186/1471-2288-12-42

28. Schulz P, Schlotz W. The Trier Inventory for the Assessment of Chronic Stress (TICS): scale construction, statistical testing, and validation of the scale work overload.. *Diagnostica* (1999) 45:8–19. doi: 10.1026//0012-1924.45.1.8

29. Flor H, Behle DJ, Birbaumer N. Assessment of pain-related cognitions in chronic pain patients. *Behav Res Ther* (1993) 31:63–73. doi: 10.1016/0005-7967(93)90044-U

30. Scholz U, Doña BG, Sud S, Schwarzer R. Is general self-efficacy a universal construct? Psychometric findings from 25 countries. *Eur J Psychol Assess* (2002) 18:242–51. doi: 10.1027//1015-5759.18.3.242

31. Craig AD. How do you feel? Interoception: the sense of the physiological condition of the body. *Nat Rev Neurosci* (2002) 3:655–66. doi: 10.1038/nrn894

32. Schulz A, Vögele C. Interoception and stress. *Front Psychol* (2015) 6:993. doi: 10.3389/fpsyg.2015.00993

33. Critchley HD, Garfinkel SN. Interoception and emotion. *Curr Opin Psychol* (2017) 17:7–14. doi: 10.1016/j.copsyc.2017.04.020

34. Pace-Schott EF, Amole MC, Aue T, Balconi M, Bylsma LM, Critchley H, et al. Physiological feelings. *Neurosci Biobehav Rev* (2019) 103:267–304. doi: 10.1016/j.neubiorev.2019.05.002

35. Zhu L, Huang D, Shi L, Liang L, Xu T, Chang M, et al. Intestinal symptoms and psychological factors jointly affect quality of life of patients with irritable bowel syndrome with diarrhea. *Health Qual Life Outcomes* (2015) 13:49. doi: 10.1186/s12955-015-0243-3

36. Mayer EA, Bradesi S, Chang L, Spiegel BMR, Bueller JA, Naliboff BD. Functional GI disorders: from animal models to drug development. *Gut* (2008) 57:384–404. doi: 10.1136/gut.2006.101675

37. Bharucha AE, Zinsmeister AR, Locke GR, Seide BM, McKeon K, Schleck CD, et al. Prevalence and burden of fecal incontinence: a population-based study in women. *Gastroenterology* (2005) 129:42–9. doi: 10.1053/j.gastro.2005.04.006

38. Labus JS, Hubbard CS, Bueller J, Ebrat B, Tillisch K, Chen M, et al. Impaired emotional learning and involvement of the corticotropin-releasing factor signaling system in patients with irritable bowel syndrome. *Gastroenterology* (2013) 145:1253. doi: 10.1053/j.gastro.2013.08.016

39. Dunckley P, Wise RG, Aziz Q, Painter D, Brooks J, Tracey I, et al. Cortical processing of visceral and somatic stimulation: differentiating pain intensity from unpleasantness. *Neuroscience* (2005) 133:533–42. doi: 10.1016/j.neuroscience.2005.02.041

40. Strigo IA, Bushnell MC, Boivin M, Duncan GH. Psychophysical analysis of visceral and cutaneous pain in human subjects. *Pain* (2002) 97:235–46. doi: 10.1016/S0304-3959(02)00023-4

41. Koenen LR, Icenhour A, Forkmann K, Pasler A, Theysohn N, Forsting M, et al. Greater fear of visceral pain contributes to differences between visceral and somatic pain in healthy women. *Pain* (2017) 158:1599–608. doi: 10.1097/j.pain.0000000000000924

42. Koenen LR, Icenhour A, Forkmann K, Theysohn N, Forsting M, Bingel U, et al. From anticipation to the experience of pain: the importance of visceral versus somatic pain modality in neural and behavioral responses to pain-predictive cues. *Psychosom Med* (2018) 80:826–35. doi: 10.1097/PSY.0000000000000612

43. Elsenbruch S, Enck P. The stress concept in gastroenterology: from Selye to today. *F1000Research* (2017) 6:2149. doi: 10.12688/f1000research.12435.1

44. Shin LM, Liberzon I. The neurocircuitry of fear, stress, and anxiety disorders. *Neuropsychopharmacology* (2010) 35:169–91. doi: 10.1038/npp.2009.83

45. Hannibal KE, Bishop MD. Chronic stress, cortisol dysfunction, and pain: a psychoneuroendocrine rationale for stress management in pain rehabilitation. *Phys Ther* (2014) 94:1816–25. doi: 10.2522/ptj.20130597

46. Engler H, Elsenbruch S, Rebernik L, Kocke J, Cramer H, Schols M, et al. Stress burden and neuroendocrine regulation of cytokine production in patients with ulcerative colitis in remission. *Psychoneuroendocrinology* (2018) 98:101–7. doi: 10.1016/j.psyneuen.2018.08.009

47. Icenhour A, Labrenz F, Roderigo T, Siebert C, Elsenbruch S, Benson S. Are there sex differences in visceral sensitivity in young healthy men and women ? *Neurogastroenterol Motil* (2019) 31:e13664. doi: 10.1111/nmo.13664

48. Mulak A, Tache Y, Larauche M. Sex hormones in the modulation of irritable bowel syndrome. *World J Gastroenterol* (2014) 20:2433–48. doi: 10.3748/wjg.v20.i10.2433

49. Oyola MG, Handa RJ. Hypothalamic-pituitary-adrenal and hypothalamic-pituitary-gonadal axes: sex differences in regulation of stress responsivity. *Stress* (2017) 20:476–94. doi: 10.1080/10253890.2017.1369523

50. Li SH, Graham BM. Why are women so vulnerable to anxiety, trauma-related

and stress-related disorders? The potential role of sex hormones. *Lancet Psychiatry* (2017) 4:73–82. doi: 10.1016/S2215-0366(16)30358-3

51. Kåhrström CT, Pariente N, Weiss U. Intestinal microbiota in health and disease. *Nature* (2016) 535:47. doi: 10.1038/535047a

52. Rieder R, Wisniewski PJ, Alderman BL, Campbell SC. Microbes and mental health: a review. *Brain Behav Immun* (2017) 66:9–17. doi: 10.1016/j.bbi.2017.01.016

53. Cryan JF, Dinan TG. Mind-altering microorganisms: the impact of the gut microbiota on brain and behaviour. *Nat Rev Neurosci* (2012) 13:701–12. doi: 10.1038/nrn3346

54. Cryan JF, O'Riordan KJ, Cowan CSM, Sandhu KV, Bastiaanssen TFS, Boehme M, et al. The Microbiota-Gut-Brain Axis. *Physiol Rev* (2019) 99:1877–2013. doi: 10.1152/physrev.00018.2018

55. Jeffery IB, Quigley EMM, Öhman L, Simrén M, O'Toole PW. The microbiota link to irritable bowel syndrome an emerging story. *Gut Microbes* (2012) 3:572–6. doi: 10.4161/gmic.21772

56. Moloney RD, Desbonnet L, Clarke G, Dinan TG, Cryan JF. The microbiome: stress, health and disease. *Mamm Genome* (2014) 25:49–74. doi: 10.1007/s00335-013-9488-5

57. Yang B, Wei J, Ju P, Chen J. Effects of regulating intestinal microbiota on anxiety symptoms: a systematic review. *Gen Psychiatry* (2019) 32:e100056. doi: 10.1136/gpsych-2019-100056

58. Valles-Colomer M, Falony G, Darzi Y, Tigchelaar EF, Wang J, Tito RY, et al. The neuroactive potential of the human gut microbiota in quality of life and depression. *Nat Microbiol* (2019) 4:623–32. doi: 10.1038/s41564-018-0337-x

59. Leclercq S, Forsythe P, Bienenstock J. posttraumatic stress disorder: does the gut microbiome hold the key? *Can J Psychiatry* (2016) 61:204–13. doi: 10.1177/0706743716635535

12

The Gut Microbiome in Psychosis from Mice to Men: A Systematic Review of Preclinical and Clinical Studies

Ann-Katrin Kraeuter [1,2,3], Riana Phillips [1,2] and Zoltán Sarnyai [1,2]*

[1] Laboratory of Psychiatric Neuroscience, Centre for Molecular Therapeutics, James Cook University, Townsville, QLD, Australia, [2] Australian Institute of Tropical Health and Medicine, James Cook University, Townsville, QLD, Australia, [3] Faculty of Health and Life Sciences, Psychology, Northumbria University, Newcastle upon Tyne, United Kingdom

*Correspondence:
Zoltán Sarnyai
zoltan.sarnyai@jcu.edu.au

The gut microbiome is rapidly becoming the focus of interest as a possible factor involved in the pathophysiology of neuropsychiatric disorders. Recent understanding of the pathophysiology of schizophrenia emphasizes the role of systemic components, including immune/inflammatory and metabolic processes, which are influenced by and interacting with the gut microbiome. Here we systematically review the current literature on the gut microbiome in schizophrenia-spectrum disorders and in their animal models. We found that the gut microbiome is altered in psychosis compared to healthy controls. Furthermore, we identified potential factors related to psychosis, which may contribute to the gut microbiome alterations. However, further research is needed to establish the disease-specificity and potential causal relationships between changes of the microbiome and disease pathophysiology. This can open up the possibility of. manipulating the gut microbiome for improved symptom control and for the development of novel therapeutic approaches in schizophrenia and related psychotic disorders.

Keywords: gut microbiota, schizophrenia, early life events, inflammation, microbiota metabolites, stress

INTRODUCTION

The gut microbiome has recently received considerable interest, due to its potential role in maintaining health and in the pathophysiology of chronic diseases (1). Our understanding of the involvement of the gut microbiome in diseases is fast increasing due to the emergence of new molecular biological techniques (2). In healthy individuals, the gut microbiome, which consists of more than 100 trillion bacteria (3, 4), has a symbiotic relationship with enteric cells to influence physiological function (5). The gut microbiome is highly variable between healthy individuals (3), with twins only sharing 50% of their species-level bacterial taxa (6). This interindividual difference is

Abbreviations: C-section, Cesarean delivery; CoR, completeness of reporting; GABA, gamma-aminobutyric acid; HPA, hypothalamic pituitary adrenal; MIA, maternal immune activation; NMDA, N-methyl-D-aspartate; OTU, operational taxonomic units; PCoA, principal coordinate analysis; PICRUSt, Phylogenetic Investigation of Communities by Reconstruction of Unobserved States; PRISM-P, Preferred Items for Reporting Systematic Reviews and Meta-analysis Protocols; RoB, risk of bias; SCFA, short-chain fatty acid; TNF, tumor necrosis factor.

shaped through host-extrinsic, host-intrinsic, and environmental factors (2, 3). Host-extrinsic factors include lifestyles, such as physical activity, cultural habits, medication, and diet (2). Environmental factors altering the microbiome include the local environment and maternal transmission (2). Host-intrinsic factors, which might shape the gut microbiota, are genetics, sex, innate, and adaptive immunity, as well as metabolic factors, i.e., body mass index (2, 7). Although interindividual differences exist in healthy individuals, studies have demonstrated clear separations of the gut microbiome in chronic diseases such as individuals with allergies (8–10), celiac disease (11), gastric cancer (12), inflammatory bowel disease (13, 14) including Crohn's disease (15) and ulcerative colitis (3, 16), obesity (3, 17, 18), anorexia (17, 19), and type 2 diabetes mellitus (20) compared to healthy controls. The functional importance of the gut microbiome was demonstrated by the transfer of the gut microbiome from obese to germ-free mice resulting in obesity (21).

Bidirectional communication has been well established between the gut and the brain and its importance for maintaining neuronal, hormonal and immunological homeostasis has been recently demonstrated (22). A damage to the integrity of the gut-brain communication results in altered brain function and behavior (23). More recently, the importance of the gut-brain axis has been highlighted as a possible contributing factor, among many others, such as genes, early environment and nutrition, in the development of neuropsychiatric disorders (5, 22).

Schizophrenia is a heterogeneous, chronic neurodevelopmental psychiatric spectrum disorder influenced by a hitherto poorly understood interaction between genetic and environmental factors (24). It affects about 1 in 100 people (1%) worldwide (25). A variety of different pathophysiological mechanisms have been proposed, such as the dopamine hyperactivity in certain brain systems (26, 27), impaired glutamate neurotransmission (28), and a disruption of the brain glucose and energy metabolism (29–32). It has been conceptualized that multiple environmental "hits" on the background of a genetic predisposition are required for its development (33, 34). Genome-wide association studies have shown that schizophrenia is a polygenic disorder with a complex array of contributing risk loci across the allelic frequency spectrum (35, 36). Environmental events throughout development and adulthood, such as viruses before birth, method of delivery, birth complications, and psychosocial traumas, are important in the pathophysiology of schizophrenia (27) and the shaping of the gut microbiome (37–39). Most recently, a study demonstrated that mice receiving feces from individuals with schizophrenia showed a behavioral phenotype that is consistent with that have been seen in animal models of schizophrenia and depression (40). This finding demonstrates that a constituent of the fecal matter have effect of brain function and behavior of the host and strengthen the suggestion that the microbiome might contribute to behavioral symptoms in psychosis (41).

In this systematic review, we summarize the most recent findings on the gut microbiome in psychosis, including animal models and clinical data. Furthermore, we identified potential factors particular to psychosis, which may contribute to the altered gut microbiome. The methodology of the studies covered was not described in details as these were extensively reviewed elsewhere (42). Compared to previous reviews (43) we provide detailed discussion of factors such as antipsychotic use, lifestyle and environmental factors as well as the potential pathological role of the microbiome in psychosis relevant to microbial changes.

METHODS

Eligibility and Inclusion Criteria
We included original articles investigating preclinical and clinical studies exploring the fecal microbiome in animal models of schizophrenia and individuals of all ages with psychosis or at high risk and schizophrenia along with respective controls. Only studies published in English were included without a date restriction throughout the database search.

Database Search Strategy
This study followed the Preferred Items for Reporting Systematic Reviews and Meta-analysis Protocols (PRISM-P) (44). One author (AKK) conducted a Scopus, Web of Science, and PubMed database searches until the cut-off date of 14/02/2019. In all databases, free-text terms included (microbiota OR gastrointestinal microbiome OR microbiome OR microbio*) AND (schizophreni* OR "Dementia Praecox" OR psychotic OR schizoaffective OR psychoses OR psychosis). The search was limited to original articles, and therefore we excluded reviews, meta-analyses, and systematic reviews. The reference lists of eligible papers were manually screened for further relevant articles.

Report Selection
One of the authors (A-KK) determined the eligibility of papers by screening titles and abstracts for relevance. Eligible documents were then read as a whole to analyze if the articles matched the inclusion criteria. Excluded articles were documented, and reasons were given for exclusion.

Data Extraction
A-KK extracted information from relevant publications such as animal and patient characteristics. Study characteristics for animal experiments included strain, sex, number, age, and weight of animals and "schizophrenia" induction method, length of study, the timing of fecal sample collection, microbiota, and other findings of the study. Human studies were characterized by the number of participants, gender, age, exclusion and inclusion criteria, microbiota findings, and other findings within the study.

SYRCLE's Risk of Bias Analysis
The overall risk of bias (RoB) was assessed in animal studies using an adapted SYRCLE's risk of bias tool (45). All ten entries of the SYRCLE's RoB tool were assessed by the authors (A-KK, RP) relating to selection, performance, detection, attrition, reporting, and other biases (45). All individual entries were

assigned as "low RoB," "high RoB," "unclear," or "not feasible." A parameter was determined "unclear" if the item was not mentioned in the publication. The only exception to this was item 8, where 'not mentioned' was scored "high RoB." For one article, it was not feasible to assess housing conditions (items 3, 4, and 5) due to the nature of that particular animal model of schizophrenia (46). Furthermore, studies were assessed for quality by answering the categories: (1) conflict of interest stated, (2) power analysis or sample size calculation, (3) experiment blinding at any level, and (4) randomization at any level.

STROBE Risk of Bias Analysis

Human studies were assessed using adapted STROBE assessment criteria, including 32 subsections, which were scored for all six studies. A-KK and RP assessed the completeness of reporting (CoR) score (*CoR (%)=(yes/(yes+no))*100*) by answering each recommendation in the STROBE statement with "yes" or "no."

Microbiome Methodological Consideration

All studies were investigate for their CoR for microbiome relevant methodology. Categories range from sample preparation, handling to analysis of samples. The CoR score was calculated as described in the previous section. The overall CoR score was calculated for all studies, animal studies alone and human studies alone.

RESULTS

Database Search

The initial search yielded 763 documents, including one additional record identified through other sources. After exclusion of duplicates, 673 articles remained and were included for evaluation of titles or abstracts, which resulted in 69 records for full-text article review. During full-text article review, 60 articles were excluded because they were not original research articles (reviews, n=43; letter to the editor, n=1; book chapter, n=1), referred to microbiomes other than the gut microbiome (oropharyngeal, n=4; blood, n=2), was not a mouse model of schizophrenia (n=4), or reported no control (n=5). One additional article was found during scanning of the references. This search resulted in nine articles included in this systematic review (**Figure 1**).

Study Characteristics
Animals

Preclinical publications included within this review used three different types of translationally validated animal models. A neurodevelopmental model, the maternal immune activation (MIA), which takes advantage of the finding that maternal infection during pregnancy increases the risk of developing schizophrenia in the offspring, by injecting pregnant females with viral mimic polyriboinosinic–polyribocytidilic acid (Poly I: C), which disrupts prenatal and early postnatal development (48). A pharmacological model, the N-methyl-D-aspartate (NMDA) receptor hypofunction model induced by administration of the NMDA receptor antagonist phencyclidine, is based on the

findings that the administration of NMDA antagonists [phencyclidine (PCP) and ketamine] induce schizophrenia-like behaviors (49, 50). Social isolation is a major "psychological" stressor that has been used over the years to induce a behavioral and neurochemical phenotype corresponding to schizophrenia (51). This alteration has long-lasting effects on the brain and behavior (48). Articles describing preclinical results included 144 male Lister-Hooded rats investigated the microbiome in a pharmacological, phencyclidine (52), and a developmental model (social isolation) (46) (**Table 1**). In the neurodevelopmental model, the gut microbiome was assessed in ten C57/Bl6 offspring in the MIA group and ten respective controls with unknown sex (53). The two studies using rats had similar size rats of 100-130 g (46, 52); only one study reported that rats were 24 days old (46). C57BL/6N mice were six weeks of age (53). All studies analyzed microbiome using 16S rRNA gene MiSeq-based high throughput sequencing (46, 52, 53). All studies were supported by various sources of funding (46, 52, 53).

Human

Six eligible studies were identified, which investigated high-risk and ultrahigh-risk (UHR) individuals (4), first-episode psychosis (54), first-episode schizophrenia (55), and individuals with chronic schizophrenia (40, 56, 57) all compared to healthy controls (**Table 2**). High-risk (or at risk) state is the clinical presentation of those considered at risk of developing psychosis or schizophrenia. Such states were formerly considered as prodromes, emerging symptoms of psychosis, but this view is no longer maintained as a prodromal period can not be confirmed unless the emergence of the condition has occurred. Individuals are considered UHR for psychosis if they meet a set of standardized criteria including presumed genetic vulnerability (Trait), or a recent history of Attenuated Psychotic Symptoms (APS) or Brief Limited Intermittent Psychotic Symptoms (BLIPS) Yung, McGorry (58, 59). First-episode and chronic schizophrenia are defined in **Table 2**. A total of 321 patients and 273 healthy controls were investigated. All studies reported no significant differences between the experimental and control group for age, sex, and weight. Age varied widely between studies due to different stages of the disorder from 20.47 ± 4.57 to 54.7 ± 10.7. Common exclusion criteria included factors potentially influencing the gut microbiome such as gastrointestinal and endocrine disorders, previous antibiotic or probiotic treatment, alcohol and substance abuse. Inclusion criteria varied greatly between studies due to different baseline diagnostic criteria.

Risk of Bias
Animals

Of the 30 SYRCLE entries of all three studies, 15 (50%) were low RoB, 2 (6.6%) were high RoB, 10 (33.3%) were unclear, and 3 (10%) were considered not feasible (**Figure 2**).

Quality Assessment

All studies were randomized and acknowledged their funding source (**Figure 3**). However, none of the studies reported how the sample size was estimated during the design of the experiment

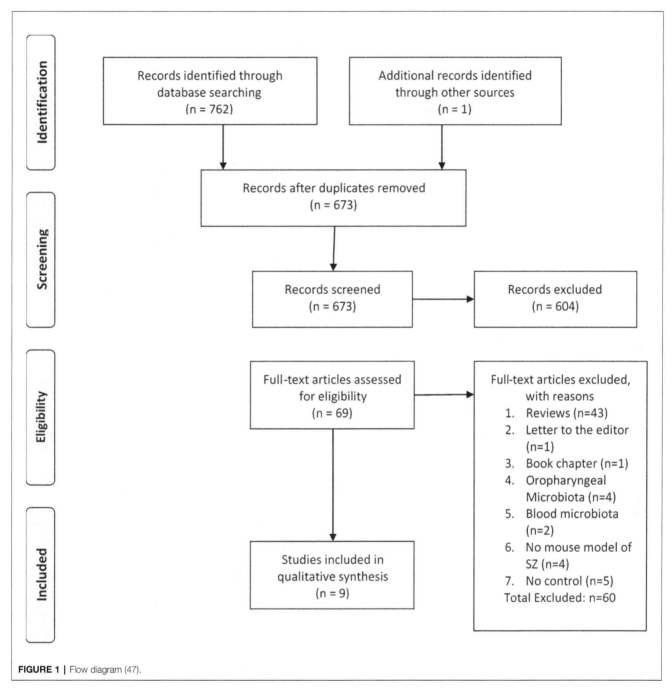

FIGURE 1 | Flow diagram (47).

(**Figure 3**). One study failed to report if the experimenter was blinded at any level.

Human Studies

The analysis included a total of 192 entries (32 STROBE entries per study). Of the 192 STROBE entries, 139 (72.4%) entries were scores "Yes" for CoR, and 53 (27.6%) were scored "No" for CoR (**Figure 4**).

Microbiome Methodological Consideration

The analysis included a total of 63 entries (7 entries per study). Of the 63 entries, 47 (74.6%) entries were scores "Yes" for CoR,

and 16 (25.4%) were scored "No" for CoR (**Figure 5**). One study within this review did not use caecum samples rather than fecal samples (46). None of the animal studies reported the amount used for microbial analysis (46, 52, 53). Reporting for the amount of fecal sample varied within human studies with two studies failing to report amount used (40, 55). Similarly, mixed results were found for storage information given with two animal studies (52, 53) and one human study (55) not reporting the storage of samples between collection and analysis. Three studies did not report target regions (53–55). All studies reported the sequencing platform used (4, 40, 46, 52–57) and all human studies reported the DNA extraction protocol and PCR primers

TABLE 1 | Gut microbiota changes in animal models of schizophrenia.

	Strain, Sex (n), Age (weight)	Disease induction and length of study	Fecal sample collection timing	Microbiota changes	Other findings	Comments
Pyndt Jørgensen, Krych (52)	EXP1-4: Lister-Hooded rats, M (24), NA (100-130g)	EXP1-4: SZ: 5 mg/kg free base PCP i.p. Control: vehicle i.p. EXP4: addition ampicillin through the drinking water Length of study EXP1: 7 days PCP and 7 day washout EXP2: 7 days PCP and 28 day washout EXP3: 7 days PCP and 49 day washout EXP4: 7 days PCP and 7 day washout	EXP1: Day 16 EXP2: Day 37 EXP3: Day 58 EXP4: Caecum: Day 19	EXP1: No difference • α-diversity Altered • β-diversity Increased • *Roseburia* (Phylum: *Firmicutes*) • *Odoribacter* (Phylum: *Bacteroidetes*) Increased Locomotor activity positively correlated with: • *Lachnospiraceae* (Phylum: *Firmicutes*) • *Clostridiaceae* (Phylum: *Firmicutes*) • *Roseburia* (Phylum: *Firmicutes*) • *Clostridium* (Phylum: *Firmicutes*) • *Odoribacter* (Phylum: *Bacteroidetes*) EXP2: No difference • α-diversity • β-diversity Increased • unclassified genus bellowing to the S24-7 family (Phylum: *Bacteroidetes*) • *Dorea* (Phylum: *Firmicutes*)	EXP1-3: Increased • Locomotion EXP1 and 2: Decreased • NOR performance EXP3: No Change • NOR performance EXP4: Improved • Reversed cognitive deficits in No change • Locomotion	EXP1 and 4: • NOR on day 15 and16 • Locomotor activity on day 18 EXP2: • NOR on day 36 and 37 • Locomotor activity on day 39 EXP3: • NOR on day 57 and 58 • Locomotor activity on day 60
Dunphy-Doherty, O'Mahony (46)	Lister-Hooded rats, M (24), 24 days (100-130g)	Social isolation Control: group housed Length of study 63 days	Caecum: Day 86/87	No difference • α-diversity • β-diversity Increased: • Phylum: Actinobacteria • *Rhodococcus* (Phylum: *Actinobacteria*) • *Negativicutes* (Phylum: *Firmicutes*) • *Corynebacteriales* (Phylum: *Actinobacteria*) • *Bacillales* (Phylum: *Firmicutes*) • *Selenomonadales* (Phylum: *Firmicutes*) • *Nocardiaceae* (Phylum: *Actinobacteria*) • *Bacillaceae* (Phylum: *Firmicutes*) • *Veillonellaceae* (Phylum: *Firmicutes*) • *Prevotellaceae UCG-001* (Phylum: *Bacteroidetes*) • *Bacillus* (Phylum: *Firmicutes*) • *Defluvitaleaceae UCG-011* (Phylum: *Firmicutes*) • *Eubacterium oxidoreducens group* (Phylum: *Firmicutes*) • *Marvinbryantia* (Phylum: *Firmicutes*) • *Veillonella* (Phylum: *Firmicutes*) Decreased • *Clostridia* (Phylum: *Firmicutes*) • *Clostridiales* (Phylum: *Firmicutes*) • *Clostridiacae group 1* (Phylum: *Firmicutes*) • *Peptostreptococcaceae* (Phylum: *Firmicutes*) • *Lachnospiraceae UCG-009* (Phylum: *Firmicutes*) • *Ocillospira* (Phylum: *Firmicutes*) • *Papillibacter* (Phylum: *Firmicutes*) *Correlations described in text	Increased • Locomotion (OF) Decreased • Defecation (OF) • Freezing first, 24,48 shocks (CFR) • Cells in dentate gyrus dual labeled for BrdU and NeuN • Il-6 and IL-10 in hippocampus No Change • Rearing (OF) • Grooming (OF) • NOR • EPM • Second shock (CFR) • Corticosterone (restrained) • IL-1b or TNF-α	• 56 rats received 5-bromo-20-deoxyuridine • Open field (day59) • Locomotor activity noval area (day 65) • NOR (day 66) • EPM (day73) • Conditioned Freezing Response (day79/80/81) • Restrained Stress and Sample collection (day 86/87)

(Continued)

TABLE 1 | Continued

	Strain, Sex (n), Age (weight)	Disease induction and length of study	Fecal sample collection timing	Microbiota changes	Other findings	Comments
Hsiao, McBride (53)	C57BL/6N offspring, Sex: unknown, Microbiota: n=10/group, Behavior: 16-75/group), 6 weeks at behavioral testing	Pregnant C57BL/6N mice were injected i.p. on E12.5 with saline or 20 mg/kg poly(I:C) Length of study 9 weeks	Unknown	No difference • α-diversity Altered • β-diversity Increased • *unclassified Bacteriodales* (Phylum: *Bacteroidetes*) • Porphyromonadaceae (Phylum: *Bacteroidetes*) • *Prevotellaceae* (Phylum: *Bacteroidetes*) • *Lachnospiraceae* (Phylum: *Firmicutes*) Decreased • *Ruminococcaceae* (Phylum: *Firmicutes*) • *Erysipelotrichaceae* (Phylum: *Firmicutes*) • *Alcaligenaceae* (Phylum: *Proteobacteria*) No change • *Clostrodia (Phylum: Firmicutes)* • *Bacteroidia (Phylum: Bacteroidetes)*	Increased • Intestinal permeability (3 week old offspring) • Gene expression (CLDN15) • IL-6 mRNA and protein • Repetitive behavior (marbles buried) Decreased • Gene expression (TJP1, TJP2, OCLN, and CLDN8) • IL-12p40/p70 • MIP-1a • Centre entries and time spent (OF) • PPI • Communication (ultrasonic vocalization) • Sociability (3CST) • Social preference (3CST)	Normalization with probiotic

SZ, schizophrenia; PCP, phencyclidine; NOR, novel object recognition; OF, open field test; CRF, conditioned freezing task; CST, chronic social defeat.

used (4, 40, 54–57). However, none of the animal studies reported the DNA extraction protocol (46, 52, 53) and one animal study failed to report PCR primers used. The major of publications within this review used 16S rRNA sequencing (4, 40, 46, 52, 53, 56, 57). Two studies used alternative techniques such as RT-qPCR for 16 s primers (54) or qPCR for 16 s primers (55). Studies, which reported target region investigated V3 or V4 regions (4, 46, 52, 56, 57). The preferred sequencing platform was the Illumina Miseq platform (4, 46, 52, 54, 56, 57).

Overall, we found a CoR score of 74.6% for all studies, which a large divide between CoR of animal (CoR: 47.6%) and human studies (CoR: 88.1%).

Microbiome Analysis and Its Relationship to Behavior

In the following sections, we summarize the taxonomic changes in validated animal models of schizophrenia (46, 52, 53) and high-risk and UHR individuals (4), first-episode psychosis (54), first-episode schizophrenia (55), and individuals with chronic schizophrenia (40, 56, 57), all compared to healthy controls. The reviewed publications consistently report OTU (operational taxonomic unit) values, alpha and beta diversity, terms not frequently used outside the field of microbiome research. OTU is used to cluster sequences based on their similarities (60). Alpha diversity (within-sample) is the species number (richness) and

distribution (evenness) within a host organism or habitat, showing "how many different species were found," i.e., how many different bacteria are in a healthy individual, which can be measured using Shannon diversity index and Faith's Phylogenetic Diversity (56). Beta diversity (between-samples) answers the question "How different is the microbial composition in one environment compared to another?", calculated using Bray-Curtis dissimilarity and unweighted UniFrac and ordinated using principal coordinate analysis (PCoA).

Within the *Results* section we will be reporting changes according to phylum levels, this structure will remain for the discussion, however we will be discussion changes at lower taxonomic units within the phylum sections of the discussion. Details of the taxonomic changes are described in **Tables 1** and **2** and **Figure 6** showing reduced abundance in orange, increased abundance in purple with lighter shades of orange and purple to signify that only preclinical evidence is available.

Animals

One study investigated the gut microbiota of C57BL/6N offspring in the neurodevelopmental MIA model (53). MIA mice, from as early as three weeks, showed increased intestinal permeability, which was shown through increased translocation of fluorescein isothiocyanate-dextran across the intestinal epithelium (53). Alpha diversity is the species richness within a

TABLE 2 | Gut microbiota changes in schizophrenic patients and at risk individuals.

Patient Characteristics (N, Gender, Age)	Exclusion/Inclusion criteria	Microbiota analysis	Microbiota findings at Baseline compared to control	Other findings	Comments
He, Kosciolek (4) • HR (41M, 40F, 21.67 ± 5.75) • UHR (15M, 4F, 20.47 ± 4.57) • HC (37M, 32F, 23.13 ± 3.89)	**Exclusion:** • Gastrointestinal and endocrine diseases • Diagnosis with psychotic disorder and corresponding treatments • Last 3 month: alcohol, antibiotics, probiotics or any other oral or injectable medications	• One measure at baseline	No difference • α-diversity Altered: • β-diversity in HR and UHR Increased in UHR: • *Clostridiales* (Phylum: *Firmicutes*) • *Lactobacillales* (Phylum: *Firmicutes*) • *Bacteroidales* (Phylum: *Bacteroidetes*) • *Lactobacillus* (Phylum: *Firmicutes*) • *Prevotella* (Phylum: *Bacteroidetes*) • *Lactobacillus ruminis* (Phylum: *Firmicutes*) No Change • HR group	No difference: • Age and gender Increased: • Symptoms in UHR • Choline levels in UHR	• HC: no family history of mental illness • 37 HC did not agree with ¹H-MRS • ¹H-MRS: 7 HR and 2 UHR excluded
Schwarz, Maukonen (54) • FEP (16M, 12, 25.9 ± 5.5) • HC (8M, 8F, 27.8 ± 6.0)	**Exclusion:** • Substance-induced psychosis and psychotic disorders due to general medical conditions **Inclusion:** • Score of at least 4 in the item assessing delusion (Usual Thought Content) and hallucinations (Brief Psychiatric rating scale)	• FEP: Morning of interview • HC: Sample at home and delivered them within a few hours to the laboratory • Baseline, 2 and 12 month	No difference • α-diversity Increased: • Phylum *Actinobacteria* • *Rhizobiales* (Phylum: *Proteobacteria*) • *Bacillales* (Phylum: *Firmicutes*) • *Lactobacillaceae* (Phylum: *Firmicutes*) • *Halothiobacillaceae* (Phylum: *Proteobacteria*) • *Brucellaceae* (Phylum: *Proteobacteria*) • unclassified *Micrococcineae* (Phylum: *Actinobacteria*) • *Lactobacillus* (Phylum: *Firmicutes*) • *Tropheryma* (Phylum: *Actinobacteria*) • *Halothiobacillus* (Phylum: *Proteobacteria*) • *Saccharophagus* (Phylum: *Proteobacteria*) • *Ochrobactrum`* (Phylum: *Proteobacteria*) • *Deferribacter* (Phylum: *"Deferribacteres"*) • *Halorubrum* (Phylum: *Euryarchaeota*) • Lactobacillus aciddophilus (Phylum: *Firmicutes*) • Lactobacillus grasser (Phylum: *Firmicutes*) • Lactobacillus saliva (Phylum: *Firmicutes*) • Lactobacillus reuter (Phylum: *Firmicutes*) • Lactobacillus fermen (Phylum: *Firmicutes*) • Desulfosporosinus acidphilus (Phylum: *Firmicutes*) • Bifidobacterium dentium (Phylum: *Actinobacteria*) • Tropheryma whipplei (Phylum: *Actinobacteria*) • Ochrobactum anthropi (Phylum: *Proteobacteria*) • Bartonella clarridgeiae (Phylum: *Proteobacteria*) • Franisella hispaniensis (Phylum: *Proteobacteria*) • Nitrosococcus halophilus (Phylum: *Proteobacteria*) • Brucella canis (Phylum: *Proteobacteria*) • Saccharophagus degradans (Phylum: *Proteobacteria*)	No difference: • Age, gender and several metabolic parameters (BMI, cholesterol, high and low density lipoproteins, glucose, insulin and triglycerides) • SZ patient less active Cofounders-no association: • Physical activity • Type of psychosis • Duration of antipsychotic treatment • Distribution of risperidone, quetiapine or olanzapine treatment • Intake of different food types over the week prior to sample collection	• Food habits and physical activity assessed • Fecal sample not collected if: antibiotic use during the past 3 months, chronic gastrointestinal disease, gastrointestinal surgery, or diagnosed celiac disease. • Microbiota clustering at intake was significantly associated with remission at follow-up

(Continued)

TABLE 2 | Continued

Patient Characteristics (N, Gender, Age)	Exclusion/Inclusion criteria	Microbiota analysis	Microbiota findings at Baseline compared to control	Other findings	Comments
			• Halothiobacillus neapolitanus (Phylum: Proteobacteria) • Deferribacter desulfuricans (Phylum: "Deferribacteres") Decreased: • Negativicutes (Phylum: Firmicutes) • Selenomondales (Phylum: Firmicutes) • Veillonellaceae (Phylum: Firmicutes) • Anabaena (Phylum: Cyanobacteria) • Nitrosospira (Phylum: Proteobacteria) • Gallionella (Phylum: Proteobacteria) • Thermococcus gammatolerans (Phylum: Euryarchaeota) • Leuconostoc gasicomitatum (Phylum: Firmicutes) • Nitrosomonas spp. (Phylum: Proteobacteria) • Anabaena variabilities (Phylum: Cyanobacteria) • Gallionella capsiferriformans (Phylum: Proteobacteria) • Chlorobium chlorochromate (Phylum: Chlorobi) • Nitrosospira multiformis (Phylum: Proteobacteria) • Xenorhabdus nematophila (Phylum: Proteobacteria) In active SZ patients Increased: • Lactobacillaceae (Phylum: Firmicutes) Decreased: • Veillonellaceae (Phylum: Firmicutes) *Correlations described in text		
Shen, Xu (57)	Exclusion: • Last 3 month: Disease that may affect the stability of gut microbiota • Last 6 months: antibiotics, glucocorticoids, cytokines, large doses of probiotics and biological agents • Gastroscopy, colonoscopy or gastrointestinal barium meal • Last 5 years: major gastrointestinal tract surgery • Activity limitation • Changes in dietary habits • Alcohol abuse or dependence Inclusion: • SZ patients were diagnosed according to ICD-10 and received antipsychotic treatment in hospital or outpatient clinic	• One measure at baseline	No difference: • α-diversity Altered: • β-diversity Increased: • Phylum Proteobacteria • Phylum Fusobacteria • Gammaproteobacteria (Phylum: Proteobacteria) • Fusobacteriia (Phylum: Fusobacteria) • Enterobacteriales (Phylum: Proteobacteria) • Fusobacteriales (Phylum: Fusobacteria) • Aeromonadales (Phylum: Proteobacteria) • Prevotellaceae (Phylum: Bacteroidetes) • Enterobacteriaceae (Phylum: Proteobacteria) • Succinivibrionaceae (Phylum: Proteobacteria) • Fusobacteriaceae (Phylum: Fusobacteria) • Veillonellaceae (Phylum: Firmicutes) • Lactobacillaceae (Phylum: Firmicutes) • Succinivibrio (Phylum: Proteobacteria) • Megasphaera (Phylum: Firmicutes) • Acidaminococcus (Phylum: Firmicutes)	No difference: • Age, BMI, sex ratio, tobacco used and alcohol intake	

SZ (M36, F28, 42 ± 11)
HC (M35, F18, 39 ± 14)

(Continued)

TABLE 2 | Continued

Patient Characteristics (N, Gender, Age)	Exclusion/Inclusion criteria	Microbiota analysis	Microbiota findings at Baseline compared to control	Other findings	Comments
	• Illness duration ≤10 years and received antipsychotic drugs treatment > 6months; psychiatric symptoms were steady >3 months, and the PANSS evaluated the rate of change ≤20% and the total score of PANSS ≤60.		Collinsella (Phylum: Actinobacteria) • Clostridium (Phylum: Firmicutes) • Klebsiella (Phylum: Proteobacteria) • Citrobacter (Phylum: Proteobacteria) • Methanobrevibacter (Phylum: Euryarchaeota) • Fusobacterium (Phylum: Fusobacteria) • Lactobacillus (Phylum: Firmicutes) • Phascolarctobacterium (Phylum: Firmicutes) • Desulfovibrio (Phylum: Firmicutes) • Collinsella aerofaciens (Phylum: Actinobacteria) • Bifidobacterium adolescentis (Phylum: Actinobacteria) • Prevotella stercorea (Phylum: Bacteroidetes) • Bacteroides fragilis (Phylum: Bacteroidetes) • Lactobacillus mucosae (Phylum: Firmicutes) • Lactobacillus ruminis (Phylum: Firmicutes) Decreased: • Phylum Firmicutes • Clostridia (Phylum: Firmicutes) • Clostridiales (Phylum: Firmicutes) • Streptococcaceae (Phylum: Firmicutes) • Alcaligenaceae (Phylum: Proteobacteria) • Lachnospiraceae (Phylum: Firmicutes) • Streptococcus (Phylum: Firmicutes) • Blautia (Phylum: Firmicutes) • Coprococcus (Phylum: Firmicutes) • Roseburia (Phylum: Firmicutes) • Roseburia faecis (Phylum: Firmicutes) • Blautia producta (Phylum: Firmicutes) • Collinsella plebeius (Phylum: Actinobacteria) • Bacteroides eggerthii (Phylum: Bacteroidetes) *Correlations described in text		
Yuan, Zhang (55) • FES (M23, F18, 23.1 ± 8.0) • HC (M20, F21, 24.7 ± 6.7)	Exclusion • Autoimmune diseases, heart diseases, hepatobiliary and gastrointestinal diseases, blood diseases, diabetes neurological diseases, or psychiatric diseases other than FES • Pregnant or lactating women • A history of using any antibiotic or anti-inflammatory agent, or probiotic in the past month • A significant change in the	• Baseline, 6,12,24 weeks of risperidone treatment	Increased: • Clostridium coccoides group (Phylum: Firmicutes) Decreased: • Bifidobacterium spp. (Phylum: Actinobacteria) • Escherichia coli (Phylum: Proteobacteria) • Lactobacillus spp. (Phylum: Firmicutes) No Change: • Bacteroides spp. (Phylum: Bacteroidetes) After 24 weeks risperidone- Increased: • Bifidobacterium spp. (Phylum: Actinobacteria) • Escherichia coli (Phylum: Proteobacteria)	After 24 weeks risperidone- Increased: • Weight • BMI • Fasting serum levels of glucose • Triglycerides • LDL • HOMA-IR • Serum levels of hs-CRP • SOD	

TABLE 2 | Continued

Patient Characteristics (N, Gender, Age)	Exclusion/Inclusion criteria	Microbiota analysis	Microbiota findings at Baseline compared to control	Other findings	Comments
	living environment or diet in the past month. • Significant diarrhea or constipation in the past month. *Healthy controls had the same exclusion criteria as patients; in addition, they had no previous history of any psychiatric diseases.* Inclusion • FES based on the DSM-IV criteria • Never been on antipsychotic medication • PANSS total score N60 points • Born through normal vaginal delivery • Normal body weight (BMI: 18.5–23.0).		Decreased: • Clostridium coccoides group (Phylum: *Firmicutes*) • *Lactobacillus* spp. (Phylum: *Firmicutes*) No Change: • *Bacteroides* spp. (Phylum: *Bacteroidetes*) *Correlations described in text		
Nguyen, Kosciolek (56) • SZ or schizoaffective disorder (14M, 11F, 52.9 ± 11.2), • HC (15M, 10F, 54.7 ± 10.7)	Exclusion • Other current major DSM-IV-TR Axis I diagnoses • Alcohol or other substance (other than tobacco) (within 3 months prior to enrollment) • Diagnosis of dementia • Intellectual disability disorder, • Major neurological disorder • Any medical disability that interfered with a subject's ability to complete study procedures	• One measure • Home stool collection kits (samples returned *via* mail)	No difference • α-diversity Altered: • β-diversity Increased: • *Anaerococcus* (Phylum: *Firmicutes*) Decreased: • Phylum *Proteobacteria* • *Haemophilus* (Phylum: *Proteobacteria*) • *Sutterella* (Phylum: *Proteobacteria*) • *Clostrodium* (Phylum: *Firmicutes*) *Correlations described in text	No difference: • Age, gender, race Increased: • BMI (however, no differences in BMI classifications) • Psychiatric symptoms • Depression levels • Anxiety levels • Smoking • Medical comorbidity (diabetes and hypertension) Decreased: • Physical well-being	• 21 patients on antipsychotics at study onset
Zheng, Zeng (40) • SZ (63) • HC (69)	Exclusion • Physical or other mental disorders • Illicit drug use • Antibiotics/probiotics within 1 month of study	•	Decreased: • α-diversity Altered: • β-diversity Increased:	No difference: • Age, gender, BMI Increased: • Serum glutamine • Hippocampal GABA Decreased:	SZ were treated with a single antipsychotic drug: • Clozapine (n = 15) • Risperidone (n = 14) • Olanzapine (n = 9) • Chlorpromazine (n = 5)

(Continued)

TABLE 2 | Continued

Patient Characteristics (N, Gender, Age)	Exclusion/Inclusion criteria	Microbiota analysis	Microbiota findings at Baseline compared to control	Other findings	Comments
			• Veillonellaceae (Phylum: *Firmicutes*) • Prevotellaceae (Phylum: *Bacteroidetes*) • Bacteroidaceae (Phylum: *Bacteroidetes*) • Coriobacteriaceae (Phylum: *Actinobacteria*) Decreased: • Lachnospiraceae (Phylum: *Firmicutes*) • Ruminococcaceae (Phylum: *Firmicutes*) • Enterobacteriaceae (Phylum: *Proteobacteria*) *Correlations described in text and comparison to depressive disorder and FMT from human to mouse	• Stool and hippocampal glutamate	• Aripiprazole (n = 3) • Quetiapine (n = 3) • Remaining patients were treated with two of the above drugs in combination (n = 9) • Unmedicated (n = 5).

SZ, schizophrenia; HR, high-risk; UHR, ultrahigh-risk; HC, healthy controls; FEP, first-episode psychosis; FES, first-episode schizophrenia; BMI, body mass index; PANSS, Positive and Negative Syndrome Scale.

host organism or habitat, showing "how many different species were found," i.e., how many different bacteria are in a healthy individual. This remains unaltered in MIA mice. Beta diversity, which reflects the species diversity to contribute to species evenness between microbial communities, i.e., how different was the diversity of bacteria between healthy controls compared to diseased individuals, was significantly altered by the MIA. PCoA (index of beta-diversity) showed that MIA samples clustered significantly differently to control samples, indicating different gut microbiome composition compared to control animals. The primary drivers of the gut microbiome changes concerning diversity were the classes *Clostridia* and *Bacteroidia*. MIA significantly altered families in the phyla *Bacteroidetes*, *Firmicutes*, and *Proteobacteria* compared to controls (53) (**Figure 6** and **Table 1**).

Subchronic administration of phencyclidine for seven days, a pharmacological model of schizophrenia, significantly separated the microbiota population compared to controls (beta-diversity) (52). Locomotor activity was increased in phencyclidine treated animals with seven days and four weeks wash-out period compared to controls, which indicates a schizophrenia-like behavioral phenotype (52) (**Table 1**). Seven days after treatment with phencyclidine, no change was found in alpha-diversity. However, a weak but significant alteration was found in beta-diversity compared to controls using the PCoA-analysis, which indicates the separation of the microbial communities. Phencyclidine-treated animals showed increased abundance in genera belonging to the phyla *Firmicutes* and *Bacteroidetes* (52) (**Figure 6** and **Table 1**). Four weeks after phencyclidine treatment, no changes in alpha-diversity and beta-diversity were found between groups. However, the abundance of genera within the phyla *Firmicutes* and *Bacteroidetes* were significantly increased in phencyclidine-treated animals (52) (**Figure 6** and **Table 1**).

Social isolation resulted in hyperactivity, anxiety-like behavior, and impaired contextual learning and memory, as well as reduced IL-6 and IL-10 levels in the hippocampus (46). Although no significant changes for alpha-diversity and beta-diversity were found, socially isolated animals showed a trend toward a decrease in alpha diversity and a trend towards differential clustering of microbial communities (beta diversity) (46) (**Figure 6** and **Table 1**). Social isolation increased the abundance of *Actinobacteria* at phylum level. At class, order, family, and genus level social isolation altered the abundance to both directions of the phyla *Firmicutes*, *Actinobacteria*, and *Bacteroidetes* (46) (**Figure 6** and **Table 1**).

In summary, the preclinical studies using translationally valid models for schizophrenia show somewhat inconsistent findings with the decreased abundance of the phylum *Proteobacteria* emerging as a partially shared feature (53). At the same time, *Actinobacteria* (46) and *Bacteroidetes* (46, 52, 53) were increased, whereas bacteria within the phylum *Firmicutes* show altered expression toward both directions.

Human Studies

High-risk and UHR individuals who have a higher likelihood of developing psychosis in the future did not differ in microbial

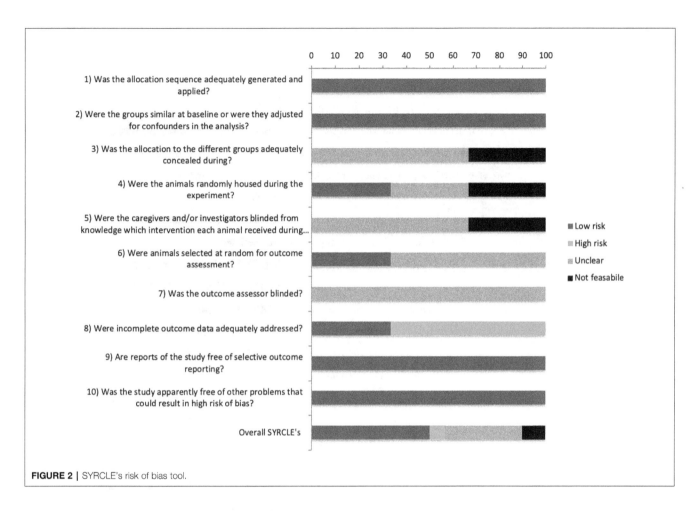

FIGURE 2 | SYRCLE's risk of bias tool.

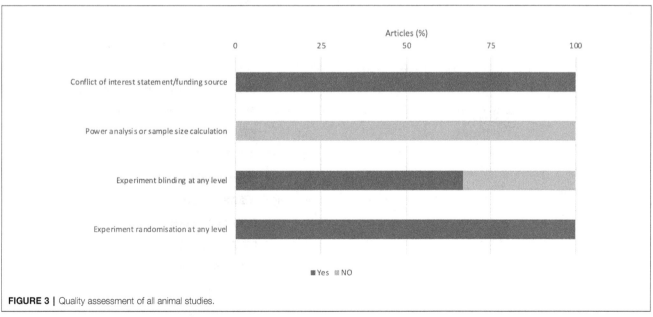

FIGURE 3 | Quality assessment of all animal studies.

richness, alpha-diversity. However, beta-diversity was altered in high-risk and UHR individual's analysis compared to controls. UHR individuals had increased bacterial abundance at order, genus, and species levels in the phyla *Firmicutes* and *Bacteroidetes* compared to the other groups (4) (**Figure 6** and **Table 2**). It is important to note that clinically, UHR individuals showed more severe symptoms and functional impairments on the Scale of Prodromal Symptoms for screening of schizophrenic

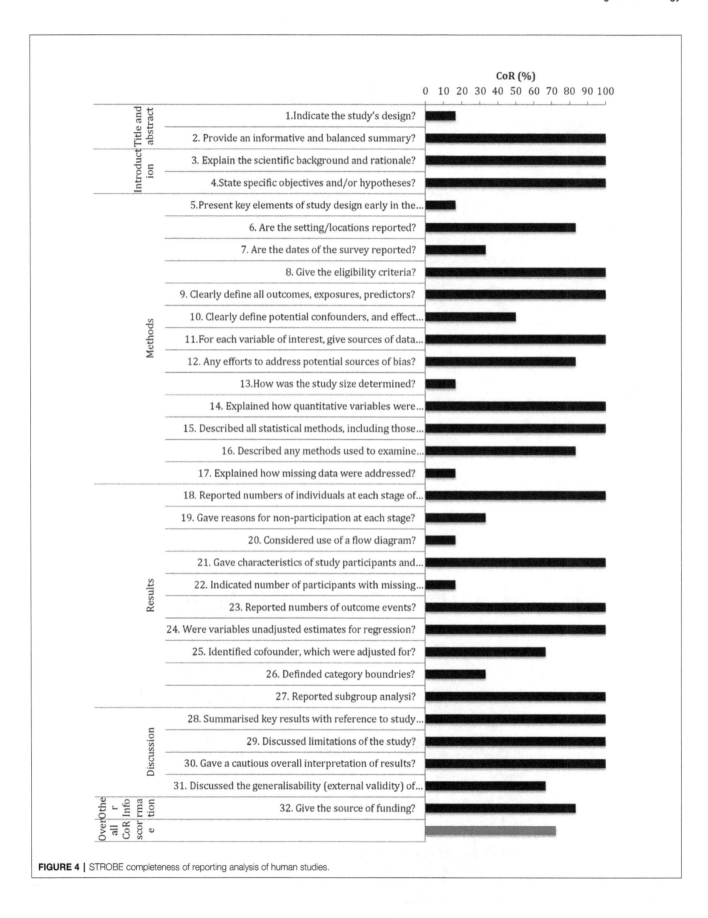

FIGURE 4 | STROBE completeness of reporting analysis of human studies.

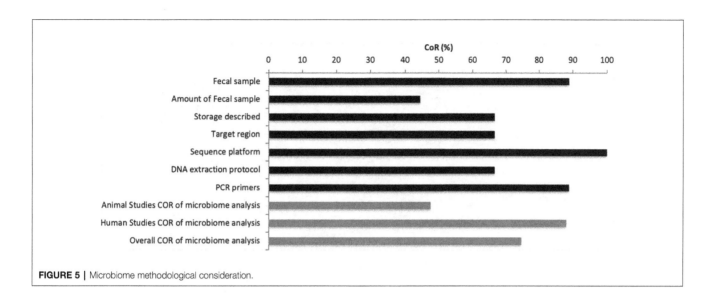

FIGURE 5 | Microbiome methodological consideration.

symptoms and the Global Assessment of Function Scale, Modified Version, respectively, than the other two groups (4). Functional profile analysis using *Phylogenetic Investigation of Communities by Reconstruction of Unobserved State*s (PICRUSt), which is a bioinformatics software for metagenomic functional predictions, predicted that short-chain fatty acids (SCFA) related to pyruvate synthesis, acetyl-CoA synthesis, and fatty acid biosynthesis initiation pathways were increased in UHR individuals compared to high-risk and controls, however only the acetyl-CoA synthesis pathway was significantly predicted (4) (**Table 2**). This profile corresponds with altered glucose metabolites, which is particularly interesting in the context of energy metabolism abnormalities that have been recently identified in schizophrenia [27-30].

Patients with first-episode psychosis, who received a relatively short antipsychotic treatment (median length of 20 days), showed no difference in alpha diversity (54) (**Figure 6** and **Table 2**). Individuals with first-episode psychosis had enrichment in the phylum Actinobacteria. At class, order, family, genus and species levels the overall abundance of bacteria were altered in the phyla *Firmicutes, Actinobacteria, Proteobacteria, "Deferribacteres," Euryarchaeota, Cyanobacteria*, and *Chlorobi* in patients with first-episode psychosis compared to healthy controls (54) (**Figure 6** and **Table 2**). Physically active patients had a reduced abundance of *Firmicutes* at family level compared to active, healthy controls.

At baseline, multiple bacteria were decreased in drug naïve first-episode schizophrenia at species level belonging to the phyla *Actinobacteria, Proteobacteria*, and *Firmicutes* compared to controls (55) (**Figure 6** and **Table 2**).

Individuals with chronic schizophrenia with over ten years of antipsychotic medication were investigated and compared to healthy controls (57). Gut microbiota samples did not differ in alpha diversity, microbial richness, and diversity, from healthy controls. However, they showed differential clustering of microbial communities of chronic schizophrenic patients compared to respective controls (beta diversity). Furthermore, healthy controls

showed more similar bacterial communities, tighter clustering, than patients with schizophrenia (57) (**Figure 6** and **Table 2**). At phylum level, *Proteobacteria* and *Fusobacteria* were significantly increased, and *Firmicutes* were less abundant in schizophrenia patients compared to controls. At class, order, family, genus, and species levels bacteria belonging to the phyla *Proteobacteria, Fusobacteria, Firmicutes, Bacteroidetes, Actinobacteria*, and *Euryarchaeota* were altered in chronic schizophrenia patients (57) (**Figure 6** and **Table 2**). Furthermore, using PICRUSt analysis, functional pathways were identified to be altered in individuals with schizophrenia, such as pathways responsible for the synthesis of vitamin B6, fatty acid, starch, sucrose, tryptophan, cysteine, methionine, and linoleic acid metabolism and the degradation of some xenobiotics (57).

Similar to the aforementioned study (57), no changes in alpha diversity were found in chronic, medicated patients with schizophrenia and schizoaffective disorder (56). However, beta diversity showed a clear separation between the patient and control populations and showed a wider distribution of schizophrenia samples (56) (**Figure 6** and **Table 2**). At phylum level, *Proteobacteria* were decreased in patients with schizophrenia. At genus level, bacterial abundance was altered bidirectional in the phyla *Proteobacteria, Proteobacteria*, and *Firmicutes* (56) (**Figure 6** and **Table 2**).

Another recent study has gone beyond just determining the bacterial abundance in the microbiome in people with schizophrenia and evaluated if behavioral phenotypes could be transferred through fecal microbial transplant from patients with schizophrenia to germ-free mice (40). The gut microbiome of patients with schizophrenia had reduced alpha diversity compared to healthy controls, suggesting a lower within-sample diversity. Furthermore, beta-diversity was also significantly altered in schizophrenia patients (40) (**Figure 6** and **Table 2**). Bacterial abundance was altered at family level belonging to the phyla *Firmicutes, Bacteroidetes, Actinobacteria*, and *Proteobacteria* (40) (**Figure 6** and **Table 2**). Animals, which received elements of the gut microbiome from patients with schizophrenia *via* fecal microbial transplants, showed

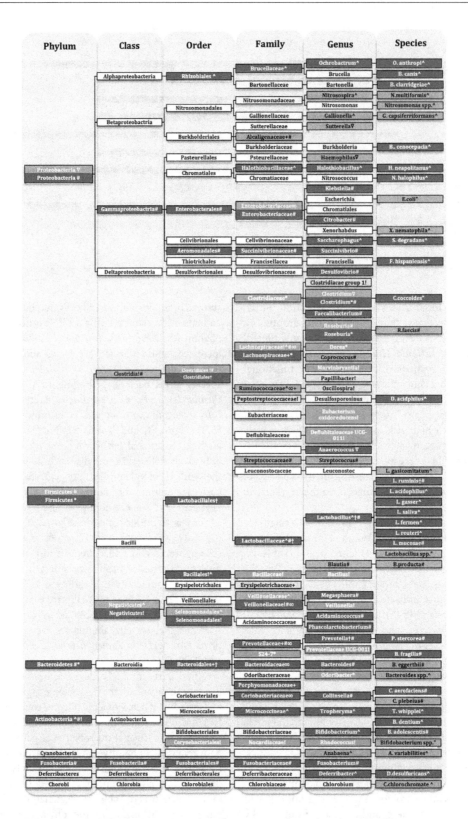

FIGURE 6 | Taxonomic tree of schizophrenia. Showing reduced abundance in orange, increased abundance in purple with lighter shades of orange and purple to signify that only preclinical evidence is available. White-no change only for representative purposes. Ultrahigh-risk individuals †(4), first episode psychosis ^ (54), first episode schizophrenia "(55), chronic schizophrenia # (57) ∇(56) ∞(40), maternal immune activation model + (53), pharmacological model * (52), social isolation! (46).

a behavioral phenotype that had some overlaps with schizophrenia-like behaviors, including locomotor hyperactivity, reduced anxiety, and decreases depression-like behavior, attributed to increased activity. However, no difference was found in cognitive behaviors and sociability. Mice, which received fecal matter from individuals with schizophrenia, showed an increased startle response at high-decibel tones; however, no difference was found in pre-pulse inhibition of startle, which has been used extensively as a translational behavioral biomarker of psychotic states. Investigators further verified that gut composition was altered through the fecal microbial transplant and found that the gut microbiome significantly differed compared to that of control mice. The most changed bacterial families were *Aerococcaceae* (Phylum: *Firmicutes*), and *Rikenellaceae* (Phylum: *Bacteroidetes)*, which was similar to changes found in patients with schizophrenia [58].

Overall, the studies highlighted in this review demonstrated differential changes for all major phyla, including *Proteobacteria*, *Firmicutes*, *Bacteroidetes*, *Actinobacteria*, and *Fusobacteria* in patients with schizophrenia compared to healthy controls (4, 40, 54–57).

DISCUSSION

Diversity of the Gut Microbiome in Schizophrenia

The diversity of the gut microbiome is unique to each individual. The majority of publications reviewed here identified no change in alpha diversity across animal and human studies (4, 46, 52–54, 56, 57). However, one study demonstrated an overall decrease in alpha diversity in individuals with chronic schizophrenia (40). The majority of patients were medicated with antipsychotics, which may have resulted in reduced microbial community diversity (40), as treatment with an atypical antipsychotic reduced microbiome community diversity in patients with bipolar disorder (alpha diversity), which was more profound in females (61). On the contrary, individuals on antipsychotic medications had no change in microbial community diversity (57). Due to conflicting results, we can only speculate that antipsychotic treatment may have resulted in a decrease in alpha diversity. Therefore, future studies should investigate the potential impact of antipsychotic treatment on the gut microbiome in schizophrenia.

The gut microbiome of patients with psychosis and animal models of schizophrenia are separated from the microbiota of healthy control individuals and control animals (beta diversity) (4, 40, 52–54, 56, 57). This clearly demonstrates that the gut microbiome in psychosis differs from that of the healthy controls. However, as there is a lack of studies comparing the microbiome between psychosis and other psychiatric and chronic, noncommunicable disorders, this does not necessary mean that the microbiome profile identified in psychosis is diagnostically specific. Nevertheless, these results, together with data showing that high-risk and UHR individuals have an altered microbiome compared to that of healthy controls (4), raise the possibility of developing the gut microbiome profiling further to be used as part of a biomarker battery to identify individuals at risk for later development of psychosis.

The studies outlined in this systematic review revealed that the phyla *Proteobacteria* (57), *Firmicutes* (52, 57), *Bacteroidetes* (52, 57) *Fusobacteria* (57), and *Actinobacteria* (46, 54, 57) were altered in patients at risk to develop schizophrenia, with chronic schizophrenia or in animal models of the disease at all different taxonomic units (**Figure 6**). First, we will individually discuss each of these phyla, within each phyla section we are discussing lower taxonomic units, and consider the functional implications that might be associated with their change.

Proteobacteria

Altered abundance, in both directions, of Proteobacteria has been associated with obesity, inflammation, and altered gut permeability (62–65). *Proteobacteria* were increased (57), as well decreased (56) in patients with chronic schizophrenia (**Figure 6** and **Table 2**) in the gut microbiome, but not in the oropharynx microbiome (66), which suggests that the imbalance of *Proteobacteria* abundance are specific to the gut microbiome. While an increased abundance of *Proteobacteria* is associated with the neonatal period (67), gastric bypass surgery (62, 68), and disease states such as metabolic disorders (69) and intestinal inflammation (70), decreased abundance of *Proteobacteria* have been found in overweight individuals (62). One study identified no difference in body mass index (57), whereas, in another study, individuals with schizophrenia had a significantly higher body mass index compared to healthy controls (56) (**Table 2**). Weight may have been a contributing factor influencing the abundance of *Proteobacteria*. Possibly, the decrease in *Proteobacteria* is more representative of patients with psychosis, because they tend to be more overweight or obese compared to mentally healthy controls (71). Therefore, future studies need to include lifestyle factors, such as diet, as potential covariates in the data analysis. At family level, both increased (57) and decreased (40) abundance of *Enterobacteriaceae* have been found (**Figure 6** and **Table 2**). An increase in *Enterobacteriaceae* have been associated with obesity (63), inflammation (64) and a "leaky gut" (65); however, obesity could not have been the driver for the change of this bacterial family as individuals with schizophrenia in both studies were in the healthy weight range based on their body mass index (40, 57). Increased gut permeability has been suggested to be related to schizophrenia (72) and may have been a contributing factor for the increase in *Enterobacteriaceae* (57). Besides, patients with schizophrenia show higher levels of proinflammatory cytokines (73). It is unclear, however, if the increased abundance of *Enterobacteriaceae* (57) was driven by proinflammatory cytokines or increased gut permeability in schizophrenia.

Firmicutes

An increased abundance of *Firmicutes* has been associated with an unhealthy dietary pattern, such as western diet and obesity (5, 74). A higher abundance of *Firmicutes* was found in the oropharynx microbiome of patients with schizophrenia (66). Animals injected with phencyclidine, a pharmacological model of schizophrenia, showed an increase in *Firmicutes* in their gut microbiome (74). In contrast, *Firmicutes* were less abundant in patients with chronic schizophrenia (57) (**Figure 6** and **Table 2**). At class, order and family levels *Negativicutes, Selenomondales,* and *Veillonellaceae* were reduced in first-episode psychosis (54) but were increased in an animal model of social isolation (46). *Veillonellaceae* were also increased in chronic schizophrenia (40, 57) (**Figure 6** and **Table 2**). Patients with chronic schizophrenia showed both an increase and a decrease in the genus *Clostridium* (56) in different studies (**Figure 6** and **Table 2**). Interestingly, an increase in this genus is associated with risperidone treatment (75). At this point, we are unable to conclude about the potential role of risperidone treatment as both studies (56, 57) report antipsychotic use, without specifying the type of medication used. Several species of *Clostridium* are precursors of 4-ethylphenylsulfate (76), which may contribute to the pathophysiology of schizophrenia, as it is important in pheromonal communication in mice under the control of testosterone levels (77). Serum 4-ethylphenylsulfate was elevated in MIA animals, a neurodevelopmental model of schizophrenia and 4-ethylphenylsulfate induced an anxiety-like behavioral phenotype, which may suggest behavioral abnormalities may be related to 4-ethylphenylsulfate produced by *Clostridium* (53). At species level, first-episode psychosis (54) and chronic schizophrenia patients (57), show similar to a study in oropharyngeal samples of schizophrenia patients, a significantly increased abundance of *Lactobacillus phage phiadh* (78) (**Figure 6** and **Table 2**).

Bacteroidetes

Bacteroidetes were increased in the pharmacological model of schizophrenia (52) and patients with chronic schizophrenia (57) (**Figure 6** and **Table 2**). Stress is involved in the pathophysiology of psychotic disorders, such as schizophrenia (79). In a mouse model of stress, mice were subjected to an aggressive male mouse within their home cage to induce stress. Investigators found elevated levels of the genus *Bacteroides* (80), which was demonstrated in chronic schizophrenia (57) (**Figure 6** and **Table 2**). Treatment with the probiotic *Bacteroides fragilis* was shown to improve anxiety-like, repetitive and communicative behaviors, and sensorimotor gating in the MIA model (53) (**Table 2**). *Bacteroides fragilis* improved anxiety-like (57), repetitive (57) and communicative behaviors (57), sensorimotor gating (57); however, *Bacteroides fragilis* do not influence social behaviors (53) (**Figure 6** and **Table 2**). Depressive-like symptoms in chronic schizophrenia patients were associated with an increased abundance of *Bacteroides* (56).

Actinobacteria

Actinobacteria are increased in first-episode psychosis, chronic schizophrenia, and socially isolated animals (46, 54, 57) (**Figure 6** and **Table 2**). *Tropheryma*, which belong to the phyla *Actinobacteria*, most studied species is *Tropheryma whipplei*, has been associated with intestinal malabsorption (81). *Tropheryma whipplei* was significantly increased in patients with first-episode psychosis (54) (**Figure 6** and **Table 2**). At genus level, *Collinsella* was elevated, which produces proinflammatory cytokines such as interleukin-17a and altered intestinal permeability in arthritis (82). Patients with schizophrenia show alter gut permeability (83). Additionally, multiple studies have found increases IL-17a plasma

concentrations in naïve first-episode schizophrenia patients (84, 85).

In conclusion, the published literature indicates that schizophrenia, both first-episode and chronic, is associated with microbiota changes, as shown by beta diversity, that will distinguish them from healthy controls. In this systematic review we included studies in which healthy controls were compared to either individuals at risk to develop psychosis or with diagnosed psychosis (either first episode or chronic). Such cross-sectional design, together with a variety of cofounding factors, which were controlled for in some, but not in all cases, precludes us from concluding about causality. However, our review of the available human literature clearly indicates the existence of an association between different stages of psychosis and the gut microbiome. Future studies will be required to identify the primary drivers of the microbiome alterations in psychosis and the potential direction of causality between gut microbiome changes in psychosis.

Methodological Considerations
Cofounding Factors

Within the reviewed publications gender was not addressed as a potential cofounding varible, which can potentially affect the gut microbiome. A review investigated gender differences in the gut microbiome and concluded that gender effects are inconsistent and identified that differences in geography, life style, diet, age, genetics, and potential other factors contribute more extensively to alterations in the gut microbiome (86). Within the reviewed articles, we reviewed populations from different geographical locations, which may have contributed to observed differences in microbiome. However, all studies demonstrated a clear separation between matched controls and psychotic individuals controlling for geographical location. Another major cofounding variable is age. We observed a broad age range in the reviewed studies, which may be expected considering that we included studies reporting on at-risk, UHR as well as on chronic schizophrenia. It has been suggested that age might be a major contributor to alterations in the gut microbiome (87). Gut microbiome changes within the elderly are associated with physiological changes within the gastrointestinal tract and has been demonstrated to reduce over time in diversity, shifts in dominant species, a decline in beneficial bacteria and decreased availability of beneficial metabolites such as short chain fatty acids (88). Older individuals have lower levels of Firmicutes and increased abundance of Proteobacteria (88). It is difficult to establish the potential cofounding effect of age on the results presented in the review. It should be noted, however, that each study contained age-matched controls, just like in the case of geographical location.

Fecal Sample Methodology Cofounders

We demonstrated that the CoR was greater in human studies allowing for greater comparability between studies. However, animal studies lacked reporting and should therefore be interpretate carefully. Overall, alterations and lack of reporting can be potential cofounding factors [further extensive review elsewhere (42)]. Methodological difference should be standardised in the future to improve translatability between animal and human studies and would allow for improved interpretation of data.

Factors Potentially Contributing to the Altered Microbiome in Psychosis

In the following section we address potential factors influencing the gut microbiome in individuals with psychosis. Due to the heterogeneous nature of psychotic disorders no specific and unique factors to leading to psychosis are known. Therefore, we considered common life-style and environmental factors, genetic susceptibility and medication use that can potentially influence the gut microbiome in psychosis, as well as in other serious mental illness.

Environmental Factors

Early Life Events

Children will receive the first inoculum from their mothers (89). Mode of delivery can influence the gut microbiome (37). Offspring will receive during vaginal birth microbes found in the maternal vagina and feces (89). Whereas, during Cesarean delivery (C-section), most microbes colonizing the gut are from external body surfaces (89). C-section significantly decreases *Bifidobacteria* spp. (90) and increases *Staphylococcus*, *Streptococcus* or *Propionibacteria* (91, 92). However, the differences in microbiota between C-section and vaginal birth gradually disappear over time (37). Preterm birth will result in an increased abundance of *Proteobacteria* and a lack of *Bifidobacterium* and *Lactobacillus* at genus level (37). It has been established that early life events are potential risk factors for schizophrenia (93, 94). C-section and preterm birth have been linked as a risk factor for schizophrenia (93, 94). *Bifidobacterium* spp., which is in line with the microbial profile of C-section and preterm birth, were decreased in first-episode psychosis patients (55) (**Figure 6** and **Table 2**). Chronic schizophrenia patients had increased levels of *Proteobacteria* at phylum level, which is related to preterm birth (57) (**Figure 6** and **Table 2**). In first-episode psychosis, UHR and chronic patients with schizophrenia *Lactobacillus*, which is again related to preterm birth, was increased (4, 54, 57) (**Figure 6** and **Table 2**).

These early life events seem to alter the gut microbiome and may influence the development of psychosis later in life, perhaps through brain development influenced by the microbiome. Future research should specifically investigate if the changes in the microbiome due to the aforementioned factors contribute to the development of psychosis.

Stress

It has long been established that stress and the activity of the hypothalamus-pituitary-adrenal (HPA) axis can alter the composition of the gut microbiome (39). Maternal separation, a model of stress, results in prolonged HPA activity, which resulted in rhesus monkeys (95), rats (96) in altered microbiome composition (95). Chronic restraint stress in adult mice resulted in differential gut microbiota composition compared to nonstressed mice (80). Stress decreased *Bacteroides* spp. and increased *Clostridium* spp., which was accompanied by an activation of the immune system and a "leaky" gut (97),

allowing for the translocation of luminal content such as lipopolysaccharides.

Stress is involved in the development of psychotic disorders such as schizophrenia (79, 98). Life events perceived as stressful can increase the occurrence of psychotic episodes (99). Individuals with schizophrenia experience stress more intensely; therefore even minor everyday stressors might exacerbate positive symptoms (100, 101). Management of day-to-day stress can be used in the management of psychosis (102); however, this intervention, in combination with antipsychotics, is only partially protective (103). This hypersensitivity to stress might be attributed to inappropriate autonomic nervous system and HPA axis function (79). Psychosis itself is a stressful event for the body, activating the stress response (98). Hypercortisolemia has been shown in patients with schizophrenia (104), which has been linked to the negative symptoms of schizophrenia (79). However, increased cortisol levels are not consistently found in individuals with schizophrenia (105). A meta-analysis found dysregulation of cortisol in psychotic patients (106). Allostatic load is the adaptation in response to stimuli such as stress (98). An increased allostatic load was seen in first-episode psychosis and schizophrenia patients compared to controls (98). This study found a positive correlation between positive symptoms with allostatic load in schizophrenia patients (98).

The genus *Clostridium* was increased in animals treated with phencyclidine (52) and chronic schizophrenia patients (57); however, Clostridium also decreased in chronic schizophrenia patients (56) (**Figure 6** and **Table 2**), consistent with a stress response. However, the stress level of schizophrenia patients was not described, and therefore it is unknown if the microbiota was altered due to increased stress or visa versa (57). A decrease in *Bacteroides* spp. is associated with stress (97), while in chronic schizophrenic patients, this genus was decreased (57) (**Figure 6** and **Table 2**).

In conclusion, based on the limited data available, it is difficult to establish if stress altered the microbiome. Future studies should assess stress levels and allostatic load to understand the impact of stress in psychosis on the gut microbiome.

Infectious Agents

Infectious agents, such as *Toxoplasma gondii*, have been suggested to contribute to the development of schizophrenia (107, 108). It has been recently demonstrated in a preclinical study that chronic *Toxoplasma gondii* infection results in an enrichment of Bacteroidetes in CD1 mice compared to noninfected controls (109). Interestingly, Bacteroidetes were also increased in a pharmacological model of schizophrenia (52) and in individuals with chronic schizophrenia (57). However, on the basis of the available evidence it is not possible to conclude about causality of the link between *Toxoplasma gondii* infection, alteration in the gut microbiome and the development of schizophrenia.

Lifestyle Factors

Diet

Diet is shaping the composition of the gut microbiome (5). The gut microbiome, in turn, is important in metabolizing the ingredients of food (18) and host fat storage, through the

156

Clinical Neurogastroenterology

absorption of monosaccharides by the gut microbiota from the lumen of the gut, promoting hepatic lipogenesis by fasting-induced adipocyte factor suppression (110). Multiple studies have demonstrated that altering diet rapidly changes the gut microbiome (5, 111) and microbial beta-diversity (112). Early life nutrition, through changing the gut microbiome, is important in the infant's development (113). Different diets in adulthood have been shown to modulate the gut microbiome, such as a high-protein, reduced carbohydrate diet (114), ketogenic diet (115), high fat, high sugar diet (western diet) (116, 117), and mediterranean diet (118). This indicates the strong impact of diet on the gut microbiome.

Nutrition is an important factor in schizophrenia due to poor dietary choices, causing obesity and secondary diseases (119). Obesity is twice as likely in schizophrenia/psychosis compared to the general population, affecting more than 50% of schizophrenic individuals (120). Drug naïve patients with schizophrenia show higher rates of obesity and type II diabetes compared to healthy individuals (120). Patients with schizophrenia consumed more fat (121, 122), saturated fat (122, 123), proteins (122), carbohydrates (122) and less fiber (121), than healthy controls. However, it was found that similar choices were made, but the overall food consumption was increased compared to healthy controls (122). Overall, people with psychosis tend to prefer unhealthy, fast food-type foods (120). This results in a dietary pattern high in saturated fats and sugars ("Western" diet). However, the gut microbiota of schizophrenia patients did not reflect that of individuals on a Western diet, characterized by a decrease in *Bifidobacteria*, *Bacteroides*, and *Prevotella* and an increase in *Firmicutes* (5). Within this review, first-episode psychosis had an increased abundance in *Bifidobacteria* (54) (**Figure 6** and **Table 2**). Different food types were not significantly associated with clustering of the microbiota (54). Increased *Prevotella* were found in UHR individuals (4); however, no conclusion can be drawn on the impact of nutrition as no metabolic or nutritional assessments were reported. In chronic schizophrenia patients, *Firmicutes* decreased, and the abundance of *Bacteroides* and *Prevotella* increased (57). It has to be noted that individuals in that study were Chinese patients, who did not show metabolic symptoms commonly seen in schizophrenia. This lack of weight gain has previously been reported in other Chinese schizophrenia patients (124). One study predicted an altered glucose metabolism (4), which is particularly interesting in the context of energy metabolism abnormalities that have been recently identified in schizophrenia [27-30]. A review investigated the link between the gut microbiome and glucose metabolism and found that the gut microbiome has substantial influence on glucose homeostasis through short chain fatty acids, bile acid metabolism, hormone secretion and synthesis of amino acids (125). However, future studies should address this point in individuals with psychosis to better understand the relationship between the gut, brain and energy metabolism.

In summary, individuals with psychosis show unhealthy dietary choices, which may influence the gut microbiome. However, the microbiome profiles described in studies on patients with psychosis do not support this notion. Nevertheless, at this point we can neither prove nor disprove the influence of diet to influence the gut microbiome in psychosis due to conflicting evidence and lack of reporting of dietary habits in these studies. Future studies should incorporate dietary patterns to be able to make a more definitive conclusion on the effects of dietary factors on the gut microbiome in individuals with psychosis.

Exercise

Exercise can impact microbial abundance in animals (126) and the human gut (127–131). The gut microbiota is different between sedentary individuals and people performing physical exercise (129, 132). Exercise reduced *Bacteroidetes* (129, 130) and *Proteobacteria* (132). Activity increased the undefined genus in the *S24-7* family (129), *Verrucomicrobia* (132), *Bifidobacteriaceae* (132), the *Streptococcaceae* family (129) and *Firmicutes* (130), compared to sedentary controls. In sedentary woman bacteria belonging to the families, *Barnesiellaceae* and *Odoribacteraceae* were more abundant compared to active women (130).

Individuals with schizophrenia and other psychotic disorders are significantly less physically active than healthy individuals, and are also less active then patients with other psychotic disorder (133, 134). Patients with chronic schizophrenia show an increased abundance in *Bacteroidetes* and *Proteobacteria* and a decreased abundance in *Streptococcaceae* and *Firmicutes* (57) (**Figure 6** and **Table 2**), which could possibly be mitigated by exercise as active individuals have opposing abundances (129, 130, 132). Further supporting this argument, *Firmicutes* were increased in phencyclidine treated animals (52), which could have been related to hyperactivity induced by the phencyclidine administration. The increase in the phylum *Bacteroidetes* is associated with a sedentary lifestyle (130). *Bacteroidetes* were increased in chronic schizophrenia patients (57) (**Figure 6** and **Table 2**); however, this increase was as well seen in the phencyclidine, hyperactive animals (52) (**Figure 6** and **Table 2**). Therefore, it is unclear at this stage if physical activity altered the gut microbiome. The activities of patients with schizophrenia are not explicit in the publications reviewed here. Nevertheless, physical activity has been considered to influence the gut microbiome composition in the context of schizophrenia Schwarz, Maukonen (54). Pateints with first-episode psychosis, stratified for amount of exercise, demonstrated an increased abundance of *Lactobacillaceae* and decreased abundance of *Veillonellaceae* at family level in physically active, first-episode psychosis individuals compared to physically active, healthy controls (54) (**Figure 6** and **Table 2**). Future studies need to assess physical activity levels as a potential cofounder to influence the gut microbiome.

Smoking

Environmental contaminants, such as smoking, influence the gut microbiota (135). Furthermore, smoking can lead to DNA damage and epithelial cell methylation (136), resulting in altered gut function and possibly altered microbiota composition. Smoking increased within-participant diversity, *Dialister invisus*, and *Megaspaera micronuciformis* were more abundant in the upper gastrointestinal tract in current smokers compared to the ones who never smoked (135). In rats, cigarette smoke decreased *Bifidobacteria* and SCFA, such as propionic and butyric acid (137), and increased *Lachnospiraceae* spp. (138). Passive smoking increases *Clostridium* spp. and reduces *Firmicutes* and *Enterobacteriaceae* in animals (139). In humans smoking increased *Clostridium* (140), *Bacteroidetes*, and *Proteobacteria* (141) and decreased *Firmicutes* and *Actinobacteria* (141).

Smoking is more prevalent in individuals with schizophrenia than in healthy individuals (142).

As reviewed above, in first-episode psychosis, *Bifidobacteria* were increased (54) (**Figure 6** and **Table 2**), whereas smoking decreased this bacteria. However, this study did not specify smoking status (54). In human studies, *Lachnospiraceae* (57) and *Firmicutes* (57) were decreased (**Figure 6** and **Table 2**). Decreased *Firmicutes* are in line with smoking; however, in patients with chronic schizophrenia, tobacco usage was not different compared to healthy control (57). At genus level contradictory results were found for *Clostridium*, however as mentioned before an increase in *Clostridium*, which is associated with smoking, was seen both in an animal model of schizophrenia (52) and in patients with chronic schizophrenia (57), where no difference in tobacco usage was seen between patients and controls. On the contrary, patients with schizophrenia, who were significantly likelier to smoke, had decreased abundance of Clostridium (56) (**Figure 6** and **Table 2**). *Enterobacteriaceae* were increased in chronic schizophrenia patients (41) (**Figure 6** and **Table 2**), which would be in line with possible tobacco usage; however, smoking status was not reported within that study.

In conclusion, according to the studies reviewed here individuals with schizophrenia either did not smoke more than the general population, or tobacco usage was not reported, except Nguyen, Kosciolek (56) where contradictory results were found with regards to smoking and the gut microbiome. Considering animal models of psychosis that do show altered gut microbiome despite the lack of smoking exposure, one can argue that the change in the gut microbiome seen in individuals with psychosis is likely to be independent of smoking status. However, most studies did not report smoking status, which predicts a firm conclusion regarding the link between smoking status and altered gut microbiome at this stage. Future studies should report smoking status and investigate if tobacco usage might be a cofounding factor influencing the gut microbiome.

Overall, although it has been widely acknowledged that life style-factors are essential in shaping the gut microbiome, the studies covered in this systematic review do not support the notion that the difference in the gut microbiome between controls and individuals with psychosis is causally related to lifestyle factors. Potentially, lifestyle factors, such as diet, exercise, and smoking may improve the gut microbiota of individuals with psychosis. Therefore, the completeness of reporting to provide a detailed account of the lifestyle factors is of great importance for future studies.

Genetics

Host genetic variation can influence the diversity of the gut microbiome (143). However, the relationship between host genetics and gut microbiota is largely unknown (143).

Although, lifestyle factors such as diet and exercise will contribute to similar gut microbiota composition of close relatives, suggesting that genetics might be an important factor (143). For example, monozygotic twins share a more similar gut microbiota profile than dizygotic twins (143).

Genetic factors are important in the etiology of psychotic disorders such as schizophrenia (144). At this stage, no studies have investigated the effect of host genetic variation in individuals with schizophrenia on the gut microbiota. Therefore, we can only speculate that variations of bacterial abundances found in this population may be due to genetic variation involved in the pathogenesis of psychosis. Future studies should incorporate genetic analysis to understand the importance of host genetic variation on the gut microbiome.

Antipsychotics

Antipsychotics are the primary medications used for the management of schizophrenia (145). However, the knowledge of the effects of antipsychotics on the gut microbiome is currently in its infancy. Antipsychotic use can cause severe metabolic side effects such as weight gain, increased visceral fat, and glucose dysregulation (146), of which the mechanism of action is not fully understood (146). It is believed that the convergence of central and peripheral mechanisms are involved in metabolic side effects (146). It has been demonstrated that the composition of the gut microbiome is linked to obesity (147). Olanzapine treatment increases body weight (146, 148) and leads to a shift of the gut microbiome, which involves the increase of the phylum *Firmicutes* (146, 148) and decreases in the phyla *Bacteriodetes* (146, 148) in rodents. In female rats, olanzapine reduced the abundance of *Actinobacteria* and *Proteobacteria* compared to controls (148). Another study found an increase in *Erysipelotrichia* and *Gammaproteobacteria* and a reduced abundance of *Bacteroidia* at class level (149). Olanzapine inhibited the growth of *Escherichia coli* NC101 (149). One study found no change in microbial composition after olanzapine treatment, which may have been due to the short duration of treatment (150). However, this study demonstrated that acetate concentration changed, suggesting that olanzapine did affect on this by-product of the microbiome function (150). Risperidone increased *Firmicutes*, where *Lactobacillus* spp. were reduced, and decreased *Bacteroidetes*, where *Bacterioides* spp. were increased and *Alistipes* spp. decreased and *Proteobacteria* in female C57BL/6J mice compared to controls (151). The most abundant genera were *Allabaculum* spp. in risperidone treated animals compared to controls (151). Risperidone treatment resulted in weight gain (151). Transplant of fecal matter of female C57BL/6J mice on risperidone treatment to naïve mice resulted in a decreased resting metabolic rate, which may have contributed to the increase in body weight (151). Donor fecal matter was analyzed for risperidone concentration, which was 10-fold less than to establish a dose-response curve (151). Therefore, investigators concluded that the microbiota of risperidone treated animals was the obesogenic factor rather than the remaining risperidone within donor fecal samples (151). In medically healthy males, risperidone treatment led to weight gain with an altered gut microbiome compared to psychiatrically ill, but untreated patients. These findings with risperidone are similar to the gut microbiota changes after olanzapine administration. Antipsychotic treatment increased the abundance of *Lachnospiraceae* and decreased the abundance of *Akkermansia* after adjustment for body mass index in patients with bipolar disorder (61). However, *Akkermansia* was less abundant in nonobese, antipsychotic-treated patients (61). One publication covered in this systematic review assessed the changes in first-episode schizophrenia after 24-weeks of risperidone treatment (55). Chronic risperidone treatment altered metabolic parameters such as an increase in weight, body mass index, fasting serum glucose levels, triglycerides, and low-density lipoproteins (**Table 2**). Risperidone treatment increased *Bifidobacterium* spp. and *Escherichia coli* and decrease the abundance of *Clostridium coccoides* and *Lactobacillus* spp. (55) (**Figure 6** and **Table 2**).

Oxytocin

As the ever evolving literature recognizes the need for new drug treatments to complement the presently used antipsychotic medication, the neuropeptide oxytocin has been suggested as a potential novel treatment approach (152). Evidence from preclinical and clinical studies suggest therapeutic effects on all symptom domains of schizophrenia, with particular improvement in the negative symptoms (152). A potential link with the microbiome is suggested by the finding that the bacterium *Lactobacillus reuteri* upregulates oxytocin (153). One study we presented in this systematic review in first episode psychosis patients showed an increased abundance of *Lactobacillus reuteri* (54). However, the exact details of the interaction between oxytocin and the microbiome are currently unknown.

In our systematic review, six articles assessed different stages of the development of schizophrenia, such as high-risk, UHR, first-episode psychosis, first-episode schizophrenia, chronic schizophrenia. High-risk, UHR, and first-episode schizophrenia, first-episode psychosis patients were at study onset drug naïve (4, 54, 55). For chronic patients, antipsychotic treatment had to be more than six months of use. Therefore, changes might be cofounded by antipsychotic treatment (40, 56, 57). More studies are needed to identify the influence of antipsychotic medication on the gut microbiome.

Functional Implication of the Change in Microbiota on the Psychopathology of Psychosis

Symptoms of Psychosis and the Gut Microbiome

Of the publications reviewed here, some have linked the gut microbiome to symptoms seen in schizophrenia. In the pharmacological model of schizophrenia, hyperactivity was associated with an increase in *Lachnospiraceae* and *Clostridiaceae* and at genus level an increase of *Roseburia*, *Clostridium*, and *Odoribacter* (52) (**Figure 6** and **Table 2**). In socially isolated animals, activity was positively correlated with the abundance of *Bacillales*. On the other hand, *Clostridales* was negatively correlated with locomotor activity (46). Socially isolated animals had increased locomotor activity in conjunction with reduced *Clostridales* (46). Furthermore, *Clostridiales* was negatively

correlated with cognitive performance (46). Additionally, taxa belonging to the order *Clostridales*, at family level *Ruminococcaceae* and genus level *Papillibacter* were positively correlated to anxiety-like behaviors (46). *Bacillales* were negatively correlated to anxiety-like behaviors. Impaired contextual fear task, which investigates the associative learning process, was associated with an increase in *Veillonella* and *Defluvitaleaceae UCG-011* (46).

In people with schizophrenia, negative symptoms were related to decreased *Ruminococcaceae*, and self-reported mental well-being was positively correlated with the phylum *Verrucomicrobia* (56). Correlation analysis revealed that age of disease onset positively correlated with *Cyanobacteria* at phylum level, indicating that the earlier the disease onset, the higher the abundance of *Cyanobacteria*. Depressive-like symptoms were associated with an increased abundance of *Bacteroides*. *Veillonellaceae* OTU191 were negatively correlated with the Positive and Negative Syndrome Scale (40). On the other hand, *Bacteroidaceae* OTU172, *Streptococcaceae* OTU834, and two *Lachnospiraceae* OTUs (477 and 629) were positively correlated with PANSS (40). Bacterial numbers of Lactobacillus group, *Lachnospiraceae*, *Ruminococcaceae*, and *Bacteroides* spp. were correlated with symptom severity, particularly for negative symptoms and poorer functioning (54). Positive symptoms were correlated with bacteria of the *Lactobacillus group* (54).

Systemic biochemical changes and their relationship with the gut microbiome have been investigated. It was identified that *Blautia*, *Coprococcus*, and *Roseburia* were negatively associated with vitamin B6, taurine, and hypotaurine metabolic pathway and positively associated with methane metabolic pathways (57). Increased inflammatory cytokines have been seen in patients with schizophrenia (73). Hippocampal IL-10 and IL-6 correlated with *Peptostreptococcaceae* positively (46), while *Bacillales* correlated negatively with hippocampal IL-6 (46, 54). Interestingly, if the microbial composition of first-episode psychosis clustered with controls, these patients were more likely to show remission (70% of patients) (54). However, patients with abnormal microbial composition at baseline showed low remission rates (28% of patients) (54). Analysis revealed that this remission was not due to symptom severity at baseline (54). Clustering was not influenced by physical activity, body mass index, type of psychosis, duration of antipsychotic treatment, and the food consumed one week before fecal sample collection (54).

In summary, the abundance of specific bacteria correlated with behaviors and biochemical changes. This raises the possibility of targeted treatment approaches, such as pre/probiotics, to alleviate individual symptoms, however at this point in time causation has not been established. Further studies are required to link individual behaviors and biochemical changes in psychosis to the gut microbiome.

Does the Microbiome Have a Pathogenic Role in Psychosis?

To address this question, we investigated retrospective studies to see if antibiotic use increased the prevalence of psychosis. A nationwide, register-based cohort study in Denmark outlined that antibiotics increased the risk of mental health disorders, which was independent of age, compared to antivirals and antimycotics (154). The risk for mental disorders increased in a dose-dependent manner, were a risk for mental disorders were more likely in individuals with more treated infections (154). The study showed that anti-infective agents were associated with an increased risk for schizophrenia spectrum disorders (154). Another study investigating the same Danish cohort identified that maternal infection during pregnancy treated with anti-infective agents increased the risk of mental disorders in the offspring, compared to offspring without maternal infection with anti-infective agents during pregnancy (155). The risk of mental health was increased if maternal infection treated with anti-infective medications occurred during the second and third trimester (155). It can be argued that maternal infection during pregnancy is known to be a risk factor to develop schizophrenia (156). However, Lydholm, Kohler-Forsberg (155) demonstrated that mental health disorder risk increased in response to maternal prescriptions during and after pregnancy. These recent studies suggest that antibiotic treatment during pregnancy and later in life may result in the later onset of schizophrenia. However, these studies are merely observational and would need further research to create causality.

Interestingly, animals, which received gut microbiome from patients with schizophrenia *via* fecal microbial transplant, showed a schizophrenia-like behavioral phenotype (40). Investigators further verified that gut composition was altered through the fecal microbial transplant and found that the gut microbiome significantly differed compared to that of control mice and was similar to that of patients with schizophrenia (40). Furthermore, the gut microbiota was altered in UHR individuals (4). Therefore, the changes in gut microbiota composition may contribute to the development of the disease pathophysiology. If confirmed, this raises the possibility to utilize the gut microbiome as an early biomarker for schizophrenia spectrum disorders.

Further research should be directed toward the understanding of bacteriophages, viruses that infect bacteria leading to the death of the bacteria or integration of the phage into the gut microbiome (78). Interestingly, a significantly increased abundance of *Lactobacillus phage phiadh* has been identified at species level in first-episode psychosis (54) and in patients with chronic schizophrenia (57), as well as in the oropharyngeal microbiome samples of patients with schizophrenia (78) (**Figure 6** and **Table 2**). However, the importance of bacteriophages is currently unknown and will require further investigation.

If alterations in the gut microbiome do indeed play a pathogenetic role in psychosis, agents, which modify the gut microbiome, can be considered as a potential modifiers of the disease process in schizophrenia. No research to date has investigated the effects of pre-or probiotics, antibiotics, fecal microbial transplant, or dietary intervention on the gut microbiome, specifically in people with schizophrenia. *Bacteroides fragilis*, a probiotic, in MIA model of schizophrenia in mice resulted in the restoration of gut permeability, gene expression, and IL-6 in the colon and normalized at family level *Lachnospiraceae* and

unclassified Bacteroidales (53). Behaviorally, *Bacteroides fragilis* improved anxiety-like, sensorimotor, repetitive and communicative behavior; however, *Bacteroides fragilis* treatment did not affect sociability and social preference in MIA mice (53). Similar behavioral effects were found with *Bacteroides thetaiotaomicron*, whereas *Enterococcus faecalis* did not improve anxiety-like and repetitive behavior (53). Therefore, probiotic treatment might be a novel treatment for schizophrenia by improving gut functioning. However, a current review comes to the conclusion that the most recent evidence does not yet support the use of probiotics for the treatment of psychiatric disorders and more research is needed (157). Fecal microbial transplant, first performed approximately 1700 years ago (158), has not yet been described in either animal models or individuals with schizophrenia, but has been trialed for multiple sclerosis, patients showing normalization of neurological symptoms (159). These promising results may open up a new area in which the therapeutic effects of the microbiome can be taken advantage of. However, clinical trails are needed as currently only speculations can be made.

The antibiotic minocycline, which exerts neuroprotective and anti-inflammatory actions through supressing microglia activation and the modulation of excitatory neurotransmission, have attracted attention as potential treatments for schizophrenia, as shown by a number of small pilot studies with encouraging results (160). Although, a recent, large, randomized, placebo controlled clinical trial has provided unequivocal results showing no measurable therapeutic benefit on negative and other symptoms in patients with schizophrenia spectrum disorders (161), it has to be emphasized that active neuroinflammation involving microglial activation and neuropathology was unlikely to be present during the first years of schizophrenia, potentially explaining the lack of effect. The involvement of the gut microbiome in the mediation of the effects of minocycline has not been investigated.

Lastly, it is feasible to assume that diet could shift and normalize the gut microbiome in individuals with psychosis. The high fat, low carbohydrate ketogenic diet modifies the gut microbiome in an animal model of autism (115). Ketogenic diet increased *Enterobacteriaceae* and decreased *Firmicutes*, *Lactobacillus* spp., and *Roseburia* (115), which were altered in schizophrenia (**Figure 6** and **Table 2**). We have recently reported that ketogenic diet improves schizophrenia-like behaviors in an animal model of schizophrenia (162, 163), which can be due to the diet-induced alterations of the gut microbiome.

CONCLUSION

Overall, the studies covered by this systematic review demonstrate that the gut microbiome in patients with schizophrenia spectrum disorders and animal models of schizophrenia is different from the microbiome of healthy controls. Once these initial findings are replicated and further extended in different patient populations the changes in the microbiome might be used as an independent biomarker of psychosis for high-risk and UHR individuals. While lifestyle factors do shape the gut microbiome, it is currently uncertain how they contribute to psychosis.

Lifestyle changes such as diet, exercise, and cessation of smoking may influence the gut microbiome positively in individuals with schizophrenia. Stress and other early life events are possible further environmental factors contributing to this change. Multiple pathways by which alterations in the gut microbiome may have occurred, such as inflammation, the vagus nerve communication, stress response, and metabolites produced by the microbiota have been reviewed elsewhere (1, 5, 22). Clearly, more research is needed to clarify the role of specific host extrinsic and intrinsic factors and to identify specific mechanistic links, if any, between the gut microbiota and psychosis. Animal and human studies showed both similarities and differences in gut microbiota composition, which reflect the well-known difficulties to translate between preclinical and clinical research in the area of psychosis. Greater understanding and reporting of methodology of the gut microbiome will improve translatability from murine to human studies.

We conclude that the gut microbiome changes may precede the appearance of the diagnostic clinical symptoms of schizophrenia spectrum disorders and may contribute to the disease pathophysiology and the development of the behavioral symptoms. Further rigorous, well reported preclinical and longitudinal, mechanistically oriented clinical studies are needed to provide more evidence to support these potential links. Normalizing the altered gut microbiome with diet, pre- or probiotics, fecal microbiome transfer, or pharmacological interventions, may lead to improved symptom control and mitigation of the metabolic side effects of antipsychotic medication. However, randomized controlled clinical trials are urgently required to substantiate the potential use of targeting the microbiome as a novel therapeutic intervention in psychotic disorders.

AUTHOR CONTRIBUTIONS

A-KK performed the data search, report selection, data extraction, and quality assessment and wrote the manuscript. RP was the independent assessor for the quality assessment and revised the final draft of the manuscript. ZS edited and revised all drafts of the manuscript.

REFERENCES

1. Cryan JF, Dinan TG. Mind-altering microorganisms: the impact of the gut microbiota on brain and behaviour. *Nat Rev Neurosci* (2012) 13(10):701–12. doi: 10.1038/nrn3346

2. Schmidt TSB, Raes J, Bork P. The human gut microbiome: from association to modulation. *Cell* (2018) 172(6):1198–215. doi: 10.1016/j.cell.2018.02.044

3. Clemente JC, Ursell LK, Parfrey LW, Knight R. The impact of the gut microbiota on human health: an integrative view. *Cell* (2012) 148(6):1258–70. doi: 10.1016/j.cell.2012.01.035

4. He Y, Kosciolek T, Tang J, Zhou Y, Li Z, Ma X, et al. Gut microbiome and magnetic resonance spectroscopy study of subjects at ultra-high risk for psychosis may support the membrane hypothesis. *Eur Psychiatry* (2018) 53:37–45. doi: 10.1016/j.eurpsy.2018.05.011

5. Sandhu KV, Sherwin E, Schellekens H, Stanton C, Dinan TG, Cryan JF. Feeding the microbiota-gut-brain axis: diet, microbiome, and neuropsychiatry. *Transl Res* (2017) 179:223–44. doi: 10.1016/j.trsl.2016.10.002

6. Turnbaugh PJ, Quince C, Faith JJ, McHardy AC, Yatsunenko T, Niazi F, et al. Organismal, genetic, and transcriptional variation in the deeply sequenced gut microbiomes of identical twins. *Proc Natl Acad Sci U S A* (2010) 107 (16):7503–8. doi: 10.1073/pnas.1002355107

7. Hall AB, Tolonen AC, Xavier RJ. Human genetic variation and the gut microbiome in disease. *Nat Rev Genet* (2017) 18(11):690–9. doi: 10.1038/nrg.2017.63

8. Arnold IC, Dehzad N, Reuter S, Martin H, Becher B, Taube C, et al. Helicobacter pylori infection prevents allergic asthma in mouse models through the induction of regulatory T cells. *J Clin Invest* (2011) 121 (8):3088–93. doi: 10.1172/JCI45041

9. Round JL, Mazmanian SK. The gut microbiota shapes intestinal immune responses during health and disease. *Nat Rev Immunol* (2009) 9(5):313–23. doi: 10.1038/nri2515

10. Round JL, Lee SM, Li J, Tran G, Jabri B, Chatila TA, et al. The Toll-like receptor 2 pathway establishes colonization by a commensal of the human microbiota. *Science* (2011) 332(6032):974–7. doi: 10.1126/science.1206095

11. Elinav E, Strowig T, Kau AL, Henao-Mejia J, Thaiss CA, Booth CJ, et al. NLRP6 inflammasome regulates colonic microbial ecology and risk for colitis. *Cell* (2011) 145(5):745–57. doi: 10.1016/j.cell.2011.04.022

12. Lathrop SK, Bloom SM, Rao SM, Nutsch K, Lio CW, Santacruz N, et al. Peripheral education of the immune system by colonic commensal microbiota. *Nature* (2011) 478(7368):250–4. doi: 10.1038/nature10434

13. Spor A, Koren O, Ley R. Unravelling the effects of the environment and host genotype on the gut microbiome. *Nat Rev Microbiol* (2011) 9(4):279–90. doi: 10.1038/nrmicro2540

14. Perry S, de la Luz Sanchez M, Yang S, Haggerty TD, Hurst P, Perez-Perez G, et al. Gastroenteritis and transmission of Helicobacter pylori infection in households. *Emerg Infect Dis* (2006) 12(11):1701–8. doi: 10.3201/eid1211.060086

15. Dicksved J, Halfvarson J, Rosenquist M, Jarnerot G, Tysk C, Apajalahti J, et al. Molecular analysis of the gut microbiota of identical twins with Crohn's disease. *ISME J* (2008) 2(7):716–27. doi: 10.1038/ismej.2008.37

16. Sekirov I, Russell SL, Antunes LC, Finlay BB. Gut microbiota in health and disease. *Physiol Rev* (2010) 90(3):859–904. doi: 10.1152/physrev.00045.2009

17. Pflughoeft KJ, Versalovic J. Human microbiome in health and disease. *Annu Rev Pathol* (2012) 7:99–122. doi: 10.1146/annurev-pathol-011811-132421

18. Ley RE, Backhed F, Turnbaugh P, Lozupone CA, Knight RD, Gordon JI. Obesity alters gut microbial ecology. *Proc Natl Acad Sci U S A* (2005) 102 (31):11070–5. doi: 10.1073/pnas.0504978102

19. Armougom F, Henry M, Vialettes B, Raccah D, Raoult D. Monitoring bacterial community of human gut microbiota reveals an increase in Lactobacillus in obese patients and Methanogens in anorexic patients. *PloS One* (2009) 4(9):e7125. doi: 10.1371/journal.pone.0007125

20. Brown LM. Helicobacter pylori: epidemiology and routes of transmission. *Epidemiol Rev* (2000) 22(2):283–97. doi: 10.1093/oxfordjournals.epirev.a018040

21. Ridaura VK, Faith JJ, Rey FE, Cheng J, Duncan AE, Kau AL, et al. Gut microbiota from twins discordant for obesity modulate metabolism in mice. *Science* (2013) 341(6150):1241214. doi: 10.1126/science.1241214

22. Cryan JF, O'Mahony SM. The microbiome-gut-brain axis: from bowel to behavior. *Neurogastroenterol Motil Off J Eur Gastrointestinal Motil Soc* (2011) 23(3):187–92. doi: 10.1111/j.1365-2982.2010.01664.x

23. Rhee SH, Pothoulakis C, Mayer EA. Principles and clinical implications of the brain-gut-enteric microbiota axis. *Nat Rev Gastroenterol Hepatol* (2009) 6(5):306–14. doi: 10.1038/nrgastro.2009.35

24. Tandon R, Keshavan MS, Nasrallah HA. Schizophrenia, "Just the Facts": What we know in 2008 Part 1: Overview. *Schizophr Res* (2008) 100:4–19. doi: 10.1016/j.schres.2008.01.022

25. Schizophrenia Fact sheet N°397 [Internet] (2014).

26. McCutcheon RA, Reis Marques T, Howes OD. Schizophrenia-An Overview. *JAMA Psychiatry* (2020) 77(2):201–10. doi: 10.1001/jamapsychiatry.2019.3360

27. van Os J, Kapur S. Schizophrenia. *Lancet* (2009) 374(9690):635–45. doi: 10.1016/s0140-6736(09)60995-8

28. Javitt DC, Zukin SR. Recent advances in the phencyclidine model of schizophrenia. *Am J Psychiatry* (1991) 148(10):1301–8. doi: 10.1176/ajp.148.10.1301

29. Fujimoto T, Takeuch K, Matsumoto T, Kamimura K, Hamada R, Nakamura K, et al. Abnormal glucose metabolism in the anterior cingulate cortex in patients with schizophrenia. *Psychiatry Res* (2007) 154(1):49–58. doi: 10.1016/j.pscychresns.2006.04.002

30. Dwyer DS, Bradley RJ, Kablinger AS, Freeman AM. 3rd. Glucose metabolism in relation to schizophrenia and antipsychotic drug treatment. *Ann Clin Psychiatry* (2001) 13(2):103–13. doi: 10.3109/10401230109148955

31. Du F, Cooper AJ, Thida T, Sehovic S, Lukas SE, Cohen BM, et al. In vivo evidence for cerebral bioenergetic abnormalities in schizophrenia measured using 31P magnetization transfer spectroscopy. *JAMA Psychiatry* (2014) 71 (1):19–27. doi: 10.1001/jamapsychiatry.2013.2287

32. Nascimento JM, Martins-de-Souza D. The proteome of schizophrenia. *NPJ Schizophr* (2015) 1:14003. doi: 10.1038/npjschz.2014.3

33. Davis J, Eyre H, Jacka FN, Dodd S, Dean O, McEwen S, et al. A review of vulnerability and risks for schizophrenia: Beyond the two hit hypothesis. *Neurosci Biobehav Rev* (2016) 65:185–94. doi: 10.1016/j.neubiorev.2016.03.017

34. Craddock N, O'Donovan MC, Owen MJ. The genetics of schizophrenia and bipolar disorder: dissecting psychosis. *J Med Genet* (2005) 42(3):193–204. doi: 10.1136/jmg.2005.030718

35. Kavanagh DH, Tansey KE, O'Donovan MC, Owen MJ. Schizophrenia genetics: emerging themes for a complex disorder. *Mol Psychiatry* (2015) 20(1):72–6. doi: 10.1038/mp.2014.148

36. Misiak B, Stramecki F, Gaweda L, Prochwicz K, Sasiadek MM, Moustafa AA, et al. Interactions Between Variation in Candidate Genes and Environmental Factors in the Etiology of Schizophrenia and Bipolar Disorder: a Systematic Review. *Mol Neurobiol* (2018) 55(6):5075–100. doi: 10.1007/s12035-017-0708-y

37. Tamburini S, Shen N, Wu HC, Clemente JC. The microbiome in early life: implications for health outcomes. *Nat Med* (2016) 22(7):713–22. doi: 10.1038/nm.4142

38. Dinan TG, Borre YE, Cryan JF. Genomics of schizophrenia: time to consider the gut microbiome? *Mol Psychiatry* (2014) 19(12):1252–7. doi: 10.1038/mp.2014.93

39. Tannock GW, Savage DC. Influences of dietary and environmental stress on microbial populations in the murine gastrointestinal tract. *Infect Immun* (1974) 9(3):591–8. doi: 10.1128/IAI.9.3.591-598.1974

40. Zheng P, Zeng B, Liu M, Chen J, Pan J, Han Y, et al. The gut microbiome from patients with schizophrenia modulates the glutamate-glutamine-GABA cycle and schizophrenia-relevant behaviors in mice. *Sci Adv* (2019) 5(2):eaau8317. doi: 10.1126/sciadv.aau8317

41. Rodrigues-Amorim D, Rivera-Baltanas T, Regueiro B, Spuch C, de Las Heras ME, Vazquez-Noguerol Mendez R, et al. The role of the gut microbiota in schizophrenia: Current and future perspectives. *World J Biol Psychiatry Off J World Fed Soc Biol Psychiatry* (2018) 19(8):571–85. doi: 10.1080/15622975.2018.1433878

42. Nguyen TT, Hathaway H, Kosciolek T, Knight R, Jeste DV. Gut microbiome in serious mental illnesses: A systematic review and critical evaluation. *Schizophr Res* (2019) S0920-9964(19):30382–2. doi: 10.1016/j.schres.2019.08.026

43. Severance EG, Yolken RH, Eaton WW. Autoimmune diseases, gastrointestinal disorders and the microbiome in schizophrenia: more than a gut feeling. *Schizophr Res* (2016) 176(1):23–35. doi: 10.1016/j.schres.2014.06.027

44. Shamseer L, Moher D, Clarke M, Ghersi D, Liberati A, Petticrew M, et al. Preferred reporting items for systematic review and meta-analysis protocols (PRISMA-P) 2015: elaboration and explanation. *BMJ* (2015) 350:g7647.

doi: 10.1136/bmj.g7647

45. Hooijmans CR, Rovers MM, de Vries RBM, Leenaars M, Ritskes-Hoitinga M, Langendam MW. SYRCLE's risk of bias tool for animal studies. *BMC Med Res Methodol* (2014) 14(1):43. doi: 10.1186/1471-2288-14-43

46. Dunphy-Doherty F, O'Mahony SM, Peterson VL, O'Sullivan O, Crispie F, Cotter PD, et al. Post-weaning social isolation of rats leads to long-term disruption of the gut microbiota-immune-brain axis. *Brain Behav Immun* (2018) 68:261–73. doi: 10.1016/j.bbi.2017.10.024

47. Moher DLA, Tetzlaff J, Altman DG. The PRISMA Group Preferred Reporting Items for Systematic Reviews and Meta-Analyses: The PRISMA Statement. *PLoS Med* (2009) 6(7):e1000097. doi: 10.1371/journal.pmed1000097

48. Li Q, Cheung C, Wei R, Hui ES, Feldon J, Meyer U, et al. Prenatal immune challenge is an environmental risk factor for brain and behavior change relevant to schizophrenia: evidence from MRI in a mouse model. *PloS One* (2009) 4(7):e6354. doi: 10.1371/journal.pone.0006354

49. Coyle JT. NMDA receptor and schizophrenia: a brief history. *Schizophr Bull* (2012) 38(5):920–6. doi: 10.1093/schbul/sbs076

50. McCutcheon RA, Krystal JH, Howes OD. Dopamine and glutamate in schizophrenia: biology, symptoms and treatment. *World Psychiatry Off J World Psychiatr Assoc (WPA)* (2020) 19(1):15–33. doi: 10.1002/wps.20693

51. Robbins TW. Neurobehavioural sequelae of social deprivation in rodents revisited: Modelling social adversity for developmental neuropsychiatric disorders. *J Psychopharmacol* (2016) 30(11):1082–9. doi: 10.1177/0269881116664450

52. Pyndt Jørgensen B, Krych L, Pedersen TB, Plath N, Redrobe JP, Hansen AK, et al. Investigating the long-term effect of subchronic phencyclidine-treatment on novel object recognition and the association between the gut microbiota and behavior in the animal model of schizophrenia. *Physiol Behav* (2015) 141:32–9. doi: 10.1016/j.physbeh.2014.12.042

53. Hsiao EY, McBride SW, Hsien S, Sharon G, Hyde ER, McCue T, et al. Microbiota modulate behavioral and physiological abnormalities associated with neurodevelopmental disorders. *Cell* (2013) 155(7):1451–63. doi: 10.1016/j.cell.2013.11.024

54. Schwarz E, Maukonen J, Hyytiäinen T, Kieseppä T, Orešič M, Sabunciyan S, et al. Analysis of microbiota in first episode psychosis identifies preliminary associations with symptom severity and treatment response. *Schizophr Res* (2018) 192:398–403. doi: 10.1016/j.schres.2017.04.017

55. Yuan X, Zhang P, Wang Y, Liu Y, Li X, Kumar BU, et al. Changes in metabolism and microbiota after 24-week risperidone treatment in drug naive, normal weight patients with first episode schizophrenia. *Schizophr Res* (2018) 201:299–306. doi: 10.1016/j.schres.2018.05.017

56. Nguyen TT, Kosciolek T, Maldonado Y, Daly RE, Martin AS, McDonald D, et al. Differences in gut microbiome composition between persons with chronic schizophrenia and healthy comparison subjects. *Schizophr Res* (2018) 204:23–9. doi: 10.1016/j.schres.2018.09.014

57. Shen Y, Xu JT, Li ZY, Huang YC, Yuan Y, Wang JX, et al. Analysis of gut microbiota diversity and auxiliary diagnosis as a biomarker in patients with schizophrenia: a cross-sectional study. *Schizophr Res* (2018) 197:470–7. doi: 10.1016/j.schres.2018.01.002

58. Yung AR, McGorry PD, McFarlane CA, Jackson HJ, Patton GC, Rakkar A. Monitoring and care of young people at incipient risk of psychosis. *Schizophr Bull* (1996) 22(2):283–303. doi: 10.1093/schbul/22.2.283

59. Yung AR. Treatment of people at ultra-high risk for psychosis. *World Psychiatry Off J World Psychiatr Assoc (WPA)* (2017) 16(2):207–8. doi: 10.1002/wps.20424

60. Nguyen NP, Warnow T, Pop M, White B. A perspective on 16S rRNA operational taxonomic unit clustering using sequence similarity. *NPJ Biofilms Microbiomes* (2016) 2:16004. doi: 10.1038/npjbiofilms.2016.4

61. Flowers SA, Evans SJ, Ward KM, McInnis MG, Ellingrod VL. Interaction Between Atypical Antipsychotics and the Gut Microbiome in a Bipolar Disease Cohort. *Pharmacotherapy* (2017) 37(3):261–7. doi: 10.1002/phar.1890

62. Graessler J, Qin Y, Zhong H, Zhang J, Licinio J, Wong ML, et al. Metagenomic sequencing of the human gut microbiome before and after bariatric surgery in obese patients with type 2 diabetes: correlation with inflammatory and metabolic parameters. *Pharmacogenomics J* (2013) 13

(6):514–22. doi: 10.1038/tpj.2012.43

63. Burcelin R, Garidou L, Pomie C. Immuno-microbiota cross and talk: the new paradigm of metabolic diseases. *Semin Immunol* (2012) 24(1):67–74. doi: 10.1016/j.smim.2011.11.011

64. Carvalho FA, Koren O, Goodrich JK, Johansson ME, Nalbantoglu I, Aitken JD, et al. Transient inability to manage proteobacteria promotes chronic gut inflammation in TLR5-deficient mice. *Cell Host Microbe* (2012) 12(2):139–52. doi: 10.1016/j.chom.2012.07.004

65. Martinez-Medina M, Denizot J, Dreux N, Robin F, Billard E, Bonnet R, et al. Western diet induces dysbiosis with increased E coli in CEABAC10 mice, alters host barrier function favouring AIEC colonisation. *Gut* (2014) 63 (1):116–24. doi: 10.1136/gutjnl-2012-304119

66. Castro-Nallar E, Bendall ML, Pérez-Losada M, Sabuncyan S, Severance EG, Dickerson FB, et al. Composition, taxonomy and functional diversity of the oropharynx microbiome in individuals with schizophrenia and controls. *PeerJ* (2015) 3(8):e1140. doi: 10.7717/peerj.1140

67. Jakobsson HE, Abrahamsson TR, Jenmalm MC, Harris K, Quince C, Jernberg C, et al. Decreased gut microbiota diversity, delayed Bacteroidetes colonisation and reduced Th1 responses in infants delivered by caesarean section. *Gut* (2014) 63(4):559–66. doi: 10.1136/gutjnl-2012-303249

68. Liou AP, Paziuk M, Luevano JMJr., Machineni S, Turnbaugh PJ, Kaplan LM. Conserved shifts in the gut microbiota due to gastric bypass reduce host weight and adiposity. *Sci Transl Med* (2013) 5(178):178ra41. doi: 10.1126/scitranslmed.3005687

69. Fei N, Zhao L. An opportunistic pathogen isolated from the gut of an obese human causes obesity in germfree mice. *ISME J* (2013) 7(4):880–4. doi: 10.1038/ismej.2012.153

70. Morgan XC, Tickle TL, Sokol H, Gevers D, Devaney KL, Ward DV, et al. Dysfunction of the intestinal microbiome in inflammatory bowel disease and treatment. *Genome Biol* (2012) 13(9):R79. doi: 10.1186/gb-2012-13-9-r79

71. Annamalai A, Kosir U, Tek C. Prevalence of obesity and diabetes in patients with schizophrenia. *World J Diabetes* (2017) 8(8):390–6. doi: 10.4239/wjd.v8.i8.390

72. Severance EG, Prandovszky E, Castiglione J, Yolken RH. Gastroenterology issues in schizophrenia: why the gut matters. *Curr Psychiatry Rep* (2015) 17 (5):27. doi: 10.1007/s11920-015-0574-0

73. Muller N, Weidinger E, Leitner B, Schwarz MJ. The role of inflammation in schizophrenia. *Front Neurosci* (2015) 9:372. doi: 10.3389/fnins.2015.00372

74. Hand TW, Vujkovic-Cvijin I, Ridaura VK, Belkaid Y. Linking the Microbiota, Chronic Disease, and the Immune System. *Trends Endocrinol Metab* (2016) 27(12):831–43. doi: 10.1016/j.tem.2016.08.003

75. Bahr SM, Tyler BC, Wooldridge N, Butcher BD, Burns TL, Teesch LM, et al. Use of the second-generation antipsychotic, risperidone, and secondary weight gain are associated with an altered gut microbiota in children. *Transl Psychiatry* (2015) 5:e652. doi: 10.1038/tp.2015.135

76. Nicholson JK, Holmes E, Kinross J, Burcelin R, Gibson G, Jia W, et al. Host-gut microbiota metabolic interactions. *Science* (2012) 336(6086):1262–7. doi: 10.1126/science.1223813

77. Lafaye A, Junot C, Ramounet-Le Gall B, Fritsch P, Ezan E, Tabet JC. Profiling of sulfoconjugates in urine by using precursor ion and neutral loss scans in tandem mass spectrometry. Application to the investigation of heavy metal toxicity in rats. *J Mass Spectrom* (2004) 39(6):655–64. doi: 10.1002/jms.635

78. Yolken RH, Severance EG, Sabunciyan S, Gressitt KL, Chen O, Stallings C, et al. Metagenomic Sequencing Indicates That the Oropharyngeal Phageome of Individuals With Schizophrenia Differs From That of Controls. *Schizophr Bull* (2015) 41(5):1153–61. doi: 10.1093/schbul/sbu197

79. Gispen-de Wied CC. Stress in schizophrenia: an integrative view. *Eur J Pharmacology* (2000) 405(1-3):375–84. doi: 10.1016/s0014-2999(00)00567-7

80. Bailey MT, Dowd SE, Galley JD, Hufnagle AR, Allen RG, Lyte M. Exposure to a social stressor alters the structure of the intestinal microbiota: implications for stressor-induced immunomodulation. *Brain Behav Immun* (2011) 25(3):397–407. doi: 10.1016/j.bbi.2010.10.023

81. Barka EA, Vatsa P, Sanchez L, Gaveau-Vaillant N, Jacquard C, Meier-Kolthoff JP, et al. Taxonomy, Physiology, and Natural Products of Actinobacteria. *Microbiol Mol Biol Rev* (2016) 80(1):1–43. doi: 10.1128/

MMBR.00019-15

82. Chen J, Wright K, Davis JM, Jeraldo P, Marietta EV, Murray J, et al. An expansion of rare lineage intestinal microbes characterizes rheumatoid arthritis. *Genome Med* (2016) 8(1):43. doi: 10.1186/s13073-016-0299-7

83. Wood NC, Hamilton I, Axon ATR, Khan SA, Quirke P, Mindham RHS, et al. Abnormal Intestinal Permeability. *Br J Psychiatry J Ment Sci* (2018) 150 (06):853–6. doi: 10.1192/bjp.150.6.853

84. Sahbaz C, Zibandeyeh N, Kurtulmuş A, Avaroglu G, Kırpınar İ, Sahin F, et al. F239. Role of Lymphocyte Subsets and T-Cell Profiles in the Immune Dysfunction of Schizophrenia. *Biol Psychiatry* (2018) 83(9):S331–S2. doi: 10.1016/j.biopsych.2018.02.853

85. Ding M, Song X, Zhao J, Gao J, Li X, Yang G, et al. Activation of Th17 cells in drug naive, first episode schizophrenia. *Prog Neuropsychopharmacol Biol Psychiatry* (2014) 51:78–82. doi: 10.1016/j.pnpbp.2014.01.001

86. Cabal A, Wassenaar TM, Ussery DW. Gender Differences in the Gut Microbiome and How These Affect Cardiovascular Diseases. *Gender Differences in the Pathogenesis and Management of Heart Disease*. (2018). p.89–100.

87. Yatsunenko T, Rey FE, Manary MJ, Trehan I, Dominguez-Bello MG, Contreras M, et al. Human gut microbiome viewed across age and geography. *Nature* (2012) 486(7402):222–7. doi: 10.1038/nature11053

88. Salazar N, Valdes-Varela L, Gonzalez S, Gueimonde M, de Los Reyes-Gavilan CG. Nutrition and the gut microbiome in the elderly. *Gut Microbes* (2017) 8(2):82–97. doi: 10.1080/19490976.2016.1256525

89. Franklin CL, Ericsson AC. Microbiota and reproducibility of rodent models. *Lab Anim (NY)* (2017) 46(4):114–22. doi: 10.1038/laban.1222

90. Penders J, Thijs C, Vink C, Stelma FF, Snijders B, Kummeling I, et al. Factors influencing the composition of the intestinal microbiota in early infancy. *Pediatrics* (2006) 118(2):511–21. doi: 10.1542/peds.2005-2824

91. Backhed F, Roswall J, Peng Y, Feng Q, Jia H, Kovatcheva-Datchary P, et al. Dynamics and Stabilization of the Human Gut Microbiome during the First Year of Life. *Cell Host Microbe* (2015) 17(5):690–703. doi: 10.1016/j.chom.2015.04.004

92. Dominguez-Bello MG, De Jesus-Laboy KM, Shen N, Cox LM, Amir A, Gonzalez A, et al. Partial restoration of the microbiota of cesarean-born infants via vaginal microbial transfer. *Nat Med* (2016) 22(3):250–3. doi: 10.1038/nm.4039

93. McGrath JJ, Féron FP, Burne THJ, Mackay-Sim A, Eyles DW. The neurodevelopmental hypothesis of schizophrenia: a review of recent developments. *Ann medicine* (2009) 35(2):86–93. doi: 10.1080/07853890310010005

94. Boksa P, El-Khodor BF. Birth insult interacts with stress at adulthood to alter dopaminergic function in animal models: possible implications for schizophrenia and other disorders. *Neurosci Biobehav Rev* (2003) 27(1-2):91–101. doi: 10.1016/s0149-7634(03)00012-5

95. Bailey MT, Coe CL. Maternal separation disrupts the integrity of the intestinal microflora in infant rhesus monkeys. *Dev Psychobiol* (1999) 35 (2):146–55. doi: 10.1002/(sici)1098-2302(199909)35:2<146::aid-dev7>3.0.co;2-g

96. O'Mahony SM, Marchesi JR, Scully P, Codling C, Ceolho AM, Quigley EM, et al. Early life stress alters behavior, immunity, and microbiota in rats: implications for irritable bowel syndrome and psychiatric illnesses. *Biol Psychiatry* (2009) 65(3):263–7. doi: 10.1016/j.biopsych.2008.06.026

97. Santos J, Yang PC, Soderholm JD, Benjamin M, Perdue MH. Role of mast cells in chronic stress induced colonic epithelial barrier dysfunction in the rat. *Gut* (2001) 48(5):630–6. doi: 10.1136/gut.48.5.630

98. Berger M, Juster RP, Westphal S, Amminger GP, Bogerts B, Schiltz K, et al. Allostatic load is associated with psychotic symptoms and decreases with antipsychotic treatment in patients with schizophrenia and first-episode psychosis. *Psychoneuroendocrinology* (2018) 90:35–42. doi: 10.1016/j.psyneuen.2018.02.001

99. Birley JLT, Brown GW. Crises and Life Changes preceding the Onset or Relapse of Acute Schizophrenia: Clinical Aspects. *Br J Psychiatry* (1970) 116 (532):327–33. doi: 10.1192/bjp.116.532.327

100. Norman RM, Malla AK. A prospective study of daily stressors and symptomatology in schizophrenic patients. *Soc Psychiatry Psychiatr Epidemiol* (1994) 29(6):244–9. doi: 10.1007/BF00802047

101. Reininghaus U, Kempton MJ, Valmaggia L, Craig TK, Garety P, Onyejiaka A, et al. Stress Sensitivity, Aberrant Salience, and Threat Anticipation in Early Psychosis: An Experience Sampling Study. *Schizophr Bull* (2016) 42 (3):712–22. doi: 10.1093/schbul/sbv190

102. Liberman RP, Mueser KT, Wallace CJ. Social skills training for schizophrenic individuals at risk for relapse. *Am J Psychiatry* (1986) 143(4):523–6. doi: 10.1176/ajp.143.4.523

103. Barrelet L, Ferrero F, Szigethy L, Giddey C, Pellizzer G. Expressed Emotion and First-Admission Schizophrenia. *Br J Psychiatry J Ment Sci* (2018) 156 (03):357–62. doi: 10.1192/bjp.156.3.357

104. Breier A, Buchanan RW. The effects of metabolic stress on plasma progesterone in healthy volunteers and schizophrenic patients. *Life Sci* (1992) 51(19):1527–34. doi: 10.1016/0024-3205(92)90563-5

105. Jansen LM, Gispen-de Wied CC, Kahn RS. Selective impairments in the stress response in schizophrenic patients. *Psychopharmacol (Berl)* (2000) 149 (3):319–25. doi: 10.1007/s002130000381

106. Berger M, Kraeuter AK, Romanik D, Malouf P, Amminger GP, Sarnyai Z. Cortisol awakening response in patients with psychosis: Systematic review and meta-analysis. *Neurosci Biobehav Rev* (2016) 68:157–66. doi: 10.1016/ j.neubiorev.2016.05.027

107. Torrey EF, Yolken RH. Toxoplasma gondii and schizophrenia. *Emerg Infect Dis* (2003) 9(11):1375–80. doi: 10.3201/eid0911.030143

108. Severance EG, Xiao J, Jones-Brando L, Sabunciyan S, Li Y, Pletnikov M, et al. Toxoplasma gondii-A Gastrointestinal Pathogen Associated with Human Brain Diseases. *Int Rev neurobiology* (2016) 131:143–63. doi: 10.1016/ bs.irn.2016.08.008

109. Prandovszky E, Li Y, Sabunciyan S, Steinfeldt CB, Avalos LN, Gressitt KL, et al. Toxoplasma gondii-Induced Long-Term Changes in the Upper Intestinal Microflora during the Chronic Stage of Infection. *Scientifica (Cairo)* (2018) 2018:2308619. doi: 10.1155/2018/2308619

110. Backhed F, Ding H, Wang T, Hooper LV, Koh GY, Nagy A, et al. The gut microbiota as an environmental factor that regulates fat storage. *Proc Natl Acad Sci U S A* (2004) 101(44):15718–23. doi: 10.1073/pnas. 0407076101

111. Kovatcheva-Datchary P, Arora T. Nutrition, the gut microbiome and the metabolic syndrome. *Best Pract Res Clin Gastroenterol* (2013) 27(1):59–72. doi: 10.1016/j.bpg.2013.03.017

112. Li H, Li T, Beasley DE, Hedenec P, Xiao Z, Zhang S, et al. Diet Diversity Is Associated with Beta but not Alpha Diversity of Pika Gut Microbiota. *Front microbiology* (2016) 7:1169. doi: 10.3389/fmicb.2016.01169

113. Blanton LV, Charbonneau MR, Salih T, Barratt MJ, Venkatesh S, Ilkaveya O, et al. Gut bacteria that prevent growth impairments transmitted by microbiota from malnourished children. *Science* (2016) 351(6275): aad3311. doi: 10.1126/science.aad3311

114. Russell WR, Gratz SW, Duncan SH, Holtrop G, Ince J, Scobbie L, et al. High-protein, reduced-carbohydrate weight-loss diets promote metabolite profiles likely to be detrimental to colonic health. *Am J Clin Nutr* (2011) 93(5):1062 72. doi: 10.3945/ajcn.110.002188

115. Newell C, Bomhof MR, Reimer RA, Hittel DS, Rho JM, Shearer J. Ketogenic diet modifies the gut microbiota in a murine model of autism spectrum disorder. *Mol Autism* (2016) 7(1):37. doi: 10.1186/s13229-016-0099-3

116. Hildebrandt MA, Hoffmann C, Sherrill-Mix SA, Keilbaugh SA, Hamady M, Chen YY, et al. High-fat diet determines the composition of the murine gut microbiome independently of obesity. *Gastroenterology* (2009) 137(5):1716 24 e1-2. doi: 10.1053/j.gastro.2009.08.042

117. Murphy EA, Velazquez KT, Herbert KM. Influence of high-fat diet on gut microbiota: a driving force for chronic disease risk. *Curr Opin Clin Nutr Metab Care* (2015) 18(5):515–20. doi: 10.1097/MCO.00000000 00000209

118. De Filippis F, Pellegrini N, Vannini L, Jeffery IB, La Storia A, Laghi L, et al. High-level adherence to a Mediterranean diet beneficially impacts the gut microbiota and associated metabolome. *Gut* (2016) 65(11):1812–21. doi: 10.1136/gutjnl-2015-309957

119. Strassnig M, Brar JS, Ganguli R. Dietary Intake of Patients with Schizophrenia. *Psychiatry (Edgmont)* (2005) 2(2):31–5.

120. Elman I, Borsook D, Lukas SE. Food intake and reward mechanisms in patients with schizophrenia: implications for metabolic disturbances and treatment with second-generation antipsychotic agents. *Neuropsychopharmacology* (2006) 31

(10):2091–120. doi: 10.1038/sj.npp.1301051

121. Brown S, Birtwistle J, Roe L, Thompson C. The unhealthy lifestyle of people with schizophrenia. *psychol Med* (1999) 29(3):697–701. doi: 10.1017/ S0033291798008186

122. Strassnig M, Brar JS, Ganguli R. Nutritional Assessment of Patients With Schizophrenia: A Preliminary Study. *Schizophr Bull* (2003) 29(2):393–7. doi: 10.1093/oxfordjournals.schbul.a007013

123. McCreadie R, Macdonald E, Blacklock C, Tilak-Singh D, Wiles D, Halliday J, et al. Dietary intake of schizophrenic patients in Nithsdale, Scotland: case-control study. *BMJ* (1998) 317(7161):784–5. doi: 10.1136/ bmj.317.7161.784

124. Zhang ZJ, Yao ZJ, Liu W, Fang Q, Reynolds GP. Effects of antipsychotics on fat deposition and changes in leptin and insulin levels. Magnetic resonance imaging study of previously untreated people with schizophrenia. *Br J Psychiatry J Ment Sci* (2004) 184:58–62. doi: 10.1192/bjp.184.1.58

125. Utzschneider KM, Kratz M, Damman CJ, Hullar M. Mechanisms Linking the Gut Microbiome and Glucose Metabolism. *J Clin Endocrinol Metab* (2016) 101(4):1445–54. doi: 10.1210/jc.2015-4251

126. Lambert JE, Myslicki JP, Bomhof MR, Belke DD, Shearer J, Reimer RA. Exercise training modifies gut microbiota in normal and diabetic mice. *Appl Physiol Nutr Metab* (2015) 40(7):749–52. doi: 10.1139/apnm-2014-0452

127. Zhao X, Zhang Z, Hu B, Huang W, Yuan C, Zou L. Response of Gut Microbiota to Metabolite Changes Induced by Endurance Exercise. *Front microbiology* (2018) 9:765:765. doi: 10.3389/fmicb.2018.00765

128. Allen JM, Mailing LJ, Niemiro GM, Moore R, Cook MD, White BA, et al. Exercise Alters Gut Microbiota Composition and Function in Lean and Obese Humans. *Med Sci Sports Exerc* (2018) 50(4):747–57. doi: 10.1249/ MSS.0000000000001495

129. Welly RJ, Liu TW, Zidon TM, Rowles JL,3, Park YM, Smith TN, et al. Comparison of Diet versus Exercise on Metabolic Function and Gut Microbiota in Obese Rats. *Med Sci Sports Exerc* (2016) 48(9):1688–98. doi: 10.1249/MSS.0000000000000964

130. Bressa C, Bailen-Andrino M, Perez-Santiago J, Gonzalez-Soltero R, Perez M, Montalvo-Lominchar MG, et al. Differences in gut microbiota profile between women with active lifestyle and sedentary women. *PloS One* (2017) 12(2):e0171352. doi: 10.1371/journal.pone.0171352

131. Clarke SF, Murphy EF, O'Sullivan O, Lucey AJ, Humphreys M, Hogan A, et al. Exercise and associated dietary extremes impact on gut microbial diversity. *Gut* (2014) 63(12):1913–20. doi: 10.1136/gutjnl-2013-306541

132. Munukka E, Ahtiainen JP, Puigbo P, Jalkanen S, Pahkala K, Keskitalo A, et al. Six-Week Endurance Exercise Alters Gut Metagenome That Is not Reflected in Systemic Metabolism in Over-weight Women. *Front microbiology* (2018) 9:2323:2323. doi: 10.3389/fmicb.2018.02323

133. Chamove AS. Positive short-term effects of activity on behavior in chronic schizophrenic pa- tients. *Br J Clin Psychol* (1986) 25:125–33. doi: 10.1111/ j.2044-8260.1986.tb00681.x

134. Vancampfort D, Stubbs B, Sienaert P, Wyckaert S, De Hert M, Soundy A, et al. A comparison of physical fitness in patients with bipolar disorder, schizophrenia and healthy controls. *Disabil Rehabil* (2016) 38(20):2047–51. doi: 10.3109/09638288.2015.1114037

135. Vogtmann E, Flores R, Yu G, Freedman ND, Shi J, Gail MH, et al. Association between tobacco use and the upper gastrointestinal microbiome among Chinese men. *Cancer Causes Control* (2015) 26 (4):581–8. doi: 10.1007/s10552-015-0535-2

136. Capurso G, Lahner E. The interaction between smoking, alcohol and the gut microbiome. *Best Pract Res Clin Gastroenterol* (2017) 31(5):579–88. doi: 10.1016/j.bpg.2017.10.006

137. Tomoda K, Kubo K, Asahara T, Andoh A, Nomoto K, Nishii Y, et al. Cigarette smoke decreases organic acids levels and population of bifidobacterium in the caecum of rats. *J Toxicol Sci* (2011) 36(3):261– doi: 10.2131/jts.36.261

138. Allais L, Kerckhof FM, Verschuere S, Bracke KR, De Smet R, Laukens D, et al. Chronic cigarette smoke exposure induces microbial and inflammatory shifts and mucin changes in the murine gut. *Environ Microbiol* (2016) 18 (5):1352–63. doi: 10.1111/1462-2920.12934

139. Wang H, Zhao JX, Hu N, Ren J, Du M, Zhu MJ. Side-stream smoking reduces intestinal inflammation and increases expression of tight junction proteins. *World J Gastroenterol* (2012) 18(18):2180–7. doi: 10.3748/wjg.v18.i18.2180

140. Rogers MA, Greene MT, Saint S, Chenoweth CE, Malani PN, Trivedi I, et al. Higher rates of Clostridium difficile infection among smokers. *PloS One* (2012) 7(7):e42091. doi: 10.1371/journal.pone.0042091

141. Biedermann L, Zeitz J, Mwinyi J, Sutter-Minder E, Rehman A, Ott SJ, et al. Smoking cessation induces profound changes in the composition of the intestinal microbiota in humans. *PloS One* (2013) 8(3):e59260. doi: 10.1371/journal.pone.0059260

142. Hartz SM, Pato CN, Medeiros H, Cavazos-Rehg P, Sobell JL, Knowles JA, et al. Comorbidity of severe psychotic disorders with measures of substance use. *JAMA Psychiatry* (2014) 71(3):248–54. doi: 10.1001/jamapsychiatry.2013.3726

143. Goodrich JK, Waters JL, Poole AC, Sutter JL, Koren O, Blekhman R, et al. Human genetics shape the gut microbiome. *Cell* (2014) 159(4):789–99. doi: 10.1016/j.cell.2014.09.053

144. Matheson SL, Shepherd AM, Pinchbeck RM, Laurens KR, Carr VJ. Childhood adversity in schizophrenia: a systematic meta-analysis. *psychol Med* (2013) 43(2):225–38. doi: 10.1017/S0033291712000785

145. Miyamoto S, Duncan GE, Marx CE, Lieberman JA. Treatments for schizophrenia: a critical review of pharmacology and mechanisms of action of antipsychotic drugs. *Mol Psychiatry* (2004) 10:79–104. doi: 10.1038/sj.mp.4001556

146. Davey KJ, Cotter PD, O'Sullivan O, Crispie F, Dinan TG, Cryan JF, et al. Antipsychotics and the gut microbiome: olanzapine-induced metabolic dysfunction is attenuated by antibiotic administration in the rat. *Transl Psychiatry* (2013) 3:e309. doi: 10.1038/tp.2013.83

147. Nadal I, Santacruz A, Marcos A, Warnberg J, Garagorri JM, Moreno LA, et al. Shifts in clostridia, bacteroides and immunoglobulin-coating fecal bacteria associated with weight loss in obese adolescents. *Int J Obes (Lond)* (2009) 33(7):758–67. doi: 10.1038/ijo.2008.260

148. Davey KJ, O'Mahony SM, Schellekens H, O'Sullivan O, Bienenstock J, Cotter PD, et al. Gender-dependent consequences of chronic olanzapine in the rat: effects on body weight, inflammatory, metabolic and microbiota parameters. *Psychopharmacol (Berl)* (2012) 221(1):155–69. doi: 10.1007/s00213-011-2555-2

149. Morgan AP, Crowley JJ, Nonneman RJ, Quackenbush CR, Miller CN, Ryan AK, et al. The Antipsychotic Olanzapine Interacts with the Gut Microbiome to Cause Weight Gain in Mouse. *PloS One* (2014) 9(12):e115225. doi: 10.1371/journal.pone.0115225

150. Kao AC, Spitzer S, Anthony DC, Lennox B, Burnet PWJ. Prebiotic attenuation of olanzapine-induced weight gain in rats: analysis of central and peripheral biomarkers and gut microbiota. *Transl Psychiatry* (2018) 8 (1):66. doi: 10.1038/s41398-018-0116-8

151. Bahr SM, Weidemann BJ, Castro AN, Walsh JW, deLeon O, Burnett CML, et al. Risperidone-induced weight gain is mediated through shifts in the gut microbiome and suppression of energy expenditure. *EBioMedicine* (2015) 2 (11):1725–34. doi: 10.1016/j.ebiom.2015.10.018

152. Shilling PD, Feifel D. Potential of Oxytocin in the Treatment of Schizophrenia. *CNS Drugs* (2016) 30(3):193–208. doi: 10.1007/s40263-016-0315-x

153. Erdman SE, Poutahidis T. Microbes and Oxytocin: Benefits for Host Physiology and Behavior. *Int Rev neurobiology* (2016) 131:91–126. doi: 10.1016/bs.irn.2016.07.004

154. Kohler-Forsberg O, Petersen L, Gasse C, Mortensen PB, Dalsgaard S, Yolken RH, et al. A Nationwide Study in Denmark of the Association Between Treated Infections and the Subsequent Risk of Treated Mental Disorders in Children and Adolescents. *JAMA Psychiatry* (2018) 76(3):271–9. doi: 10.1001/jamapsychiatry.2018.3428

155. Lydholm CN, Kohler-Forsberg O, Nordentoft M, Yolken RH, Mortensen PB, Petersen L, et al. Parental Infections Before, During, and After Pregnancy as Risk Factors for Mental Disorders in Childhood and Adolescence: A Nationwide Danish Study. *Biol Psychiatry* (2019) 85(4):317–25. doi: 10.1016/j.biopsych.2018.09.013

156. Mednick SA, Machon RA, Huttunen MO, Bonett D. Adult schizophrenia following prenatal exposure to an influenza epidemic. *Arch Gen Psychiatry* (1988) 45(2):189–92. doi: 10.1001/archpsyc.1988.01800260109013

157. Ng QX, Soh AYS, Venkatanarayanan N, Ho CYX, Lim DY. Yeo WS. A Systematic Review of the Effect of Probiotic Supplementation on Schizophrenia Symptoms. *Neuropsychobiology* (2019) 78(1):1–6. doi: 10.1159/000498862

158. Zhang F, Luo W, Shi Y, Fan Z, Ji G. Should we standardize the 1,700-year-old fecal microbiota transplantation? *Am J gastroenterology* (2012) 107(11):1755. doi: 10.1038/ajg.2012.251. author reply p -6.

159. Borody T, Leis S, Campbell J, Torres M, Nowak A. Fecal microbiota transplantation (FMT) in multiple sclerosis (MS). *Am J gastroenterology* (2011) 106:S352. doi: 10.14309/00000434-201110002-00942

160. Oya K, Kishi T, Iwata N. Efficacy and tolerability of minocycline augmentation therapy in schizophrenia: a systematic review and meta-analysis of randomized controlled trials. *Hum Psychopharmacol* (2014) 29 (5):483–91. doi: 10.1002/hup.2426

161. Deakin B, Suckling J, Barnes TRE, Byrne K, Chaudhry IB, Dazzan P, et al. The benefit of minocycline on negative symptoms of schizophrenia in patients with recent-onset psychosis (BeneMin): a randomised, double-blind, placebo-controlled trial. *Lancet Psychiatry* (2018) 5(11):885–94. doi: 10.1016/s2215-0366(18)30345-6

162. Kraeuter AK, Loxton H, Lima BC, Rudd D, Sarnyai Z. Ketogenic diet reverses behavioral abnormalities in an acute NMDA receptor hypofunction model of schizophrenia. *Schizophr Res* (2015) 169(1-3):491–3. doi: 10.1016/j.schres.2015.10.041

163. Kraeuter AK, van den Buuse M, Sarnyai Z. Ketogenic diet prevents impaired prepulse inhibition of startle in an acute NMDA receptor hypofunction model of schizophrenia. *Schizophr Res* (2019) 206:244–50. doi: 10.1016/j.schres.2018.11.011

13

The Role of Diet in Functional Dyspepsia Management

Henri Duboc [1,2,3], Sofya Latrache [1,2], Nicoleta Nebunu [2] and Benoit Coffin [1,2]*

[1] Université de Paris, Paris, France, [2] AP-HP, Gastroenterology Unit, Hopital Louis Mourier, Colombes, France, [3] INSERM UMR 1149, Université de Paris, Paris, France

*Correspondence:
Benoit Coffin
benoit.coffin@aphp.fr

Functional dyspepsia is a common functional gastrointestinal disease that is characterized by postprandial fullness, early satiation, epigastric pain, and/or epigastric burning. Eating a meal is a key factor in the occurrence of symptoms during functional dyspepsia, and patients frequently request dietary advice that could relieve these symptoms. Eating behaviors, irregular meal patterns, and moderate-to-fast eating rates are significantly associated with functional dyspepsia. The role of diet is complex; fat ingestion increases the occurrence of symptoms in dyspeptic patients, which might be affected by cognitive factors and palatability. Data concerning the role of carbohydrates are conflicting. Wheat may induce symptoms in patients with nonceliac gluten/wheat sensitivity, and gluten-free diets might be beneficial. Data concerning the role of FODMAPs (Fructo, Oligo, Di-, Monosaccharides, And Polyols) in functional dyspepsia are lacking; however, as there is a frequent overlap between functional dyspepsia and irritable bowel syndrome, a diet that is low in FODMAPs might be useful in relieving some symptoms. Data concerning alcohol are also conflicting. Adherence to a Mediterranean diet seems to be associated with a decrease in dyspepsia symptoms. Finally, data concerning diet modifications are conflicting, and the impact of diet modifications on symptom intensity or frequency has never been reported in randomized prospective studies. Common sense dietary recommendations, such as eating slowly and regularly, as well as decreasing the fat content of meals, can be provided in daily clinical practice.

Keywords: functional dyspepsia, diet, eating behaviour, fat, gluten, FODMAPs, alcohol

INTRODUCTION

Functional dyspepsia is a common functional disease that affects up to 20% of the population, and it is believed to originate from the gastro-duodenal region (1). According to the Rome IV criteria, functional dyspepsia is defined by one or more of the following symptoms: bothersome postprandial fullness, bothersome early satiation, bothersome epigastric pain, and/or bothersome epigastric burning, with no evidence of structural diseases, including the use of an upper endoscopy (if necessary), according to age, past history, or presence of alarm symptoms in the patient (2). Symptoms must be present for at least 3 days a week during the last 3 months and must be chronic, with an onset of at least 6 months before the diagnosis. Two subgroups of dyspepsia have been identified. Postprandial distress syndrome is defined by bothersome postprandial fullness, such as fullness that is severe enough to have an impact on typical activities, and/or bothersome early satiation, such as satiation that is severe enough to prevent the completion of a regular size meal. Epigastric pain syndrome is defined by bothersome epigastric pain and/or epigastric burning, which are both severe enough to have an impact on usual activities (2). In most patients, there is a temporal relationship between meal ingestion and the occurrence of symptoms during postprandial distress syndrome and during epigastric pain syndrome, but also symptoms are not necessarily associated with a meal, as pain can be induced or relieved by the ingestion of a meal or may occur during fasting (2).

FUNCTIONAL DYSPEPSIA AND MEAL INGESTION

Meal ingestion is clearly a triggering factor of the symptoms in dyspeptic patients. In a cohort of 218 patients with functional dyspepsia, Bisschops et al. demonstrated that the intensity of dyspeptic symptoms occurred rapidly (within 15 min) after ingestion of a test meal and remained elevated until the end of the measurement period (4 h) (3). The time course of the development of the individual symptoms varied, with early peaks for fullness and bloating, intermediate peaks for nausea and belching, and late peaks for pain and burning (3). Meal-induced aggravation of symptoms was reported by 79% of patients and was not associated with a decrease in the gastric-emptying rate, as only 20% of the patients had a delayed gastric emptying. These results suggest that factors other than gastric motility may explain the development of symptoms. Hypersensitivity to gastric distension has been demonstrated as one of the key pathophysiological factors in patients with functional dyspepsia during fasting and during the postprandial period (4, 5). In this latter, gastric distension was demonstrated to induce more intense symptoms in patients than in control individuals and to reproduce spontaneous symptoms. The highest symptom severity scores were obtained for postprandial fullness and bloating, whereas the lowest score was obtained for epigastric burning (5). Gastric distension was also associated with impaired gastric accommodation to meals (5). Finally, Di Stefano et al. demonstrated that, in comparison to healthy controls, gastric postprandial hypersensitivity and relationship between symptoms intensity and postprandial discomfort threshold were significant only in patients with postprandial distress syndrome and not in patients with epigastric pain syndrome (6). As eating a meal is a key factor in the occurrence of symptoms during functional dyspepsia, patients frequently request dietary advice that could relieve these symptoms.

EATING BEHAVIOR AND FUNCTIONAL DYSPEPSIA

In normal conditions, meal ingestion induces fundic accommodation with subsequently slow contractions, antral contractions, and finally, gastric emptying. As it has been previously reported, gastric fundic accommodation, as measured by an electronic barostat, is significantly impaired in patients with functional dyspepsia (5). A rapid drinking test, which is a noninvasive test, has been proposed as a diagnostic method to evoke the symptoms of functional dyspepsia, and it has been shown that the occurrence of dyspeptic symptoms is related to impaired gastric accommodation (7). In the daily lives of patients, abnormal eating behaviors, such as rapid or large volume meal ingestion (conditions that are reproduced during the rapid drinking test), may overload the gastric accommodation process, thus generating symptoms. In small cohorts of patients, the results have been conflicting, with some authors observing a relationship with dietary patterns, such as eating quickly, and the occurrence of symptoms (8, 9), whereas other authors have not observed this relationship (10). Recently, in a large cohort of 4,763 Iranian adults, and through the use of the technique known as latent class analysis (which is a person-centered approach that provides a unique opportunity to classify individuals according to behavioral subclasses), Keshteli et al. (11) found a prevalence of dyspepsia of 15.2%. Furthermore, these authors could identify that irregular meal patterns [odds ratio (OR): 1.42; 95% CI: 1.12–1.78] and moderate-to-fast eating rates (OR: 1.42; 95% CI: 1.15–1.75) were significantly associated with chronic uninvestigated dyspepsia. Meal-to-sleep intervals and intrameal fluid intake, which were the other two domains that were investigated, were not associated with dyspepsia (11). This study has some limitations as the evaluation of patients was made only by questionnaire, the use of translated modified Rome III questionnaire, and the lack of systematic endoscopic evaluation, but it confirms the observations that were made during the provocative tests. The physiology of food intake is complex; besides gastric distension induced by volume of meal ingestion, meal temperature may also modify gastric perception as cold temperature may induce smooth muscle contraction (12). In a small study of patient with epigastric pain syndrome, Wang et al. (13) demonstrated that gastric perfusion with an 8°C liquid induced significant gastric contraction and decreased gastric sensory threshold in comparison to a 37°C liquid infusion. Even if no interventional studies have been reported so far, we can still recommend that patients eat slowly (which is probably more important in the subgroup of patients with delayed gastric emptying) and regularly and probably avoid cold liquid ingestion.

NUTRIENTS AND FUNCTIONAL DYSPEPSIA

Fat

Dietary fat is ingested in a number of different forms, depending on the type of food that is eaten (i.e., extracellular vs. intracellular fat), the meal temperature (solid fat vs. oil), and the proportion of fat ingested with other macronutrients. A high-fat diet is frequently associated with high carbohydrate content or high protein content. In normal conditions, a high-fat meal is associated with a decrease in the gastric emptying rate (14). A prospective cross-sectional study that was performed in delegates attending a conference on four consecutive days demonstrated that a low-fat, low-calorie dinner induced significantly fewer symptoms than a high-calorie dinner (15). During a mechanistic study with gastric distension, intraduodenal fat infusion, but not an infusion with carbohydrates, induced a greater intensity of symptoms in dyspeptic patients (16). In an experimental condition with a similar calorie intake, a high-fat meal induced more symptoms than a high-carbohydrate meal in dyspeptic patients, with symptoms including nausea, bloating, postprandial fullness, and epigastric pain (17). Carvalho et al. (18) reported no differences in the total caloric intake between 41 patients with functional dyspepsia and 30 healthy controls; however, these authors found a significant reduction in fat intake (28% vs. 34%). These results were not confirmed by other authors (19). Cognitive factors may also contribute to the occurrence of symptoms by fat ingestion in patients with functional dyspepsia. In a randomized study, Feinle-Bisset et al. demonstrated that high-fat foods elicited more symptoms than low-fat foods; however, low-fat foods elicited similar symptoms if the patients perceived these foods to be high-fat foods even if they were not (20). Finally, meal palatability may also interfere with the occurrence of symptoms (21). No interventional study testing the long-term effects of a low-fat diet on symptoms has been reported so far. It is likely that dyspeptic patients, especially patients with severe symptoms, have determined for themselves that lipids can increase their typical symptoms. Therefore, these patients will spontaneously decrease their degree of fat ingestion; if they do not adjust their diet, then a low-fat diet could be recommended.

Proteins and Gluten

No study has reported a relationship between symptoms and the intake of proteins. Functional symptoms, irritable bowel syndrome (IBS), and dyspepsia are frequent occurrences in patients with celiac disease, with an OR of 4.48 for biopsy-proven celiac disease in patients fulfilling the Rome criteria for IBS (95% CI: 2.33–8.60) (22). However, the risk of celiac disease in patients with functional dyspepsia does not seem to be increased (23). Conversely, during an observational study in a cohort of 85 patients with diagnosed celiac disease, 27% of the patients fulfilled the criteria of functional dyspepsia upon inclusion, and only 8% of the patients remained dyspeptic after consuming a gluten-free diet for 1 year (24). More recently, the concept of nonceliac gluten/wheat sensitivity has emerged in the literature (25). Nonceliac gluten/wheat sensitivity is a syndrome that is characterized by intestinal and extra-intestinal symptoms related to the ingestion of gluten-containing food, and this syndrome occurs in subjects who are not affected by either celiac disease or wheat allergies (26). Dyspeptic symptoms are frequent in patients with nonceliac gluten/wheat sensitivity, with approximately 50% of patients having reported nausea or epigastric pain in an Italian cohort (27) and 31.3% in an Australian cohort (28). Patients having dyspepsia reported more frequently symptoms of postprandial distress syndrome (26%) than epigastric pain syndrome (17%), and differences for both subtypes were significant in comparison to the control

group (postprandial distress syndrome: OR 2.98, CI 95%: 2.34–3.79; epigastric pain syndrome: OR 3.17, CI 95%: 1.31–3.50) (28). In these patients, Elli et al. demonstrated that, during a double-blind crossover study, gluten-free diets induced a significant decrease in postprandial fullness, early satiety, and epigastric pain (29). However, this study has some limits as symptoms were evaluated by visual analogic scale and not specific questionnaire, and also in the whole group of patients and not only in those identified with isolated dyspeptic symptoms. However, there is increasing popularity in the general population that a gluten-free diet may be "healthier," despite a lack of evidence to support this notion, as 8%–16% of the western population adheres to a gluten-free diet, which has resulted in a gluten-free food industry boom of an estimated $6 billion per year (25). The long-term nutritional impact of a gluten-free diet is still a matter of debate; adults adhering to a gluten-free diet did not consume enough nutrient-dense foods to meet all nutritional recommendations (30). Also, some patients who begin avoiding dietary gluten with the intention of improving their health and well-being may ultimately progress to develop pathologically obsessive behaviors regarding their diet (30). Results of well–conducted, randomized, controlled clinical trials testing the effects of gluten-free diet in dyspeptic patients are still lacking to clearly recommend such diet in patients. In daily clinical practice, if a diagnosis of celiac disease has been ruled out with a negative test of anti-transglutaminase antibodies and if a dyspeptic patient asks for the efficacy of gluten-free diet, then a short (4–8 weeks) gluten-free diet test period could be suggested, but this diet should be continued only if the symptoms decrease significantly according to patient's perception with a good clinical evaluation.

Carbohydrates

Only three studies have examined the relationships between carbohydrates and dyspeptic symptoms, with conflicting results. One study reported a lower carbohydrate intake being associated with the occurrence of symptoms (31), which was possibly related to the lower energy intake that was reported in this study. Another study reported a daily intake of carbohydrates in dyspeptic patients in comparison to controls (230 vs. 199 g/day), but the difference was not significant (18), and one study reported no relationship between symptoms and a high-carbohydrate meal (17). Thus, no specific recommendation can be made.

FODMAPS AND FUNCTIONAL DYSPEPSIA

FODMAPs (Fructo, Oligo, Di-, Monosaccharides And Polyols) are poorly absorbable and highly fermentable substances that may induce bloating and gas sensations, which are common symptoms in dyspepsia, even if they do not specifically appear in the Rome IV diagnostic criteria. By using specific dietary questionnaires, it has been shown in several studies that dyspepsia is associated with grain/pasta/wheat products, soft drinks/carbonated drinks, fruit/fruit juice/watermelon, milk, and takeout/processed foods (e.g., pizza/fried foods) (32). Most of these foods contain a large proportion of FODMAPs. Several studies have clearly demonstrated that a low-FODMAPs diet significantly decreases symptoms in IBS patients (33). The overlap between IBS and dyspepsia is frequent and, in daily clinical settings, the overlap of both of these syndromes has occurred in 64% in patient questionnaires vs. 23% in routine clinical documentations (34). Thus, this overlap appears to be a normal occurrence, rather than an exception. However, the intensity of dyspeptic symptoms has never been specifically reported during the clinical studies that reported a beneficial effect of a low-FODMAPs diet in IBS patients (33). Indeed, further randomized studies that are specifically performed with dyspeptic patients are needed to recommend a low-FODMAPs diet in dyspeptic patients as during IBS. However, it could be suggested in some dyspeptic patients with IBS symptoms and/or bloating, with a 4- to 8-week test period.

ULTRA-PROCESSED FOODS AND FUNCTIONAL DYSPEPSIA

Ultra-processed foods (UPFs) are industrial formulations that are usually made from substances derived from foods and additives by using a multitude of sequential processes to create the final product (hence the term "ultra-processed"). UPFs are typically branded, convenient (durable and ready to consume), and hyperpalatable food products that tend to displace fresh or minimally processed foods, as well as freshly prepared dishes and meals. UPFs are characterized by a high density of saturated fatty acids, sugars, and sodium, as well as a low content of fiber. In a large cohort of 33,343 subjects from the web-based NutriNet-Santé cohort who responded to dietary and Rome III questionnaires, Schnabel et al. demonstrated that the proportion of UPFs in the diets was not associated with symptoms in subjects who had pure functional dyspepsia (OR: 1.066; 95% CI: 0.97–1.16), whereas it was significantly associated with symptoms in patients who had IBS (OR: 1.09; 95% CI: 1.04–1.14) and in patients with associations of both IBS and functional dyspepsia (OR: 1.14; 95% CI: 1.05–1.24) (35). No interventional studies have been reported; however, we can recommend that not only patients but also the whole population should decrease the intake of UPFs, which also include additives, contact material, or neo-formed contaminants frequently not or poorly detailed in their formula (35), and should increase the intake of fresh and tasty foods.

ALCOHOL AND FUNCTIONAL DYSPEPSIA

Alcohol interferes with normal gastric physiology. Alcohol can increase gastric acid secretion, with low doses accelerating gastric emptying and high doses delaying gastric emptying (36). When considering the effects of alcohol on dyspepsia, the results are also conflicting. Some studies have not demonstrated any relationship between the occurrence of new dyspeptic symptoms and the severity of dyspepsia, postprandial distress syndrome, or epigastric pain syndrome (regardless of the subgroups) (37, 38). On the other hand, a large cohort study demonstrated that in 4,390 subjects, there was a relationship between the consumption of greater than seven alcoholic drinks a week and dyspeptic symptoms (OR: 2.3; CI 95%: 1.1–5.0) (39). Thus, it is difficult to determine if alcohol induces or not dyspeptic symptoms. As chronic alcohol consumption is not healthy, we can recommend decreasing the level of alcohol consumption in dyspeptic patients, as in all other conditions, with a maximum intake of 10 units a week in both men and women according to the WHO recommendations (40).

SPICY FOODS

Capsaicin is the active component of spicy foods (chili, red pepper …). It has a dual effect with first activation of C-afferent fibers, sensitization that increases symptoms, followed by desensitization that decreases symptoms. Capsaicin test, that is, ingestion of 0.75 mg capsule of capsaicin, has been proposed as a simple diagnostic test to reproduce symptoms in the subgroup of dyspeptic patients with gastric chemosensitivity (41, 42). A randomized study with only 30 patients (15 in each group) demonstrated that oral supplements with 2.5 g red pepper powder during 5 weeks induced a significant decrease in dyspeptic symptoms overall and also epigastric pain or fullness; two patients of the red pepper group had to rapidly stop the study because of an increase of abdominal pain (43). There is no sufficient convincing clinical data to recommend the chronic ingestion of spicy foods to decrease symptoms in dyspeptic patients; however, we can strongly recommend avoiding occasional intake of spicy foods, which probably could increase symptoms.

COFFEE AND FUNCTIONAL DYSPEPSIA

Coffee consumption increases gastric acid secretion (44). Coffee consumption has also been found to induce dyspeptic symptoms (8, 18, 44), whereas in one study, no association was found (37). Thus, it is difficult to conclude on the effects of coffee consumption on dyspeptic symptoms, but patients have been observed to frequently and spontaneously decrease coffee consumption.

IS THERE A GOOD DIET FOR DYSPEPTIC PATIENTS?

The relationships between diet and dyspepsia complaints are complex and, except for fat, no clear recommendations based on randomized trials can be proposed to patients. Common sense advice can be provided to the patients, with recommendations

TABLE 1 | Common sense dietary recommendations that could be provided to patients with functional dyspepsia.

Eat slowly and regularly.
Decrease fat intake.
Try to observe a diet that is more similar to a Mediterranean diet or increase the intake of fresh foods and decrease the intake of ultra-processed foods.
Decrease coffee and alcohol consumption.
A gluten-free diet and a low-FODMAPs diet could be tested over a short time period (4–8 weeks) and must be stopped if there is no efficacy.
Be careful in providing strong recommendations to obsessive patients, and avoid the recommendation of very restrictive diets.

No interventional studies have been reported thus far.

including slow and regular eating, decreasing fat intake, possibly testing a gluten-free diet or a low-FODMAPs diet over short-term periods, avoiding coffee, and having a low alcohol intake (**Table 1**). Recommendations in observing a Mediterranean diet could also likely be performed. A Mediterranean diet is considered to be a complex set of eating habits adopted by people in countries bordering the Mediterranean Sea. This diet includes a high consumption of olive oil, fiber-rich foods, milk, or dairy products, in addition to a low consumption of meat or meat-based products. In the last few years, this dietary regimen has been proposed as a health-protective diet because populations who have adopted it exhibit a remarkable reduction in all-cause mortality, especially from cardiovascular diseases and cancer, and when compared to the United States or Northern European countries. Recently, *via* the use of a questionnaire that measured adherence to a Mediterranean diet, Zito et al. (45) demonstrated that in a population of 1,134 subjects, a lower adherence to a Mediterranean diet was significantly associated with the occurrence of dyspepsia (adherence score: 0.56 ± 0.24) and of IBS (adherence score: 0.57 ± 0.23), in comparison to controls (adherence score: 0.62 ± 0.21), mainly in the 17–24 and 25–34 age groups. With increasing age, patients have tended to adopt dietary regimens that are more similar to Mediterranean diets and, consequently, have fewer symptoms. From this observational study, it cannot be concluded if Mediterranean diet will decrease symptoms by itself or if it has a preventive effect on the occurrence of dyspeptic symptoms.

LIMITS OF DIETETIC RECOMMENDATIONS IN PATIENTS WITH FUNCTIONAL DYSPEPSIA

In patients with functional dyspepsia, weight loss is considered an alarm sign that much leads to complementary examinations (2). However, in dyspeptic patients referred to tertiary referral centers, weight loss >5% is not exceptional as it can occur in around 40% of patients with epigastric pain syndrome as well as postprandial distress syndrome (46). In this study, weight loss was significantly higher in patients with early satiety and vomiting. It is highly probable that weight loss occurred because patients limit, consciously or unconsciously, their oral intake to decrease symptom intensity. In this condition, dietetic approach is limited, and specialized advice with dietician must be performed in order to try to regain weight.

CONCLUSION

Food is clearly a triggering factor for dyspeptic symptoms in the majority of patients. However, the relationships between nutrients, except for fat, or other specific foods and the onset or intensity of dyspeptic symptoms have been poorly evaluated, and there is a lack of high-quality evidence to guide dietary therapies in functional dyspepsia. The effects of a gluten-free diet or a low-FODMAPs diet could be tested during interventional studies. Large cohort studies are also necessary to better identify the relationships between food and dyspepsia. As no clear recommendations are available, only common sense dietetic recommendations can be provided during daily clinical practice (**Table 1**). However, we must be very cautious, as some obsessive patients may observe very restrictive diets inducing nutritional deficiency.

AUTHOR CONTRIBUTIONS

HD and BC wrote the manuscript. SL and NN made the literature review.

REFERENCES

1. Ford AC. Aetiopathogenesis of functional dyspepsia. *Gut* (2015) 64:1182–3. doi: 10.1136/gutjnl-2014-308959
2. Stanghellini V, Chan FKL, Hasler WL, Malagelada JR, Suzuki H, Tack J, et al. Gastroduodenal Disorders. *Gastroenterology* (2016) 150:1380–92. doi: 10.1053/j.gastro.2016.02.011
3. Bisschops R, Karamanolis G, Arts J, Caenepeel P, Verbeke K, Janssens J, et al. Relationship between symptoms and ingestion of a meal in functional dyspepsia. *Gut* (2008) 57:1495–503. doi: 10.1136/gut.2007.137125
4. Coffin B, Azpiroz F, Guarner F, Malagelada JR. Selective gastric hypersensitivity and reflex hyporeactivity in functional dyspepsia. *Gastroenterology* (1994) 107:1345–51. doi: 10.1016/0016-5085(94)90536-3
5. Farre R, Vanheel H, Vanuytsel T, Masaoka T, Tornblom H, Simren M, et al.

In functional dyspepsia, hypersensitivity to postprandial distention correlates with meal-related symptom severity. *Gastroenterology* (2013) 145:566–73. doi: 10.1053/j.gastro.2013.05.018
6. Di Stefano M, Miceli E, Tana P, Mengoli C, Bergonzi M, Pagani E, et al. Fasting and postprandial gastric sensorimotor activity in functional dyspepsia: postprandial distress vs. epigastric pain syndrome. *Am J Gastroenterol* (2014) 109:1631–9. doi: 10.1038/ajg.2014.231
7. van den Elzen BD, Bennink RJ, Holman R, Tytgat GN, Boeckxstaens GE. Impaired drinking capacity in patients with functional dyspepsia: intragastric distribution and distal stomach volume. *Neurogastroenterol Motil* (2007) 19:968 –76. doi: 10.1111/j.1365-2982.2007.00971.x
8. Filipovic BF, Randjelovic T, Kovacevic N, Milinic N, Markovic O, Gajic M, et al. Laboratory parameters and nutritional status in patients with functional dyspepsia. *Eur J Intern Med* (2011) 22:300–4. doi: 10.1016/j.ejim.2011.01.012
9. Sinn DH, Shin DH, Lim SW, Kim K-M, Son HJ, Kim JJ, et al. The speed of

eating and functional dyspepsia in young women. *Gut Liver* (2010) 4:173–8. doi: 10.5009/gnl.2010.4.2.173

10. Cuperus P, Keeling PW, Gibney MJ. Eating patterns in functional dyspepsia: a case control study. *Eur J Clin Nutr* (1996) 50:520–3.

11. Keshteli AH, Feizi A, Esmaillzadeh A, Zaribaf F, Feinle-Bisset C, Talley NJ, et al. Patterns of dietary behaviours identified by latent class analysis are associated with chronic uninvestigated dyspepsia. *Br J Nutr* (2015) 113:803–12. doi: 10.1017/S0007114514004140

12. Villanova N, Azpiroz F, Malagelada JR. Perception and gut reflexes induced by stimulation of gastrointestinal thermoreceptors in humans. *J Physiol* (1997) 502:215–22. doi: 10.1111/j.1469-7793.1997.215bl.x

13. Wang R-F, Wang Z-F, Ke M-Y, Fang X-C, Sun X-H, Zhu L-M, et al. Temperature can influence gastric accommodation and sensitivity in functional dyspepsia with epigastric pain syndrome. *Dig Dis Sci* (2013) 58:2550–5. doi: 10.1007/s10620-012-2363-5

14. Feinle-Bisset C, Azpiroz F. Dietary lipids and functional gastrointestinal disorders. *Am J Gastroenterol* (2013) 108:737–47. doi: 10.1038/ajg.2013.76

15. Parker HL, Curcic J, Heinrich H, Sauter M, Hollenstein M, Schwizer W, et al. What to eat and drink in the festive season: a pan-European, observational, cross-sectional study. *Eur J Gastroenterol Hepatol* (2017) 29:608–14. doi: 10.1097/MEG.0000000000000829

16. Barbera R, Feinle C, Read NW. Nutrient-specific modulation of gastric mechanosensitivity in patients with functional dyspepsia. *Dig Dis Sci* (1995) 40:1636–41. doi: 10.1007/BF02212683

17. Pilichiewicz AN, Feltrin KL, Horowitz M, Holtmann G, Wishart JM, Jones KL, et al. Functional dyspepsia is associated with a greater symptomatic response to fat but not carbohydrate, increased fasting and postprandial CCK, and diminished PYY. *Am J Gastroenterol* (2008) 103:2613–23. doi: 10.1111/j.1572-0241.2008.02041.x

18. Carvalho RVB, Lorena SLS, Almeida JR de S, Mesquita MA. Food intolerance, diet composition, and eating patterns in functional dyspepsia patients. *Dig Dis Sci* (2010) 55:60–5. doi: 10.1007/s10620-008-0698-8

19. Pilichiewicz AN, Horowitz M, Holtmann GJ, Talley NJ, Feinle-Bisset C. Relationship between symptoms and dietary patterns in patients with functional dyspepsia. *Clin Gastroenterol Hepatol* (2009) 7:317–22. doi: 10.1016/j.cgh.2008.09.007

20. Feinle-Bisset C, Meier B, Fried M, Beglinger C. Role of cognitive factors in symptom induction following high and low fat meals in patients with functional dyspepsia. *Gut* (2003) 52:1414–8. doi: 10.1136/gut.52.10.1414

21. Pribic T, Hernandez L, Nieto A, Malagelada C, Accarino A, Azpiroz F. Effects of meal palatability on postprandial sensations. *Neurogastroenterol Motil* (2018) 30:e13248. doi: 10.1111/nmo.13248

22. Irvine AJ, Chey WD, Ford AC. Screening for celiac disease in irritable bowel syndrome: an updated systematic review and meta-analysis. *Am J Gastroenterol* (2017) 112:65–76. doi: 10.1038/ajg.2016.466

23. Lasa J, Spallone L, Gandara S, Chaar E, Berman S, Zagalsky D. Celiac disease prevalence is not increased in patients with functional dyspepsia. *Arq Gastroenterol* (2017) 54:37–40. doi: 10.1590/s0004-2803.2017v54n1-07

24. Silvester JA, Graff LA, Rigaux L, Bernstein CN, Leffler DA, Kelly CP, et al. Symptoms of functional intestinal disorders are common in patients with celiac disease following transition to a gluten-free diet. *Dig Dis Sci* (2017) 62:2449–54. doi: 10.1007/s10620-017-4666-z

25. Potter MDE, Walker MM, Keely S, Talley NJ. What's in a name? « Non-coeliac gluten or wheat sensitivity »: controversies and mechanisms related to wheat and gluten causing gastrointestinal symptoms or disease. *Gut* (2018) 67:2073–7. doi: 10.1136/gutjnl-2018-316360

26. Catassi C, Elli L, Bonaz B, Bouma G, Carroccio A, Castillejo G, et al. Diagnosis of non-celiac gluten sensitivity (NCGS): the salerno experts' criteria. *Nutrients* (2015) 7:4966–77. doi: 10.3390/nu7064966

27. Volta U, Bardella MT, Calabro A, Troncone R, Corazza GR. An Italian prospective multicenter survey on patients suspected of having non-celiac gluten sensitivity. *BMC Med* (2014) 12:85. doi: 10.1186/1741-7015-12-85

28. Potter MDE, Walker MM, Jones MP, Koloski NA, Keely S, Talley NJ. Wheat intolerance and chronic gastrointestinal symptoms in an australian population-based study: association between wheat sensitivity, celiac disease and functional gastrointestinal disorders. *Am J Gastroenterol* (2018) 113:1036–44. doi: 10.1038/s41395-018-0095-7

29. Elli L, Tomba C, Branchi F, Roncoroni L, Lombardo V, Bardella MT, et al. Evidence for the presence of non-celiac gluten sensitivity in patients with functional gastrointestinal symptoms: results from a multicenter randomized double-blind placebo-controlled gluten challenge. *Nutrients* (2016) 8:84. doi: 10.3390/nu8020084

30. Niland B, Cash BD. Health benefits and adverse effects of a gluten-free diet in non-celiac disease patients. *Gastroenterol Hepatol* (2018) 14:82–91.

31. Mullan A, Kavanagh P, O'Mahony P, Joy T, Gleeson F, Gibney MJ. Food and nutrient intakes and eating patterns in functional and organic dyspepsia. *Eur J Clin Nutr* (1994) 48:97–105.

32. Duncanson KR, Talley NJ, Walker MM, Burrows TL. Food and functional dyspepsia: a systematic review. *J Hum Nutr Diet* (2018) 31:390–407. doi: 10.1111/jhn.12506

33. Dionne J, Ford AC, Yuan Y, Chey WD, Lacy BE, Saito YA, et al. A systematic review and meta-analysis evaluating the efficacy of a gluten-free diet and a low FODMAPs diet in treating symptoms of irritable bowel syndrome. *Am J Gastroenterol* (2018) 113:1290–300. doi: 10.1038/s41395-018-0195-4

34. von Wulffen M, Talley NJ, Hammer J, McMaster J, Rich G, Shah A, et al. Overlap of irritable bowel syndrome and functional dyspepsia in the clinical setting: prevalence and risk factors. *Dig Dis Sci* (2019) 64:480–6. doi: 10.1007/s10620-018-5343-6

35. Schnabel L, Buscail C, Sabate J-M, Bouchoucha M, Kesse-Guyot E, Alles B, et al. Association between ultra-processed food consumption and functional gastrointestinal disorders: results from the french nutrinet-sante cohort. *Am J Gastroenterol* (2018) 113:1217–28. doi: 10.1038/s41395-018-0137-1

36. Bujanda L. The effects of alcohol consumption upon the gastrointestinal tract. *Am J Gastroenterol* (2000) 95:3374–82. doi: 10.1111/j.1572-0241.2000.03347.x

37. Talley NJ, McNeil D, Piper DW. Environmental factors and chronic unexplained dyspepsia. Association with acetaminophen but not other analgesics, alcohol, coffee, tea, or smoking. *Dig Dis Sci* (1988) 33:641–8. doi: 10.1007/BF01540424

38. Talley NJ, Weaver AL, Zinsmeister AR. Smoking, alcohol, and nonsteroidal anti-inflammatory drugs in outpatients with functional dyspepsia and among dyspepsia subgroups. *Am J Gastroenterol* (1994) 89:524–8.

39. Halder SLS, Locke GR3rd, Schleck CD, Zinsmeister AR, Talley NJ. Influence of alcohol consumption on IBS and dyspepsia. *Neurogastroenterol Motil* (2006) 18:1001–8. doi: 10.1111/j.1365-2982.2006.00815.x

40. World Health Organization. *Global status reports on Alcohol and Health*. Geneva, Switzerland: World Health Organization; (2014).

41. Hammer J. Identification of individuals with functional dyspepsia with a simple, minimally invasive test: a single center cohort study of the oral capsaicin test. *Am J Gastroenterol* (2018) 113:584–92. doi: 10.1038/ajg.2018.16

42. Hammer J, Fuhrer M. Clinical characteristics of functional dyspepsia depending on chemosensitivity to capsaicin. *Neurogastroenterol Motil* (2017) 29:1–12. doi: 10.1111/nmo.13103

43. Bortolotti M, Coccia G, Grossi G, Miglioli M. The treatment of functional dyspepsia with red pepper. *Aliment Pharmacol Ther* (2002) 16:1075–82. doi: 10.1046/j.1365-2036.2002.01280.x

44. Elta GH, Behler EM, Colturi TJ. Comparison of coffee intake and coffee-induced symptoms in patients with duodenal ulcer, nonulcer dyspepsia, and normal controls. *Am J Gastroenterol* (1990) 85:1339–42.

45. Zito FP, Polese B, Vozzella L, Gala A, Genovese D, Verlezza V, et al. Good adherence to mediterranean diet can prevent gastrointestinal symptoms: a survey from Southern Italy. *World J Gastrointest Pharmacol Ther* (2016) 7:564–71. doi: 10.4292/wjgpt.v7.i4.564

46. Karamanolis G, Caenepeel P, Arts J, Tack J. Association of the predominant symptom with clinical characteristics and pathophysiological mechanisms in functional dyspepsia. *Gastroenterology* (2006) 130:296–303. doi: 10.1053/j.gastro.2005.10.019

14

Herbal Therapies in Functional Gastrointestinal Disorders

Yong Sung Kim [1,2], Jung-Wook Kim [3], Na-Yeon Ha [4,5], Jinsung Kim [5]
and Han Seung Ryu [1,6*]

[1] Wonkwang Digestive Disease Research Institute, Gut and Food Healthcare, Wonkwang University School of Medicine, Iksan, South Korea, [2] Good Breath Clinic, Gunpo, South Korea, [3] Department of Gastroenterology, Kyung Hee University College of Medicine, Seoul, South Korea, [4] Department of Clinical Korean Medicine, College of Korean Medicine, Graduate School, Kyung Hee University, Seoul, South Korea, [5] Department of Gastroenterology, College of Korean Medicine, Kyung Hee University, Seoul, South Korea, [6] Brain-Gut Stress Clinic, Division of Gastroenterology, Wonkwang University Hospital, Iksan, South Korea

*Correspondence:
Han Seung Ryu
hanseung43@naver.com;
hanseung@wku.ac.kr

The pathophysiology of functional gastrointestinal disorders (FGIDs) is still unclear and various complex mechanisms have been suggested to be involved. In many cases, improvement of symptoms and quality of life (QoL) in patients with FGIDs is difficult to achieve with the single-targeted treatments alone and clinical application of these treatments can be challenging owing to the side effects. Herbal preparations as complementary and alternative medicine can control multiple treatment targets of FGIDs simultaneously and relatively safely. To date, many herbal ingredients and combination preparations have been proposed across different countries and together with a variety of traditional medicine. Among the herbal therapies that are comparatively considered to have an evidence base are iberogast (STW-5) and peppermint oil, which have been mainly studied and used in Europe, and rikkunshito and motilitone (DA-9701), which are extracted from natural substances in traditional medicine, are the focus of this review. These herbal medications have multi-target pharmacology similar to the etiology of FGIDs, such as altered intestinal sensory and motor function, inflammation, neurohormonal abnormality, and have displayed comparable efficacy and safety in controlled trials. To achieve the treatment goal of refractory FGIDs, extensive and high quality studies on the pharmacological mechanisms and clinical effects of these herbal medications as well as efforts to develop new promising herbal compounds are required.

Keywords: herbal, functional dyspepsia, irritable bowel syndrome, STW 5, peppermint

INTRODUCTION

Functional gastrointestinal disorders (FGIDs) are a group of diseases with variable combinations of chronic or recurrent gastrointestinal (GI) symptoms not explained by structural or biochemical abnormalities (1). FGIDs include diseases that are commonly found in daily practice, such as gastroesophageal reflux disease (GERD), functional dyspepsia (FD), irritable bowel syndrome (IBS), and functional constipation (FC), and show various symptom presentation throughout the GI tract. They impair the quality of life (QoL) of patients and entail a huge expenditure of medical resources (2, 3). Although the possible pathological mechanisms involved in these diseases have been studied and proposed from various perspectives, their etiologies are still not fully understood. Numerous factors such as GI dysmotility, visceral hypersensitivity, altered immune function, stress, central nervous system dysregulation, intestinal dysbiosis, and genetic predispositions seem to affect the clinical expressions of these diseases, but the mechanisms or complex crosstalk between the pathways have not been clearly elucidated (4).

In spite of treatments have been attempted for FGIDs in the past decades by controlling specific etiologies determined from preclinical and human studies, the positive therapeutic yields of these treatments were unsatisfactory in many cases. Various single-drug treatments with a single target site have been used, but cases that showed complete improvement of symptoms are rare, except for a few in which the treatment showed a marginal effect. Despite the advances on the understanding of the pathophysiology of FGIDs and the development of drugs targeting novel pathways, agents that display satisfactory therapeutic effects on various FGIDs according to both patients and physicians are still limited (5).

Herbal medications have been used in many countries by various races since ancient times and are still used by some physicians or as home remedies. They can be used as complementary and alternative medicine for patients with FGIDs when primary therapeutic approaches fail and are recommended by treatment guidelines for FGIDs in certain countries (6–8). As the various FGIDs overlap in many cases or show a wide range of symptoms even if they occur as a single disease entity (9, 10), herbal medications with multiple mechanisms of action in virtue of diverse components can potentially regulate various, complex etiologies simultaneously and comprehensively improve symptoms of FGIDs. Furthermore, herbal medication will have fewer adverse effects owing to its proven safety from long-term use. Thus, it can be a more desirable therapeutic agent for FGIDs.

A variety of herbs can be used as therapeutic agents for FGIDs and are presumed to target the GI system, as proposed by traditional medicines in numerous countries. However, this paper only discusses drugs whose mechanism of action was demonstrated by various preclinical studies and proved effective by clinical trials. Herbs with potential indications not covered in this review require further research and validation.

METHODS

A PubMed literature search was performed using the following terms individually or in combination: STW, STW-5, Iberogast, peppermint, peppermint oil, menthol, Mentha, Rikkunshito, Yukgunja-tang, Liu-Jun-Zi-Tang, DA-9701, Motilitone, esophagus, stomach, small intestine, colon, dyspepsia, nausea, abdominal pain, gastroesophageal reflux disease, esophagitis, irritable bowel syndrome, constipation, and functional gastrointestinal disorders. In the case of motilitone, published in Korean were additionally searched. More than 250 references were initially reviewed. Following removal of references that overlapped between searches and those lacking original data, the authors agreed on inclusion of 111 references based on which the information has been presented within this manuscript. The Jadad score were calculated by two investigators (YSK and HSR) independently to assess the quality of each included study (10).

RESULTS

STW-5 (IBEROGAST®)

STW-5 is liquid preparation made from extracts of nine well-known herbs, obtained using alcohol and combined at a fixed ratio. It has been used clinically in German-speaking countries for over several decades and is sold in Europe as an over-the-counter medication (11). The liquid extract contains unique constituents, including fresh plant extract of bitter candytuft (*Iberis amara*) and extracts from eight dried herbs, including angelica roots (*Angelicae radix*), chamomile flowers (*Matricariae flos*), caraway fruit (*Carvi fructus*), St. Mary's thistle fruit (*Cardui mariae fructus*), balm leaves (*Melissae folium*), peppermint leaves (*Menthae x piperitae*), greater celandine (*Chelidonii herba*), and licorice root (*Liquiritiae radix*), generated using a defined extraction method with fixed amounts of components (12). Various plant components display single effects, and their interactions have also been predicted. Therefore, STW-5 has shown therapeutic effects through multiple mechanisms in several preclinical studies and clinical trials for a wide range of symptoms.

Mechanisms of Action

Effects on Gastrointestinal Motility and Sensation

In an animal study that used stomach muscle strips of guinea pigs, STW-5 was shown to act directly on muscles rather than exert neural mechanisms of action, as it was not affected by concomitant treatment with tetrodotoxin, capsaicin, or N-nitro-l-arginine methyl ester (L-NAME). STW-5 inhibited and relaxed muscle activity dose dependently in the fundus area of the stomach but enhanced the amplitude of phasic contraction in the antrum area (13, 14). In a study with healthy volunteers, administration of STW-5 1.1 ml (20 drops) in nine subjects led to a significant increase in proximal gastric volume measured with a gastric barostat. It also increased the antral pressure wave from

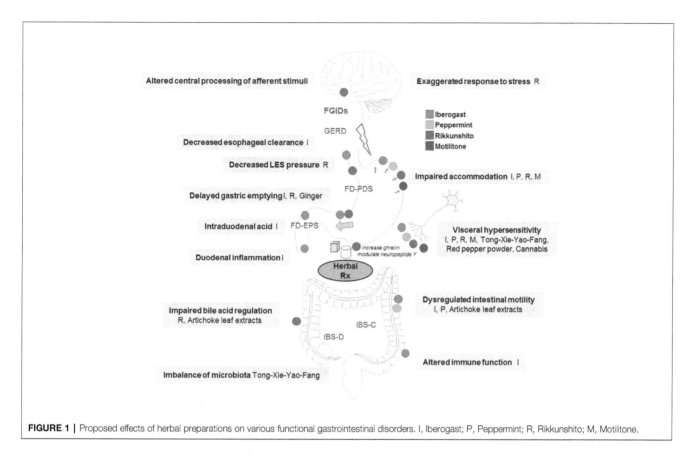

FIGURE 1 | Proposed effects of herbal preparations on various functional gastrointestinal disorders. I, Iberogast; P, Peppermint; R, Rikkunshito; M, Motilitone.

antroduodenal manometry using 16-channel catheter in 12 subjects, but did not cause any change in pyloric or duodenal pressures and gastric emptying (GE) measured by scintigraphy (12). In an experiment that used an ileal muscle strip isolated from guinea pigs, STW-5 showed spasmolytic properties by reducing acetylcholine- and histamine-induced contractions. However it increased the basal resting tone and contraction of the atonic segment through its component *Iberis amara* extract. Thus, STW-5 exerted dual activity with spasmolytic and tonic effects depending on the basal tone of the intestine and these effects were also observed in the duodenum, jejunum, and colon (15). In the large and small intestines of mice, STW-5 reduced the amplitude and frequency of slow waves (16). The target sites in the intestine were 5-HT$_4$, 5-HT$_3$, muscarinic M$_3$, and opioid receptors (17).

In an *in vivo* experiment that used Wister rats, extracellular multi-unit intestinal afferent nerve recordings were performed in anesthetized animals. When the afferent nerve discharge was measured after applying stimuli such as ramp distension, bradykinin, or serotonin, STW-5 reduced the afferent nerve discharge that occurred in response to the chemical and mechanical stimuli without affecting the baseline discharge (18).

Effects on Inflammation and Mucosal Function

STW-5 reduced the incidence of gastric ulcer and inflammation by reducing the indomethacin-induced acid hyper-production and increasing leukotrienes, mucin secretion, and prostaglandin E$_2$ release in Wistar rats (19). Its inhibitory effects on intestinal inflammation were also validated in the dextran sulfate sodium-

and trinitrobenzenesulfonic acid (TNBS)-induced colitis models (20, 21). In the Ussing chamber study that used human intestinal tissues, STW-5 exerted a pro-secretory effect by increasing epithelial chloride fluxes through the cystic fibrosis transmembrane conductance regulator and calcium-activated chloride channels, showing therapeutic potential for constipation symptoms (22).

Clinical Studies

Functional Dyspepsia

In a multicenter placebo-controlled double-blind study conducted in Germany, either STW-5 or placebo was administered in 315 patients with FD by Rome II criteria for 8 weeks after a 7-day washout period. The validated GI symptom (GIS) scale that incorporated 10 dyspeptic symptoms was used to assess symptom severity using a 5-point Likert scale. After 4 and 8 weeks, the GIS score significantly decreased ($p < 0.05$) in the STW-5 group as compared with the placebo, and this effect was independent of *Helicobacter pylori* (*H. pylori*) status. However, no primary efficacy parameters were used except for the GIS score, and the percentage of responders (based on the improvement of the GIS scores by ≥40%) was very high in the placebo group (78%) (23) (**Table 1**). In a multicenter placebo-controlled double-blind study with 103 patients with FD by Rome II criteria, the GIS score decreased after 4 weeks of STW-5 administration and the percentage of treatment responders by STW-5 was 75%, which was higher than the 54% in the placebo group ($p = 0.03$). However, the difference in mean GIS score was

TABLE 1 | Summary of clinical trials of STW-5.

Subject	Design	County	Comparison	Number	Outcome	Ref.	Jadad score
FD by Rome II	Multi-center, randomized, double-blind, placebo-controlled	Germany	STW-5 1.1 ml (20 drops) t.i.d., 8 weeks vs. placebo	158:157	• Improvement of GIS score ($p < 0.05$) • H. pylori did not influence the results	von Arnim et al. (23)	5
FD by Rome II	Multi-center, randomized, double-blind, placebo-controlled	Germany	STW-5 1.1 ml (20 drops) t.i.d., 4 weeks vs. placebo	44:42	• Improvement of GIS score ($p = 0.08$) and the proportion of patients with a treatment response ($p = 0.03$) • Effects of STW-5 were not mediated by accelerating GE	Braden et al. (24)	4
IBS by Rome II	Multi-center, randomized, double-blind, placebo-controlled	Germany	STW-5 1.1 ml (20 drops) t.i.d., 4 weeks vs. STW-5-II 1.1 ml (20 drops) t.i.d., 4 weeks vs. bitter candytuft mono-extract 1.1 ml (20 drops) t.i.d., 4 weeks vs. placebo	51:52:53:52	• STW 5 and STW 5-II were significantly better than placebo in reducing the total abdominal pain score (STW 5, $p = 0.0009$; STW 5-II, $p = 0.0005$) and the irritable bowel syndrome symptom score (STW 5, $p = 0.001$; STW 5-II, $p = 0.0003$)	Madisch et al. (25)	5

FD, functional dyspepsia; GIS, gastrointestinal symptom; t.i.d., three times a day; GE, gastric emptying.

only 2.2 point, and no correlation was observed between symptom improvement and GE measured using the ^{13}C-octanoic acid breath test (24).

Irritable Bowel Syndrome
In a randomized, double-blind placebo-controlled multicenter trial conducted in Germany, STW-5 and STW-5-II were administered to 208 patients with IBS by Rome II criteria. Changes in total abdominal pain scores and IBS symptom score, which incorporated eight symptoms (flatulence/meteorism, sensation of tension or fullness, sensation of incomplete evacuation, changes in bowel habit) defined by the authors, were measured using a 4-point Likert scale. The results showed that the total abdominal pain score (STW-5, $p = 0.0009$; STW-5-II, $p = 0.0005$) and the IBS symptom score (STW-5, $p = 0.001$; STW-5-II, $p = 0.0003$) improved after 4 weeks (25).

Safety
In a clinical study with 315 patients with FD that was conducted in Germany, no significant difference in overall tolerability was observed after the administration of STW-5 for 8 weeks as compared with the placebo group. Adverse effects such as abdominal pain, pruritus, sore throat, alopecia, hypersensitivity, hypertension, and GI pain were observed in five patients (23). In a study with 103 patients with FD, 8 adverse events showed possible or probable relationships, including 3 adverse events (stomatitis, abdominal pain, and diarrhea) in the STW-5 group and 5 adverse events (rhinitis, diarrhea, dyspepsia, vomiting, and genitourinary tract infection) in the placebo group (24). In a study with 208 patients with IBS, only 2 minor adverse events (headache and constipation) were reported, and the treatment was continued (25). However, there were recent reports of severe hepatotoxicity associated with the use of this drug (26, 27), which is possibly related with greater celandine, one of the extracts used in STW-5 (28).

Usage
A commercially available STW-5 preparation (Iberogast®, Steigerwald GmbH, Darmstadt, Germany) is a dark brown, clear to lightly cloudy liquid supplied in a brown glass bottle and administered at the recommended dose of 1.1 ml (20 drops), three times daily (24, 25).

Peppermint Oil
Mint plants have a long history of medicinal use as stomach soothers and anecdotal evidence of its purported efficacy abounds to this day (29, 30). Peppermint is a perennial herb (*Mentha* x *piperita*) that grows throughout Europe and North America. Usually, peppermint is a sterile hybrid of two mints, spearmint (*Mentha spicata*) and water mint (*Mentha aquatica*) (31). Peppermint oil (PMO) is obtained by steam distillation from the fresh leaves of peppermint (30). It contains a large number (> 80) of components including menthol (35–55%), menthone (20–31%), menthyl acetate (3–10%), cineol, and several other volatile oils (31–33). Its major constituent and active ingredients appear to be menthol that in nature exists as a pure stereoisomer (32). Owing to the various constituents of peppermint, it has a variety uses, including topical application as an antiseptic and analgesic, inhalation as aromatherapy, and oral formulation for treatment of headache and various FGIDs such as IBS.

Mechanisms of Action
Effects on Gastrointestinal Motility
Many lines of evidence to date suggest that PMO acts as a smooth muscle relaxant of the GI tract (32). *In vitro* research has indicated that both PMO and its constituent menthol exert calcium channel blocking properties in guinea pig ileal smooth muscle, contributing to intestinal smooth muscle relaxation (34). Another study also suggested that PMO markedly attenuated contractile responses in the guinea pig tenia coli to acetylcholine, histamine, 5-hydroxytryptamine, and substance P (35). They suggested that the PMO relaxes GI smooth muscle by its ability to decrease the influx of extracellular calcium ions through voltage-dependent channels (32, 35). In addition, PMO may affect the enteric nerve system directly. In an experiment using the mouse small intestine, menthol induced membrane potential

depolarization in a concentration-dependent manner using cultured interstitial cells of Cajal (ICC), the pacemaker cells of the GI tract (36). The authors also identified that PMO acts on ICC by a G-protein-, Ca^{2+}-, Rho-kinase-, COX-, and thromboxane A_2 dependent manner *via* transient receptor potential ankyrin 1 (TRPA1), which may explain the promoting effect on GI motility.

In addition, there is also evidence indicating that PMO decreases small bowel contractility and attenuates orocecal transit. Both duodenally instilled and given orally PMO decreased duodenal contractions in a double contrast barium study and manometry (37–39). Furthermore, a study using hydrogen breath testing showed that the PMO combination with caraway oil had delayed orocecal transit in healthy volunteers (40). Similarly, PMO decreased colonic spasm and/or peristalsis. A randomized trial of endoscopy evaluated inhibition effect of intraluminally administered PMO on colonic motility during colonoscopy using the barostat balloon and endoscopic evaluation (41). Although the duration of relaxation was short, about 20 minutes, the authors found peristalsis and spasm of the colon were diminished after administration of PMO.

Effects on Visceral Sensitivity

Peppermint (*via* menthol) is a well-known topical analgesic. Some studies show that PMO can attenuate visceral pain in animal models (42, 43). An animal study showed that the combined treatment of peppermint and caraway oil had a significant effect on the reduction of post-inflammatory visceral hyperalgesia in rats that had been pretreated with TNBS/ethanol (43). Recent studies have suggested that the reduction of visceral pain by menthol is mediated through the TRPM8 and/or TRPA1 receptor (42, 44).

Effects on Esophageal and Gastric Function

An early study demonstrated that PMO decreased esophageal body and lower esophageal sphincter (LES) pressure based on esophageal manometry in healthy adults (45). Likewise, orally administered PMO reduced spasm of the esophagus in double-contrast barium meal examination (37). Another study using esophageal manometry demonstrated that PMO did not affect the esophageal body and LES pressures in patients with diffuse esophageal spasm despite improvement of manometric findings (46). Given orally or topically sprayed PMO also decreased spasm of the sto mach (37, 47). Some studies using manometry and/or barostat have demonstrated various effects on the gastric physiology such as decreased intragastric pressure, decreased gastric motility index, with no change in gastric accommodation (38, 39, 48). However, studies addressing the effects of PMO on GE have shown mixed results (40, 49).

Psychological Effects

Although there have been no studies in humans demonstrating the mood modulating effects, some studies in rodents have suggested that menthol has dose-dependent anxiolytic effects by acting on dopamine signaling pathways (50–52). A study in rodents demonstrated that menthone, a constituent of PMO, promotes ambulation in mice and dopamine might be involved

effects inducing mental excitation and thereby reducing mental fatigue (50). Thus, PMO could help change mood by reducing mental fatigue. This may be another mechanism through which PMO activity targets the brain-gut axis in the common pathogenesis of various FGIDs.

Clinical Studies

Irritable Bowel Syndrome

A prospective, double blind, placebo-controlled randomized trial with 57 patients with IBS by Rome II criteria showed that 64% of patients receiving enteric-coated PMO and 34% of placebo users experienced a reduction in the total IBS symptom score at 4 weeks of ≥50% ($p < 0.002$) in the intention-to-treat population (54) (**Table 2**). They also assessed the symptom score at 4 weeks after the end of treatment (8 weeks) and found a persisting beneficial effect at 8 weeks ($p < 0.05$). Another randomized double-blind placebo-controlled study on 90 outpatients with IBS by Rome II criteria was conducted to demonstrate the efficacy of PMO on QoL (55). Patients were randomly assigned to receive one capsule of Colpermin® (Tillotts Pharma, Ziefen, Switzerland) or a placebo three times daily for 8 weeks. They examined the effectiveness of PMO in terms of relieving symptoms and improving QoL using a questionnaire addressing six IBS symptoms and the 36-item Short Form Health Survey (SF-36) for QoL. At week 8, 42.5% of patients receiving PMO and 22.2% of patients receiving placebo were free from abdominal pain or discomfort ($p < 0.001$). However, there were no significant between-group differences detected in other IBS symptoms such as abdominal distension, flatulence, loose stool, hard stool, urgency, and incomplete evacuation. Although overall scores of SF-36 for the two groups were not significantly different, patients in the PMO group showed improvements in the SF-36 domains of bodily pain, general health, social functioning, and role limitations due to emotional problems.

A recent study reported the findings of a 4-week randomized controlled trial which tested a novel formulation of PMO designed for sustained release in the small intestine (IBgard®, IM HealthScience, Boca Raton, FL, USA) for its efficacy and tolerability in reducing IBS symptoms in 72 patients with mixed IBS (IBS-M) or IBS with diarrhea (IBS-D) by Rome III criteria (56). The specialized enteric-coating utilized in their trial consisted of a solid-state matrix that was triple-coated and designed to deliver PMO with sustained release to the small intestine with fewer potential adverse effects. At trial completion, there was a 40% reduction in the total IBS symptom score in the PMO group compared to baseline *vs.* 24.3% with placebo ($p = 0.0246$). Moreover, there was an increased improvement in multiple individual GI symptoms, as well as in severe or unbearable symptoms compared to the placebo.

Similarly, some meta-analyses have shown PMO to be effective in IBS, the number needed to treat (NNT) ranged between 2 and 3 (60–62). In most recent meta-analysis of 12 randomized controlled trials with 835 patients with IBS, the risk ratio (RR) for the effect of PMO (n = 253) *versus* placebo (n = 254) on global symptoms was 2.39 (95% CI 1.93–2.97, $p < 0.00001$) (63). Overall, there were no differences in the

TABLE 2 | Summary of clinical trials of peppermint oil.

Subject	Design	County	Comparison	Number		Outcome	Ref.	Jadad score
IBS based on symptoms	Single center, randomized, double-blind, placebo-controlled	Taiwan	Peppermint oil 137 mg t.i.d. or q.i.d., a.c., 4 weeks vs. placebo	25:49	•	Symptom improvements after peppermint oil therapy were significantly better than after placebo.	Liu et al. (53)	4
IBS by Rome II	Single center, randomized, double-blind, placebo-controlled	Italy	Peppermint oil 450 mg b.i.d., a.c., 4 weeks vs. placebo	28:29	•	A 4-week treatment with peppermint oil is more effective than placebo in reducing abdominal symptoms related to IBS.	Cappello et al. (54)	4
IBS by Rome II	Single center, randomized, double-blind, placebo-controlled	Iran	Peppermint oil 187 mg t.i.d., a.c., 8 weeks vs. placebo	33:27	• •	Severity of abdominal pain and discomfort were reduced significantly in the peppermint oil group. Peppermint oil significantly improved the QoL.	Merat et al. (55)	5
IBS by Rome III	Multicenter, randomized, double-blind, placebo-controlled	USA	Peppermint oil 180 mg t.i.d., 4 weeks vs. placebo	35:37	•	Patients treated with peppermint oil experienced greater improvement in multiple individual gastrointestinal symptoms as well as in severe or unbearable symptoms, compared to placebo.	Cash et al. (56)	5
Childhood IBS by Manning or Rome II	Multicenter, randomized, double-blind, placebo-controlled	USA	Peppermint oil 374 mg or 187 mg t.i.d., 2 weeks vs. placebo	21:21	•	After 2 weeks, improvements in the change of symptom scale were reported in 71% of the patients receiving peppermint oil compared with 43% receiving placebo with statistical significance.	Kline et al. (57)	3
FD based on symptoms	Single center, randomized, double-blind, placebo-controlled	Germany	Peppermint oil 90 mg and caraway oil 50 mg b.i.d., 4 weeks vs. placebo	48:48	•	For the major symptoms (intensity of pain, sensation of pressure, heaviness and fullness, and global improvement), the superiority of combination therapy of peppermint oil and caraway oil over placebo was statistically significant.	May et al. (58)	5
FD by Rome III	Multicenter, randomized, double-blind, placebo-controlled	Germany	Peppermint oil 90 mg and caraway oil 50 mg b.i.d., 4 weeks vs. placebo	58:56	•	Compared to placebo, 4-week treatment with peppermint oil and caraway oil therapy significantly reduced symptoms of epigastric pain and postprandial distress and improved the participants' QoL.	Rich et al. (59)	5

IBS, irritable bowel syndrome; t.i.d., three times a day; q.i.d., four times a day; b.i.d., two times a day; a.c., before meal; QoL, quality of life; FD, functional dyspepsia.

reported adverse effects, PMO (9.3%) *versus* placebo (6.1%). The NNT with PMO was three for global symptoms and four for abdominal pain.

Functional Dyspepsia
To our knowledge, no study has determined whether PMO alone is useful in patients with FD. However, some randomized controlled trials have shown PMO to be effective for FD when used in combination with other herbal remedies such as STW5-II and caraway oil (58, 59, 64). Recently, a randomized placebo-controlled trial with 114 outpatients with chronic or recurrent FD demonstrated that a fixed peppermint and caraway- oil combination (Menthacarin) treatment is effective for the relief of FD symptoms and improvement of disease-specific QoL (59). After 4 weeks of treatment, pain and discomfort scores improved by 7.6 ± 4.8 and 3.6 ± 2.5 points for Menthacarin and by 3.4 ± 4.3 and 1.3 ± 2.1 points for placebo (all $p < 0.001$), respectively.

Safety
PMO has been used safely for various conditions in short-term clinical trials. Menthol, the major constituent of PMO, is also listed as generally regarded as safe by the US Food and Drug Administration. In a randomized controlled trial with 90 patients with IBS, the most common adverse events of PMO treatment

group were heartburn, headache, and dizziness. However, these were not significantly different in the two groups (55). However, PMO is relatively contraindicated in patients with hiatal hernia or significant GERD, because its effects on the lower esophageal sphincter can lead to exacerbation of symptoms (31). Especially, when non-coated PMO is taken orally, it can cause heartburn, nausea, and vomiting. The effective delivery method to the target organ by enteric coating is believed to prevent or reduce these upper GI symptoms as well as improve PMO efficacy (31). Even in the enteric coated formulation, heartburn could develop because of the premature rupture of capsules containing PMO (41). High concentrations of PMO have been reported to cause anal burning (65). Other minor adverse effects of PMO reported in clinical trials include allergic reactions and blurred vision. Because PMO may inhibit the cytochrome P450 system, it theoretically could lead to increased serum levels of drugs such as amitriptyline, haloperidol, and cyclosporine which are metabolized by this enzyme (66, 67). However, this interaction has not been proven in humans.

Usage
The dosage of PMO for the treatment of GI diseases usually ranges from 0.2 to 0.4 ml, three times a day. The oral dosage

range studied in most IBS trials was 187 to 500 mg (0.2–0.4 ml) administered two or three times daily for 2 to 8 weeks (53–55). To secure the availability of unmetabolized PMO at the target organ, a lower digestive tract in IBS, enteric-coated formation such as Colpermin® and Mintoil® (Cadigroup, Rome, Italy) capsules have been developed and have been widely used in clinical trials or real-world practice (54, 55). Each capsule of Colpermin® and Mintoil® contains 187 mg and 225 mg PMO, respectively. These formulated capsules are usually administered 30 to 60 min before meals in order to guarantee low gastric pH which prevents untimely capsule dissolution with premature release of PMO into the stomach (54). In FD, most trials used a dose of 90 mg of PMO in combination with 50 mg of caraway oil (58, 59).

Rikkunshito

Rikkunshito (RKT; *Rikkunshi-to* in Japan, *Yukgunja-tang* in Korea, *Liu-Jun-Zi-Tang* in China) is one of the more famous herbal formulas in traditional medicine. It has been prescribed for hundreds of years to alleviate abdominal discomfort due to indigestion (68). In Japan, RKT has been widely used and marketed to treat various symptoms of the GI tract (69). The Japanese Ministry of Health and Welfare gave RKT approval for medical use (TJ-43, Tsumura & Co., Tokyo, Japan) (70).

RKT is a form of extracted granules for oral intake, containing 4.0 g of dried mixture consisting of eight crude herbs in fixed proportions (71): *Pinelliae* tuber (18.6%), *Ginseng* radix (18.6%), *Atractylodis lanceae* rhizoma (18.6%), *Hoelen* (18.6%), *Aurantii nobilis* pericarpium (9.3%), *Ziziphi* fructus (9.3%), *Glycyrrhizae* radix (4.7%), and *Zingiberis* rhizoma (2.3%) (72, 73). RKT has been shown to reduce GI symptoms including dyspeptic or reflux symptoms, as well as improve fundic relaxation, GE, and antral contractions (74). It has been suggested that RKT shows synergetic effects through a complex interactive pathway by each component (75, 76).

Mechanisms of Action

Effects on Esophageal Sensory and Motor Function
RKT has been shown to suppress dilation of the intercellular space and to improve the barrier function of esophageal mucosa in an experimental rat esophagitis model (77). In a study with eight children with symptomatic gastroesophageal reflux, a 7-day administration of RKT reduced clinical symptoms and acid exposure time in the distal esophagus in 24-h esophageal pH monitoring tests, by activating esophageal acid clearance mechanisms (78). In a pilot study of 30 patients with proton pump inhibitor (PPI)-refractory non-erosive reflux disease (NERD), 8 weeks of RKT treatment improved esophageal clearance by reducing the residual LES pressure during swallows, and increasing complete bolus transit rate and peristaltic contractions rate in esophageal multichannel impedance and manometry (79).

Effects on Plasma Ghrelin Level
RKT, an endogenous ghrelin enhancer (80), exerts orexigenic effects by ghrelin secretion to stimulate food intake (71). It has been prescribed to treat nausea, vomiting, and anorexia (73).

Moreover, RKT prevents plasma acylated-ghrelin levels from decreasing against cisplatin and increases appetite and food intake in the rat (81). RKT likely has an effect on activating ghrelin secretion and also reduces inactivation of ghrelin (82). A study with FD patients showed that a lower plasma des-acyl ghrelin level at baseline were associated with the higher efficacy of RKT (83). Also, RKT alleviated dyspeptic symptoms in FD patients with an increase of acylated-ghrelin levels (84). In addition, RKT was beneficial for aging-related decrease in food intake *via* ghrelin activity (85).

Effects on Gastric Motor Function
The effect of RKT on gastric relaxation is mediated by β_2- and β_3-adrenergic pathways, which are associated with smooth muscle relaxation (86, 87). Furthermore, RKT had a relaxant effect on fundus smooth muscles of isolated rat stomach, triggered by activation of the Ca^{2+}-activated K^+ channel (88). RKT has been shown to enhance gastric adaptive relaxation in the isolated guinea pig stomach (89).

RKT was shown to ameliorate delayed GE induced by N(G)-nitro-L-arginine (L-NNA), a nitric oxide (NO) synthase inhibitor, in rat. The hesperidin and L-arginine was identified as an active ingredient of RKT contributing to the increase in GE (90). Moreover, hesperidin, the major active component of RKT, was identified to stimulate contraction of intestinal smooth muscle mediated *via* 5-HT$_3$ receptor pathway and acetylcholine release (75). The administration of RKT on normal and vagotomized dogs activated GI contractions during the interdigestive state and enhanced GE (91). In patients with FD, RKT improved gastric accommodation reflex and GE rate assessed by extracorporeal ultrasonography. In summary, RKT may be beneficial for treating GI dysmotility disorders, acting as a prokinetic agent (74).

Effects on Bile Salts
RKT showed a great binding capacity for bile salts and may prevent esophageal mucosal damage by bile acid exposure. It can be useful for the treatment of refractory GERD and duodeno-gastroesophageal reflux (92). This observation suggests that RKT may alleviate bile acid-induced mucosal hypersensitivity (93).

Effects on Stress-Induced Gastrointestinal Dysfunction
RKT can alleviate both GI and psychological symptoms in FD patients (94). First of all, physical or psychological stress can cause an imbalance in plasma ghrelin levels and decreasing gastric motility (95, 96). RKT may be beneficial for delayed GE induced by stress (97). Anxiety and stress can also induce dysfunction of the GI tract such as impairment of gastric accommodation (98, 99). RKT can modulate stress-induced gastric hypersensitivity and improving gastric accommodation (94). Moreover, it was shown that RKT improved GE through antagonistic activities on corticotropin-releasing factor receptor 1, 5-HT$_{2B/2C}$ receptors, and 5-HT$_3$ receptor in rats with delayed GE and anorexia model (75, 81, 100).

In a healthy human study to verify the effects of RKT on the hypothalamo-pituitary-adrenal (HPA) axis, RKT significantly suppressed plasma levels of adrenocorticotropic hormone (ACTH) and cortisol under continual stress, and improved the mental component of QoL (101). FD patients have an imbalance of autonomic nervous system function (102). RKT suppressed increased plasma levels of neuropeptide Y, a neurotransmitter of the sympathetic nervous system, under venipuncture stress (103). RKT also increased the activity of efferent vagus nerve and decreased the afferent activity of gastric vagus nerve, meanwhile, its active ingredient atractylodin stimulated ghrelin binding activity (104).

Clinical Studies
Functional Dyspepsia
In a randomized, placebo-controlled trial with 42 chronic idiopathic dyspepsia patients in Japan, RKT had a prokinetic action to improve GE, evaluated by the acetaminophen absorption method, and reduced upper GI symptoms (epigastric fullness, heartburn, belching, and nausea) compared to placebo (105) (**Table 3**). The first randomized, double-blind, placebo-controlled trial in Japan, 247 patients with FD by Rome III criteria, the administration of RKT for 8 weeks ameliorated symptoms of FD, especially epigastric pain and postprandial fullness. In addition, it showed a tendency whereby RKT was more effective among *H. pylori*-infected patients than the uninfected, providing a basis for different mechanisms of each

symptom and treatment strategy depending on the of *H. pylori* infection (69). The Japanese DREAM study, a multi-center, randomized, double-blind, placebo-controlled trial, showed that RKT significantly improved dyspeptic but also psychological symptoms in 128 FD patients by Rome III criteria without *H. pylori* infection. After an 8 week RKT treatment, significant improvement was reported compared to placebo. RKT reduced upper GI symptoms especially postprandial fullness, early satiety, and bloating but also anxiety. Interestingly, the improvements of psychological symptoms were correlated with those of upper GI symptoms (106). In conclusion, RKT can be more useful for postprandial distress syndrome (PDS)-type of FD (110).

Gastroesophageal Reflux Disease
A randomized, parallel comparative trial in Japan with 104 PPI-refractory GERD patients showed that the effect of RKT with standard dose of PPI on decreasing acid-related dysmotility symptom and reflux symptom was similar to that of a double dose of PPI. Particularly, this effect was greater in male NERD patients and in NERD patients with low body mass index (BMI < 22) (107). In a multi-center, randomized, double-blind, placebo-controlled study with 242 Japanese PPI-refractory NERD

TABLE 3 | Summary of clinical trials of rikkunshito.

Subject	Design	County	Comparison	Number		Outcome	Ref	Jadad score
Chronic idiopathic dyspepsia	Single-center, randomized, placebo-controlled	Japan	Rikkunshito 2.5 g t.i.d., a.c., 7 days vs. placebo (Combizym)	22:20	• •	Rikkunshito increased gastric emptying. Rikkunshito reduced gastrointestinal symptoms.	Tatsuta et al. (105)	1
FD by Rome III	Multi-center, randomized, double-blind, placebo-controlled	Japan	Rikkunshito 2.5 g t.i.d., a.c., 8 weeks vs. placebo 2.5 g t.i.d., a.c., 8 weeks	125:122	•	Rikkunshito improved dyspeptic symptoms, such as epigastric pain and postprandial fullness.	Suzuki et al. (69)	5
FD by Rome III without *H. pylori* infection, severe heartburn, and depression	Multi-center, randomized, double-blind, placebo-controlled	Japan	Rikkunshito 2.5 g t.i.d., 8 weeks vs. placebo 2.5 g t.i.d., 8 weeks	64:61	•	Rikkunshito alleviated dyspeptic and psychological symptoms at the same time.	Tominaga et al. (106)	4
PPI-refractory GERD	Multi-center, randomized, parallel comparative	Japan	Rikkunshito 2.5 g t.i.d. + rabeprazole 10 mg q. d. 4 weeks vs. rabeprazole 20 mg qD 4 weeks	48:51	•	Improvement effect of rikkunshito combined with a standard dose of PPI was similar with double dose of PPI.	Tominaga et al. (107)	3
PPI-refractory NERD	Multi-center, randomized, double-blind, placebo-controlled	Japan	Rikkunshito 2.5 g t.i.d. + rabeprazole 10 mg q.d. 8 weeks vs. placebo 2.5 g t.i.d. + rabeprazole 10 mg q.d. 8 weeks	109:108	•	Rikkunshito combined with PPI improved mental health in non-obese patients and acid-related dysmotility symptoms in female and the elderly.	Tominaga et al. (73)	5
PPI-refractory GERD	Multi-center, open-labeled	Japan	Rikkunshito 2.5 g t.i.d. + PPI (rabeprazole 20 mg q.d. lansoprazole 30 mg q.d. omeprazole 20 mg q.d.) 6–8 weeks	47	•	Rikkunshito combined with PPI reduced dyspeptic symptoms and improved QoL on eating and sleep.	Kawai et al. (108)	0
PPI-refractory LPR	Single-center, randomized, parallel comparative	Japan	Rikkunshito 2.5 g t.i.d. 4 weeks vs. Rikkunshito 2.5 g t.i.d. + lansoprazole 30 mg q.d. 4 weeks	11:11	• •	Rikkunshito reduced globus sensation. Rikkunshito enhanced delayed gastric emptying.	Tokashiki et al. (109)	2

FD, functional dyspepsia; GERD, gastroesophageal reflux disorder; PPI, proton pump inhibitor; NERD, non-erosive reflux disease ;q.d., once a day;t.i.d., three times a day; a.c., before meal; QoL, quality of life; LPR, laryngopharyngeal reflux.

patients, the RKT combination group (standard dose of PPI plus RKT) improved the mental QoL component compared to the placebo group (standard dose of PPI plus placebo) at 4 weeks. However, the improvements of GERD symptoms were not significantly different between these groups. Through subgroup analysis, it was especially noteworthy that the mental-related scores in non-obese patients (BMI < 22) and acid-related dysmotility symptoms in female and the elderly ($\geq$ 65 years) were more improved in the 8 week RKT group (73). It can also be suggested that RKT is more effective with postprandial symptoms (heavy feeling in stomach, sick feeling, and heartburn after meals) in elderly NERD patients (111). In addition, a clinical study conducted in 47 Japanese patients with PPI-refractory GERD treated for more than 8 weeks showed that the addition of RKT to PPI therapy for 6–8 weeks improved heartburn, fullness, abdominal discomfort, and abdominal pain as well as QoL for meals and sleep (108). Meanwhile, a randomized, parallel comparative trial conducted in 22 Japanese patients with PPI-refractory laryngopharyngeal reflux showed that the 4 week RKT treatment alleviated globus sensation, regardless of PPI co-administration. In addition, RKT enhanced delayed GE in positive correlation with the improvement of globus sensation (109).

Safety

In a meta-analysis of randomized controlled trials, there were few drug-related severe adverse events reported in the included studies (112). However, it is important to note that RKT should be administered by taking into account symptoms, age, pregnancy potential, and concomitant medications of the patient.

Usage

The standard RKT dose for adults in general practice is 7.5 g/day is containing 4.0 g of dried mixture consisting of eight crude herbs in fixed proportions. In Japan and several clinical trials, the standard RKT dose for adults in general practice is 7.5 g/day (2.5 g three times a day) with a proper volume of water before or between meals for 8 weeks (73, 74, 107). The dosage may be adjusted according to the patient's age, body weight, and symptoms (106).

DA-9701 (Motilitone®)

DA-9701 is a new herbal drug developed in South Korea that received New Drug Application approval in May 2011 from the Korean Food and Drug Administration (113). It is formulated with ethanolic extracts of Pharbitidis semen from the seeds of *Pharbitis nil* Choisy and Corydalis tuber from the roots of *Corydalis yanhusuo* W. T. Wang (114) These two herbs have been commonly used in traditional medicine in China, Korea, and Japan for abdominal and gynecological symptoms. Pharbitidis semen has been used as an analgesic for the abdomen and a stimulant of intestinal peristalsis (114). Corydalis tuber has been used as an analgesic or anti-spasmodic agent for the GI tract (115). Moreover, it has been known to have an effect on gastric secretion

and prevention of ulcer (116). The active ingredients of DA-9701 include chlorogenic acid in Pharbitidis semen and corydaline and tetrahydropalmatine in Corydalis tuber. The pharmacological study has demonstrated that DA-9701 has dopamine D_2 antagonistic activity, adrenergic α_2 agonist activity, 5-HT_{1A} agonist activity, and 5-HT_4 agonist activity (113, 114).

Mechanisms of Action
Effects on Gastrointestinal Motility

The oral administration of DA-9701 significantly increased semi-solid or solid GE in normal rat and mice (117, 118). Moreover, DA-9701 restored semi-solid or liquid GE in the apomorphine or cisplatin-induced delayed GE rat model (117). Immobilization induced delayed GE was also reversed by oral administration of DA-9701. A study with strain gauge force transducer in the antrum of rat showed that oral administration of DA-9701 improved the clonidine-induced hypomotility of the gastric antrum, but it showed no effect on antral motility in normal conditions (119).

The effect of GE in healthy volunteers was investigated using gastric magnetic resonance imaging in a randomized, double-blind, placebo-controlled trial (120). After administration of 60 mg of DA-9701 or placebo t.i.d. for 7 days, GE was significantly enhanced in DA-9701 group compared to the placebo group. In another randomized, double-blind, controlled trial with patients with Parkinson's disease, 30 mg of DA-9701 three times per day before meals for 4 weeks significantly increased GE, while domperidone showed no effect (121). The concentration of plasma levodopa was increased in the DA-9701 group only, though it was not statistically significant.

DA-9701 also increased small intestinal motility in an animal study. *In vitro* study with ileal muscle strip of guinea pig showed that DA-9701 increased contractility in normal condition as well as morphine pre-treated hypomotility state (122). In postoperative ileus or atropine-induced delayed GI transit model of rat and guinea pig, oral administration of DA-9701 restores delayed transit (117, 122, 123). In contrast to the pathologic condition, only high dose of DA-9701 increased GI motility in the normal condition (117, 123). The DA-9701 seemed to influence active ghrelin levels in the stress or postoperative ileus rat model (123, 124). In addition, the central corticotropin-releasing factor pathway may mediate the improvement in GI transit and the inhibition of plasma ACTH levels by DA-9701 in the postoperative ileus guinea pig model (125).

Effects on Gastric Accommodation

An *in vivo* study with Beagle dogs showed that oral administration of DA-9701 induced proximal gastric relaxation and shift the pressure-volume curve to left similar to the intravenous administration of cisapride (117). Another study with Beagle dog showed that oral administration of DA-9701 induced gastric accommodation dose-dependently during the postprandial phase similar to the oral administration of sumatriptan (126). Restraint stress-induced feeding inhibition was reversed by oral DA-9701, and this effect was blocked by a 5-HT_{1A} antagonist in a rat study (127). A tissue bath study using rat gastric muscle strip suggested that the nitrergic rather than the purinergic pathway was involved in gastric accommodation by DA-9701 (128).

Effects on Colonic Contractility

In a tissue bath study, DA-9701 did not influence the contractility of normal colonic muscle strips; however, it increased the motility of distal colonic muscle strips of a morphine pre-treated hypomotility state (122). DA-9701 increased fecal pellet output in the *in vivo* morphine-induced constipation guinea pig model and improved defecatory dysfunction in acute spinal shock state in spinal cord injury rat model (122, 129).

Effect on Visceral Sensitivity

DA-9701 did not affect visceral perception in the normal rat. However, in the rat with visceral hypersensitivity, which was induced by neonatal colonic irritation, DA-9701 significantly decreased pain threshold in a dose-dependent manner (130).

Clinical Studies
Functional Dyspepsia

Two large multicenter clinical trials for FD of DA-9701 have been conducted in South Korea using different Rome criteria for FD and efficacy assessment methods (131, 132) (**Table 4**). A randomized, controlled, multi-center study with 462 Korean FD patients by Rome II criteria showed that the effect of 30 mg DA-9701 three times a day on the FD symptom was similar to 50 mg itopride hydrochloride three times a day (131). The overall responder rates were 37% for DA-9701 and 36% for the itopride group at 4 weeks. DA-9701 and itopride significantly reduced the score of all individual symptoms (upper abdominal pain, upper abdominal discomfort, epigastric burning, inability to finish a regular meal, fullness after eating, pressure in the upper abdomen, bloating, and nausea) from baseline. Another randomized, double-blind, multi-center study with 389 Korean FD patients by Rome III criteria showed that the effect of 30 mg DA-9701 three times a day on the FD symptom was similar to 40 mg pantoprazole once-daily (132). The global symptom improvement rates were 60.5 and 65.6% in the DA-9701 and pantoprazole groups at 4 weeks, respectively. Both DA-9701 and

TABLE 4 | Summary of clinical trials of DA-9701.

Subject	Design	County	Comparison	Number		Outcome	Ref.	Jadad score
FD by modified Rome II	Multi-center, randomized, double-blind, controlled	Korea	DA-9701 30 mg t.i.d., a.c., 4 weeks vs. Itopride 50 mg t.i.d., a.c., 4 weeks	228:227	• •	DA-9701 and itopride significantly improved symptoms and QoL. DA-9701 was not inferior to itopride for symptom improvement.	Choi et al. (131)	5
FD by Rome III	Multi-center, randomized, double-blind, controlled	Korea	Placebo PPI q.d. a.c. + Motilitone 30 mg t.i.d., a.c., 4 weeks vs. Pantoprazole 40 mg q.d. a.c. + Placebo t.i.d., a.c., 4 weeks vs. Pantoprazole 40 mg q.d. a.c.+ Motilitone 30 mg t.i.d. a.c. 4 weeks	131:131:127	•	Symptoms and QoL were significantly improved with no significant difference among three groups.	Jung et al. (132)	5
FD by Rome III with *H. pylori*-positive	Multi-center, randomized, double-blind, placebo-controlled	Korea	DA-9701 30 mg t.i.d., a.c., 12 weeks vs. Eradication therapy 1 week + placebo 11 weeks	12:18	•	Effect of DA-9701 therapy on FD symptom was not different from the eradication group.	Park et al. (133)	5
Minimal change with reflux and dyspeptic symptoms	Bi-center, randomized, double-blind, placebo-controlled	Korea	DA-9701 30 mg t.i.d. 4 weeks vs. placebo	42:39	•	Symptoms and QoL were improved; however, DA-9701 was not superior to placebo.	Park et al. (134)	4
Parkinson's disease	Single center, randomized, double-blind, controlled	Korea	DA-9701 30 mg t.i.d., a.c., 4 weeks vs. Domperidone 10 mg t.i.d., a.c., 4 weeks	19:19	• •	DA-9701 significantly increased GE, but not domperidone. The concentration of plasma levodopa was increased in DA-9701 group only, but not significant.	Shin et al. (121)	5
FC by Rome III	Single center, open-labeled	Korea	DA-9701 30 mg t.i.d., a.c., 24 days	33	• •	Constipation-related symptoms were all significantly improved after treatment. Right and rectosigmoid colon transit time was significantly decreased.	Kim et al. (135)	1

FD, functional dyspepsia; FC, functional constipation; q.d., once a day; t.i.d., three times a day; a.c., before meal; QoL, quality of life; GE, gastric emptying.

pantoprazole significantly reduced the score of all individual symptoms (epigastric pain epigastric soreness score, early satiety score, and postprandial fullness) from baseline. Interestingly, combination therapy of DA-9701 and pantoprazole did not increase the response rate compared with DA-9701 or pantoprazole monotherapy. Both studies demonstrated that DA-9701 therapy significantly improved symptom-related QoL in patients with FD.

H. pylori infection is considered a possible cause of FD symptoms. In sub-analysis for the H. pylori-positive group in the above clinical trial comparing DA-9701 and pantoprazole, the response rate was significantly higher in the pantoprazole alone and combination therapy group compared with the DA-9701 alone group (132). While in a small study with 30 patients with FD by Rome III criteria and H. pylori-positive, DA-9701 therapy group showed higher symptom improvement rates at 12 weeks compared with eradication group (73.3 and 60%, respectively); however, it was not statistically different because of the small sample number (133).

Gastroesophageal Reflux Disorder

A randomized, double-blind, placebo-controlled study for the effect of DA-9701 on GERD was conducted in 81 patients with minimal change esophagitis presenting with reflux and dyspeptic symptoms (134). Although the Nepean dyspepsia index and QoL were improved after 4 weeks, 30 mg DA-9701 three times a day was not superior to placebo. The outcome might have been associated with the high placebo response in patients with NERD or FD (134). In subgroup analysis, DA-9701 significantly improved the reflux symptom score compared to the placebo in patients aged 65 years or older (134).

Constipation

DA-9701 has an affinity for the 5-HT$_4$ receptor, and some animal studies have showed it increases colonic motility (122, 129). A prospective and single-center study investigated the efficacy of DA-9701 in 27 patients with functional constipation by Rome III criteria (135). After administration of 30 mg DA-9701 three times a day for 24 days, spontaneous bowel movement, stool form, and constipation-related subjective symptoms were improved. Moreover, right and rectosigmoid colon transit time significantly decreased. However, this study was an open-labeled, uncontrolled study, and most participants were young-aged women (mean age 36.1 ± 15.4 years, 93% female).

Safety

The incidence of adverse events of DA-9701 was not different from itopride or pantoprazole in clinical trials. The reported adverse events include nausea, diarrhea, vomiting, constipation, pruritus, and increased alanine aminotransferase or prolactin levels with mild severity (131, 132). There was no clinically significant cardiovascular events in clinical studies.

Usage

In two large clinical trials, the standard dose of DA-9701 (Motilitone®, Dong-A ST, Seoul, Korea) for adults was 30 mg three times a day before meals.

SUMMARY AND CONCLUSIONS

STW-5 normalizes the stomach and intestinal motility and reduces inflammation and gastric acid production. These effects partially influence the pathophysiology of the FGIDs and their therapeutic effects have been proven in several clinical studies. However, despite the animal experiments that showed fundal relaxation and improvement in antral hypomotility by STW-5, at least ≥50% of patients with FD did not have delayed gastric emptying, and more patients had no abnormalities of gastric accommodation. Although STW-5 reduces the secretion of gastric acid, gastric acid hypersecretion is not always observed in patients with FD. Therefore, such therapeutic effects on the motility and other functions of the GI tract may not necessarily lead to improvement of FGID symptoms, and well-designed clinical studies are still lacking. However, as STW-5 has multiple mechanisms of action and show favorable safety profiles, further studies on their roles on pathophysiology of FGIDs will allow the use of STW-5 as a promising alternative treatment for FGIDs, especially FD and IBS.

Evidence from in vitro studies and clinical trials indicate that PMO seems to alleviate IBS symptoms, mainly abdominal pain, by relaxing smooth muscles in the gut. A recent meta-analysis examining 12 randomized controlled trials showed that PMO was beneficial in the management of IBS and an Asian consensus on IBS mentioned its potential efficacy in treating IBS with a high level of agreement (8, 63). However, any benefit of PMO remains unclear in other FGIDs such as FD owing to the paucity of reliable preclinical and clinical data. Furthermore, relatively unclear mechanisms of action of the active ingredients, unstandardized formulation, and unidentified adverse events are currently significant challenges for its use in the treatment of FGIDs. Relevant evidence based on rigorous studies supporting the efficacy and safety of PMO is needed.

According to a meta-analysis of randomized controlled trials (112), the effects of RKT on the treatment of FD were better than prokinetic drugs, though there was lack of clinically significant evidence due to poor quality of the included studies such as selection bias. Nevertheless, basic research and clinical studies have elucidated that RKT improves esophageal clearance and motility, and promotes gastric motor activity including gastric accommodation and emptying. It also increases ghrelin secretion and food intake. Moreover, RKT attenuates stress-induced injury on the GI tract via the brain-gut axis and balancing the autonomic nervous system. Consequently, it is possible and clinically meaningful to target RKT for subtypes of FD (e.g., PDS type) or specific symptoms (e.g., postprandial fullness), and co-administration with PPI to resolve symptoms of refractory GERD that do not respond to conventional PPI treatment may be more effective.

Several preclinical and human studies have demonstrated that DA-9701 increased gastric emptying and antral motility in normal or diseased states. In addition, DA-9701 improved gastric accommodation as well as feeding inhibition by stress. Based on these results, subsequent clinical trials in patients with FD demonstrated that DA-9701 was not inferior compared with itopride or PPI to improve FD symptoms. It was also suggested that DA-9701 could improve symptoms of GERD and constipation in the specific patient population. However, most studies for the effect of DA-9701 on FD and other FGIDs have performed only in one country. Moreover, the clinical trials for FD recruited a large number of participants but were non-inferiority studies. Therefore, well-designed clinical trials in different countries and more detailed mechanical studies should be performed in the future.

The role of herbal therapies in FGIDs is still unclear. The active ingredients and mechanisms of action have not been fully identified and well-designed clinical trials are insufficient.

However, herbal therapies play a role as a complementary and alternative medicine and may find suitable application in refractory patients. The development of various promising herbal medications in the near future may help to improve the QoL of patients with FGIDs.

AUTHOR CONTRIBUTIONS

YK, J-WK, JK and HR conceptualized the study. YK, J-WK, N-YH and HR wrote the first draft of the manuscript. YK, J-WK and JK critically revised the manuscript. HR received the grant. All authors contributed to the article and approved the submitted version.

REFERENCES

1. Drossman DA. The functional gastrointestinal disorders and the Rome II process. *Gut* (1999) 45(Suppl 2):1–5. doi: 10.1136/gut.45.2008.ii1
2. Sperber AD, Gwee KA, Hungin AP, Corazziari E, Fukudo S, Gerson C, et al. Conducting multinational, cross-cultural research in the functional gastrointestinal disorders: issues and recommendations. A Rome Foundation working team report. *Aliment Pharmacol Ther* (2014) 40:1094–102. doi: 10.1111/apt.12942
3. Koloski NA, Talley NJ, Boyce PM. Epidemiology and health care seeking in the functional GI disorders: a population-based study. *Am J Gastroenterol* (2002) 97:2290–9. doi: 10.1111/j.1572-0241.2002.05783.x
4. Drossman DA, Hasler WL. Rome IV-Functional GI Disorders: Disorders of Gut-Brain Interaction. *Gastroenterology* (2016) 150:1257–61. doi: 10.1053/j.gastro.2016.03.035
5. Camilleri M. Pharmacological agents currently in clinical trials for disorders in neurogastroenterology. *J Clin Invest* (2013) 123:4111–20. doi: 10.1172/JCI70837
6. Magge S, Lembo A. Complementary and alternative medicine for the irritable bowel syndrome. *Gastroenterol Clin North Am* (2011) 40:245–53. doi: 10.1016/j.gtc.2010.12.005
7. Miwa H, Ghoshal UC, Gonlachanvit S, Gwee KA, Ang TL, Chang FY, et al. Asian consensus report on functional dyspepsia. *J Neurogastroenterol Motil* (2012) 18:150–68. doi: 10.5056/jnm.2012.18.2.150
8. Gwee KA, Gonlachanvit S, Ghoshal UC, Chua ASB, Miwa H, Wu J, et al. Second Asian Consensus on Irritable Bowel Syndrome. *J Neurogastroenterol Motil* (2019) 25:343–62. doi: 10.5056/jnm19041
9. Jang SH, Ryu HS, Choi SC, Lee SY. Psychological factors influence the overlap syndrome in functional gastrointestinal disorders and their effect on quality of life among firefighters in South Korea. *J Dig Dis* (2016) 17:236–43. doi: 10.1111/1751-2980.12330
10. Jadad AR, Moore RA, Carroll D, Jenkinson C, Reynolds DJ, Gavaghan DJ, et al. Assessing the quality of reports of randomized clinical trials: is blinding necessary? *Control Clin Trials* (1996) 17:1–12. doi: 10.1016/0197-2456(95)00134-4
11. Malfertheiner P. STW 5 (Iberogast) Therapy in Gastrointestinal Functional Disorders. *Dig Dis* (2017) 35(Suppl 1):25–9. doi: 10.1159/000485410
12. Pilichiewicz AN, Horowitz M, Russo A, Maddox AF, Jones KL, Schemann M, et al. Effects of Iberogast on proximal gastric volume, antropyloroduodenal motility and gastric emptying in healthy men. *Am J Gastroenterol* (2007) 102:1276–83. doi: 10.1111/j.1572-0241.2007.01142.x
13. Hohenester B, Ruhl A, Kelber O, Schemann M. The herbal preparation STW5 (Iberogast) has potent and region-specific effects on gastric motility. *Neurogastroenterol Motil* (2004) 16:765–73. doi: 10.1111/j.1365-2982.2004.00548.x
14. Schemann M, Michel K, Zeller F, Hohenester B, Rühl A. Region-specific effects of STW 5 (Iberogast) and its components in gastric fundus, corpus

and antrum. *Phytomedicine* (2006) 13(Suppl 5):90–9. doi: 10.1016/j.phymed.2006.03.020
15. Ammon HP, Kelber O, Okpanyi SN. Spasmolytic and tonic effect of Iberogast (STW 5) in intestinal smooth muscle. *Phytomedicine* (2006) 13 (Suppl 5):67–74. doi: 10.1016/j.phymed.2006.08.004
16. Sibaev A, Yuece B, Kelber O, Weiser D, Schirra J, Göke B, et al. STW 5 (Iberogast) and its individual herbal components modulate intestinal electrophysiology of mice. *Phytomedicine* (2006) 13(Suppl 5):80–9. doi: 10.1016/j.phymed.2006.03.015
17. Simmen U, Kelber O, Okpanyi SN, Jaeggi R, Bueter B, Weiser D. Binding of STW 5 (Iberogast) and its components to intestinal 5-HT, muscarinic M3, and opioid receptors. *Phytomedicine* (2006) 13(Suppl 5):51–5. doi: 10.1016/j.phymed.2006.03.012
18. Liu CY, Muller MH, Glatzle J, Weiser D, Kelber O, Enck P, et al. The herbal preparation STW 5 (Iberogast) desensitizes intestinal afferents in the rat small intestine. *Neurogastroenterol Motil* (2004) 16:759–64. doi: 10.1111/j.1365-2982.2004.00576.x
19. Khayyal MT, Seif-El-Nasr M, El-Ghazaly MA, Okpanyi SN, Kelber O, Weiser D. Mechanisms involved in the gastro-protective effect of STW 5 (Iberogast) and its components against ulcers and rebound acidity. *Phytomedicine* (2006) 13(Suppl 5):56–66. doi: 10.1016/j.phymed.2006.03.019
20. Wadie W, Abdel-Aziz H, Zaki HF, Kelber O, Weiser D, Khayyal MT. STW 5 is effective in dextran sulfate sodium-induced colitis in rats. *Int J Colorectal Dis* (2012) 27:1445–53. doi: 10.1007/s00384-012-1473-z
21. Michael S, Kelber O, Hauschildt S, Spanel-Borowski K, Nieber K. Inhibition of inflammation-induced alterations in rat small intestine by the herbal preparations STW 5 and STW 6. *Phytomedicine* (2009) 16:161–71. doi: 10.1016/j.phymed.2008.10.011
22. Allam S, Krueger D, Demir IE, Ceyhan G, Zeller F, Schemann M. Extracts from peppermint leaves, lemon balm leaves and in particular angelica roots mimic the pro-secretory action of the herbal preparation STW 5 in the human intestine. *Phytomedicine* (2015) 22:1063–70. doi: 10.1016/j.phymed.2015.08.008
23. von Arnim U, Peitz U, Vinson B, Gundermann KJ, Malfertheiner P. STW 5, a phytopharmacon for patients with functional dyspepsia: results of a multicenter, placebo-controlled double-blind study. *Am J Gastroenterol* (2007) 102:1268–75. doi: 10.1111/j.1572-0241.2006.01183.x
24. Braden B, Caspary W, Borner N, Vinson B, Schneider AR. Clinical effects of STW 5 (Iberogast) are not based on acceleration of gastric emptying in patients with functional dyspepsia and gastroparesis. *Neurogastroenterol Motil* (2009) 21:632-8:e25. doi: 10.1111/j.1365-2982.2008.01249.x
25. Madisch A, Holtmann G, Plein K, Hotz J. Treatment of irritable bowel syndrome with herbal preparations: results of a double-blind, randomized, placebo-controlled, multi-centre trial. *Aliment Pharmacol Ther* (2004) 19:271–9. doi: 10.1111/j.1365-2036.2004.01859.x
26. Saez-Gonzalez E, Conde I, Diaz-Jaime FC, Benlloch S, Prieto M, Berenguer M. Iberogast-induced severe hepatotoxicity leading to liver transplantation. *Am J Gastroenterol* (2016) 111:1364 5. doi: 10.1038/ajg.2016.260

27. Gerhardt F, Benesic A, Tillmann HL, Rademacher S, Wittekind C, Gerbes AL, et al. Iberogast-induced acute liver failure-reexposure and in vitro assay support causality. *Am J Gastroenterol* (2019) 114:1358–9. doi: 10.14309/ajg.0000000000000300

28. Teschke R, Frenzel C, Glass X, Schulze J, Eickhoff A. Greater celandine hepatotoxicity: a clinical review. *Ann Hepatol* (2012) 11:838–48. doi: 10.1016/S1665-2681(19)31408-5

29. Ulbricht C, Costa D, JMGS, Guilford J, Isaac R, Seamon E, et al. An evidence-based systematic review of spearmint by the natural standard research collaboration. *J Diet Suppl* (2010) 7:179–215. doi: 10.3109/19390211.2010.486702

30. Kearns GL, Chumpitazi BP, Abdel-Rahman SM, Garg U, Shulman RJ. Systemic exposure to menthol following administration of peppermint oil to paediatric patients. *BMJ Open* (2015) 5:e008375. doi: 10.1136/bmjopen-2015-008375

31. Haber SL, El-Ibiary SY. Peppermint oil for treatment of irritable bowel syndrome. *Am J Health Syst Pharm* (2016) 73:22, 24, 26. passim. doi: 10.2146/ajhp140801

32. Grigoleit HG, Grigoleit P. Pharmacology and preclinical pharmacokinetics of peppermint oil. *Phytomedicine* (2005) 12:612–6. doi: 10.1016/j.phymed.2004.10.007

33. Blumenthal M, Goldberg A, Brinckmann J. Herbal medicine: expanded Commission E monographs (2000).

34. Hawthorn M, Ferrante J, Luchowski E, Rutledge A, Wei XY, Triggle DJ. The actions of peppermint oil and menthol on calcium channel dependent processes in intestinal, neuronal and cardiac preparations. *Aliment Pharmacol Ther* (1988) 2:101–18. doi: 10.1111/j.1365-2036.1988.tb00677.x

35. Hills JM, Aaronson PI. The mechanism of action of peppermint oil on gastrointestinal smooth muscle. An analysis using patch clamp electrophysiology and isolated tissue pharmacology in rabbit and guinea pig. *Gastroenterology* (1991) 101:55–65. doi: 10.1016/0016-5085(91)90459-X

36. Kim HJ, Wie J, So I, Jung MH, Ha KT, Kim BJ. Menthol modulates pacemaker potentials through TRPA1 channels in cultured interstitial cells of Cajal from murine small intestine. *Cell Physiol Biochem* (2016) 38:1869–82. doi: 10.1159/000445549

37. Mizuno S, Kato K, Ono Y, Yano K, Kurosaka H, Takahashi A, et al. Oral peppermint oil is a useful antispasmodic for double-contrast barium meal examination. *J Gastroenterol Hepatol* (2006) 21:1297–301. doi: 10.1111/j.1440-1746.2006.04131.x

38. Micklefield G, Jung O, Greving I, May B. Effects of intraduodenal application of peppermint oil (WS(R) 1340) and caraway oil (WS(R) 1520) on gastroduodenal motility in healthy volunteers. *Phytother Res* (2003) 17:135–40. doi: 10.1002/ptr.1089

39. Micklefield GH, Greving I, May B. Effects of peppermint oil and caraway oil on gastroduodenal motility. *Phytother Res* (2000) 14:20–3. doi: 10.1002/(SICI)1099-1573(200002)14:1<20::AID-PTR542>3.0.CO;2-Z

40. Goerg KJ, Spilker T. Effect of peppermint oil and caraway oil on gastrointestinal motility in healthy volunteers: a pharmacodynamic study using simultaneous determination of gastric and gall-bladder emptying and orocaecal transit time. *Aliment Pharmacol Ther* (2003) 17:445–51. doi: 10.1046/j.1365-2036.2003.01421.x

41. Asao T, Mochiki E, Suzuki H, Nakamura J, Hirayama I, Morinaga N, et al. An easy method for the intraluminal administration of peppermint oil before colonoscopy and its effectiveness in reducing colonic spasm. *Gastrointest Endosc* (2001) 53:172–7. doi: 10.1067/mge.2000.108477

42. Karashima Y, Damann N, Prenen J, Talavera K, Segal A, Voets T, et al. Bimodal action of menthol on the transient receptor potential channel TRPA1. *J Neurosci* (2007) 27:9874–84. doi: 10.1523/JNEUROSCI.2221-07.2007

43. Adam B, Liebregts T, Best J, Bechmann L, Lackner C, Neumann J, et al. A combination of peppermint oil and caraway oil attenuates the post-inflammatory visceral hyperalgesia in a rat model. *Scand J Gastroenterol* (2006) 41:155–60. doi: 10.1080/00365520500206442

44. Liu B, Fan L, Balakrishna S, Sui A, Morris JB, Jordt SE, et al. TRPM8 is the principal mediator of menthol-induced analgesia of acute and inflammatory pain. *Pain* (2013) 154:2169–77. doi: 10.1016/j.pain.2013.06.043

45. Sigmund CJ, McNally EF. The action of a carminative on the lower esophageal sphincter. *Gastroenterology* (1969) 56:13–8. doi: 10.1016/S0016-5085(69)80061-2

46. Pimentel M, Bonorris GG, Chow EJ, Lin HC. Peppermint oil improves the manometric findings in diffuse esophageal spasm. *J Clin Gastroenterol* (2001) 33:27–31. doi: 10.1097/00004836-200107000-00007

47. Imagawa A, Hata H, Nakatsu M, Yoshida Y, Takeuchi K, Inokuchi T, et al. Peppermint oil solution is useful as an antispasmodic drug for esophagogastroduodenoscopy, especially for elderly patients. *Dig Dis Sci* (2012) 57:2379–84. doi: 10.1007/s10620-012-2194-4

48. Papathanasopoulos A, Rotondo A, Janssen P, Boesmans W, Farre R, Vanden Berghe P, et al. Effect of acute peppermint oil administration on gastric sensorimotor function and nutrient tolerance in health. *Neurogastroenterol Motil* (2013) 25:e263–71. doi: 10.1111/nmo.12102

49. Dalvi SS, Nadkarni PM, Pardesi R, Gupta KC. Effect of peppermint oil on gastric emptying in man: a preliminary study using a radiolabelled solid test meal. *Indian J Physiol Pharmacol* (1991) 35:212–4.

50. Umezu T. Evidence for dopamine involvement in ambulation promoted by menthone in mice. *Pharmacol Biochem Behav* (2009) 91:315–20. doi: 10.1016/j.pbb.2008.07.017

51. Umezu T, Morita M. Evidence for the involvement of dopamine in ambulation promoted by menthol in mice. *J Pharmacol Sci* (2003) 91:125–35. doi: 10.1254/jphs.91.125

52. da Silveira NS, de Oliveira-Silva GL, Lamanes Bde F, Prado LC, Bispo-da-Silva LB. The aversive, anxiolytic-like, and verapamil-sensitive psychostimulant effects of pulegone. *Biol Pharm Bull* (2014) 37:771–8. doi: 10.1248/bpb.b13-00832

53. Liu JH, Chen GH, Yeh HZ, Huang CK, Poon SK. Enteric-coated peppermint-oil capsules in the treatment of irritable bowel syndrome: a prospective, randomized trial. *J Gastroenterol* (1997) 32:765–8. doi: 10.1007/BF02936952

54. Cappello G, Spezzaferro M, Grossi L, Manzoli L, Marzio L. Peppermint oil (Mintoil) in the treatment of irritable bowel syndrome: a prospective double blind placebo-controlled randomized trial. *Dig Liver Dis* (2007) 39:530–6. doi: 10.1016/j.dld.2007.02.006

55. Merat S, Khalili S, Mostajabi P, Ghorbani A, Ansari R, Malekzadeh R. The effect of enteric-coated, delayed-release peppermint oil on irritable bowel syndrome. *Dig Dis Sci* (2010) 55:1385–90. doi: 10.1007/s10620-009-0854-9

56. Cash BD, Epstein MS, Shah SM. A novel delivery system of peppermint oil is an effective therapy for irritable bowel syndrome symptoms. *Dig Dis Sci* (2016) 61:560–71. doi: 10.1007/s10620-015-3858-7

57. Kline RM, Kline JJ, Di Palma J, Barbero GJ. Enteric-coated, pH-dependent peppermint oil capsules for the treatment of irritable bowel syndrome in children. *J Pediatr* (2001) 138:125–8. doi: 10.1067/mpd.2001.109606

58. May B, Kohler S, Schneider B. Efficacy and tolerability of a fixed combination of peppermint oil and caraway oil in patients suffering from functional dyspepsia. *Aliment Pharmacol Ther* (2000) 14:1671–7. doi: 10.1046/j.1365-2036.2000.00873.x

59. Rich G, Shah A, Koloski N, Funk P, Stracke B, Köhler S, et al. A randomized placebo-controlled trial on the effects of Menthacarin, a proprietary peppermint- and caraway-oil-preparation, on symptoms and quality of life in patients with functional dyspepsia. *Neurogastroenterol Motil* (2017) 29:e13132. doi: 10.1111/nmo.13132

60. Pittler MH, Ernst E. Peppermint oil for irritable bowel syndrome: a critical review and metaanalysis. *Am J Gastroenterol* (1998) 93:1131–5. doi: 10.1111/j.1572-0241.1998.00343.x

61. Ford AC, Talley NJ, Spiegel BM, Foxx-Orenstein AE, Schiller L, Quigley EM, et al. Effect of fibre, antispasmodics, and peppermint oil in the treatment of irritable bowel syndrome: systematic review and meta-analysis. *BMJ* (2008) 337:a2313. doi: 10.1136/bmj.a2313

62. Khanna R, MacDonald JK, Levesque BG. Peppermint oil for the treatment of irritable bowel syndrome: a systematic review and meta-analysis. *J Clin Gastroenterol* (2014) 48:505–12. doi: 10.1097/MCG.0b013e3182a88357

63. Alammar N, Wang L, Saberi B, Nanavati J, Holtmann G, Shinohara RT, et al. The impact of peppermint oil on the irritable bowel syndrome: a meta-analysis of the pooled clinical data. *BMC Complement Altern Med* (2019) 19:21. doi: 10.1186/s12906-018-2409-0

64. Madisch A, Holtmann G, Mayr G, Vinson B, Hotz J. Treatment of functional dyspepsia with a herbal preparation. A double-blind, randomized, placebo-controlled, multicenter trial. *Digestion* (2004) 69:45–52. doi: 10.1159/000076546

65. Weston CF. Anal burning and peppermint oil. *Postgrad Med J* (1987) 63:717. doi: 10.1136/pgmj.63.742.717-a

66. Dresser GK, Wacher V, Wong S, Wong HT, Bailey DG. Evaluation of peppermint oil and ascorbyl palmitate as inhibitors of cytochrome P4503A4 activity in vitro and in vivo. *Clin Pharmacol Ther* (2002) 72:247–55. doi: 10.1067/mcp.2002.126409

67. Kligler B, Chaudhary S. Peppermint oil. *Am Fam Physician* (2007) 75:1027–30.

68. Zhang WD, Wei BH, Chen ZS. [Schedule for diagnosis and treatment of functional indigestion syndrome with intergrative Chinese and Western medicine]. *Zhongguo Zhong Xi Yi Jie He Za Zhi* (2005) 25:559–61.

69. Suzuki H, Matsuzaki J, Fukushima Y, Suzaki F, Kasugai K, Nishizawa T, et al. Randomized clinical trial: rikkunshito in the treatment of functional dyspepsia–a multicenter, double-blind, randomized, placebo-controlled study. *Neurogastroenterol Motil* (2014) 26:950–61. doi: 10.1111/nmo.12348

70. Tominaga K, Arakawa T. Kampo medicines for gastrointestinal tract disorders: a review of basic science and clinical evidence and their future application. *Gastroenterol* (2013) 48:452–62. doi: 10.1007/s00535-013-0788-z

71. Takeda H, Muto S, Nakagawa K, Ohnishi S, Asaka M. Rikkunshito and ghrelin secretion. *Curr Pharm Des* (2012) 18:4827–38. doi: 10.2174/138161212803216933

72. Cremonini F. Standardized herbal treatments on functional bowel disorders: moving from putative mechanisms of action to controlled clinical trials. *Neurogastroenterol Motil* (2014) 26:893–900. doi: 10.1111/nmo.12384   *J*

73. Tominaga K, Kato M, Takeda H, Shimoyama Y, Umegaki E, Iwakiri R, et al. A randomized, placebo-controlled, double-blind clinical trial of rikkunshito for patients with non-erosive reflux disease refractory to proton-pump inhibitor: the G-PRIDE study. *J Gastroenterol* (2014) 49:1392–405. doi: 10.1007/s00535-013-0896-9

74. Kusunoki H, Haruma K, Hata J, Ishii M, Kamada T, Yamashita N, et al. Efficacy of Rikkunshito, a traditional Japanese medicine (Kampo), in treating functional dyspepsia. *Intern Med* (2010) 49:2195–202. doi: 10.2169/internalmedicine.49.3803

75. Tominaga K, Kido T, Ochi M, Sadakane C, Masa A, Okazaki H, et al. The traditional japanese medicine rikkunshito promotes gastric emptying via the antagonistic action of the 5-HT(3) receptor pathway in rats. *Evid Based Complement Alternat Med* (2011) 2011:248481. doi: 10.1093/ecam/nep173

76. Kitagawa H, Munekage M, Matsumoto T, Sadakane C, Fukutake M, Aoki K, et al. Pharmacokinetic profiles of active ingredients and its metabolites derived from rikkunshito, a ghrelin enhancer, in healthy Japanese volunteers: a cross-over, randomized study. *PloS One* (2015) 10:e0133159. doi: 10.1371/journal.pone.0133159

77. Miwa H, Koseki J, Oshima T, Kondo T, Tomita T, Watari J, et al. Rikkunshito, a traditional Japanese medicine, may relieve abdominal symptoms in rats with experimental esophagitis by improving the barrier function of epithelial cells in esophageal mucosa. *J Gastroenterol* (2010) 45:478–87. doi: 10.1007/s00535-009-0180-1

78. Kawahara H, Kubota A, Hasegawa T, Okuyam H, Ueno T, Ida S, et al. Effects of rikkunshito on the clinical symptoms and esophageal acid exposure in children with symptomatic gastroesophageal reflux. *Pediatr Surg Int* (2007) 23:1001–5. doi: 10.1007/s00383-007-1986-7

79. Odaka T, Yamato S, Yokosuka O. Esophageal motility and rikkunshito treatment for proton pump inhibitor-refractory nonerosive reflux disease: a prospective, uncontrolled, open-label pilot study trial. *Curr Ther Res Clin Exp* (2017) 84:37–41. doi: 10.1016/j.curtheres.2017.03.007

80. Yakabi K, Sadakane C, Noguchi M, Ohno S, Ro S, Chinen K, et al. Reduced ghrelin secretion in the hypothalamus of rats due to cisplatin-induced anorexia. *Endocrinology* (2010) 151:3773–82. doi: 10.1210/en.2010-0061

81. Takeda H, Sadakane C, Hattori T, Katsurada T, Ohkawara T, Nagai K, et al. Rikkunshito, an herbal medicine, suppresses cisplatin-induced anorexia in rats via 5-HT2 receptor antagonism. *Gastroenterology* (2008) 134:2004–13. doi: 10.1053/j.gastro.2008.02.078

82. Masuy I, Van Oudenhove L, Tack J. Review article: treatment options for functional dyspepsia. *Aliment Pharmacol Ther* (2019) 49:1134–72. doi: 10.1111/apt.15191

83. Togawa K, Matsuzaki J, Kobayakawa M, Fukushima Y, Suzaki F, Kasugai K, et al. Association of baseline plasma des-acyl ghrelin level with the response to rikkunshito in patients with functional dyspepsia. *J Gastroenterol Hepatol* (2016) 31:334–41. doi: 10.1111/jgh.13074

84. Arai M, Matsumura T, Tsuchiya N, Sadakane C, Inami R, Suzuki T, et al. Rikkunshito improves the symptoms in patients with functional dyspepsia, accompanied by an increase in the level of plasma ghrelin. *Hepatogastroenterology* (2012) 59:62–6. doi: 10.5754/hge11246

85. Takeda H, Muto S, Hattori T, Sadakane C, Tsuchiya K, Katsurada T, et al. Rikkunshito ameliorates the aging-associated decrease in ghrelin receptor reactivity via phosphodiesterase III inhibition. *Endocrinology* (2010) 151:244–52. doi: 10.1210/en.2009-0633

86. Mondal A, Takehara A, Aizawa S, Tanaka T, Fujitsuka N, Hattori T, et al. Rikkunshito induces gastric relaxation via the beta-adrenergic pathway in Suncus murinus. *Neurogastroenterol Motil* (2015) 27:875–84. doi: 10.1111/nmo.12564

87. Scheid CR, Honeyman TW, Fay FS. Mechanism of beta-adrenergic relaxation of smooth muscle. *Nature* (1979) 277:32–6. doi: 10.1038/277032a0

88. Kito Y, Suzuki H. Properties of Rikkunshi-to (TJ-43)-induced relaxation of rat gastric fundus smooth muscles. *Am J Physiol Gastrointest Liver Physiol* (2010) 298:G755–63. doi: 10.1152/ajpgi.00333.2009

89. Hayakawa T, Arakawa T, Kase Y, Akiyama S, Ishige A, Takeda S, et al. Liu-Jun-Zi-Tang, a kampo medicine, promotes adaptive relaxation in isolated guinea pig stomachs. *Drugs Exp Clin Res* (1999) 25:211–8.

90. Kido T, Nakai Y, Kase Y, Sakakibara I, Nomura M, Takeda S, et al. Effects of rikkunshi-to, a traditional Japanese medicine, on the delay of gastric emptying induced by N(G)-nitro-L-arginine. *J Pharmacol Sci* (2005) 98:161–7. doi: 10.1254/jphs.FPJ04056X

91. Yanai M, Mochiki E, Ogawa A, Morita H, Toyomasu Y, Ogata K, et al. Intragastric administration of rikkunshito stimulates upper gastrointestinal motility and gastric emptying in conscious dogs. *J Gastroenterol* (2013) 48:611–9. doi: 10.1007/s00535-012-0687-8

92. Araki Y, Mukaisho KI, Fujiyama Y, Hattori T, Sugihara H. The herbal medicine rikkunshito exhibits strong and differential adsorption properties for bile salts. *Exp Ther Med* (2012) 3:645–9. doi: 10.3892/etm.2012.478

93. Tominaga K, Arakawa T. Clinical application of kampo medicine (rikkunshito) for common and/or intractable symptoms of the gastrointestinal tract. *Front Pharmacol* (2015) 6:7. doi: 10.3389/fphar.2015.00007

94. Shiratori M, Shoji T, Kanazawa M, Hongo M, Rukudo S, et al. Effect of rikkunshito on gastric sensorimotor function under distention. *Neurogastroenterol Motil* (2011) 23:323–9e155–6. doi: 10.1111/j.1365-2982.2010.01648.x

95. Tanaka C, Asakawa A, Ushikai M, Sakoguchi T, Amitani H, Mutsumi T, et al. Comparison of the anorexigenic activity of CRF family peptides. *Biochem Biophys Res Commun* (2009) 390:887–91. doi: 10.1016/j.bbrc.2009.10.069

96. Saegusa Y, Takeda H, Muto S, Nakagawa K, Ohnishi S, Sadakane C, et al. Decreased plasma ghrelin contributes to anorexia following novelty stress. *Am J Physiol Endocrinol Metab* (2011) 301:E685–96. doi: 10.1152/ajpendo.00121.2011

97. Nahata M, Saegusa Y, Sadakane C, Yamada C, Nakagawa K, Okubo N, et al. Administration of exogenous acylated ghrelin or rikkunshito, an endogenous ghrelin enhancer, improves the decrease in postprandial gastric motility in an acute restraint stress mouse model. *Neurogastroenterol Motil* (2014) 26:821–31. doi: 10.1111/nmo.12336

98. Hu WH, Wong WM, Lam CL, Lam KF, Hui WM, Lai KH, et al. Anxiety but not depression determines health care-seeking behaviour in Chinese patients with dyspepsia and irritable bowel syndrome: a population-based study. *Aliment Pharmacol Ther* (2002) 16:2081–8. doi: 10.1046/j.1365-2036.2002.01377.x

99. Miwa H, Koseki J, Oshima T, Hattori T, Kase Y, Kondo T, et al. Impairment of gastric accommodation induced by water-avoidance stress is mediated by 5-HT2B receptors. *Neurogastroenterol Motil* (2016) 28:765–78. doi: 10.1111/nmo.12775

100. Mogami S, Sadakane C, Nahata M, Mizuhara Y, Yamada C, Hattori T, et al. CRF receptor 1 antagonism and brain distribution of active components contribute to the ameliorative effect of rikkunshito on stress-induced anorexia. *Sci Rep* (2016) 6:27516. doi: 10.1038/srep27516

101. Naito T, Itoh H, Takeyama M. Some gastrointestinal function regulatory Kampo medicines have modulatory effects on human plasma adrenocorticotropic hormone and cortisol levels with continual stress exposure. *Biol Pharm Bull* (2003) 26:101–4. doi: 10.1248/bpb.26.101

102. Tominaga K, Higuchi K, Kadouchi K, Sasaki E, Shiba M, Watanabe T, et al. Disorder of circadian rhythm of autonomic nervous system activity and its correlation with abdominal symptoms in functional dyspepsia. *Gastroenterology* (2003) 124:A225. doi: 10.1016/S0016-5085(03)81132-0

103. Sato Y, Katagiri F, Itoh H, Takeyama M. Effects of some kampo medicines on plasma levels of neuropeptide Y under venipuncture stress. *Biol Pharm Bull* (2005) 28:1757 61. doi: 10.1248/bpb.28.1757

104. Fujitsuka N, Asakawa A, Uezono Y, Minami K, Yamaguchi T, Niijima A, et al. Potentiation of ghrelin signaling attenuates cancer anorexia-cachexia and prolongs survival. *Transl Psychiatry* (2011) 1:e23. doi: 10.1038/tp.2011.25

105. Tatsuta M, Iishi H. Effect of treatment with liu-jun-zi-tang (TJ-43) on gastric emptying and gastrointestinal symptoms in dyspeptic patients. *Aliment Pharmacol Ther* (1993) 7:459–62. doi: 10.1111/j.1365-2036.1993.tb00120.x

106. Tominaga K, Sakata Y, Kusunoki H, Odaka T, Sakurai K, Kawamura O, et al. Rikkunshito simultaneously improves dyspepsia correlated with anxiety in patients with functional dyspepsia: A randomized clinical trial (the DREAM study). *Neurogastroenterol Motil* (2018) 30:e13319. doi: 10.1111/nmo.13319

107. Tominaga K, Iwakiri R, Fujimoto K, Fujiwara Y, Tanaka M, Shimoyama Y, et al. Rikkunshito improves symptoms in PPI-refractory GERD patients: a prospective, randomized, multicenter trial in Japan. *J Gastroenterol* (2012) 47:284–92. doi: 10.1007/s00535-011-0488-5

108. Kawai T, Hirayama Y, Oguchi A, Ishii F, Matushita M, Kitayama N, et al. Effects of rikkunshito on quality of life in patients with gastroesophageal reflux disease refractory to proton pump inhibitor therapy. *J Clin Biochem Nutr* (2017) 60:143–5. doi: 10.3164/jcbn.16-77

109. Tokashiki R, Okamoto I, Funato N, Suzuki M. Rikkunshito improves globus sensation in patients with proton-pump inhibitor-refractory laryngopharyngeal reflux. *World J Gastroenterol* (2013) 19:5118–24. doi: 10.3748/wjg.v19.i31.5118

110. Yamawaki H, Futagami S, Wakabayashi M, Sakasegawa N, Agawa S, Higuchi K, et al. Management of functional dyspepsia: state of the art and emerging therapies. *Ther Adv Chronic Dis* (2018) 9:23–32. doi: 10.1177/2040622317725479

111. Sakata Y, Tominaga K, Kato M, Takeda H, Shimoyama Y, Takeuchi T, et al. Clinical characteristics of elderly patients with proton pump inhibitor-refractory non-erosive reflux disease from the G-PRIDE study who responded to rikkunshito. *BMC Gastroenterol* (2014) 14:116. doi: 10.1186/1471-230X-14-116

112. Xiao Y, Liu YY, Yu KQ, Ouyang MZ, Luo R, Zhao XS. Chinese herbal medicine liu jun zi tang and xiang sha liu jun zi tang for functional dyspepsia: meta-analysis of randomized controlled trials. *Evid Based Complement Alternat Med* (2012) 2012:936459. doi: 10.1155/2012/936459

113. Kwon YS, Son M. DA-9701: a new multi-acting drug for the treatment of functional dyspepsia. *Biomol Ther (Seoul)* (2013) 21:181–9. doi: 10.4062/biomolther.2012.096

114. Jin M, Son M. DA-9701 (Motilitone): a multi-targeting botanical drug for the treatment of functional dyspepsia. *Int J Mol Sci* (2018) 19(12):4035. doi: 10.3390/ijms19124035

115. Jung JW, Kim JM, Jeong JS, Son M, Lee HS, Lee MG, et al. Pharmacokinetics of chlorogenic acid and corydaline in DA-9701, a new botanical gastroprokinetic agent, in rats. *Xenobiotica* (2014) 44:635–43. doi: 10.3109/00498254.2013.874610

116. Soji Y, Kadokawa T, Masuda Y, Kawashima K, Nakamura K. Effects of Corydalis alkaloid upon inhibition of gastric juice secretion and prevention of gastric ulcer in experimental animals. *Nihon Yakurigaku Zasshi* (1969) 65:196–209. doi: 10.1254/fpj.65.196

117. Lee TH, Choi JJ, Kim DH, Choi S, Lee KR, Son M, et al. Gastroprokinetic effects of DA-9701, a new prokinetic agent formulated with Pharbitis Semen and Corydalis Tuber. *Phytomedicine* (2008) 15:836–43. doi: 10.1016/j.phymed.2008.02.019

118. Lim CH, Choi MG, Park H, Baeg MK, Park JM. Effect of DA-9701 on gastric emptying in a mouse model: assessment by (1)(3)C-octanoic acid breath test. *World J Gastroenterol* (2013) 19:4380–5. doi: 10.3748/wjg.v19.i27.4380

119. Kang JW, Han DK, Kim ON, Lee KJ. Effect of DA-9701 on the Normal Motility and Clonidine-induced Hypomotility of the Gastric Antrum in Rats. *J Neurogastroenterol Motil* (2016) 22:304–9. doi: 10.5056/jnm15131

120. Min YW, Min BH, Kim S, Choi D, Rhee PL. Effect of DA-9701 on gastric motor function assessed by magnetic resonance imaging in healthy volunteers: a randomized, double-blind, placebo-controlled trial. *PloS One* (2015) 10:e0138927. doi: 10.1371/journal.pone.0138927

121. Shin CM, Lee YJ, Kim JM, Lee JY, Kim KJ, Choi YJ, et al. DA-9701 on gastric motility in patients with Parkinson's disease: A randomized controlled trial. *Parkinsonism Relat Disord* (2018) 54:84–9. doi: 10.1016/j.parkreldis.2018.04.018

122. Hussain Z, Rhee KW, Lee YJ, Park H. The effect of DA-9701 in opioid-induced bowel dysfunction of guinea pig. *J Neurogastroenterol Motil* (2016) 22:529–38. doi: 10.5056/jnm15194

123. Lee SP, Lee OY, Lee KN, Lee HL, Choi HS, Yoon BC, et al. Effect of DA-9701, a novel prokinetic agent, on post-operative ileus in rats. *J Neurogastroenterol Motil* (2017) 23:109–16. doi: 10.5056/jnm16003

124. Jung YS, Kim MY, Lee HS, Park SL, Lee KJ. Effect of DA-9701, a novel prokinetic agent, on stress-induced delayed gastric emptying and hormonal changes in rats. *Neurogastroenterol Motil* (2013) 25:254–9. e166. doi: 10.1111/nmo.12053

125. Jo SY, Hussain Z, Lee YJ, Park H. Corticotrophin-releasing factor-mediated effects of DA-9701 in postoperative Ileus guinea pig model. *Neurogastroenterol Motil* (2018) 30:e13385. doi: 10.1111/nmo.13385

126. Kim ER, Min BH, Lee SO, Lee TH, Son M, Rhee PL. Effects of DA-9701, a novel prokinetic agent, on gastric accommodation in conscious dogs. *J Gastroenterol Hepatol* (2012) 27:766–72. doi: 10.1111/j.1440-1746.2011.06924.x

127. Kim YS, Lee MY, Park JS, Choi ES, Kim MS, Park SH, et al. Effect of DA-9701 on feeding inhibition induced by acute restraint stress in rats. *Korean J Helicobacter Up Gastrointest Res* (2018) 18:50–5. doi: 10.7704/kjhugr.2018.18.1.50

128. Min YW, Ko EJ, Lee JY, Min BH, Lee JH, Kim JJ, et al. Nitrergic pathway is the major mechanism for the effect of DA-9701 on the rat gastric fundus relaxation. *J Neurogastroenterol Motil* (2014) 20:318–25. doi: 10.5056/jnm13098

129. Kim YS, Ryu HS, Joo MC, OH JT, Choi ES, Choi SC. Effect of DA-9701, new prokinetic, on colonic function of spinal cord injured rat model. in *Abstracts of the Joint International Neurogastroenterology and Motility Meeting*; 6–8 September 2012; Bologna, Italy. (2012) 24(Supple 2):148. Available at: https://onlinelibrary.wiley.com/toc/13652982/2012/24/s2

130. Kim ER, Min BH, Lee TH, Son M, Rhee PL. Effect of DA-9701 on colorectal distension-induced visceral hypersensitivity in a rat model. *Gut Liver* (2014) 8:388–93. doi: 10.5009/gnl.2014.8.4.388

131. Choi MG, Rhee PL, Park H, Lee OY, Lee KJ, Choi SC, et al. Randomized, controlled, multi-center trial: comparing the safety and efficacy of DA-9701 and itopride hydrochloride in patients with functional dyspepsia. *J Neurogastroenterol Motil* (2015) 21:414–22. doi: 10.5056/jnm14117

132. Jung HK, Lee KJ, Choi MG, Park H, Lee JS, Rhee PL, et al. Efficacy of DA-9701 (Motilitone) in functional dyspepsia compared to pantoprazole: a multicenter, randomized, double-blind, non-inferiority study. *J Neurogastroenterol Motil* (2016) 22:254–63. doi: 10.5056/jnm15178

133. Park JY, Kim JG, Hong SJ, Jeon SW, Kim GH, Kim HS, et al. A randomized double-blind comparative study of the efficacy of helicobacter pylori eradication therapy and motilitone® for functional dyspepsia. *Korean J Helicobacter Up Gastrointest Res* (2019) 19:106–14. doi: 10.7704/kjhugr.2019.19.2.106

134. Park CH, Kim HS, Lee SK. Effects of the new prokinetic agent DA-9701 formulated with corydalis tuber and pharbitis seed in patients with minimal change esophagitis: a bicenter, randomized, double blind, placebo-controlled study. *J Neurogastroenterol Motil* (2014) 20:338–46. doi: 10.5056/jnm14019

135. Kim SY, Woo HS, Kim KO, Choi SH, Kwon KA, Chung JW, et al. DA-9701 improves colonic transit time and symptoms in patients with functional constipation: A prospective study. *J Gastroenterol Hepatol* (2017) 32:1943–8. doi: 10.1111/jgh.13807

15

Anxiety and Depression Profile is Associated with Eating Disorders in Patients with Irritable Bowel Syndrome

Chloé Melchior [1,2*], Charlotte Desprez [1,3], Ghassan Riachi [2], Anne-Marie Leroi [1,3,5], Pierre Déchelotte [1,4], Najate Achamrah [1,4], Philippe Ducrotté [1,2], Marie-Pierre Tavolacci [1,5] and Guillaume Gourcerol [1,3]

[1] INSERM U1073, UNIROUEN, Normandie University, Rouen, France, [2] Department of Gastroenterology, Rouen University Hospital, Rouen, France, [3] Department of Physiology, Rouen University Hospital, Rouen, France, [4] Department of Nutrition, Rouen University Hospital, Rouen, France, [5] INSERM CIC-CRB 1404, Rouen University Hospital, Rouen, France

*Correspondence:
Chloé Melchior
chloe.melchior@chu-rouen.fr

Objective: To compare the prevalence of anxiety and depression states and eating disorders (EDs) between patients with irritable bowel syndrome (IBS) and healthy volunteers without IBS.

Methods: IBS patients according to Rome III criteria referred to our tertiary care center for therapeutic management and matched volunteers without IBS were prospectively included. EDs were screened by Sick, Control, One stone, Fat, Food—French version (SCOFF-F) questionnaire. IBS symptom severity (IBS symptom severity score), stool consistency (Bristol stool scale), anxiety and depression levels (Hospital Anxiety and Depression scale), and quality of life (validated Gastrointestinal Quality of Life Index) were assessed by validated self-questionnaires.

Results: IBS (228) patients and healthy volunteers (228) were included. Mean age was 42.5 ± 13.9 years with mainly women (76.7%). Among IBS patients, 25.4% had positive SCOFF-F compared to 21.1% of volunteers. IBS patients more frequently had a lower body mass index (BMI) than volunteers ($p < 0.0001$). IBS patients with ED had poorer quality of life and more stressful life events ($p = 0.02$) than IBS patients without ED. The prevalence of anxiety and depression was significantly higher in IBS patients with ED than in volunteers without ED, respectively (19.0% vs 1.9%, p=0.00, and 60.3% vs 19.7%, $p < 0.0001$).

Conclusions: The prevalence of ED assessed with positive SCOFF-F questionnaire was not significantly different between IBS patients and healthy volunteers. The combination of IBS and ED was associated with higher levels of anxiety or depression and poorer quality of life.

Keywords: healthy volunteers, quality of life, Rome III criteria, body mass index (BMI), stressful life events, validated self-questionnaires

INTRODUCTION

Irritable bowel syndrome (IBS) is the main functional intestinal disorder with a prevalence of about 5% in Western Europe (1). IBS is characterized by chronic abdominal pain associated with transit disorders (diarrhea, constipation, or both). The disease significantly impairs patients' quality of life and is a significant burden on health care resources (1).

Many IBS patients consider that food is either the cause or an important trigger of their intestinal symptoms (2) and that their intestinal discomfort is related to food intolerance. This possible relationship often promotes significant changes in diet with food restriction. In some patients, restriction leads to an increased risk of undernutrition (3). The risk of food restriction is probably higher in the subgroup of IBS patients in whom IBS symptoms are associated with upper gastrointestinal (GI) symptoms, mainly functional dyspepsia but also gastro-esophageal reflux disease (3).

In clinical practice, it is sometimes difficult to determine whether this food restriction is only related to the triggering role of food intake on the onset of IBS symptoms or if it is also related to an underlying eating disorder (ED) associated with IBS. Indeed, GI symptoms are frequently reported by patients with ED (4, 5). If we consider specifically IBS, epidemiological studies have reported that 41% to 52% of ED patients also suffer from IBS (6, 7), while the severity of IBS is associated with poorer quality of life in ED patients (8). In these series, patients seemed to develop ED prior to IBS suggesting that ED may increase the risk of developing IBS (9). Whereas data exist on the prevalence of IBS symptoms in patients treated for ED, conversely the frequency of an underlying ED in patients with IBS remains poorly documented (10).

IBS is commonly associated with high anxiety and depression levels (11). ED is also associated with anxiety, depression, and other mood disorders (12). The combined presence of IBS and ED could be associated with worse treatment outcomes (13). Psychological treatments are associated with improvement in IBS symptoms as well as in quality of life in IBS (14, 15).

The aims of this prospective study were: 1) to compare the prevalence of ED between patients with IBS and healthy volunteers without IBS, matched for age and sex, and 2) to compare anxiety and depression levels according to the presence of IBS, ED, or a combination of both.

METHODS

Design

A case–control study was carried out.

Cases had IBS (IBS+) according to Rome III criteria (16) and were 18 to 75 years old. Patients were recruited in the physiology department of our tertiary care center between 2012 and 2013.

During this period, French legislation (Huriet-Sérusclat law) allowed patients to be interviewed in current care without obtaining written informed consent. The use of informatics data was declared to the Commission Nationale de l'Informatique et des Libertés (CNIL) (n° 817.917).

Controls had no IBS (IBS–), and were recruited later from the healthy volunteer registry of the Clinical Investigation Center of Rouen University Hospital in 2017. IBS– were matched on sex and age with IBS+ (1:1). Controls and IBS+ cases filled out an anonymous self-administered questionnaire comprising the SCOFF-F (Sick, Control, One stone, Fat, Food—French version) questionnaire and the Hospital Anxiety and Depression scale (HAD). IBS was assessed using Rome III criteria. Volunteers with a positive Rome III score were excluded. For healthy volunteers, in agreement with the Ethics Committee, their response to the self-questionnaire was considered as written consent. Subjects who did not complete the questionnaire were presented with information on the study. All subjects gave their tacit informed consent. The study was approved by the Ouest III Ethics Committee (2013-AOO512-53).

No patients or controls were under the age of 16.

Data Collection

Self-reported height and weight were used to calculate body mass index (BMI) using the standard formula [BMI (kg/m^2) = weight (kg)/height (m^2) and classified as: underweight (BMI below 18.5); normal (BMI between 18.5 and 24.9); overweight (BMI between 25.0 and 29.9), and obese (BMI above 30) (according to Centers for Disease Control and Prevention)].

Irritable Bowel Syndrome

IBS clinical phenotypes were characterized by validated self-questionnaires. IBS severity was quantified by the IBS symptom severity score (IBS-SSS) (17), and transit disorders were characterized using the Bristol stool scale from 1 to 7 (18). IBS-SSS is composed of five questions: 1) How severe is your abdominal pain? 2) Please enter the number of days that you get the pain every 10 days. 3) How severe is your abdominal distension? 4) How satisfied are you with your bowel habits? 5) Please indicate how much your IBS is affecting or interfering with your life in general. Each of the five questions generates a maximum score of 100 using prompted visual analog scales, leading to a total possible score of 500. Quality of life was assessed using the validated 36-item Gastrointestinal Quality of Life Index (GIQLI), with a maximum score of 144 (19). Items are about symptoms, physical status, emotions, social dysfunction, and effects of medical treatment. In addition, IBS patients were questioned about a possible history of acute gastroenteritis prior to onset of IBS, suggestive of post-infectious IBS. A stressful life event (as sexual abuse) prior to the beginning of symptoms was reported.

Eating Disorders

The self-administered French version of the SCOFF questionnaire (SCOFF-F) (20) was used as a screening test for ED. This screening test does not allow a diagnosis and does not distinguish between different EDs. The score is composed of five dichotomous questions. One point is given for each "yes" answer.

Abbreviations: BMI, body mass index; ED, eating disorder; GIQLI, Gastrointestinal Quality of Life Index; HAD, Hospital Anxiety and Depression scale; IBS, irritable bowel syndrome; IBS-SSS, IBS symptom severity score; SCOFF-F, Sick, Control, One stone, Fat, Food—French version.

At least two positive answers indicate a positive SCOFF score with a sensitivity of 88.2% and a specificity of 92.5% (21). ED prevalence could be overestimated using this test.

Anxiety and Depression

Levels of anxiety and depression were calculated using the HAD scale (22, 23) with a score of 10 out of 21 defining anxiety and depression. Patients were divided into four groups for depression and anxiety analysis: IBS+ with positive SCOFF-F (IBS+/ED+), IBS+ with negative SCOFF-F (IBS+/ED−), IBS− with positive SCOFF-F (IBS−/ED+) and IBS− with negative SCOFF-F (IBS−/ED−).

Statistical Analysis

Data are expressed as percentage (95% confidence interval) and mean ± SD. Characteristics were compared using Fisher's exact test for qualitative variables and Student t test for continuous variables. Fisher's test was used to compare groups of unequal size when variances were not different. Associations were considered statistically significant when p < 0.05. The analysis was carried out using XlstatBiomed 19.5 2017.

RESULTS

Characteristics of IBS+ and IBS−

A total of 456 adults between 18 and 75 years old were included, with 228 IBS+ and 228 IBS−: 53 men and 175 women in each group. Mean age was 42.5 ± 13.9 years.

In IBS+, the mean Bristol stool scale score was 4.4 ± 1.8. IBS was post-infectious in 14.9% and occurred after a stressful life event in 64.5%. The mean IBS-SSS was 248.9 ± 101.3, and quality of life was altered with a mean GIQLI score of 78.9 ± 21.8.

Comparisons of IBS+ and IBS−

SCOFF-F questionnaire was positive in 25.4% (20.0–31.7) of IBS+ and in 21.1% (16.1–27.0) of IBS− (p = 0.27) (**Table 1**). A positive SCOFF-F was more frequent in women than in men, 29.4% and 15.1% respectively, (p = 0.02). A low BMI was more frequent in IBS+ than in IBS− while normal BMI was more frequent in volunteers than in IBS patients (p < 0.0001, **Table 1**). Prevalence of anxiety and depression was significantly higher in IBS+ [43% (36.5–49.7) and 14.0% (9.9–19.4) respectively] than in IBS− [24.7% (19.0–31.5) and 4.0% (1.9–8.1)] ($<10^{-3}$) (**Table 1**).

TABLE 1 | Characteristics of the 228 IBS+ and 228 IBS−.

	IBS + n = 228	IBS− n = 228	p
BMI (%)			<0.0001
<18.5	15.7	1.3	
18.5–24.9	50.9	64.0	
25–29.9	17.5	24.1	
≥30	15.8	10.5	
Positive SCOFF-F (%)	25.4	21.1	0.27
Male	17.0	13.2	0.59
Female	28.0	23.4	0.33
Anxiety (%)	43.0	24.7	<0.0001
Depression (%)	14.0	4.0	<0.0001

BMI, body mass index; IBS, irritable bowel syndrome; SCOFF-F, the French version of SCOFF (Sick, Control, One stone, Fat, Food).

TABLE 2 | Comparison between IBS+ with positive and negative SCOFF-F.

	IBS+/ED+ (n = 58)	IBS+/ED− (n = 170)	p
Age (years) mean (SD)	42.4 (14.6)	42.9 (14.5)	0.80
Female (%)	84.5	74.1	0.15
Acute gastroenteritis prior to onset of IBS (%)	12.1	15.9	0.67
Stressful life events (%)	**77.6**	**60.0**	**0.02**
IBS-SSS mean (SD)	264.5 (106.3)	243.4 (99.2)	0.19
GIQLI mean (SD)	**73.1 (19.7)**	**80.8 (22.2)**	**0.02**

IBS-SSS, IBS symptom severity score; GIQLI, validated Gastrointestinal Quality of Life Index; IBS+/ED+, IBS with positive SCOFF-F; IBS+/ED−, IBS with negative SCOFF-F.

Comparison of IBS+ With or Without ED (IBS+/ED+ Vs IBS+/ED−)

Age, gender, and symptomatic IBS profile were not significantly different between IBS+ with positive or negative SCOFF-F (**Table 2**). IBS patients with positive SCOFF-F had a significantly poorer quality of life and more stressful life events (p = 0.02 and p = 0.02) (**Table 2**).

Comparison of Depression and Anxiety Prevalence According to the Presence of IBS, ED, or Both

In our study, we analyzed four groups: IBS+/ED+ (n = 58), IBS+/ED− (n = 170), IBS−/ED+ (n = 48), and IBS−/ED− (n = 180). The prevalence of anxiety and depression was significantly higher in IBS+/ED+ than in IBS−/ED−, respectively (19.0% vs 1.9%, p = 0.0003, **Figure 1**, and 60.3% vs 19.7%, p < 0.0001, **Figure 2**). There was no difference for anxiety and depression between IBS+/ED− and IBS−/ED+.

DISCUSSION

To our knowledge, this is the first study, conducted in a large IBS population, highlighting a similar prevalence of SCOFF-F screened ED between IBS patients and healthy volunteers. The presence of ED in IBS is associated with the risk of a previous stressful life event. However, the SCOFF-F questionnaire, selected in this study for

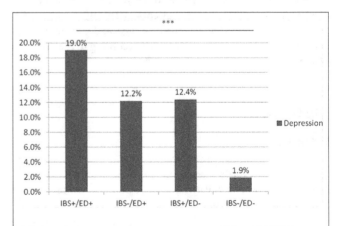

FIGURE 1 | Prevalence of depression according to IBS and SCOFF-F status. IBS+/ED+, IBS with positive SCOFF-F; IBS+/ED−, IBS with negative SCOFF-F; IBS−/ED−, Volunteers without IBS with negative SCOFF-F; IBS−/ED+, Volunteers without IBS with positive SCOFF-F.

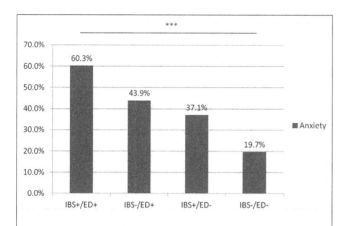

FIGURE 2 | Prevalence of anxiety according to IBS and SCOFF-F status. IBS+/ED+, IBS with positive SCOFF-F; IBS+/ED-, IBS with negative SCOFF-F; IBS-/ED-, Volunteers without IBS with negative SCOFF-F; IBS-/ED+, Volunteers without IBS with positive SCOFF-F.

practical reasons because it is simple, self-administered, and easy to use, is a tool mainly for the detection of patients at risk of an ED, but it is not a test for the formal diagnosis of an ED. Nevertheless, we have previously demonstrated a correlation between positive SCOFF-F and the criteria of the *Diagnostic and Statistical Manual of Mental Disorders (DSM)-IV* which is the validated diagnostic classification for ED (20).

Our results are consistent with previous data reported in students (24) showing no difference in the prevalence of ED between IBS patients and healthy volunteers. This result suggests that the prevalence of ED is not increased in IBS patients.

Our IBS population, with a predominance of women and middle-aged patients, is comparable to that of published series. In IBS patients, age, gender, and symptomatic IBS profile were not predictive of a possible underlying ED. The lack of correlation between age, gender, and risk of ED is an unexpected result since young women are recognized as having an increased risk of ED, at least in a population of students (25). The well-established overrepresentation of women in the IBS population and the low number of young patients in our series could explain this lack of correlation. Nevertheless, in our IBS patients, high levels of anxiety or depression and poor quality of life were associated with the presence of ED. These results are in accordance with those already reported in patients with ED (26). In this latter population, both high anxiety levels and psychological abnormalities are common and associated with functional GI disorders, particularly IBS (5, 6). In ED patients, the presence of IBS was also correlated with poorer quality of life (8).

Our study did not allow us to explain why the prevalence of ED was similar in IBS+ and IBS− populations. Indeed, studies of patients with ED have reported that an ED in childhood increases the risk of further development of IBS (27). In the Perkins' study, most patients were treated for an ED prior to IBS, with a mean delay of 10 years between the ED and the onset of IBS (9).

Nevertheless, we have demonstrated that IBS patients with ED had impaired mental health with higher levels of depression and anxiety than healthy volunteers. This result is in accordance with observations made separately in IBS and ED studies.

Psychopathological profiles have already been associated with the presence of digestive symptoms in ED (5, 6). IBS patients are well known to have higher levels of anxiety and depression than controls (11, 28). Anxiety and depression are able to increase GI symptoms (29). In particular, depression has been shown to increase postprandial symptoms (29). In these IBS and ED populations and especially in patients with a combination of both IBS and ED, anxiety and depression should be systematically suspected and treated to allow better patient outcomes.

Our study has several important weaknesses: the SCOFF-F questionnaire did not allow the complete characterization of ED; there was a lack of prospective identification of IBS patients who self-imposed severe food restriction, and a possible overestimation of any association between ED and IBS as our results were obtained in a tertiary care center. Nevertheless, its strength lies in the fact that our data are based on a large cohort of IBS patients.

The present study serves as a warning not to overlook an underlying ED, especially in IBS patients who are anxious or depressed and who report previous stressful life events. This seems particularly important in clinical practice when some regimens (i.e. low-FODMAP diet, gluten-free diet) are increasingly discussed as a first-line therapeutic option in IBS management (30). Indeed in a recent IBS study, greater adherence to a low-Fermentable Oligo-, Di-, Mono-saccharides And Polyols (FODMAP) diet was associated with a positive SCOFF (31). Further investigation is required to explore suitable therapeutic options for these patients with a combination of IBS and underlying EDs associated with anxiety or depression and poor quality of life.

ETHICS STATEMENT

The study was approved by the Ouest III Ethics Committee (2013-AOO512-53). Written informed consent for participation was not required for this study in accordance with the national legislation and the institutional requirements.

AUTHOR CONTRIBUTIONS

GG and M-PT designed the research. CM, CD, A-ML, PDu, M-PT, and GG performed the research. NA, PDe, and GR contributed new reagents/analytic tools. CM, CD, M-PT, and GG analyzed the data. CM, M-PT, and GG wrote the paper.

ACKNOWLEDGMENTS

This work is dedicated to the memory of Professor Philippe Ducrotté, who passed away during the completion of the study. The authors wish, however, to acknowledge his contribution to this work. The authors are grateful to Nikki Sabourin-Gibbs, Rouen University Hospital, for her help in editing the manuscript.

REFERENCES

1. Dapoigny M. Irritable bowel syndrome: epidemiology/economic burden. *Gastroenterol Clin Biol* (2009) 33 Suppl 1:S3–8. doi: 10.1016/S0399-8320 (09)71519-2

2. Bohn L, Storsrud S, Tornblom H, Bengtsson U, Simren M. Self-reported food-related gastrointestinal symptoms in IBS are common and associated with more severe symptoms and reduced quality of life. *Am J Gastroenterol* (2013) 108(5):634–41. doi: 10.1038/ajg.2013.105

3. Hayes P, Corish C, O'Mahony E, Quigley EM. A dietary survey of patients with irritable bowel syndrome. *J Hum Nutr Diet.* (2014) 27 Suppl 2:36–7. doi: 10.1111/jhn.12114

4. Abraham S, Kellow JE. Do the digestive tract symptoms in eating disorder patients represent functional gastrointestinal disorders? *BMC Gastroenterol* (2013) 13:38. doi: 10.1186/1471-230X-13-38

5. Salvioli B, Pellicciari A, Iero L, Di Pietro E, Moscano F, Gualandi S, et al. Audit of digestive complaints and psychopathological traits in patients with eating disorders: a prospective study. *Dig. Liver Dis* (2013) 45(8):639–44. doi: 10.1016/j.dld.2013.02.022

6. Boyd C, Abraham S, Kellow J. Psychological features are important predictors of functional gastrointestinal disorders in patients with eating disorders. *Scand J Gastroenterol* (2005) 40(8):929–35. doi: 10.1080/00365520510015836

7. Wang X, Luscombe GM, Boyd C, Kellow J, Abraham S. Functional gastrointestinal disorders in eating disorder patients: altered distribution and predictors using Rome III compared to ROME II criteria. *World J Gastroenterol* (2014) 20(43):16293–9. doi: 10.3748/wjg.v20.i43.16293

8. Abraham S, Kellow J. Exploring eating disorder quality of life and functional gastrointestinal disorders among eating disorder patients. *J Psychosom. Res* (2011) 70(4):372–7. doi: 10.1016/j.jpsychores.2010.11.009

9. Perkins SJ, Keville S, Schmidt U, Chalder T. Eating disorders and irritable bowel syndrome: is there a link? *J Psychosom. Res* (2005) 59(2):57–64. doi: 10.1016/j.jpsychores.2004.04.375

10. Tang TN, Toner BB, Stuckless N, Dion KL, Kaplan AS, Ali A. Features of eating disorders in patients with irritable bowel syndrome. *J Psychosom. Res* (1998) 45(2):171–8. doi: 10.1016/S0022-3999(97)00300-0

11. Fond G, Loundou A, Hamdani N, Boukouaci W, Dargel A, Oliveira J, et al. Anxiety and depression comorbidities in irritable bowel syndrome (IBS): a systematic review and meta-analysis. *Eur Arch Psychiatry Clin Neurosci* (2014) 264(8):651–60. doi: 10.1007/s00406-014-0502-z

12. Marucci S, Ragione LD, De Iaco G, Mococci T, Vicini M, Guastamacchia E, et al. Anorexia nervosa and comorbid psychopathology. *Endocr Metab Immune Disord Drug Targets* (2018) 18(4):316–24. doi: 10.2174/1871530318666180213111637

13. Fewell LK, Levinson CA, Stark L. Depression, worry, and psychosocial functioning predict eating disorder treatment outcomes in a residential and partial hospitalization setting. *Eat Weight Disord* (2017) 22(2):291–301. doi: 10.1007/s40519-016-0357-6

14. Pinto-Sanchez MI, Hall GB, Ghajar K, Nardelli A, Bolino C, Lau JT, et al. Probiotic bifidobacterium longum NCC3001 reduces depression scores and alters brain activity: a pilot study in patients with irritable bowel syndrome. *Gastroenterology* (2018) 153(2):448–59. doi: 10.1053/j.gastro.2017.05.003

15. Thakur ER, Holmes HJ, Lockhart NA, Carty JN, Ziadni MS, Doherty HK, et al. Emotional awareness and expression training improves irritable bowel syndrome: a randomized controlled trial. *Neurogastroenterol Motil* (2017) 29 (12). doi: 10.1111/nmo.13143

16. Longstreth GF, Thompson WG, Chey WD, Houghton LA, Mearin F, Spiller RC. Functional bowel disorders. *Gastroenterology* (2006) 130(5):1480–91. doi: 10.1053/j.gastro.2005.11.061

17. Spiller RC, Humes DJ, Campbell E, Hastings M, Neal KR, Dukes GE, et al. The Patient Health Questionnaire 12 Somatic Symptom scale as a predictor of symptom severity and consulting behaviour in patients with irritable bowel syndrome and symptomatic diverticular disease. *Aliment Pharmacol Ther* (2010) 32(6):811–20. doi: 10.1111/j.1365-2036.2010.04402.x

18. Heaton KW, Radvan J, Cripps H, Mountford RA, Braddon FE, Hughes AO. Defecation frequency and timing, and stool form in the general population: a prospective study. *Gut* (1992) 33(6):818–24. doi: 10.1136/gut.33.6.818

19. Slim K, Bousquet J, Kwiatkowski F, Lescure G, Pezet D, Chipponi J. First validation of the French version of the Gastrointestinal Quality of Life Index (GIQLI). *Gastroenterol Clin Biol* (1999) 23(1):25–31. doi: GCB-01-1999-23-1-0399-8320-101019-ART2

20. Garcia FD, Grigioni S, Allais E, Houy-Durand E, Thibaut F, Dechelotte P. Detection of eating disorders in patients: validity and reliability of the French version of the SCOFF questionnaire. *Clin Nutr* (2010) 30(2):178–81. doi: 10.1016/j.clnu.2010.09.007

21. Botella J, Sepulveda AR, Huang H, Gambara H. A meta-analysis of the diagnostic accuracy of the SCOFF. *Span. J Psychol* (2013) 16:E92. doi: 10.1017/sjp.2013.92

22. Cho HS, Park JM, Lim CH, Cho YK, Lee IS, Kim SW, et al. Anxiety, depression and quality of life in patients with irritable bowel syndrome. *Gut Liver* (2011) 5(1):29–36. doi: 10.5009/gnl.2011.5.1.29

23. Zigmond AS, Snaith RP. The hospital anxiety and depression scale. *Acta Psychiatr Scand* (1983) 67(6):361–70. doi: 10.1111/j.1600-0447.1983.tb09716.x

24. Tavolacci MP, Ladner J, Grigioni S, Richard L, Villet H, Dechelotte P. Prevalence and association of perceived stress, substance use and behavioral addictions: a cross-sectional study among university students in France, 2009-2011. *BMC Public Health* (2013) 13:724. doi: 10.1186/1471-2458-13-724

25. Costarelli V, Demerzi M, Stamou D. Disordered eating attitudes in relation to body image and emotional intelligence in young women. *J Hum Nutr Diet.* (2009) 22(3):239–45. doi: 10.1111/j.1365-277X.2009.00949.x

26. Tavolacci MP, Grigioni S, Richard L, Meyrignac G, Dechelotte P, Ladner J. Eating disorders and associated health risks among university students. *J Nutr Educ Behav* (2015) 47(5):412–20. doi: 10.1016/j.jneb.2015.06.009

27. Svedberg P, Johansson S, Wallander MA, Hamelin B, Pedersen NL. Extra-intestinal manifestations associated with irritable bowel syndrome: a twin study. *Aliment Pharmacol Ther* (2002) 16(5):975–83. doi: 10.1046/j.1365-2036.2002.01254.x

28. Lee C, Doo E, Choi JM, Jang SH, Ryu HS, Lee JY, et al. The increased level of depression and anxiety in irritable bowel syndrome patients compared with healthy controls: systematic review and meta-analysis. *J Neurogastroenterol. Motil.* (2017) 23(3):349–62. doi: 10.5056/jnm16220

29. Van Oudenhove L, Tornblom H, Storsrud S, Tack J, Simren M. Depression and somatization are associated with increased postprandial symptoms in patients with irritable bowel syndrome. *Gastroenterology* (2016) 150(4):866–74. doi: 10.1053/j.gastro.2015.11.010

30. Spiller R, Aziz Q, Creed F, Emmanuel A, Houghton L, Hungin P, et al. Guidelines on the irritable bowel syndrome: mechanisms and practical management. *Gut* (2007) 56(12):1770–98. doi: 10.1136/gut.2007.119446

31. Mari A, Hosadurg D, Martin L, Zarate-Lopez N, Passananti V, Emmanuel A. Adherence with a low-FODMAP diet in irritable bowel syndrome: are eating disorders the missing link? *Eur J Gastroenterol Hepatol* (2019) 31(2):178–82. doi: 10.1097/MEG.0000000000001317

16

Small Intestinal Bacterial Overgrowth and Irritable Bowel Syndrome

*Will Takakura[1] and Mark Pimentel[1,2]**

[1] Department of Medicine, Medically Associated Science and Technology (MAST) Program, Cedars-Sinai Medical Center, Los Angeles, CA, United States, [2] Department of Medicine, Division of Digestive and Liver Diseases, Cedars-Sinai Medical Center, Los Angeles, CA, United States

Correspondence:
Mark Pimentel
mark.pimentel@cshs.org

Small intestinal bacterial overgrowth (SIBO) is one manifestation of gut microbiome dysbiosis and is highly prevalent in IBS (Irritable Bowel Syndrome). SIBO can be diagnosed either by a small bowel aspirate culture showing $\geq 10^3$ colony-forming units (CFU) per mL of aspirate, or a positive hydrogen lactulose or glucose breath test. Numerous pathogenic organisms have been shown to be increased in subjects with SIBO and IBS, including but not limited to *Enterococcus, Escherichia coli*, and *Klebsiella*. In addition, *Methanobrevibacter smithii*, the causal organism in a positive methane breath test, has been linked to constipation predominant irritable bowel syndrome (IBS-C). As *M. smithii* is an archaeon and can overgrow in areas outside of the small intestine, it was recently proposed that the term intestinal methanogen overgrowth (IMO) is more appropriate for the overgrowth of these organisms. Due to gut microbiome dysbiosis, patients with IBS may have increased intestinal permeability, dysmotility, chronic inflammation, autoimmunity, decreased absorption of bile salts, and even altered enteral and central neuronal activity. As a consequence, SIBO and IBS share a myriad of symptoms including abdominal pain, distention, diarrhea, and bloating. Furthermore, gut microbiome dysbiosis may be associated with select neuropsychological symptoms, although more research is needed to confirm this connection. This review will focus on the role of the gut microbiome and SIBO in IBS, as well as novel innovations that may help better characterize intestinal overgrowth and microbial dysbiosis.

Keywords: small intestinal bacterial overgrowth, irritable bowel syndrome, gut dysbiosis, breath test, methane, archaea, hydrogen, hydrogen sulfide

INTRODUCTION

Irritable bowel syndrome (IBS) is a functional bowel disorder defined by recurrent abdominal pain for at least 1 day per week in the last 3 months that is associated with 2 or more of the following: related to defecation, associated with a change in stool form, or associated with a change in stool frequency (1). Symptom onset must occur at least 6 months prior to diagnosis, but many patients suffer long-term chronic symptoms as a result of this disorder. Patients may experience various comorbidities including, but not limited to, bloating, constipation, diarrhea, incontinence, and psychological disturbances.

Historically, IBS has been associated with stress and anxiety, and the brain-gut axis has been widely described as important in understanding IBS (2). Because of this, many treatments focus on antidepressants and neurobehavioral intervention (3). Although these treatments can be effective, newer studies have demonstrated more complex, organic etiologies specific to the gut that have led to novel therapeutic options. The complex network of etiologies likely represents various pathophysiological states that may be unique to the patient and include visceral hyperalgesia, intestinal permeability, immune activation, altered gastrointestinal motility, autoimmunity, and alteration of the gut microbiome. The last category, the gut microbiome, has seen an exponential growth in interest over the last few years. One manifestation of dysbiosis, small intestinal bacterial overgrowth (SIBO), is linked to IBS and will be the focus of this review.

DEFINITION OF SIBO

While a diagnosis of IBS is based on clinical symptoms, the gold standard for a diagnosis of SIBO is the presence of $\geq 10^3$ colony forming units per milliliter (CFU/mL) of jejunal aspirate by culture (4, 5). However, aspiration is invasive and expensive, requiring a skilled gastroenterologist. Also, there may be sampling errors given that only a small segment of the small bowel can be aspirated, leaving the rest unexplored. Alternatively, a breath test can be used to assess microbial overgrowth in the gut. Hydrogen (H_2) and methane (CH_4) are exclusively produced by microbial metabolism and are exhaled on the breath (6–8). The North American consensus defines a rise in $H_2 \geq 20$ parts per million (ppm) from baseline within 90 min of substrate ingestion as positive for the H_2 breath test, and a CH_4 level ≥ 10 ppm at any time is defined as positive for the CH_4 breath test (4). Two of the most common carbohydrate substrates used for the breath test are glucose and lactulose. Glucose is a monosaccharide that is readily absorbed in the proximal small intestine, whereas lactulose is a disaccharide and has more limited absorbability (9). SIBO is associated with a myriad of symptoms including, but not limited to bloating, abdominal pain, nausea, constipation, and diarrhea. A positive H_2 breath test is diagnostic of SIBO, which has been associated with diarrhea-predominant IBS (IBS-D) and IBS with mixed bowel habits (IBS-M) (10). A positive CH_4 breath test is indicative of methanogen overgrowth, which has been associated with constipation predominant IBS (IBS-C) (5, 11, 12). Of note, the recent SIBO guidelines have reclassified CH_4 positive breath test as intestinal methanogen overgrowth (IMO), as methanogenesis is likely not limited to the small intestine (5, 13–15). In addition, although measurement of CH_4 is not always included, the North American consensus and the recent SIBO guidelines both recommend that CH_4 be measured concurrently with H_2 during breath testing (4, 5).

PREVALENCE OF SIBO IN IBS

The relationship between SIBO and IBS was described in a 2020 meta-analysis of 25 case-control studies involving 3,192 IBS

subjects and 3,320 controls, that showed that the prevalence of SIBO in IBS was 31.0% (95% CI 29.4–32.6) with an OR of 3.7 (95% CI 2.3–6.0, p = 0.001) compared to controls (16). This meta-analysis included studies with healthy controls and non-IBS patient controls. When comparing SIBO rates with only healthy controls the OR increased to 4.9 (95% CI 2.8–8.6, p = 0.001). This meta-analysis included studies that had several definitions of SIBO, as well as several IBS diagnostic criteria. The Rome IV diagnostic criteria for IBS were published in 2016, and the meta-analysis did not include any studies utilizing the newer Rome IV criteria. A funnel plot evaluating publication bias showed some asymmetry, although after including only the top 15 high-quality studies with low risk of bias, the asymmetry was no longer observed. Interestingly, this increased the OR for SIBO in IBS with an OR of 4.1 (95% CI 3.0–5.6, p < 0.001). Slightly higher rates of SIBO were seen in studies that utilized breath testing as opposed to small intestinal aspiration (35.5 vs. 33.5%, respectively). The two most common breath test utilized were glucose breath test (n = 9) and lactulose breath test (n = 8). The prevalence of SIBO in IBS subjects vs controls was 62.3 vs 33.5% for the lactulose breath test, and 20.7 vs 4.4% for glucose. The association between SIBO and IBS seemed to be the strongest for IBS-D vs IBS-C or IBS-M, at 35.5% (95% CI 32.7–40.3) vs 22.5% (95% CI 18.1–26.9) or 25.2% (95% CI 22.2–28.4), respectively. Since this meta-analysis, one study utilizing the newer Rome IV diagnostic criteria for IBS has shown that the prevalence of SIBO is increased in subjects with IBS (51.7 vs. 16.7%, p ≤ .001) (17). **Figure 1** summarizes the prevalence of SIBO in IBS vs controls from case-control studies (n>80) using Rome III and the latest Rome IV criteria for IBS (17–29). Our analysis of these 13 studies shows that the pooled SIBO rate is significantly higher in IBS subjects than in controls (30 vs 9%, n = 2,494, p < 0.0001). The number of healthy subjects with SIBO likely reflects the complex relationship between SIBO and symptoms. A balance of specific bacterial strains with different adaptive host factors may produce asymptomatic, or mildly symptomatic patients with SIBO.

In contrast to SIBO (based on a positive H_2 breath test), which is more strongly associated with IBS-D, IMO has been linked to IBS-C (5, 11, 16, 30, 31). Unlike H_2, which has not been shown to directly induce diarrhea, CH_4 has been shown to directly slow intestinal transit and causes constipation, both in

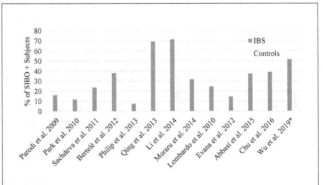

FIGURE 1 | SIBO positive rates in Rome III or IV IBS. Overall SIBO is highly prevalent in IBS. *Used Rome IV definition, all other studies used Rome III (16–28).

humans (32) and in animal models (33). Pimentel et al. showed that direct infusion of CH_4 in animals slows intestinal transit, and also showed that segments of guinea pig ileum exhibit increased contractile impulses when bathed in CH_4 (33). CH_4 appears to cause dysregulation in motility by amplifying neuronal activity in the intestine through the anticholinergic pathway (34). In humans, a study showed that the degree of constipation correlated with breath CH_4 levels in subjects with IBS (31). Of note, for patients with constipation without IBS, the percentage of CH_4 positive patients also correlated with constipation (35). In this study, those with decreased motility in the colon had higher levels of total and maximum CH_4 (35). Two strict anaerobic methanogens have been isolated from the human gut, *Methanosphaera stadtmaniae* (36) and *Methanobrevibacter smithii* (37), with the latter being the predominant source of methanogenesis and associated with constipation (38). Supporting this, another study found that higher levels of *M. smithii* correlated with higher CH_4 on breath test (12). These studies shed light on a causal relationship between methanogen overgrowth and at least a subset of IBS-C. Interestingly, bile acids are a proposed etiology of functional diarrhea and IBS-D, and have been shown to decrease methanogenesis in human feces (39).

Only a few studies have attempted to characterize the small bowel microbiome in subjects with SIBO and IBS. A North American study found that SIBO subjects had a 7–8-fold increase in *Klebsiella* and *Escherichia/Shigella* compared to non SIBO patients (40). One Indian study, on jejunal aspirate of SIBO and IBS subjects, found that 40% of subjects had *Pseudomonas aeruginosa*, 6.7% had *Acinetobacter baumannii*, 13.3% had *Acinetobacter lwoffii*, 13.3% had *Staphylococcus spp*, 6.7% had *Enterococcus faecalis*, 20% had *Escherichia coli*, 6.7% had *Enterococcus faecium*, 13.3% had *Klebsiella pneumoniae*, and 6.7% had *Streptococcus spp.* by culture (41). This study also noted an increase in *Acinetobacter lwoffii*, *Staphylococcus* spp., *Enterococcus faecalis*, *Escherichia coli*, and *Klebsiella pneumoniae* in IBS subjects with SIBO vs. those without SIBO. Similarly, a Swedish study found that IBS subjects with SIBO had a high prevalence of Gram-negative *Bacilli* and *Enterobacter* on jejunal aspirate (42). Lastly, a study from Athens found high prevalence of *Escherichia coli*, *Enterococcus spp*, and *Klebsiella pneumoniae* in duodenal aspirates from subjects with SIBO (43). Given the highly variable results of microbiome studies arising from different sampling locations, geography, and definitions of SIBO, caution should be exercised when generalizing these results.

GUT MICROBIOME DYSBIOSIS, IBS AND SIBO—FOCUS ON POST-INFECTIOUS IBS MODELS

SIBO only comprises a subset of gut microbiome dysbiosis, and this review would not be complete without discussing how microbial dysbiosis in general contributes to IBS. Previous

studies have shown that infectious etiologies such as infectious gastroenteritis (44, 45) and diverticulitis (46) are associated with the development of IBS, which have been termed post-infectious IBS (PI-IBS). A recent systemic review has shown that roughly 10% of patients with enteritis develop PI-IBS within the following year and the prevalence of PI-IBS seems to increase with time (47) These infections are thought to induce changes through long-lasting low-grade inflammation, an increase in intestinal permeability, and autoimmunity, ultimately leading to the symptoms of IBS (**Figure 2**). Given that roughly 10% of the population has IBS (48) and the that an estimated 10 million food-borne illnesses occur each year (49), it is possible that a significant portion of patients with IBS may have had gastroenteritis in the past that they cannot recall and may have PI-IBS. Interestingly, a mathematical model has shown that infectious gastroenteritis may contribute to a large proportion of IBS (50). Therefore, we hypothesize that studies of PI-IBS may be relevant to many subjects with IBS.

Infectious diarrhea has been known to cause intestinal permeability (51, 52), and a similar phenomenon is seen in patients with IBS (52, 53). This is thought to be partially mediated through bacterial effects on tight junctions (54). Although the mechanism(s) underlying how intestinal permeability persists after the acute infection is not entirely clear, there are many hypotheses centered on gut microbiome dysbiosis. Butyrate, a microbial metabolite, is a key player in maintaining a healthy epithelial barrier by regulating cell turnover, antioxidants, and energy maintenance in the gut lining (55, 56). Interestingly, one study found lower levels of butyrate-producing bacterial families such as Ruminococcaceae, an unknown family from the order Clostridiales, and Erysipelotrichaceae in subjects with IBS-D (57). Butyrate appears to mediate cell turnover through inhibition of histone deacetylase (HDAC), which causes apoptosis of the luminal cells (56). Interestingly, in a rodent model of IBS, inhibition of HDAC alleviated symptoms of visceral hypersensitivity (58). In addition, another candidate important in the maintenance of intestinal permeability has recently gained interest in IBS. A double-blind placebo-controlled randomized control trial in 2019 evaluated glutamine, a key amino acid that helps gut epithelial integrity (59), and found that an 8-week course significantly alleviated IBS symptoms (60). The improvement in symptoms was correlated with improvement in intestinal permeability. Interestingly, glutamine-enriched total parenteral nutrition did not improve intestinal permeability in malnourished surgical subjects undergoing gastrointestinal surgery (61), which may suggest additional mechanisms are needed to maintain the gut epithelial barrier which are not present in these subjects. Given that these subjects had poor oral intake coupled with severe gastrointestinal disease which necessitated surgery, their microbiome dysbiosis should be further investigated.

Secondly, inflammation seems to play a role in the pathophysiology of IBS. Previous studies have shown that rectal biopsies from subjects who had acute *Campylobacter enteritis* and diarrhea exhibit persistently elevated T-lymphocytes and

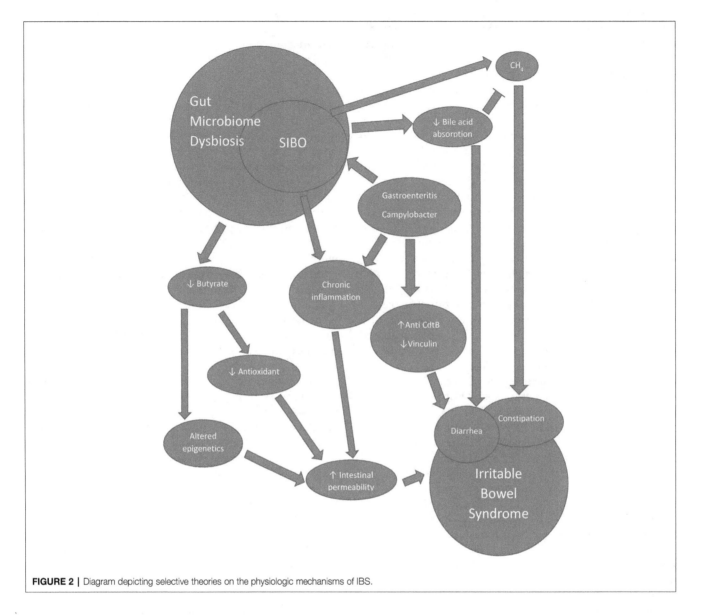

FIGURE 2 | Diagram depicting selective theories on the physiologic mechanisms of IBS.

enteroendocrine cells, and that similar elevations are seen in subjects with post-infectious IBS (52). Another study found an increase in enterochromaffin cells and T-lymphocytes in subjects with new-onset post-infectious IBS following *Campylobacter* infection compared to both subjects who were asymptomatic following infection and to healthy controls (62). The increase in lymphocytes appears to be present in the general IBS population as well, as one study found a 1.8-fold increase in intraepithelial lymphocytes in IBS subjects as compared to asymptomatic controls (63). This is not surprising since a large proportion of IBS is suspected to be due to a previous infection (50). A mouse model of post-infectious IBS developed using *Trichinella spiralis* (64) found similar results, with enterochromaffin cells being persistently elevated in the bowel long after clearance of the acute infection, as well as an increase in intraepithelial cells and a decrease in intestinal cells of Cajal in mice that developed SIBO (65). In addition, a post-*Campylobacter* rat model of IBS exhibited persistent alterations in stool consistency and in rats that

exhibited SIBO, intraepithelial lymphocytes in the rectum and the left colon were also increased (66).

Autoimmunity may also play a significant role in the development of IBS as it relates to the gut microbiome. In a post-infectious IBS model, rats who were exposed to *Campylobacter* with an insertional deletion of the bacterial toxin cytolethal distending toxin B (CdtB) exhibited significantly fewer intraepithelial lymphocytes and less alterations in stool form (67). Antibodies to CdtB were found to have a high affinity to the neuronal protein vinculin, and a decrease in vinculin expression correlated with the number of times the rats were exposed to *Campylobacter* (68). Vinculin is a key cytoskeletal protein that plays an essential role in cell-matrix and cell-cell adhesion (69). In humans, numerous studies have found that these two biomarkers (antibodies to CdtB and vinculin) can differentiate between IBS-D/M (70–73) and other bowel diseases and conditions that cause diarrhea, although one study in Australia failed to show such relationship (74). A longitudinal observation of a single patient who developed IBS after an episode of infectious diarrhea demonstrated a subsequent elevation in anti-CdtB, followed by an elevation in anti-vinculin, each coinciding with symptoms (44). A thorough evaluation failed to find an "organic" gastrointestinal disorder in this patient. In humans, this pathway seems to be specific to patients with IBS-D and IBS-M but not IBS-C (71), which is consistent with findings in the rat model.

Finally, SIBO and malabsorption has also been proposed as a mechanism underlying the development of diarrhea. It is thought that deconjugation of bile salts in the upper gut induces a decrease in absorption of fat and lipophilic vitamins, leading to the production of lithocholic acid, which is poorly absorbed and thought to be enterotoxic (75). In subjects with malabsorption syndrome with and without SIBO, subjects who had SIBO exhibited significantly elevated unconjugated bile salts, acetate, lactate, and formate than those without SIBO (76).

MICROBIOME-TARGETED TREATMENT OF SIBO, IMO, AND IBS

There are treatments for both SIBO and IBS which target the microbiome, including treatment with a non-absorbable oral antibiotic, rifaximin. A meta-analysis which evaluated normalization of breath test in response to antibiotics for SIBO found that of the 10 studies included, rifaximin was the most common and was used in 8 studies. They found a pooled normalization rate of 49.5%, 95% CI 44.0–55.1 with rifaximin vs. 9.8%, 95% CI 4.6–17.8 with placebo (77). Rifaximin was compared against placebo in only 3 studies and had a favorable response with an effectiveness ratio of 1.97, 95% CI 0.93–4.17, p = 0.08. although this did not reach statistical significance. Four studies directly compared antibiotics to placebo and found an effectiveness ratio of 2.55, 95% CI 1.29–5.04, p = 0.03 favoring antibiotics.

Similarly, multiple large randomized controlled trials have shown that rifaximin can improve symptoms in subjects with IBS without constipation (78, 79). Currently this is the only FDA-approved therapy to treat IBS by directly affecting the gut microbiome. Unlike other medications on the market for the treatment of IBS, the effects of this treatment outlasted the duration of treatment by weeks to months. This is thought to be due to the effects of rifaximin on the gut microbiome which persist after the treatment is over. Unfortunately, a subset of subjects experience a relapse of their symptoms, but repeat dosing with rifaximin appears to be safe and effective (79, 80). The mechanism of action for this drug is not entirely clear, but it appears to induce a small, transient reduction in Shannon index as well as a decrease in the relative abundance of 7 taxa including Enterobacteriaceae, Verrucomicrobiaceae, Peptosteptococcaceae, Pasteuellaceae, Synergistaceae, Eubacteriaceae, and Enterococcaceae (81), as determined from stool samples. These transient effects are consistent with clinical observations. Whether the reductions in these taxa are directly linked to the improvements in IBS symptoms is yet to be determined. Further studies are needed to also evaluate changes in small bowel and proximal colon.

A metanalysis by Shah et al. found 7 studies which evaluated patients with SIBO in IBS and found that antibiotics relieve symptoms in 81.6% of patients. Only 5 studies reported eradication of SIBO and 93% of patients with a glucose breath test achieved normalization while 71.4% of patients who were diagnosed *via* small bowel aspirate culture reached normalization (16).

Furthermore, treatment with specific antibiotics results in decreased CH_4 levels that correlate with improvements in constipation (82, 83). Of note, while neomycin and rifaximin can each reduce constipation in IBS-C, using a combination of both appears to be most effective (84). Currently only a small number of studies with limited sample sizes have evaluated the use of antibiotics in the treatment of IMO, and larger, multicentered randomized control trials are needed to further characterize their efficacies and potential adverse events.

Perhaps the largest clinical indication of the overlap between SIBO and IBS was demonstrated by Rezaie et al, who showed that a positive lactulose breath test predicted a favorable response to rifaximin (59.7 vs 25.8%, p = 0.002) (85) than patients who had a negative lactulose breath test. Given this finding, patients with IBS should undergo a lactulose breath test to rule out SIBO, as this may have treatment implications (86).

Finally, probiotics have also been evaluated in the treatment of IBS. A systemic review by Ford et al. (87) found that certain combinations of probiotics may be helpful in IBS, although there was significant heterogeneity between the studies with possible publication bias. In this study, combination probiotics LacClean Gold and VSL#3 had some efficacy with RR = 0.59; 95% CI 0.37–0.93 (n = 130) and RR = 0.82; 95% CI 0.52–1.30 (n = 78), respectively. Interpretation of metanalyses of probiotic studies is difficult since different strains are studied in different combinations assessing various endpoints. Many studies also have small sample sizes, making it difficult to generalize the results.

NEUROPSYCHOLOGICAL SYMPTOMS, SIBO, AND IBS

IBS patients can experience significant effects on their mental health with increased rates of comorbid psychological conditions such as stress and anxiety, as well as decreased energy and disruptions in sleep and functioning (88–90). Whether these conditions are part of the IBS-SIBO overlap remains a focus of research. A recent study by Rao et al. found that subjects with brain fog had increased rates of SIBO (91), and also found an association between brain fog and probiotic use as well as D-lactic acidosis, a condition found in patients with short bowel syndrome (92). Although the participants in this study were all referred from a gastrointestinal clinic, none were classified as having IBS, although the study did exclude subjects with "organic" gastrointestinal diseases. Furthermore, although this study was not placebo-controlled, an improvement was seen with initiation of antibiotics and the cessation of probiotics. Given this, probiotics may have subtle effects on health and despite their accessibility as an over-the-counter medication, should be taken cautiously. Similarly, in subjects with chronic fatigue syndrome, another disease which carries an enigmatic pathophysiology, erythromycin was shown to have a significant effect on sleep duration but only in those that exhibited significant effects on the gut microbiome, specifically a decrease in *Streptococcus* levels (93). It is unclear whether the promotility effect of erythromycin or its antimicrobial effect played a greater role in these findings.

Finally, one study has demonstrated a possible connection from the gut microbiome to the brain *via* the vagus nerve. In this study, mice supplemented with *Lactobacillus rhamnosus* exhibited decreased stress-related behaviors and altered expression of gamma-aminobutyric acid (GABA) receptor in the brain (94). Interestingly, this effect was decreased in rodents who underwent vagotomy, suggesting a direct neuronal effect *via* the 10th cranial nerve. Unfortunately, many of these studies have methodological issues concerning blinding, open-labeled design, and small sample size, to name a few potential biases. Whether alterations in the gut microbiome can directly affect the central nervous system and whether further modification *via* antibiotics or probiotics can have beneficial effects on humans requires further research.

FUTURE DIRECTIONS

Currently there is no consensus on the use of lactulose or glucose in breath testing (5). The lactulose breath test is limited by its potential false positive rates in patients with high motility, and the glucose breath test may not adequately detect SIBO in the distal bowel as it gets readily absorbed in the proximal small intestine (9). More validation studies are needed for standardization. As a potential solution, an ingestible capsule that can directly measure gas in the intestine is being developed. This may potentially improve the diagnostic accuracy over current methods which utilize breath testing.

There are several other innovations that may significantly influence the field of SIBO and IBS. A new study by Leite et al. has found that the use of dithiothreitol, a mucolytic, can significantly increase bacterial yield from small intestinal aspirates by approximately 3-fold (95). This will allow a more complete and thorough sampling of the small bowel which may lead to novel discoveries. As noted above, aspiration techniques

can vary and this may explain why one recent study did not find any correlation between symptoms and SIBO defined by CFU/mL in a duodenal aspirate (96). Further studies will be needed to optimize sampling methods for the intestinal microbiome but until then the breath test, which has potential clinical implications and can evaluate a larger section of the bowel (85), should be utilized in the diagnosis of SIBO (4).

Interestingly, another potential marker of bacterial overgrowth on a breath test, the exhaled gas hydrogen sulfide (H_2S), has recently been explored. H_2S appears to have implications for multiple gastrointestinal disorders, and can relax smooth muscle and have pro- and anti-inflammatory properties (97). Singer-Englar et al. described an association between diarrhea and levels of exhaled H_2S (98). Whether there is also an association with IBS-D (the definition of which requires pain in addition to diarrhea) remains to be seen.

Lastly, given that dysbiosis does not necessarily mean an overall overgrowth in the number of CFU and that changes in the relative abundances of specific microbial strains or taxa can cause symptoms, a reliance on measuring the overall abundance of bacteria may not be suitable in the era of 16S rRNA sequencing and breath testing.

CONCLUSION

IBS and SIBO appear to be intertwined. The methods for measuring SIBO still need further optimization. SIBO and other forms of gut microbiome dysbiosis are likely responsible for some symptoms in a subset of patients with IBS and can help guide treatment options. Given its therapeutic potential, further research in IBS and SIBO is needed.

AUTHOR CONTRIBUTIONS

MP and WT contributed to the concept, design, and writing of the review article.

REFERENCES

1. Lacy BE, Mearin F, Chang L, Chey WD, Lembo AJ, Simren M, et al. Bowel Disorders. *Gastroenterology* (2016) 150:1393–1407.e5. doi: 10.1053/j.gastro.2016.02.031
2. Drossman DA, Camilleri M, Mayer EA, Whitehead WE. AGA technical review on irritable bowel syndrome. *Gastroenterology* (2002) 123(6):2108–31. doi: 10.1053/gast.2002.37095
3. Ford AC, Lacy BE, Harris LA, Quigley EMM, Moayyedi P. Effect of Antidepressants and Psychological Therapies in Irritable Bowel Syndrome: An Updated Systematic Review and Meta-Analysis. *Am J Gastroenterol* (2019) 114(1):21–39. doi: 10.1038/s41395-018-0222-5
4. Rezaie A, Buresi M, Lembo A, Lin H, McCallum R, Rao S, et al. Hydrogen and Methane-Based Breath Testing in Gastrointestinal Disorders: The North American Consensus. *Am J Gastroenterol* (2017) 112(5):775–84.

doi: 10.1038/ajg.2017.46
5. Pimentel M, Saad RJ, Long MD, Rao SSC. ACG Clinical Guideline: Small Intestinal Bacterial Overgrowth. *Am J Gastroenterol* (2020) 115:165–78. doi: 10.14309/ajg.0000000000000501
6. Levitt MD. Volume and composition of human intestinal gas determined by means of an intestinal washout technic. *N Engl J Med* (1971) 284(25):1394–8. doi: 10.1056/NEJM197106242842502
7. Bond JH, Engel RR, Levitt MD. Factors influencing pulmonary methane excretion in man. An indirect method of studying the in situ metabolism of the methane-producing colonic bacteria. *J Exp Med* (1971) 133(3):572–88. doi: 10.1084/jem.133.3.572
8. Christl SU, Murgatroyd PR, Gibson GR, Cummings JH. Production, metabolism, and excretion of hydrogen in the large intestine. *Gastroenterology* (1992) 102(4 Pt 1):1269–77. doi: 10.1016/0016-5085(92)90765-Q
9. Romagnuolo J, Schiller D, Bailey RJ. Using breath tests wisely in a gastroenterology practice: an evidence-based review of indications and

pitfalls in interpretation. *Am J Gastroenterol* (2002) 97(5):1113–26. doi: 10.1111/j.1572-0241.2002.05664.x

10. Chen B, Kim JJ, Zhang Y, Du L, Dai N. Prevalence and predictors of small intestinal bacterial overgrowth in irritable bowel syndrome: a systematic review and meta-analysis. *J Gastroenterol* (2018) 53(7):807–18. doi: 10.1007/s00535-018-1476-9

11. Hwang L, Low K, Khoshini R, Melmed G, Sahakian A, Makhani M, et al. Evaluating breath methane as a diagnostic test for constipation-predominant IBS. *Dig Dis Sci* (2010) 55(2):398–403. doi: 10.1007/s10620-009-0778-4

12. Ghoshal U, Shukla R, Srivastava D, Ghoshal UC. Irritable Bowel Syndrome, Particularly the Constipation-Predominant Form, Involves an Increase in Methanobrevibacter smithii, Which Is Associated with Higher Methane Production. *Gut Liver* (2016) 10(6):932–8. doi: 10.5009/gnl15588

13. Takakura WR, Oh SJ, Singer-Englar T, Leite G, Pimentel M, Fridman A, et al. Patients with Appendectomy Have Significantly Less Methane in Their Exhaled Breath: is the Appendix a Vestigial Organ Or an Important Reservoir for Methanogens? *Gastroenterology* (2019) 156(6):S-1161. doi: 10.1016/S0016-5085(19)39870-1

14. Weaver GA, Krause JA, Miller TL, Wolin MJ. Incidence of methanogenic bacteria in a sigmoidoscopy population: an association of methanogenic bacteria and diverticulosis. *Gut* (1986) 27(6):698–704. doi: 10.1136/gut.27.6.698

15. Eckburg PB, Bik EM, Bernstein CN, Purdom E, Dethlefsen L, Sargent M, et al. Diversity of the human intestinal microbial flora. *Science* (2005) 308 (5728):1635–8. doi: 10.1126/science.1110591

16. Shah A, Talley NJ, Jones M, Kendall BJ, Koloski N, Walker MM, et al. Intestinal Bacterial Overgrowth in Irritable Bowel Syndrome: A Systematic Review and Meta-Analysis of Case-Control Studies. *Am J Gastroenterol* (2020) 115:190–201. doi: 10.14309/ajg.0000000000000504

17. Wu KQ, Sun WJ, Li N, Chen YQ, Wei YL, Chen DF. Small intestinal bacterial overgrowth is associated with Diarrhea-predominant irritable bowel syndrome by increasing mainly Prevotella abundance. *Scand J Gastroenterol* (2019) 54:1–7. doi: 10.1080/00365521.2019.1694067

18. Parodi A, Dulbecco P, Savarino E, Giannini EG, Bodini G, Corbo M, et al. Positive glucose breath testing is more prevalent in patients with IBS-like symptoms compared with controls of similar age and gender distribution. *J Clin Gastroenterol* (2009) 43(10):962–6. doi: 10.1097/MCG.0b013e3181a099a5

19. Park JS, Yu JH, Lim HC, Kim JH, Yoon YH, Park HJ, et al. [Usefulness of lactulose breath test for the prediction of small intestinal bacterial overgrowth in irritable bowel syndrome]. *Korean J Gastroenterol* (2010) 56(4):242–8. doi: 10.4166/kjg.2010.56.4.242

20. Sachdeva S, Rawat AK, Reddy RS, Puri AS. Small intestinal bacterial overgrowth (SIBO) in irritable bowel syndrome: frequency and predictors. *J Gastroenterol Hepatol* (2011) 26 Suppl 3:135–8. doi: 10.1111/j.1440-1746.2011.06654.x

21. Bertelè A, Papadia C, Bosi S, Marcucci F, Corrente V, Ciarleglio A, et al. P.07.16 Bacterial Overgrowth In Irritable Bowel Syndrome: A Cohort Study. *Digest Liver Dis* (2012) 44:S132. doi: 10.1016/S1590-8658(12)60365-X

22. Philip AJV, Mukunda M, Krishnadas D, Sobhana Devi R. SI-11 Prevalence of small intestinal bacterial overgrowth in patients with irritable bowel syndrome using lactulose hydrogen breath test. *Indian J Gastroenterol* (2013) 32(1):1–132. doi: 10.1007/s12664-013-0417-z

23. Qing Y. Relationship betweeen the irritable bowel syndrome and small intestinal bacterial. *J Gastroenterol Hepatol* (2013) 28(S3):23–693.

24. Li N, Wang Z, Fei G, Zhu L, Chen W, Li X, et al. Measurement of methane and hydrogen on lactulose breath test detects small intestinal bacterial overgrowth in patients with irritable bowel syndrome. *Neurogastroenterol Motil* (2014) 26 (s1):11–82.

25. Moraru IG, Moraru AG, Andrei M, Iordache T, Drug V, Diculescu M, et al. Small intestinal bacterial overgrowth is associated to symptoms in irritable bowel syndrome. Evidence from a multicentre study in Romania. *Rom J Intern Med* (2014) 52(3):143–50.

26. Lombardo L, Foti M, Ruggia O, Chiecchio A. Increased incidence of small intestinal bacterial overgrowth during proton pump inhibitor therapy. *Clin Gastroenterol Hepatol Off Clin Pract J Am Gastroenterol Assoc* (2010) 8 (6):504–8. doi: 10.1016/j.cgh.2009.12.022

27. Evans K, Lunn E, Raza S, Sanders DS, Higham S. PWE-050 Does small intestine bacterial overgrowth cause neurodysmotility in IBS and coeliac disease? *Gut* (2012) 61(Suppl 2):A317–A. doi: 10.1136/gutjnl-2012-302514d.50

28. Abbasi MH, Zahedi M, Darvish Moghadam S, Shafieipour S, HayatBakhsh Abbasi M. Small bowel bacterial overgrowth in patients with irritable bowel syndrome: the first study in iran. *Middle East J Dig Dis* (2015) 7 (1):36–40.

29. Chu H, Fox M, Zheng X, Deng Y, Long Y, Huang Z, et al. Small Intestinal Bacterial Overgrowth in Patients with Irritable Bowel Syndrome: Clinical Characteristics, Psychological Factors, and Peripheral Cytokines. *Gastroenterol Res Pract* (2016) 2016:3230859. doi: 10.1155/2016/3230859

30. Pimentel M, Mayer AG, Park S, Chow EJ, Hasan A, Kong Y. Methane production during lactulose breath test is associated with gastrointestinal disease presentation. *Dig Dis Sci* (2003) 48(1):86–92. doi: 10.1023/A:1021738515885

31. Chatterjee S, Park S, Low K, Kong Y, Pimentel M. The degree of breath methane production in IBS correlates with the severity of constipation. *Am J Gastroenterol* (2007) 102(4):837–41. doi: 10.1111/j.1572-0241.2007.01072.x

32. Suri J, Kataria R, Malik Z, Parkman HP, Schey R. Elevated methane levels in small intestinal bacterial overgrowth suggests delayed small bowel and colonic transit. *Med (Baltimore)* (2018) 97(21):e10554. doi: 10.1097/MD.0000000000010554

33. Pimentel M, Lin HC, Enayati P, van den Burg B, Lee HR, Chen JH, et al. Methane, a gas produced by enteric bacteria, slows intestinal transit and augments small intestinal contractile activity. *Am J Physiol Gastrointest Liver Physiol* (2006) 290(6):G1089–95. doi: 10.1152/ajpgi.00574.2004

34. Park YM, Lee YJ, Hussain Z, Lee YH, Park H. The effects and mechanism of action of methane on ileal motor function. *Neurogastroenterol Motil Off J Eur Gastrointest Motil Soc* (2017) 29(9):e13077. doi: 10.1111/nmo.13077

35. Attaluri A, Jackson M, Valestin J, Rao SS. Methanogenic flora is associated with altered colonic transit but not stool characteristics in constipation without IBS. *Am J Gastroenterol* (2010) 105(6):1407–11. doi: 10.1038/ajg.2009.655

36. Miller TL, Wolin MJ. Methanosphaera stadtmaniae gen. nov., sp. nov.: a species that forms methane by reducing methanol with hydrogen. *Arch Microbiol* (1985) 141(2):116–22. doi: 10.1007/BF00423270

37. Miller TL, Wolin MJ, Conway de Macario E, Macario AJ. Isolation of Methanobrevibacter smithii from human feces. *Appl Environ Microbiol* (1982) 43(1):227–32. doi: 10.1128/AEM.43.1.227-232.1982

38. Kim G, Deepinder F, Morales W, Hwang L, Weitsman S, Chang C, et al. Methanobrevibacter smithii is the predominant methanogen in patients with constipation-predominant IBS and methane on breath. *Dig Dis Sci* (2012) 57 (12):3213–8. doi: 10.1007/s10620-012-2197-1

39. Florin TH, Woods HJ. Inhibition of methanogenesis by human bile. *Gut* (1995) 37(3):418–21. doi: 10.1136/gut.37.3.418

40. Leite G, Morales W, Weitsman S, Celly S, Parodi G, Mathur R, et al. The microbiome in small intestinal bacterial overgrowth: the REIMAGINE study. *PloS One* (2020).

41. Ghoshal UC, Srivastava D, Ghoshal U, Misra A. Breath tests in the diagnosis of small intestinal bacterial overgrowth in patients with irritable bowel syndrome in comparison with quantitative upper gut aspirate culture. *Eur J Gastroenterol Hepatol* (2014) 26(7):753–60. doi: 10.1097/MEG.0000000000000122

42. Posserud I, Stotzer PO, Bjornsson ES, Abrahamsson H, Simren M. Small intestinal bacterial overgrowth in patients with irritable bowel syndrome. *Gut* (2007) 56(6):802–8. doi: 10.1136/gut.2006.108712

43. Pyleris E, Giamarellos-Bourboulis EJ, Tzivras D, Koussoulas V, Barbatzas C, Pimentel M. The prevalence of overgrowth by aerobic bacteria in the small intestine by small bowel culture: relationship with irritable bowel syndrome. *Dig Dis Sci* (2012) 57(5):1321–9. doi: 10.1007/s10620-012-2033-7

44. Rezaie A, Pimentel M, Cohen E. Autoimmunity as a Potential Cause of Post-Infectious Gut Dysmotility: A Longitudinal Observation. *Am J Gastroenterol* (2017) 112(4):656–7. doi: 10.1038/ajg.2017.8

45. Thabane M, Kottachchi DT, Marshall JK. Systematic review and meta-analysis: The incidence and prognosis of post-infectious irritable bowel syndrome. *Aliment Pharmacol Ther* (2007) 26(4):535–44. doi: 10.1111/j.1365-2036.2007.03399.x

46. Cohen E, Fuller G, Bolus R, Modi R, Vu M, Shahedi K, et al. Increased risk for irritable bowel syndrome after acute diverticulitis. *Clin Gastroenterol Hepatol* (2013) 11(12):1614–9. doi: 10.1016/j.cgh.2013.03.007

47. Klem F, Wadhwa A, Prokop LJ, Sundt WJ, Farrugia G, Camilleri M, et al. Prevalence, Risk Factors, and Outcomes of Irritable Bowel Syndrome After Infectious Enteritis: A Systematic Review and Meta-analysis. *Gastroenterology* (2017) 152(5):1042–54. doi: 10.1053/j.gastro.2016.12.039

48. Lovell RM, Ford AC. Global prevalence of and risk factors for irritable bowel syndrome: a meta-analysis. *Clin Gastroenterol Hepatol* (2012) 10(7):712–21. doi: 10.1016/j.cgh.2012.02.029

49. Scallan E, Hoekstra RM, Angulo FJ, Tauxe RV, Widdowson MA, Roy SL, et al. Foodborne illness acquired in the United States–major pathogens. *Emerg Infect Dis* (2011) 17(1):7–15. doi: 10.3201/eid1701.P11101

50. Shah ED, Riddle MS, Chang C, Pimentel M. Estimating the contribution of acute gastroenteritis to the overall prevalence of irritable bowel syndrome. *J Neurogastroenterol Motil* (2012) 18(2):200–4. doi: 10.5056/jnm.2012.18.2.200

51. Zuckerman MJ, Watts MT, Bhatt BD, Ho H. Intestinal permeability to [51Cr] EDTA in infectious diarrhea. *Dig Dis Sci* (1993) 38(9):1651–7. doi: 10.1007/BF01303174

52. Spiller RC, Jenkins D, Thornley JP, Hebden JM, Wright T, Skinner M, et al. Increased rectal mucosal enteroendocrine cells, T lymphocytes, and increased gut permeability following acute Campylobacter enteritis and in post-dysenteric irritable bowel syndrome. *Gut* (2000) 47(6):804–11. doi: 10.1136/gut.47.6.804

53. Dunlop SP, Hebden J, Campbell E, Naesdal J, Olbe L, Perkins AC, et al. Abnormal intestinal permeability in subgroups of diarrhea-predominant irritable bowel syndromes. *Am J Gastroenterol* (2006) 101(6):1288–94. doi: 10.1111/j.1572-0241.2006.00672.x

54. Zhang Q, Li Q, Wang C, Liu X, Li N, Li J. Enteropathogenic Escherichia coli changes distribution of occludin and ZO-1 in tight junction membrane microdomains in vivo. *Microb Pathog* (2010) 48(1):28–34. doi: 10.1016/j.micpath.2009.10.002

55. Hamer HM, Jonkers D, Venema K, Vanhoutvin S, Troost FJ, Brummer RJ. Review article: the role of butyrate on colonic function. *Aliment Pharmacol Ther* (2008) 27(2):104–19. doi: 10.1111/j.1365-2036.2007.03562.x

56. Hullar MA, Fu BC. Diet, the gut microbiome, and epigenetics. *Cancer J* (2014) 20(3):170–5. doi: 10.1097/PPO.0000000000000053

57. Pozuelo M, Panda S, Santiago A, Mendez S, Accarino A, Santos J, et al. Reduction of butyrate- and methane-producing microorganisms in patients with Irritable Bowel Syndrome. *Sci Rep* (2015) 5:12693. doi: 10.1038/srep12693

58. Moloney RD, Stilling RM, Dinan TG, Cryan JF. Early-life stress-induced visceral hypersensitivity and anxiety behavior is reversed by histone deacetylase inhibition. *Neurogastroenterol Motil Off J Eur Gastrointest Motil Soc* (2015) 27(12):1831–6. doi: 10.1111/nmo.12675

59. Rapin JR, Wiernsperger N. Possible links between intestinal permeability and food processing: A potential therapeutic niche for glutamine. *Clinics (Sao Paulo)* (2010) 65(6):635–43. doi: 10.1590/S1807-59322010000600012

60. Zhou Q, Verne ML, Fields JZ, Lefante JJ, Basra S, Salameh H, et al. Randomised placebo-controlled trial of dietary glutamine supplements for postinfectious irritable bowel syndrome. *Gut* (2019) 68(6):996–1002. doi: 10.1136/gutjnl-2017-315136

61. Hulsewe KW, van Acker BA, Hameeteman W, van der Hulst RR, Vainas T, Arends JW, et al. Does glutamine-enriched parenteral nutrition really affect intestinal morphology and gut permeability? *Clin Nutr* (2004) 23(5):1217–25. doi: 10.1016/j.clnu.2004.04.002

62. Dunlop SP, Jenkins D, Neal KR, Spiller RC. Relative importance of enterochromaffin cell hyperplasia, anxiety, and depression in postinfectious IBS. *Gastroenterology* (2003) 125(6):1651–9. doi: 10.1053/j.gastro.2003.09.028

63. Chadwick VS, Chen W, Shu D, Paulus B, Bethwaite P, Tie A, et al. Activation of the mucosal immune system in irritable bowel syndrome. *Gastroenterology* (2002) 122(7):1778–83. doi: 10.1053/gast.2002.33579

64. Bercik P, Wang L, Verdu EF, Mao YK, Blennerhassett P, Khan WI, et al. Visceral hyperalgesia and intestinal dysmotility in a mouse model of postinfective gut dysfunction. *Gastroenterology* (2004) 127(1):179–87. doi: 10.1053/j.gastro.2004.04.006

65. Chen B, Zhu S, Du L, He H, Kim JJ, Dai N. Reduced interstitial cells of Cajal and increased intraepithelial lymphocytes are associated with development of small intestinal bacterial overgrowth in post-infectious IBS mouse model. *Scand J Gastroenterol* (2017) 52(10):1065–71. doi: 10.1080/00365521.2017.1342141

66. Pimentel M, Chatterjee S, Chang C, Low K, Song Y, Liu C, et al. A new rat model links two contemporary theories in irritable bowel syndrome. *Dig Dis Sci* (2008) 53(4):982–9. doi: 10.1007/s10620-007-9977-z

67. Pokkunuri V, Pimentel M, Morales W, Jee SR, Alpern J, Weitsman S, et al. Role of Cytolethal Distending Toxin in Altered Stool Form and Bowel Phenotypes in a Rat Model of Post-infectious Irritable Bowel Syndrome. *J Neurogastroenterol Motil* (2012) 18(4):434–42. doi: 10.5056/jnm.2012.18.4.434

68. Pimentel M, Morales W, Pokkunuri V, Brikos C, Kim SM, Kim SE, et al. Autoimmunity Links Vinculin to the Pathophysiology of Chronic Functional Bowel Changes Following Campylobacter jejuni Infection in a Rat Model. *Dig Dis Sci* (2015) 60(5):1195–205. doi: 10.1007/s10620-014-3435-5

69. Bays JL, DeMali KA. Vinculin in cell-cell and cell-matrix adhesions. *Cell Mol Life Sci* (2017) 74(16):2999–3009. doi: 10.1007/s00018-017-2511-3

70. Schmulson M, Balbuena R, Corona de Law C. Clinical experience with the use of anti-CdtB and anti-vinculin antibodies in patients with diarrhea in Mexico. *Rev Gastroenterol Mex* (2016) 81(4):236–9. doi: 10.1016/j.rgmxen.2016.07.002

71. Rezaie A, Park SC, Morales W, Marsh E, Lembo A, Kim JH, et al. Assessment of Anti-vinculin and Anti-cytolethal Distending Toxin B Antibodies in Subtypes of Irritable Bowel Syndrome. *Dig Dis Sci* (2017) 62(6):1480–5. doi: 10.1007/s10620-017-4585-z

72. Morales W, Rezaie A, Barlow G, Pimentel M. Second-Generation Biomarker Testing for Irritable Bowel Syndrome Using Plasma Anti-CdtB and Anti-Vinculin Levels. *Dig Dis Sci* (2019) 64(11):3115–21. doi: 10.1007/s10620-019-05684-6

73. Pike BL, Paden KA, Alcala AN, Jaep KM, Gormley RP, Maue AC, et al. Immunological Biomarkers in Postinfectious Irritable Bowel Syndrome. *J Travel Med* (2015) 22(4):242–50. doi: 10.1111/jtm.12218

74. Talley NJ, Holtmann G, Walker MM, Burns G, Potter M, Shah A, et al. Circulating Anti-cytolethal Distending Toxin B and Anti-vinculin Antibodies as Biomarkers in Community and Healthcare Populations With Functional Dyspepsia and Irritable Bowel Syndrome. *Clin Transl Gastroenterol* (2019) 10 (7):e00064. doi: 10.14309/ctg.0000000000000064

75. Gasbarrini A, Lauritano EC, Gabrielli M, Scarpellini E, Lupascu A, Ojetti V, et al. Small intestinal bacterial overgrowth: diagnosis and treatment. *Dig Dis* (2007) 25(3):237–40. doi: 10.1159/000103892

76. Bala L, Ghoshal UC, Ghoshal U, Tripathi P, Misra A, Gowda GA, et al. Malabsorption syndrome with and without small intestinal bacterial overgrowth: a study on upper-gut aspirate using 1H NMR spectroscopy. *Magn Reson Med* (2006) 56(4):738–44. doi: 10.1002/mrm.21041

77. Shah SC, Day LW, Somsouk M, Sewell JL. Meta-analysis: antibiotic therapy for small intestinal bacterial overgrowth. *Aliment Pharmacol Ther* (2013) 38 (8):925–34. doi: 10.1111/apt.12479

78. Pimentel M, Lembo A, Chey WD, Zakko S, Ringel Y, Yu J, et al. Rifaximin therapy for patients with irritable bowel syndrome without constipation. *N Engl J Med* (2011) 364(1):22–32. doi: 10.1056/NEJMoa1004409

79. Lembo A, Pimentel M, Rao SS, Schoenfeld P, Cash B, Weinstock LB, et al. Repeat Treatment With Rifaximin Is Safe and Effective in Patients With Diarrhea-Predominant Irritable Bowel Syndrome. *Gastroenterology* (2016) 151(6):1113–21. doi: 10.1053/j.gastro.2016.08.003

80. Pimentel M, Cash BD, Lembo A, Wolf RA, Israel RJ, Schoenfeld P. Repeat Rifaximin for Irritable Bowel Syndrome: No Clinically Significant Changes in Stool Microbial Antibiotic Sensitivity. *Dig Dis Sci* (2017) 62(9):2455–63. doi: 10.1007/s10620-017-4598-7

81. Fodor AA, Pimentel M, Chey WD, Lembo A, Golden PL, Israel RJ, et al. Rifaximin is associated with modest, transient decreases in multiple taxa in the gut microbiota of patients with diarrhoea-predominant irritable bowel syndrome. *Gut Microbes* (2019) 10(1):22–33. doi: 10.1080/19490976.2018.1460013

82. Low K, Hwang L, Hua J, Zhu A, Morales W, Pimentel M. A combination of rifaximin and neomycin is most effective in treating irritable bowel syndrome patients with methane on lactulose breath test. *J Clin Gastroenterol* (2010) 44 (8):547–50. doi: 10.1097/MCG.0b013e3181c64c90

83. Pimentel M, Chatterjee S, Chow EJ, Park S, Kong Y. Neomycin improves constipation-predominant irritable bowel syndrome in a fashion that is dependent on the presence of methane gas: subanalysis of a double-blind randomized controlled study. *Dig Dis Sci* (2006) 51(8):1297–301. doi: 10.1007/s10620-006-9104-6

84. Pimentel M, Chang C, Chua KS, Mirocha J, DiBaise J, Rao S, et al. Antibiotic treatment of constipation-predominant irritable bowel syndrome. *Dig Dis Sci* (2014) 59(6):1278–85. doi: 10.1007/s10620-014-3157-8

85. Rezaie A, Heimanson Z, McCallum R, Pimentel M. Lactulose Breath Testing as a Predictor of Response to Rifaximin in Patients With Irritable Bowel Syndrome With Diarrhea. *Am J Gastroenterol* (2019) 114(12):1886–93. doi: 10.14309/ajg.0000000000000444

86. Gupta A, Chey WD. Breath Testing for Small Intestinal Bacterial Overgrowth: A Means to Enrich Rifaximin Responders in IBS Patients? *Am J Gastroenterol* (2016) 111(3):305–6. doi: 10.1038/ajg.2016.32

87. Ford AC, Harris LA, Lacy BE, Quigley EMM, Moayyedi P. Systematic review with meta-analysis: the efficacy of prebiotics, probiotics, synbiotics and antibiotics in irritable bowel syndrome. *Aliment Pharmacol Ther* (2018) 48 (10):1044–60. doi: 10.1111/apt.15001

88. Luscombe FA. Health-related quality of life and associated psychosocial factors in irritable bowel syndrome: a review. *Qual Life Res* (2000) 9 (2):161–76. doi: 10.1023/A:1008970312068

89. Gaynes BN, Drossman DA. The role of psychosocial factors in irritable bowel syndrome. *Baillieres Best Pract Res Clin Gastroenterol* (1999) 13(3):437–52. doi: 10.1053/bega.1999.0038

90. Drossman DA, McKee DC, Sandler RS, Mitchell CM, Cramer EM, Lowman BC, et al. Psychosocial factors in the irritable bowel syndrome. A multivariate study of patients and nonpatients with irritable bowel syndrome. *Gastroenterology* (1988) 95(3):701–8. doi: 10.1016/S0016-5085(88)80017-9

91. Rao SSC, Rehman A, Yu S, Andino NM. Brain fogginess, gas and bloating: a link between SIBO, probiotics and metabolic acidosis. *Clin Transl Gastroenterol* (2018) 9(6):162. doi: 10.1038/s41424-018-0030-7

92. Thompson JS, Rochling FA, Weseman RA, Mercer DF. Current management of short bowel syndrome. *Curr Probl Surg* (2012) 49(2):52–115. doi: 10.1067/j.cpsurg.2011.10.002

93. Jackson ML, Butt H, Ball M, Lewis DP, Bruck D. Sleep quality and the treatment of intestinal microbiota imbalance in Chronic Fatigue Syndrome: A pilot study. *Sleep Sci* (2015) 8(3):124–33. doi: 10.1016/j.slsci.2015.10.001

94. Bravo JA, Forsythe P, Chew MV, Escaravage E, Savignac HM, Dinan TG, et al. Ingestion of Lactobacillus strain regulates emotional behavior and central GABA receptor expression in a mouse via the vagus nerve. *Proc Natl Acad Sci U.S.A.* (2011) 108(38):16050–5. doi: 10.1073/pnas.1102999108

95. Leite GGS, Morales W, Weitsman S, Celly S, Parodi G, Mathur R, et al. Optimizing microbiome sequencing for small intestinal aspirates: validation of novel techniques through the REIMAGINE study. *BMC Microbiol* (2019) 19(1):239. doi: 10.1186/s12866-019-1617-1

96. Saffouri GB, Shields-Cutler RR, Chen J, Yang Y, Lekatz HR, Hale VL, et al. Small intestinal microbial dysbiosis underlies symptoms associated with functional gastrointestinal disorders. *Nat Commun* (2019) 10(1):2012. doi: 10.1038/s41467-019-09964-7

97. Linden DR. Hydrogen sulfide signaling in the gastrointestinal tract. *Antioxid Redox Signal* (2014) 20(5):818–30. doi: 10.1089/ars.2013.5312

98. Singer-Englar T, Rezaie A, Gupta K, Pichetshote N, Sedighi R, Lin E, et al. 182 - Competitive Hydrogen Gas Utilization by Methane- and Hydrogen Sulfide-Producing Microorganisms and Associated Symptoms: Results of a Novel 4-Gas Breath Test Machine. *Gastroenterology* (2018) 154(6):S-47. doi: 10.1016/S0016-5085(18)30625-5

17

High Rates of Non-Response Across Treatment Attempts in Chronic Irritable Bowel Syndrome: Results from a Follow-Up Study in Tertiary Care

Yuanjun Dong*, David Baumeister, Sabrina Berens, Wolfgang Eich and Jonas Tesarz

Department of General Internal Medicine and Psychosomatics, University Hospital Heidelberg, Heidelberg, Germany

*Correspondence:
Yuanjun Dong
Yuanjun.Dong@med.uni-heidelberg.de

Objective: Despite a wealth of treatment options for irritable bowel syndrome (IBS), data on the subjective experience of treatments in ongoing clinical practice are sparse. This follow-up study assessed the individual usage of treatment modalities by IBS patients over time and investigated the patients' subjective experience of therapeutic impact.

Methods: The study was conducted at the Specialty Clinic for Functional Gastrointestinal Disorders of the Heidelberg University Hospital. All patients who fulfilled the Rome III criteria for IBS and treated in our outpatient clinic between January 2012 and December 2016 were invited to the assessment. The primary outcome variables were individual usage of treatment modalities and the Patient Global Impression of Change (PGIC) with treatments.

Results: Three hundred and sixty-six patients fulfilled the Rome III criteria for IBS and thus were eligible for this study. Two hundred and seven patients dropped out from the study. The study could include 159 patients (43.7 ± 17.1 years; 71.1% female). The mean time since the first visit to the clinic was 2.8 ± 1.3 years (median 3.0 years). The mean time of symptom duration was 14.1 ± 11.1 years (median 10 years). The average number of treatment attempts was 12, ranging from 2 to 39). With respect to the subjective experience of therapeutic impact, there were no significant differences in the PGIC scores among different treatments ($p = 0.183$). The rates of non-response rates (minimally improved, no change, or minimally worse) ranged from 63.0% to 83.9%. The PGIC score was correlated negatively with the mean number of treatment attempts ($r = -0.316$, $p < 0.01$). The mean number of treatment attempts was correlated negatively with quality of life ($r = -0.262$, $p < 0.01$).

Conclusion: A multidisciplinary treatment approach of IBS is characterized by high rates of non-response and a high number of frustrating treatment attempts. The connection between the various treatment attempts and the frustrating subjective experience of therapeutic impact puts a substantial burden on IBS patients.

Keywords: irritable bowel syndrome, treatment modalities, subjective experience, therapeutic impact, response rate

INTRODUCTION

Irritable bowel syndrome (IBS) is a distressing chronic gastrointestinal disorder characterized by abdominal pain and changes in bowel habits (1). With a global prevalence of 9% to 12%, IBS is one of the most common functional gastrointestinal disorders in the world (2) and is associated with a substantial socioeconomic impact on the individual (3) as well as on society (4, 5). As the exact origin of IBS remains poorly understood, there are neither causal therapeutic approaches nor single-treatment interventions suitable and effective for all patients (6, 7). Accordingly, guidelines for the diagnosis and treatment of functional gastrointestinal diseases emphasize the combination of different therapies in a multimodal interdisciplinary treatment approach (8), including non-specific therapeutic recommendations (e.g., physical activity) as well as more specific recommendations, such as dietary advices, psychological interventions, and symptom-targeting medications. Although current guidelines (9) included a variety of different treatment options, adequate symptom control is still one of the greatest challenges in the treatment of IBS.

Against this background, a combination of several different treatment approaches is usually recommended in guidelines. However, Halder et al. (10) found that even after 10 years of treatment, patients with IBS are still plagued by various kinds of symptoms. In addition, more than half of IBS primary care counseling is due to patients being dissatisfied with previous treatments (11). Indeed, there is evidence that patients often use numerous treatments (12).

Despite a broad spectrum of IBS treatment options, few data have been published so far on the subjective experience of engagement with these treatment modalities and their performance under actual clinical conditions. While the superiority of several different treatment modalities over placebo was supported by a multitude of clinical trials (13), there is only limited evidence (14) for which treatments patients are engaged in and which are experienced as helpful by patients. Therefore, the aims of this study were 1) to determine the individual usage of treatment modalities by IBS patients over time and 2) to assess the patients' subjective experience of therapeutic impact.

MATERIALS AND METHODS

Study Design

This cross-sectional study was carried out at the Specialty Clinic for Functional Gastrointestinal Disorders at the Department of General Internal Medicine and Psychosomatics of Heidelberg University Hospital in tertiary care. This study was approved by the Ethics Committee of Heidelberg University (S-071/2017) and carried out in accordance with the Declaration of Helsinki and the Regulations for the Physicians of the Baden-Württemberg Chamber of Physicians in the latest versions. All patients who fulfilled the Rome III criteria for IBS and treated in our outpatient clinic between January 2012 and December 2016 were invited to the study. Patients received the study questionnaire package *via* mail, together with study invitation and consent forms, in October 2017. The study used the approach of the Dillman Total Design Method (15) to increase response rates.

There were 366 patients who fulfilled the Rome III criteria for IBS and thus were eligible for this study. Two hundred and four (55.7%) patients did not respond (including those whose new addresses were unknown), and three (0.8%) patients actively refused to participate in the study. Percentages of IBS subgroups, i.e., constipation predominant (IBS-C), diarrhea predominant (IBS-D), alternating or mixed (IBS-M), and undetermined (IBS-U), were also calculated in the patient cohort. The flowchart of patients' responses and reasons for non-participation is shown in **Figure 1**.

Inclusion/exclusion criteria: All patients had to be ≥18 years of age and had to provide signed informed consent. Patients were only included if they fulfilled the Rome III criteria for the diagnosis of IBS (16). Patients with illiteracy were excluded.

Measures

In addition to the treatment modalities and the subjective experience of therapeutic impact, the sociodemographic data, symptom severity, psychological comorbidities, and quality of life were assessed by a set of general and functional gastrointestinal disorder–specific questionnaires.

Sociodemographic Data

Sociodemographic data including age, gender, family status, education level, duration of symptoms, and treatments were collected using the Psychosomatic Basis Documentation Questionnaire (Psy-BaDo) according to Heuft and Senf (17).

Symptomatic Characteristics

To assess the patients' current symptomatic characteristics, symptom severity, quality of life, and psychological comorbidities were measured:

Symptom severity: Symptom severity was evaluated using the IBS Symptom Severity Scale (IBS-SSS, range 0–500) (18, 19). High values indicate greater symptom burden, and the following cutoff values have been suggested: <75 healthy, 75–174 mild, 175–300 moderate, and >300 severe IBS (20).

Quality of life: Quality of life was measured by the quality-of-life questionnaire for functional digestive disorders (FDDQL, range 0–100) (21, 22). FDDQL is a form of 48 items over eight domains (i.e., daily activity, disease-related anxiety, diet, sleep, discomfort, health perception, coping with disease, and impact of stress). Higher scores indicate better quality of life.

Psychological comorbidities: Depression was measured using the nine-item depression module of the Patient Health Questionnaire (PHQ-9, range 0–27) (23). A cutoff value of ≥10 was interpreted as clinically relevant depressive comorbidity. Anxiety was assessed using the Generalized Anxiety Disorder seven-item questionnaire (GAD-7, range 0–21) (24). A cutoff value of ≥10 was used to indicate clinically relevant anxiety comorbidity. Disease-related fear was measured with the brief Whitley Index-7 (WI-7, range 0–28) (25). A cutoff value of >3 was interpreted as the presence of a clinically relevant level of disease-related fear.

Usage of Treatment Modalities and Subjective Experience of Therapeutic Impact

To explore the usage of treatment modalities and patients' subjective experience of therapeutic impact, an additional questionnaire set

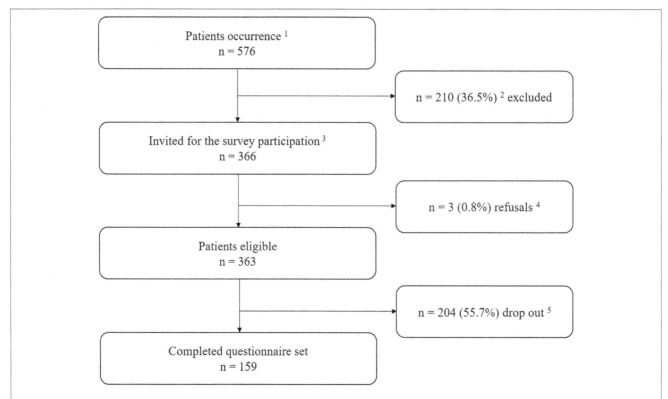

FIGURE 1 | Flowchart of the study.[1]All patients treated within our functional gastrointestinal disorders (FGIDs) specialty care unit from January 2012 to December 2016 were screened for eligibility. [2]Patients who did not meet the Rome III criteria for irritable bowel syndrome (IBS). [3]The invitation period was from September 2017 to December 2017. [4]Declared their refusal to participate by email or phone. [5]Not available (e.g., missing contact data, did not respond).

was developed based on the German IBS treatment guidelines (9, 26) and the Patient Global Impression of Change (PGIC) scale (27).

To assess the individual usage of treatment modalities, participants were asked about their previous therapy experiences. Referring to the previous experience in this field (28), therefore, a structured and comprehensive list of different treatment modalities was developed. To develop this list, an initial focus group was employed. Next to the authors of the present work, the study involved 1) clinicians involved in the daily work with IBS patients, 2) clinical experts involved in the development of the German treatment guidelines for IBS, and 3) a methodologist. Based on the official German IBS guidelines (9, 26), an initial item pool was developed by this focus group, including all the treatment options generally recommended for IBS. This item pool was supplemented by various additional treatment options frequently reported by patients (e.g., complementary medicine, over-the-counter drugs). To assess the patients' subjective experience of therapeutic impact for each treatment modality, we combined the treatment list with the seven-point Likert scale of the PGIC rating. Patients were asked to rate their subjective treatment satisfaction and global ratings of change of the overall situation using the following items: 1) very much improved, 2) much improved, 3) minimally improved, 4) no change, 5) minimally worse, 6) much worse, and 7) very much worse. Patients who rated PGIC with treatment as very much improved and much improved were treated as "improved"; minimally

improved, no change, and minimally worse were treated as "non-response"; and very much worse and much worse were classified as "worsened" (29–31). After two rounds of piloting the comprehensibility, clarity, and comprehensiveness of this preliminary assessment, the treatment modalities were stratified according to five different treatment classes: non-specific general therapeutic recommendations (Cronbach's $\alpha_{\text{non-specific general therapeutic recommendations}} = 0.582$, e.g., physical activity, herbal tea, symptom diary); dietary recommendations (Cronbach's $\alpha_{\text{dietary recommendations}} = 0.617$, e.g., avoiding fructose, avoiding lactose, nutritional counseling); psychosocial interventions (Cronbach's $\alpha_{\text{psychosocial interventions}} = 0.669$, e.g., abdominal hypnotherapy, relaxation therapy, stress management); symptom-targeting medications (Cronbach's $\alpha_{\text{symptom-targeting medications}} = 0.706$, e.g., antidiarrhea drugs, antispasmodic drugs, acid inhibitor drugs); and complementary interventions (Cronbach's $\alpha_{\text{complementary interventions}} = 0.847$, e.g., homoeopathy, manual therapy, integrative mind–body therapy). The Cronbach's α_{overall} coefficient in this study was 0.853.

Statistical Analyses

All statistical analyses were performed using IBM SPSS Statistics 22.0 for Windows. Partial correlation was used to assess the relationship between the number of treatment attempts and the PGIC score. The average PGIC score for all treatments ever used was used in the analysis. Additionally, dropout analyses were performed to explore the impact of patients who completed the IBS diagnostic criteria at the initial visit but who dropped out in this study. For characterization of dropouts, data/medical records from the initial visit were used. All tests were two-sided. *P*-values less than 0.05 indicated statistical significance for all analyses. All analyses were explorative and not of a confirmatory nature; thus, no specific hypotheses were formulated.

RESULTS

Sociodemographic and Symptomatic Characteristics

The study could include 159 (43.4%) patients (43.7 ± 17.1 years of age; 71.1% female). Of the patient cohort, 47.8% were classified as IBS-D, 43.4% were classified as IBS-M, and 6.3% were classified as IBS-C. As shown in **Table 1**, the mean time since the first visit to the clinic was 2.8 ± 1.3 years (median 3.0 years). The mean time of symptom duration was 14.1 ± 11.1 years (median 10.0 years). The mean level of symptom severity of these patients was 225.5 ± 101.8. Of all patients, 48.4% reported scores at moderate severity levels, 9.4% showed scores above the cutoff of value for severe symptom severity, and 32.1% showed scores at mild severity levels. Categorizing participants according to the validated cutoff values, the prevalence was 16.1% for depressive syndrome, 27.6% for anxiety syndrome, and 44.9% for disease-related fear. When considering the subgroups of IBS, there was no significant differences among the demographic and clinical characteristics, subjective experience of therapeutic impact, and number of treatment attempts between IBS-D and IBS-M. For more details, see **Table S1**.

Usage of Treatment Modalities and Subjective Experience of Therapeutic Impact

Patients reported on average experiences with treatments from at least two different treatment classes. The most-often-used treatment classes were symptom-targeting medications (98.7%, 157) and non-specific general therapeutic recommendations (95.0%, 151). The least-used class was complementary treatments (46.5%, 74). The average number of treatment attempts by patients was 12, ranging from 2 to 39. The five most-often-used treatment modalities were 1) soluble fibers (e.g., psyllium seed husks); 2) herbal teas (e.g., fennel anise caraway tea); 3) physical activity; 4) hot-water bottle; and 5) liquid nine herbs (e.g., STW-5). For more details of the usage of treatment modalities within each class, see **Figure 2**.

With respect to the subjective experience of therapeutic impact, there were no significant differences in the PGIC scores among different treatments ($p = 0.183$). The rates of non-response (minimally improved, no change, or minimally worse) ranged from 63.0% to 83.9%. According to different treatment modalities, between 15% and 30% of all patients reported significant benefits (very much improved and much improved), and less than 5.0% reported that treatments have worsened their symptoms. For more details of the subjective experience of therapeutic impact within each class, see **Figure 3**. **Table S2** of the **Supplementary Material** presents the top five of the different treatment modalities stratified according to usage rate and subjective experience of therapeutic impact. **Figure S1** of the **Supplementary Material** presents the most-often-used treatments in general (treatments reported by <25% of the sample are not listed).

TABLE 1 | Demographic characteristics, symptom burden, and quality of life of the study cohort.

			IBS patients (n = 159)
Age		Mean ± SD	43.4 ± 17.1
		(range)	(18, 77)
Female		% (n)	71.1 (113)
Family status	Single	% (n)	47.4 (63)
	Stable cohabitation[1]		45.1 (60)
	Divorced or widowed		7.5 (10)
Education level above high school		% (n)	72.6 (106)
IBS subtypes	IBS-C	% (n)	6.3 (10)
	IBS-D		47.8 (76)
	IBS-M		43.4 (69)
Number of treatment attempts		Median (range)	12 (2, 39)
First onset of symptoms in years		Mean ± SD	14.1 ± 11.1
Clinic treatment period[2] in years		Mean ± SD	2.8 ± 1.3
Symptom severity (IBS-SSS)		Mean ± SD	225.5 ± 101.8
Depression (PHQ-9)		Mean ± SD	5.4 ± 4.6
Anxiety (GAD-7)		Mean ± SD	6.7 ± 5.0
Disease-related fear (WI-7)		Mean ± SD	8.7 ± 6.5
Quality of life (FDDQL)		Mean ± SD	56.8 ± 11.2

[1]Stable cohabitation, i.e., married/unmarried cohabitation. [2]Clinic treatment period: the mean period of time since the first visit in the specialty care outpatient clinic and follow-up assessment.

IBS, irritable bowel syndrome; IBS-C, IBS with constipation; IBS-D, IBS with diarrhea; IBS-M, IBS with mixed bowel habits; IBS-SSS, IBS Symptom Severity Scale; GAD-7, Generalized Anxiety Disorder seven-item questionnaire; PHQ-9, nine-item depression module of the Patient Health Questionnaire; WI-7, brief Whitley Index-7; FDDQL, quality-of-life questionnaire for functional digestive disorders; SD, standard deviation.

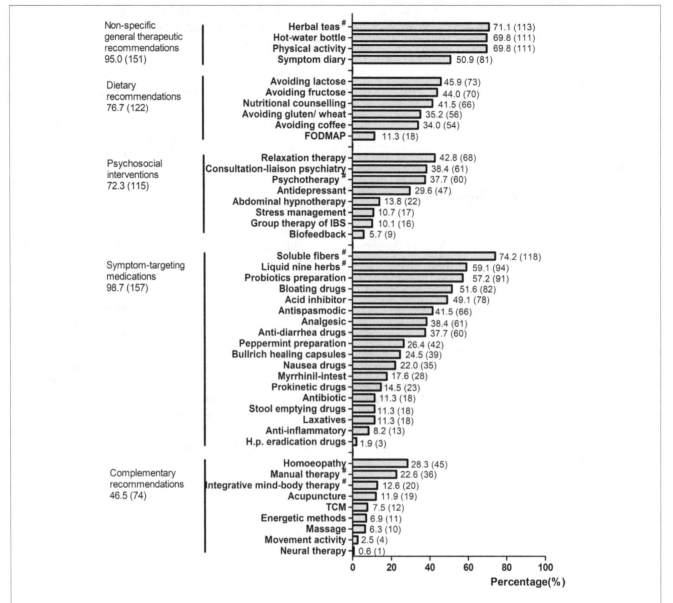

FIGURE 2 | The usage of treatment modalities within each class. All values are shown as % (n). The set of five different treatment classes were based on the German IBS treatment guidelines and clinic practices; values represent the percentage of participants who reported previous treatment attempts with the treatment classes. FODMAP, fermentable oligo-, di-, mono-saccharides and polyols; TCM, traditional Chinese medicine. #Herbal teas, e.g., fennel anise caraway tea; psychotherapy, e.g., cognitive behavioral therapy; soluble fibers, e.g., psyllium seed husks; liquid nine herbs, e.g., STW-5; manual therapy, e.g., osteopathy, chiropractic; integrative mind–body therapy, e.g., yoga, tai chi.

Correlations Among the Subjective Experience of Impact, Number of Treatment Attempts, Symptom Severity, Psychological Comorbidities, and Quality of Life

The average PGIC score for all treatments ever used was used in the correlation analysis. Controlling the mean time of symptom duration and the mean period of time since the first visit, the PGIC score was correlated negatively with the mean number of treatment attempts ($r = -0.320$, $p < 0.01$). A similar relationship was found between PGIC score and the symptom severity ($r = -0.381$, $p < 0.01$). The mean number of treatment attempts also

correlated negatively with quality of life ($r = -0.263$, $p < 0.01$). Depression, anxiety, and disease-related fear were all negatively correlated with PGIC score ($r = -0.354, -0.279, -0.257$, all $p < 0.01$). Meanwhile, depression and anxiety were both positively correlated with the number of attempted treatments ($r = 0.184$, 0.170, all $p < 0.05$). For more details, see **Table 2**.

Dropout Analyses

Of the 207 dropouts, 67.1% (139) were female. The mean age was 36.8 ± 14.5 years (range 18–77 years). The study compared initial visit clinical questionnaire data between the

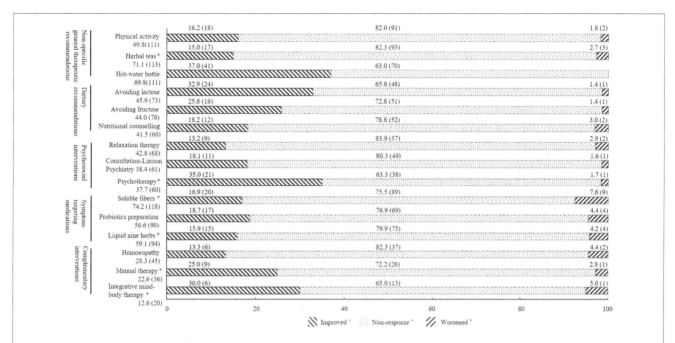

FIGURE 3 | Subjective experience of therapeutic impact of the three most-often-used treatment modalities within each treatment class. All values are shown as % (n); *Improved, patients who rated Patient Global Impression of Change (PGIC) as very much improved or much improved; non-response, patients who rated PGIC as minimally improved, no change, or minimally worse; worsened, patients who rated PGIC as very much worse or much worse. #Herbal teas, e.g., fennel anise caraway tea; psychotherapy, e.g., cognitive behavioral therapy; soluble fibers, e.g., psyllium seed husks; liquid nine herbs, e.g., STW-5; manual therapy, e.g., osteopathy, chiropractic; integrative mind–body therapy, e.g., yoga, tai chi.

TABLE 2 | Partial correlation matrix among the subjective experience of therapeutic impact, number of treatment attempts, symptom severity, psychological comorbidities, and quality of life.

	1)	2)	3)	4)	5)	6)	7)
1) Overall PGIC[1]	1.000						
2) Treatment number[2]	−0.320**	1.000					
3) Symptom severity (IBS-SSS)	−0.381**	0.254**	1.000				
4) Depression (PHQ-9)	−0.354**	0.184*	0.461**	1.000			
5) Anxiety (GAD-7)	−0.279**	0.170*	0.504**	0.806**	1.000		
6) Disease-related fear (WI-7)	−0.257**	0.062	0.473**	0.552**	0.641**	1.000	
7) Quality of life (FDDQL)	0.427**	−0.263**	−0.725**	−0.472**	−0.558**	−0.584**	1.000
Sub-analyses							
PGIC number non-specific general therapeutic recommendations			−0.056				
PGIC number dietary recommendations			−0.212*				
PGIC number psychosocial interventions			0.012				
PGIC number symptom-targeting medications			−0.313**				
PGIC number complementary interventions			−0.261*				

*p < 0.05; **p < 0.01. [1]Overall PGIC was used to measure the subjective experience of impact by all treatments ever used. [2]Treatment number, i.e., number of attempted treatments ever used. Control variables were the duration of symptoms and the mean period of time since the first visit in the analyses. PGIC, Patient Global Impression of Change. IBS-SSS, IBS Symptom Severity Scale; GAD-7, Generalized Anxiety Disorder seven-item questionnaire; PHQ-9, nine-item depression module of the patient health questionnaire; WI-7, brief Whitley Index-7; FDDQL, quality of life questionnaire for functional digestive disorders.

participants who completed the study and those who dropped out. There were no statistically significant differences in regard to sociodemographic and symptomatic characteristics between participants and dropouts except the variables of age and IBS subtypes. For more details, see **Table S3** of the **Supplementary Material**.

DISCUSSION

Findings

To our knowledge, this is the first study to evaluate specialty treatment practice variation among IBS patients at a tertiary care center in Germany. The study found that 1) IBS patients used an average of 12 different treatment modalities; 2) patients' subjective experience of therapeutic impact (i.e., PGIC) scores with these treatments were characterized by high non-response rates, and there were no significant differences among different treatment modalities; and 3) the number of treatment attempts was negatively correlated with the subjective experience of therapeutic impact and the quality of life.

The most-often-used treatment classes in the study cohort were symptom-targeting medications (98.7%), such as soluble fibers (e.g., psyllium seed husks) and liquid nine herbs (e.g., STW-5), as well as non-specific general therapeutic recommendations (95.0%), such as physical activity and herbal teas (e.g., fennel anise caraway tea) for symptom reduction. This finding is in line with current guidelines, in which symptom-targeting medications are an important pillar for the treatment of IBS patients (9). As most patients suffer from more than one symptom, the use of numerous treatments is understandable. The treatments that patients in the study used are quite similar to those of a previous study from 2002 for the standard treatment of IBS (32). This study showed dietary advice, education, exercise advice, stress management and antispasmodic medications to be the most frequently used treatment modalities. This finding indicates that there have been no relevant changes in the medical care of IBS over the last 15 years.

In light of the unclear etiology of IBS and the resulting lack of causal therapies (33–35), it is not surprising that most patients use different treatment modalities. Accordingly, guidelines for the diagnosis and treatment of functional gastrointestinal diseases emphasize the combination of different therapies in a multimodal interdisciplinary treatment approach (8), including non-specific therapeutic recommendations as well as more specific recommendations, such as dietary advice, psychological interventions, and symptom-targeting medications. However, the number of treatment attempts with, on average, more than 12 different treatment modalities per patient was substantial in the study. In the face of this high number in combination with the high non-response rates, most treatments would be classified ineffective based on current clinical standards. Further, most treatment modalities were similar in terms of the perceived therapeutic impact. The rates of non-response were high in the study cohort, ranging on average from 63.0% to 83.9%. Most patients reported that previous treatments had hardly affected their symptoms so far. In line with this, almost two-thirds of the participants reported moderate to severe complaints and reduced quality of life despite multiple treatment attempts. These data are in agreement with those obtained by a French survey (36), which found that even though 87% of IBS patients reported using some form of medication, almost half of them considered their therapy to be ineffective. Similarly, a survey carried out at a large US health maintenance organization working in primary and secondary care found that a symptom reduction of more than 50% could be achieved only in approximately 22% of IBS patients (32). The study indicates that, at least with regard to the IBS patients seen at a tertiary IBS specialty clinic, no significant progress seems to have been achieved. One possibility is that IBS is a heterogeneous disorder in which clinical symptoms vary from person to person (37). What's more, with varieties of symptoms and clinical features, IBS patients reflect many potential pathophysiological mechanisms (38). There were no significant relationships found when considering the correlation coefficient for PGIC number in non-specific general recommendations and psychosocial intervention. However, compared with other categories of treatment, psychosocial interventions and non-specific general recommendations are more susceptible to subjective conditions (e.g., cognition, personality, hypnosis), which means the responses to treatment vary more individually.

Although a high non-response rate was found, some mechanisms have also been reported. A possible mechanism to be discussed is the influence of previous negative treatment experiences on future therapy response. It is well known from nocebo research that negative expectations of a therapy have a strong potential to reduce future therapeutic effects (39). Given that the average IBS patient experiences a large number of frustrating therapy attempts, there is a risk that negative therapy expectations turn into a vicious cycle, with previous treatment failures leading to future treatment failures. Of note, anxiety was associated with an exacerbated nocebo response (40), and 44.9% of IBS patients in our study showed meaningful levels of disease-related fear, potentially indicating increased susceptibility to nocebo effects. However, these assumptions remain speculative, and further research is needed to better understand the underlying mechanisms.

Limitations and Strengths

Several limitations of this study should also be considered. First, this was a single-center study in tertiary care; our findings therefore may not be representative of practice at other centers or hospitals but instead may reflect our clinic's experience. The study cohort represents the outpatient patients, with higher disease burden and more psychological comorbidities than the primary care sample. Thus, the findings cannot be generalized. However, this long-term study shows what the current IBS patients are facing. Second, not all the subjects could be followed up, although we used repeated mailings to lower the dropout rate. However, our response rate is similar to those of other studies in this field (41–43). Moreover, dropout analyses did not indicate any obvious selection bias, at least concerning sociodemographic and symptomatic characteristics. This study used a retrospective design to measure the relationship between the usage of treatment modalities and the subjective experience of therapeutic impact. Therefore, there is a risk of a potential bias associated with self-report only. In addition to random measurement error, self-reports may be systematically biased if respondents have imperfect recall or deliberately provide misleading answers (44). The resolution of risks, which might generate spurious positive or null findings, requires large sample sizes in the future. Third, we did not assess the data of dose, duration, frequency, or order of therapies, as they may limit the efficacy to some extent. Using less effective treatments first may increase symptom severity and the opportunity for developing psychosocial distress. However, this research gap in the field of treatment still needs to be focused on in the future.

Despite those limitations, the strengths of this study should not be neglected. First, the IBS diagnosis was confirmed by a medical examination. Moreover, the treatment modalities were based on the German IBS treatment guidelines (9, 26). To capture the daily clinical perspectives in the best possible manner and to combine the scientific, clinical, and methodical experience, we used the method of focus group by including clinicians who work with IBS patients, clinical experts who are familiar with the German treatment guidelines for IBS, and a methodologist. It is well known that there is a high degree of variability among guidelines in the determination of need and type of IBS treatment in different countries. With this perspective, the findings on the subjective experience of therapeutic impact would be that IBS patients are often treated with therapies in clinic. Second, although there are many studies on efficacy and efficiency for a wide spectrum of different single treatment modalities, data on the patients' subjective experience of therapeutic impact under actual clinical conditions in IBS are rather sparse (32, 45). In an attempt to close this gap, our results present data with a large sample size on individual treatment attempts and subjective experience of impact on a wide range of different treatment modalities embedded in an interdisciplinary tertiary care clinic of IBS treatment.

Conclusions and Implications

To conclude, the multidisciplinary treatment approach of IBS is characterized by high rates of non-response and frustrating treatment attempts. Overall, IBS imposes a substantial burden on patients. This study demonstrates a complex treatment reality that is characterized by various treatment attempts and frustrating subjective experience of therapeutic impact.

to any qualified researcher. Requests for data should be sent to yuanjun.dong@med.uniheidelberg.de.

ETHICS STATEMENT

All subjects gave written informed consent in accordance with the Declaration of Helsinki. The protocol was approved by the Ethics Committee of Heidelberg University (S-071/2017).

AUTHOR CONTRIBUTIONS

The study concept and design were made by YD and JT. Acquisition of data was carried out by YD. Statistical analysis and interpretation of data were done by YD, DB, and SB. Drafting of the paper was done by YD. Critical revision of the content was by JT, DB, WE, and SB. WE was responsible for administrative or material support. Study supervision was held by JT.

SUPPLEMENTARY MATERIAL

FIGURE S1 | Subjective experience of therapeutic impact of the most often used treatments in general. Treatments reported by <25% of the sample are not listed; All values are shown as % (n); *Improved, patients who rated PGIC as very much improved or much improved; Non-response, patients who rated PGIC as minimally improved, no change or minimally worse; Worsened, patients who rated PGIC as very much worse or much worse; #Soluble fibres, e.g., psyllium seed husks; Herbal teas, e.g. fennel anise caraway tea; Liquid nine herbs, e.g., STW-5; Psychotherapy, e.g., cognitive behavioural therapy.

REFERENCES

1. Canavan C, West J, Card T. The epidemiology of irritable bowel syndrome. *Clin Epidemiol* (2014) 6:71–80. doi: 10.2147/CLEP.S40245
2. Lovell RM, Ford AC. Global prevalence of and risk factors for irritable bowel syndrome: a meta-analysis. *Clin Gastroenterol Hepatol* (2012) 10:712–21. e714 doi: 10.1016/j.cgh.2012.02.029
3. Agarwal N, Spiegel BM. The effect of irritable bowel syndrome on health-related quality of life and health care expenditures. *Gastroenterol Clin* (2011) 40:11–9. doi: 10.1016/j.gtc.2010.12.013
4. Canavan C, West J, Card T. The economic impact of the irritable bowel syndrome. *Aliment Pharmacol Ther* (2014) 40:1023–34. doi: 10.1111/apt.12938
5. Longstreth GF, Wilson A, Knight K, Wong J, Chiou C, Barghout V, et al. Irritable bowel syndrome, health care use, and costs: a US managed care perspective. *Am J Gastroenterol* (2003) 98:600–7. doi: 10.1016/S0002-9270(02)06018-5
6. Palsson OS, Baggish JS, Turner MJ, Whitehead WE. IBS patients show frequent fluctuations between loose/watery and hard/lumpy stools: implications for treatment. *Am J Gastroenterol* (2012) 107:286. doi: 10.1038/ajg.2011.358
7. Hauser G, Pletikosic S, Tkalcic M. Cognitive behavioral approach to understanding irritable bowel syndrome. *World J Gastroenterol* (2014) 20:6744. doi: 10.3748/wjg.v20.i22.6744
8. Drossman DA. Functional gastrointestinal disorders: history, pathophysiology, clinical features, and Rome IV. *Gastroenterology* (2016) 150:1262–79. e1262 doi: 10.1053/j.gastro.2016.02.032
9. Layer P, Andresen V, Pehl C, Allescher H, Bischoof SC, Classen M, et al. Irritable bowel syndrome: German consensus guidelines on definition, pathophysiology and management. *Z. Gastroenterol* (2011) 49:237. doi: 10.3238/arztebl.2011.0751
10. Halder SL, Locke GR, III, Schleck CD, Zinsmeister AR, Melton LJ, Talley NJ. Natural history of functional gastrointestinal disorders: a 12-year longitudinal population-based study. *Gastroenterology* (2007) 133:799–807. doi: 10.1053/j.gastro.2007.06.010
11. Williams R, Black C, Kim HY, Andrews EB, Mangel AW, Bud JJ, et al. Determinants of healthcare-seeking behaviour among subjects with irritable bowel syndrome. *Aliment Pharmacol Ther* (2006) 23:1667–75. doi: 10.1111/j.1365-2036.2006.02928.x
12. Camilleri M, Di Lorenzo C. The brain–gut axis: from basic understanding to treatment of irritable bowel syndrome and related disorders. *J Pediatr Gastroenterol Nutr* (2012) 54:446. doi: 10.1097/MPG.0b013e31823d34c3
13. Ford AC, Moayyedi P, Lacy BE, Lembo AJ, Saito YA, Schiller LR, et al. American College of Gastroenterology monograph on the management of irritable bowel syndrome and chronic idiopathic constipation. *Am J Gastroenterol* (2014) 109:S2. doi: 10.1038/ajg.2014.187
14. Usai-Satta P, Bellini M, Lai M, Oppia F, Cabras F. Therapeutic approach for irritable bowel syndrome: old and new strategies. *Curr Clin Pharmacol* (2018)13:164–172. doi: 10.2174/1574884713666180807143606
15. Dillman DA. The importance of adhering to details of the Total Design Method (TDM) for mail surveys. *New Dir Prog Eval* (1984) 21:49–64. doi: 10.1002/ev.1359
16. Drossman DA. The functional gastrointestinal disorders and the Rome III process. *Gastroenterology.* (2006) 130:1377–90 doi: 10.1053/j.gastro.2006.03.008
17. Heuft G, Senf W. *Practice of quality management in psychotherapy: manual for the Psy-BaDo [psychotherapeutic basis documentation].* Stuttgart, Germany: Thieme (1998). doi: 10.1007/s002780050099
18. Francis CY, Morris J, Whorwell PJ. The irritable bowel severity scoring

system: a simple method of monitoring irritable bowel syndrome and its progress. *Aliment Pharmacol Ther* (1997) 11:395–402. doi: 10.1046/j.1365-2036.1997.142318000.x

19. Betz C, Mannsdörfer K, Bischoff S. Validation of the IBS-SSS. *Z. Gastroenterol* (2013) 51:1171–6. doi: 10.1055/s-0033-1335260

20. Saigo T, Tayama J, Ogawa S, Bernick PJ, Takeoka A, Hayashida M, et al. Increased risk of irritable bowel syndrome in university students due to gastrointestinal symptom–specific anxiety. *Acta Medica Nagasakiensia* (2018) 61:137–43. doi: 10.11343/amn.61.137

21. Chassany O, Marquis P, Scherrer B, Read NW, Finger T, Bergmann JF, et al. Validation of a specific quality of life questionnaire for functional digestive disorders. *Gut* (1999) 44:527–33. doi: 10.1136/gut.44.4.527

22. Yacavone RF, Locke GR III, Provenzale DT, Eisen GM. Quality of life measurement in gastroenterology: what is available? *Am J Gastroenterol* (2001) 96:285–97. doi: 10.1111/j.1572-0241.2001.03509.x

23. Kroenke K, Spitzer RL, Williams JB. The PHQ-9: validity of a brief depression severity measure. *J Gen Intern Med* (2001) 16:606–13. doi: 10.1046/j.1525-1497.2001.016009606.x

24. Spitzer RL, Kroenke K, Williams GB, Löwe B. A brief measure for assessing generalized anxiety disorder: the GAD-7. *Arch Intern Med* (2006) 166:1092–7. doi: 10.1001/archinte.166.10.1092

25. Fink P, Ewald H, Jensen J, Sørensen L, Engberg M, Holm M, et al. Screening for somatization and hypochondriasis in primary care and neurological in-patients: a seven-item scale for hypochondriasis and somatization. *J Psychosom Res* (1999) 46:261–73. doi: 10.1016/S0022-3999(98)00092-0

26. Hausteiner-Wiehle C. Umgang mit Patienten mit nicht-spezifischen, funktionellen und somatoformen Körperbeschwerden: S3-Leitlinien mit Quellentexten, Praxismaterialien und Patientenleitlinie, Schattauer Verlag, 2013.

27. Geisser ME, Clauw DJ, Strand V, Gendreau RM, Palmer R, Williams D. A. Contributions of change in clinical status parameters to Patient Global Impression of Change (PGIC) scores among persons with fibromyalgia treated with milnacipran. *Pain®* (2010) 149:373–8. doi: 10.1016/j.pain.2010.02.043

28. Berens S, Kraus F, Gauss A, Tesarz J, Herzog W, Niesler B, et al. A specialty clinic for functional gastrointestinal disorders in tertiary care: concept and patient population. Clinical gastroenterology and hepatology. *Off Clin Pract J Am Gastroenterol Assoc* (2017) 15:1127. doi: 10.1016/j.cgh.2017.02.039

29. Middel B, Stewart R, Bouma J, Sonderen E, Heuvel WJA. How to validate clinically important change in health-related functional status. Is the magnitude of the effect size consistently related to magnitude of change as indicated by a global question rating? *J Eval Clin Pract* (2001) 7:399–410. doi: 10.1046/j.1365-2753.2001.00298.x

30. Wyrwich KW, Nienaber NA, Tierney WM, Wolinsky FD. Linking clinical relevance and statistical significance in evaluating intra-individual changes in health-related quality of life. *Med Care* (1999) 37: 469–478. doi: 10.1097/00005650-199905000-00006

31. Farrar JT, Young JP Jr, LaMoreaux L, Werth JL, Poole RM. Clinical importance of changes in chronic pain intensity measured on an 11-point numerical pain rating scale. *Pain* (2001) 94:149–58. doi: 10.1016/S0304-3959(01)00349-9

32. Whitehead WE, Levy RL, Von Korff M, Feld AD, Palsson OS, Turner M, et al. The usual medical care for irritable bowel syndrome. *Aliment Pharmacol Ther* (2004) 20:1305–15. doi: 10.1111/j.1365-2036.2004.02256.x

33. Halland M, Almazar A, Lee R, Atkinson E, Larson J, Talley NJ, et al. A case–control study of childhood trauma in the development of irritable bowel syndrome. *Neurogastroenterol Motility* (2014) 26:990–8. doi: 10.1111/nmo.12353

34. Barbara G, Feinle-Bisset C, Ghoshal UC, Quigley EM, Santos J, Vanner S, et al. The intestinal microenvironment and functional gastrointestinal disorders. *Gastroenterology* (2016) 150:1305–18. doi: 10.1053/j.gastro.2016.02.028

35. Shanahan F, Quigley EM. Manipulation of the microbiota for treatment of IBS and IBD—challenges and controversies. *Gastroenterology* (2014) 146:1554–63. doi: 10.1053/j.gastro.2014.01.050

36. Dapoigny M, Bellanger J, Bonaz B, Bruley des Varannes S, Bueno L, Coffin B, et al. Irritable bowel syndrome in France: a common, debilitating and costly disorder. *Eur J Gastroenterol Hepatol* (2004) 16:995–1001. doi: 10.1097/00042737-200410000-00008

37. Mujagic Z, Ludidi S, Keszthelyi D, Hesselink MA, Kruimel JW, Lenaerts K, et al. Small intestinal permeability is increased in diarrhoea predominant IBS, while alterations in gastroduodenal permeability in all IBS subtypes are largely attributable to confounders. *Aliment Pharmacol Ther* (2014) 40:288–97. doi: 10.1111/apt.12829

38. Gazouli M, Wouters MM, Kapur-Pojskić L, Bengtson MB, Friedman E, Nikčević G, et al. Lessons learned—resolving the enigma of genetic factors in IBS. *Nat Rev Gastroenterol Hepatol* (2016) 13:77. doi: 10.1038/nrgastro.2015.206

39. Enck P, Benedetti F, Schedlowski M. New insights into the placebo and nocebo responses. *Neuron* (2008) 59:195–206. doi: 10.1016/j.neuron.2008.06.030

40. Staats PS, Staats A, Hekmat H. The additive impact of anxiety and a placebo on pain. *Pain Med* (2001) 2:267–79. doi: 10.1046/j.1526-4637.2001.01046.x

41. Zernicke KA, Campbell TS, Blustein PK, Fung TS, Johnson JA, Bacon SL, et al. Mindfulness-based stress reduction for the treatment of irritable bowel syndrome symptoms: a randomized wait-list controlled trial. *Int J Behav Med* (2013) 20:385–96. doi: 10.1007/s12529-012-9241-6

42. Abdul-Baki H, El Hajj II, Elzahabi L, Azar C, Aoun E, Skoury A, et al. A randomized controlled trial of imipramine in patients with irritable bowel syndrome. *World J Gastroenterol* (2009) 15:3636. doi: 10.3748/wjg.15.3636

43. Mazzawi T, Hausken T, Gundersen D, El-Salhy M. Effect of dietary management on the gastric endocrine cells in patients with irritable bowel syndrome. *Eur J Clin Nutr* (2015) 69:519. doi: 10.1038/ejcn.2014.151

44. Bauhoff S. Systematic self-report bias in health data: impact on estimating cross-sectional and treatment effects. *Health Serv Outcomes Res Methodol* (2011) 11:44–53. doi: 10.1007/s10742-011-0069-3

45. Törnblom H, Goosey R, Wiseman G, Baker S, Emmanuel A. Understanding symptom burden and attitudes to irritable bowel syndrome with diarrhoea: results from patient and healthcare professional surveys. *United Eur Gastroenterol J* (2018) 6:1417–27. doi: 10.1177/2050640618787648

18

Imaging of Morphological Background in Selected Functional and Inflammatory Gastrointestinal Diseases in fMRI

Katarzyna Skrobisz[1]*, Grazyna Piotrowicz[2], Patrycja Naumczyk[3], Agnieszka Sabisz[4], Karolina Markiet[4], Grazyna Rydzewska[5] and Edyta Szurowska[4]

[1] Department of Radiology, Medical University of Gdansk, Gdansk, Poland, [2] Department of Gastroenterology, Self-Dependent Health Care Unit of Ministry of Interior, Gdansk, Poland, [3] Institute of Psychology, University of Gdansk, Gdansk, Poland, [4] II Department of Radiology, Medical University of Gdansk, Gdansk, Poland, [5] Central Clinical Hospital of the Ministry of Interior, Warsaw, Poland

*Correspondence:
Katarzyna Skrobisz
kskrobisz@gumed.edu.pl

The study focuses on evaluation of the Default Mode Network (DMN) activity in functional magnetic resonance imaging (fMRI) in resting state in patients with functional dyspepsia (FD) and irritable bowel syndrome (IBS), Crohn's disease and colitis ulcerosa (IBD) in comparison to healthy volunteers. We assume that etiology of both functional and non-specific inflammatory bowel diseases is correlated with disrupted structure of axonal connections. We would like to identify the network of neuronal connections responsible for presentation of symptoms in these diseases. 56 patients (functional dyspepsia, 18; Crohn's disease and colitis ulcerosa, 18; irritable bowel syndrome, 20) and 18 healthy volunteers underwent examination in MRI of the brain with assessment of brain morphology and central nervous system activity in functional imaging in resting state performed in 3T scanner. Compared to healthy controls' DMN in patients with non-specific digestive tract diseases comprised additional areas in superior frontal gyrus of left hemisphere, in left cingulum and in the left supplementary motor area. Discovered differences in the DMNs can be interpreted as altered processing of homeostatic stimuli. Our study group involved patients suffering from both functional and non-specific inflammatory bowel diseases. Nevertheless a spectrum of changes in the study group (superior frontal gyrus of the left hemisphere, in the left cingulum and in the left supplementary motor area) we were able to find common features, differentiating the whole study group from the healthy controls.

Keywords: functional magnetic resonance imaging (fMRI), irritable bowel syndrome (IBS), inflammatory bowel diseases, functional dyspepsia (fd), resting-state

INTRODUCTION

Functional disorders of the gastrointestinal tract (FGIDs) may explain from 25% up to 40% gastrointestinal tract (GI) derived symptoms in young adults (1). In recent years, an increase in incidence of non-specific inflammatory bowel diseases (IBDs), especially in people in their 20s to 40s, has been observed. Epidemiological data prove that chronic stress disorders underlie both FGIDs and IBDs (2, 3). Non-specific inflammatory bowel diseases, such as Crohn's disease or colitis ulcerosa, are characterized by chronic inflammation of GI tract. Stress seems not only to be a factor in exacerbation of symptoms in course of IBDs, but is considered an initiating agent as well (4).

Functional disorders of the gastrointestinal tract are diagnosed after exclusion of so called alert symptoms and structural diseases on bases of Rome III Criteria (5, 6). Etiology of FGIDs is elusive, pathogenesis theories include alteration in enteric motility, celiac hypersensitivity, intestinal barrier dysfunction, and underlying stress. FGIDs are often described as immunohormonal mucosal disorders or functional mucosal syndromes and symptoms seem to derive from a disturbance of balance between inflammatory cytokines released from intraepithelial lymphocytes and cytokines inhibiting inflammatory processes (7–9). There are ample data supporting theory that stress and other psychological disorders are factors in development of FIGDs. Patients present with increased levels of anxiety (fear), signs of depression (pessimism), and emotional tension (10–12). Moreover, the newest research in functional magnetic resonance imaging (fMRI) in resting state underline regional disturbances in brain activity in pathophysiology of functional dyspepsia. There is also extensive research into the role of disturbance of brain-gut-axis, which refers to bi-directional communication between the gut and the central nervous system, in etiology of functional gastrointestinal disorders (13, 14).

A number of studies contributed to the knowledge of neural underpinning of patients' sensations in gastric diseases and show two major findings. Abnormal interhemispheric interactions have been encountered in patients with FGIDs (15–17). The second finding focuses on mapping the brain regions—part of Default Mode Network (DMN)—connected to gastric sensations, including those involved in cognitive and emotional regulation (anterior cingulate cortex—ACC, prefrontal cortex—PFC, insula, temporal cortex, parahippocampal gyrus, and orbitofrontal cortex—OFC) (17–21) and associated with the "homeostatic afferent network" as described by Mayer Naliboff and Craig (22). Our study explored the common mechanisms underpinning different FGIDs. It is suggested that these disorders origin in central processing of the visceral stimuli (23–25). Patients with FGIDs and IBDs suffer from chronic visceral pain which is strongly connected with DMN. Studies reported that chronic pain is causing functional reorganization in the default mode network (26–28).

There is a limited number of studies which examined the role of DMN in inflammatory bowel diseases, among others, Liu et al. (29) reported disrupted local and global topological patterns of functional neural networks, including DMN in CD patients.

Another study presented aberrantly activated regions in DMN in patients with ulcerative colitis (UC) (30).

We decided to focus on the default mode network as the one most activated during processing the self-specific stimuli (31).

MATERIALS AND METHODS

All patients gave written consent to participate in the study. Study has been approved by The Bioethical Committee of The Military Medical Council (Street Koszykowa 78, 00-909 Warsaw) (document 107/12 dated 22.06.2012).

Functional Magnetic Resonance Imaging

Study group included patients with functional dyspepsia (FD), irritable bowel syndrome (IBS), and with non-specific inflammatory bowel diseases (IBDs) (Crohn's disease and ulcerative colitis)—FD, 18 (K, 13; M, 5; age range, 20–40 years; mean age, 33.28 years); IBS, 20 (K, 14; M, 6; age range, 23–44 years; mean age, 33.1 years); IBD, 18 (K, 10; M, 8; age range, 21–43 years; mean age, 26.83 years).

Patients suffering from FGIDs have been enrolled according to Rome III Criteria summarized in **Table 1** (5, 6). Patients with

TABLE 1 | Summary of Rome III Criteria on FGIDs.

	Diagnostic criteria*
1. Functional dyspepsia	Must include one or more of the following: –Bothersome postprandial fullness, –Early satiation, –Epigastric pain and/or burning. 　No evidence of structural disease (including at upper endoscopy) likely to explain the symptoms should be found.
1a. Epigastric pain syndrome (EPS)	Must include all of the following: –Pain or burning localized to the epigastrium of at least moderate severity, at least once a week, –Intermittent character of pain/burning, –Pain/burning should not be generalized or localized to other abdominal or chest regions, –Pain/burning should not be relieved by defecation or passage of flatus. 　Criteria for gallbladder and sphincter of Oddi disorders should not be fulfilled.
1b. Postprandial distress syndrome (PDS)	Must include one or both of the following: –Bothersome postprandial fullness, occurring after ordinary-sized meals, at least several times a week, –Early satiation that prevents completing a regular meal, at least several times a week
2. Irritable bowel syndrome (IBS)	Recurrent abdominal pain or discomfort** at least 3 days/ month in the last 3 months associated with two or more of the following: –Improvement with defecation, –Onset associated with a change in frequency of stool, –Onset associated with a change in form (appearance) of stool.

*Criteria fulfilled for the last 3 months with symptom onset at least 6 months prior to diagnosis.
***Discomfort" stands for uncomfortable sensation, not described as pain.

non-specific inflammatory bowel diseases have been qualified according to the anamnesis and results of additional tests, which included colonoscopy with histopathological assessment, gastrofiberoscopy, capsule endoscopy, and/or magnetic resonance enterography (MRE). To exclude stress associated with diagnosis a minimum period of three years from diagnosis has been established.

The control group of 18 healthy volunteers consisted of nine women and nine men (age range, 24–47 years; mean age, 34.27 years).

The exclusion criteria comprised lack of fulfillment of Rome III Criteria for FGIDs, head trauma in anamnesis, severe additional diseases, depression, mental disorders, pregnancy, and/or lactation and well established contraindications to MRI.

Patients from both study and control group underwent a GAST questionnaire developed by one of the authors (GP). GAST questionnaire focuses on type of functional GI disease, anamnesis with emphasis on history of symptoms and concomitant diseases as well as sociodemographic data.

All patients subjected to research have been thoroughly introduced to its principles and given detailed information on examination procedures, especially on MR, also in order to reduce stress levels and avoid potential panic or claustrophobic attacks.

Scanning Protocol

Functional and anatomical data sets were acquired in a 3T Achieva TX Scanner (Philips Healthcare, Best, the Netherlands) with the use of the eight-channel head coil. To evaluate brain morphology and exclude subjects with brain pathology standard T1 and T2 sequences were applied. No contrast agent was administered. T2* Gradient Echo-Planar Imaging (FFE-EPI: TR, 1,500 ms; TE, 27 ms; flip angle, 60°; matrix, 80 × 80; slice thickness, 3 mm with 0-mm gap, 210 volumes in series; TA 5 min 15 s; FOV, 240 mm × 240 mm), and 3D high-resolution T1 sequence (T1-TFE: TR, 7.44 ms; TE, 3.6 ms; slice thickness, 1 mm; matrix, 260 × 240; FOV, 260 mm × 240 mm) were applied for functional imaging and anatomical reference, respectively. During the resting state, acquisition subjects were asked to consciously attend to the fixation point presented in the center of the visual field and not to think of anything specific. The fixation point was presented *via* MRI-compatible goggles (NNL fMRI VisualSystem).

Statistical Analyses

Data analyses were performed using the SPM12 toolbox (Wellcome Department of Imaging Neuroscience, London, UK, www.fil.ion.ucl.ac.uk/spm) implemented in MATLAB (Mathworks Inc., Sherborn, MA, USA). Single-subject data were pre-processed with Data Processing Assistant for Resting State fMRI (DPARSF v2.3, Chao-Gan & Yu-Feng 2010). The first five fMRI volumes were discarded to allow the BOLD signal to reach steady state. Functional scans were corrected for slice timing, realigned to the first image of the time series, and normalized at 3 mm × 3 mm × 3 mm in reference to a standard brain atlas (SPM12 MNI space). Participants with movement exceeding a 2-mm vector of translation were excluded from further analyses (eight subjects met the criteria

—2 form CON group, 2 from FD group, 3 from IBD group, and 1 from IBS group). Subsequently the T1 anatomical images were segmented and the signal from the white matter and cerebrospinal fluid was extracted. Resting state data were further denoised using head motion scrubbing regressors and additional nuisance regressors that included white matter and cerebrospinal fluid signals. Finally, the data were low-pass filtered (with 0.1 Hz cut-off) and smoothed with 4-mm full width at half maximum Gaussian kernel. The purpose of the pre-processing was to remove various kinds of artifacts (i.e. the physiological noise), and to condition the data, to maximize the sensitivity of later statistical analyses, and to increase statistical validity.

In group resting state data analysis, the Group ICA of fMRI Toolbox [GIFT v4.0, icatb.sourceforge.net] (32) and a natural gradient (infomax) algorithm were used. The number of independent components was set at 20 to avoid anterior-posterior split of the Default Mode Network. Also, an ICASSO spell method was introduced (with ten times repeating of the ICA analysis) to increase the validity of the analysis. After subject-wise data concatenations, ICA was performed for all groups (CON, FD, IBD, IBS) in three stages:

- principal component analysis (PCA), which reduced each of the subject's fMRI data to predefined number of components;
- ICA algorithm (Infomax) application;
- back reconstruction for each individual subject's data, resulting in time courses and spatial maps of components.

For each of the groups 20 components were resembled. The Default Mode Network was identified with the use of spatial matching to the GIFT's binary DMN template. All independent components were converted to z-maps (32, 33). Each z-score represented the fit of a specific voxel BOLD time course to the time course of the group averaged component. The z-maps of the reconstructed subjects' DMN networks were further compared in SPM12 second-level one-way ANOVA with age as an additional covariate. Each of the group of interest (FD, IBS, IBD) DMN was contrasted with the control group using two sample t-test. Additionally, some joint intergroup comparisons including "the gastroenterological diseases vs control" (all 3 groups—FD, IBS, IBD) and "functional gastroenterological diseases vs control" (2 groups—FD and IBS) were performed with F-test. The results were all masked with the GIFTS's binary DMN template. Due to our *a priori* hypothesis whole-brain analysis was restricted to the DMN only (defined by the GIFT's template). For that purpose, a small volume correction was applied on cluster level. Clusters were regarded as significant when falling below an initial uncorrected voxel threshold of 0.001 and a topological False Discovery Rate corrected threshold of .05 adjusted for the small volume.

RESULTS

The automated matching of the Default Mode Network resulted in a component replicable amongst groups as shown in **Figure 1B**. No anterior-posterior split of the DMN was observed.

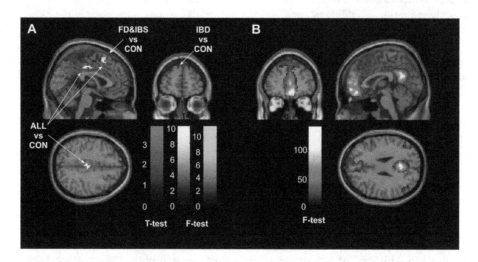

FIGURE 1 | (A) Significant (cluster corrected p_{FDR} < .05) clusters of intergroup comparisons in contrast with the control group. The red cluster defines area of additional DMN connectivity of the IBD group, the green cluster represents a region of auxiliary connectivity of the DMN shared by both FD and IBS groups, whereas the yellow clusters underpin regions of increased DMN connectivity shared by all of the gastrointestinal diseases. **(B)** A map of the main effect of the Default Mode Network as reconstructed during the Independent Component Analysis across all of the subjects—patients and controls combined (p_{FWE} < 0.05). CON, the control group; FD, the functional dyspepsia group; IBS, the irritable bowel syndrome group; IBD, the inflammatory bowel disease group; ALL, all diseases (FD, IBS, and IBD).

DMN of Given Diseases

The two-sample t-test comparisons revealed significant effect only when contrasting the IBD group with the CON group. The IBD group showed auxiliary area of DMN connectivity in one cluster in the superior frontal gyrus of the left hemisphere (peak coordinates = −18, 57, 30, Z = 3.64, k = 28, corrected cluster p_{FDR} = 0.030). The cluster is visualized in red in **Figure 1A** (the "IBD vs CON").

Joint Group Comparisons

When comparing all the patients and the controls, two clusters reached significance. First one located in the left cingulum (peak coordinates = 3, −15, 39; Z = 4.17; k = 23; corrected cluster p_{FDR} = 0.004), second one located in the left supplementary motor area (peak coordinates 0 15 54, Z=3.77, k=14, corrected cluster p_{FDR}=0.021). In both cases the DMN of the patients showed increased connectivity in those areas. The clusters are visualized in yellow in **Figure 1A** (the "ALL vs CON").

When restricting the comparison to functional gastroenterological diseases only—one cluster reached significance. It was located in left supplementary motor area (peak coordinates = −3, 12, 57; Z = 3.87; k = 14; cluster corrected p_{FDR} = 0.043) and roughly overlaps with one of the clusters of "the gastroenterological diseases vs control" reported in previous paragraph. The direction of the alternation remained unchanged (the DMN of the functional gastrointestinal patients was increased in the area as compared with the controls). The cluster is visualized in green in **Figure 1A** (the "FD and IBS vs CON").

All results are summarized in **Table 2**.

DISCUSSION

Functional diseases of gastrointestinal tract, frequently encountered worldwide, have a negative influence on the

TABLE 2 | Summary results of the intergroup comparisons.

		X	y	z	No. of voxels	T-test/ F-test	Z	Cluster corrected p_{FDR}
IBD vs CON	LH superior frontal gyrus	−18	57	30	28	3.86	3.64	.030
ALL vs CON	LH cingulum	3	−15	39	23	10.18	4.17	.004
	LH supplementary motor area	0	15	54	14	8.51	3.77	.021
FD and IBS vs CON	LH supplementary motor area	−3	12	57	14	11.54	3.87	.043

Anatomical labels according to Automated Anatomical Labeling tool. All reported clusters are significant at cluster p < .05 threshold with topological False Discovery Rate small volume correction.

CON, the control group; FD, the functional dyspepsia group; IBS, the irritable bowel syndrome group; IBD, the inflammatory bowel disease group; ALL, all diseases (FD, IBS and IBD); x, y, z, peak coordinates in MNI space; Z, Z-score.

quality of life and cause significant costs in health care systems. Diagnostic criteria are based on Rome III Criteria (5, 34). Functional dyspepsia is the most common of FIGDs, diagnosed in approx. 25% of population. In 15% to 24% of western world population irritable bowel syndrome is encountered. Functional diseases of gastrointestinal tract are more common in young women, in case of IBS 2 to 3 times in comparison to men (35).

Patients suffering from FIGDs more often present with emotional distress and lower stress tolerance. Patient's constitution and response to stress may influence biological processes within the central nervous system and through autonomic nervous system trigger somatic reactions from digestive tract, leading to decrease in quality of life (36). Brain-gut axis disorders are also taken into account in etiology of FIGDs symptoms, mainly with regard to lowering the pain threshold (37). Correlation between anxiety and lowering the pain threshold, epigastric discomfort, burning, and early satiation has been proven. Patients suffering from FIGDs are also prone to guilt, increased self-criticism, catastrophical thoughts, and focusing on failure, they are said to cope worse with everyday problems. However, no correlation between FIGDs and lifespan has been reported (38).

Since 1937 when Papez first described neural pathway in the brain thought to be involved in the cortical control of emotion, the limbic system has been under scrutiny. At first brain studies have been mainly based on observation of its response to damage or stimulation. New possibilities emerged with introduction and development of imaging techniques, such as single-photon emission computed tomography (SPECT), positron emission tomography (PET), and functional magnetic resonance imaging (fMRI). Ample research has been conducted in order to investigate neuroanatomy and recognize which areas of the brain activate while different emotional states are being induced in healthy individuals. Phan et al. (39) in their meta-analysis of 55 studies with the use of PET and fMRI in healthy subjects showed that fear is associated with increase of activity in amygdalae, while sadness with activation of the perigenual anterior cingulate cortex. Medial part of prefrontal cortex plays a significant role in evaluation and processing of emotional data.

Our results showed that DMNs in study and the control group differed in left superior frontal gyrus, left cingulum and in the left supplementary motor area. Number of studies focused on functioning of the brain in FIGDs (15, 40–42). The study of Liu at al. (2013) focused on orbitofrontal cortex (OFC), parietal cortex, pregenual anterior cingulate cortex (pACC), and dorsomedial prefrontal cortex (dmPFC) (43). There are several factors that may contribute to the discrepancies between our studies. Most important one is the study population. In our research we focused on the joint effect of the different FIGDs which may have covered different brain responses specific for the each of the group of patients separately. Also the image analysis proposed by Liu at al. did not include detrending and filtering of the data which may resulted in different SNR ratio (signal-to-

noise ratio) and also affect the results. We interpret our results with reference to the model of the brain-gut axis as explained by Mayer (2005) (44). The author describes the homeostatic afferent processing network as the one responsible for processing visceral and somatic stimuli (both painful and non-painful). What is most important in the model, is a broad understanding of homeostasis which includes responding to emotional stimuli as well. This point of view seems to be crucial for FGIDs patients description. Discovered differences in the DMNs can be interpreted as altered processing of homeostatic stimuli.

Despite that the Default Mode Network in gastric diseases is not yet well examined, there are multiple research explaining role of brain regions, which could give ideas of psychological functioning of this group of patients. Results of our study showed differences in three regions i.e. superior frontal gyrus of the left hemisphere, left cingulum, left supplementary motor area (see **Figure 1**) between particular groups. All diseases groups differed from control group in Default Mode Network pattern in left cingulum. Functions of cingulum are widely described, as a part of a limbic system it was always connected with emotions (including social interactions), motivation, and cognitive processes, such as memory and executive functions (45). However if the greater emphasis will be put on particular parts of cingulum, then its frontal connections are more likely consider as a attenuating in cognitive control, attention processes as well as pain, motor mechanisms, and reward signaling (46). Looking at cingulum in aspects of gastric diseases the role in amplifying emotional responses to pain signals described by Cohen et al. (47) seems to be the most important. As mentioned above, patients with gastric diseases often have lower stress tolerance and higher anxiety level. Thus different Default Mode Network pattern in cingulum region might be linked with often pain presence in examined gastric diseases.

Different DMN activation of superior frontal gyrus (SFG) was found in IBD group comparing to control. Functional brain imaging studies focused on chronic pain emphasis that chronic pain conditions involve mostly medial prefrontal cortical areas as well as subcortical limbic regions. Apkarian et al. (48) suggest that in majority of chronic pain diseases a shift away from brain areas engaged in sensory processing of pain to regions involved in emotional and motivational subjective states is observed. This observation would explain differences in DMN in SFG between IBD individuals and control group. Activation of these limbic/emotional structures related to subjective pain in IBD might result in psychological symptoms such as anxiety or dissatisfaction.

Last DMN with statistically relevant differences in region of supplementary motor area was noticed in comparison of functional gastric diseases (functional dyspepsia group, irritable bowel syndrome) and control groups. This brain area is considered to play role in facilitating spontaneous motor responses to auditory stimuli, and in supporting a flexible engagement of sensorimotor processes to enable auditory perception and imaginary (49). Reflecting these findings to our results may explain why symptoms of FD and IBS can appear as a react to particular sound or image.

The psychological description of the patients corresponds with this explanation. Patients are characterized as anxious and depressive; also, the comorbidity of the FGIDs and the psychiatric disorders regard mostly the mood and anxiety disorders (50), thus suggesting altered emotional processing as well.

In conclusion, it needs to be stressed that our study group involved patients suffering from both functional and non-specifi inflammatory bowel diseases. Nevertheless, with a spectrum of changes in the study group (superior frontal gyrus of the left hemisphere, in the left cingulum and in the left supplementary motor area), we were able to find common features, differentiating the whole study group from the healthy controls.

ETHICS STATEMENT

The studies involving human participants were reviewed and approved by The Bioethical Committee of The Military Medical Council. The patients/participants provided their written informed consent to participate in this study.

AUTHOR CONTRIBUTIONS

KS: planning and conducting the study, collecting data, drafting the manuscript. GP: collecting the patients and conducting the study. PN and AS: analysis and interpretation of data. KM: drafting the article it critically for important intellectual content. GR: conception and design. ES: final approval of the version to be published.

ACKNOWLEDGMENTS

We would like to thank Professor Edyta Szurowska for inspiration and scientific guidance.

REFERENCES

1. Mearin F, Calleja JL. Defining functional dyspepsia. *Rev Esp Enferm Dig* (2011) 103(12):640–7. doi: 10.4321/S1130-01082011001200006
2. Clauwaert N, Jones MP, Holvoet L, Vandenberghe J, Vos R, Tack J, et al. Associations between gastric sensorimotor function, depression, somatization, and symptom-based subgroups in functional gastroduodenal disorders: are all symptoms equal? *Neurogastroenterol* (2012) 24(12):1088–e565. doi: 10.1111/j.1365-2982.2012.01985.x
3. Kopczynska W, Mokros L, Pietras T, Malecka-Panas E. Quality of life and depression in patients with irritable bowel syndrome. *Gastroenterology Rev* (2018) 13(2):102–8. doi: 10.5114/pg.2018.75819
4. Häuser W, Moser G, Klose P, Mikocka-Walus A. Psychosocial issues in evidence-based guidelines on inflammatory bowel diseases: A review. *World J Gastroenterol* (2014) 20(13):3663–71. doi: 10.3748/wjg.v20.i13.3663
5. Tack J, Talley NJ. Functional dyspepsia–symptoms, definitions and validity of the Rome III criteria. *Nat Rev Gastroenterol Hepatol* (2013) 10(3):134. doi: 10.1038/nrgastro.2013.14
6. Waśko-Czopnik D, Mulak A, Paradowski L. Functional disorders of upper gastrointestinal tract according to Rome III functional Gastrointestinal Disorders. *Gastroenterol Polska* (2006) 13(6):469–72.
7. Philpott H, Gibson P, Thien F. Irritable bowel syndrome - An inflammatory disease involving mast cells. *Asia Pac Allergy* (2011) 1(1):36–42. doi: 10.5415/apallergy.2011.1.1.36
8. Taché Y, Perdue MH. Role of peripheral CRF signalling pathways in stress-related alterations of gut motility and mucosal function. *Neurogastroenterol Motil* (2004) 16 Suppl 1:137–42. doi: 10.1111/j.1743-3150.2004.00490.x
9. Vanheel H, Vicario M, Vanuytsel T, Van Oudenhove L, Martinez C, Keita AV, et al. Impaired duodenal mucosal integrity and low-grade inflammation in functional dyspepsia. *Gut* (2014) 63(2):262–71. doi: 10.1136/gutjnl-2012-303857
10. Haug TT, Wilhelmsen I, Ursin H, Berstad A. What are the real problems for patients with functional dyspepsia? *Scand J Gastroenterol* (1995) 30(2):97–100. doi: 10.3109/00365529509093244
11. Van Oudenhove L, Azziz Q. The role of psychosocial factors and psychiatric disorders in functional dyspepsia. *Nat Rev Gastroenterol Hepatol* (2013) 10 (3):158–67. doi: 10.1038/nrgastro.2013.10
12. Naliboff BD, Kim SE, Bolus R, Bernstein CN, Mayer EA, Chang L. Gastrointestinal and psychological mediators of health-related quality of life in IBS and IBD: a structural equation modeling analysis. *Am J Gastroenterol* (2012) 107(3):451–9. doi: 10.1038/ajg.2011.377
13. Zeng F, Qin W, Liang F, Liu J, Tang Y, Liu X, et al. Abnormal Resting Brain Activity in Patients With Functional Dyspepsia Is Related to Symptom Severity. *Gastroenterology* (2011) 141(2):499–506. doi: 10.1053/j.gastro.2011.05.003
14. Van Oudenhove L, Vandenberghe J, Dupont P, Geeraerts B, Vos R, Dirix S, et al. Regional Brain Activity in Functional Dyspepsia: A H215O-PET Study on the Role of Gastric Sensitivity and Abuse History. *Gastroenterology* (2010) 139(1):36–47. doi: 10.1053/j.gastro.2010.04.015
15. Zhou G, Liu P, Zeng F, Yuan K, Yu D, von Deneen KM, et al. Increased interhemispheric resting-state functional connectivity in functional dyspepsia: a pilot study. *NMR Biomed* (2012) 26(4):410–15. doi: 10.1002/nbm.2878
16. Vandenberghe J, Dupont P, Van Oudenhove L, Bormans G, Demyttenaere K, Fischler B, et al. Regional cerebral blood flow during gastric balloon distention in functional dyspepsia. *Gastroenterology* (2007) 132(5):1684–93. doi: 10.1053/j.gastro.2007.03.037
17. Vandenberghe J, DuPont P, Fischler B, Bormans G, Persoons P, Janssens J, et al. Regional brain activation during proximal stomach distention in humans: a positron emission tomography study. *Gastroenterology* (2005) 128(3):564–73. doi: 10.1053/j.gastro.2004.11.054
18. Liu P, Zeng F, Zhou G, Wang J, Wen H, von Deneen KM, et al. Alterations of the default mode network in functional dyspepsia patients: a resting-state fmri study. *Neurogastroenterol Motil* (2013) 25(6):382–8. doi: 10.1111/nmo.12131
19. Ladabaum U, Minoshima S, Hasler WL, Cross D, Chey WD, Owyanq C. Gastric distention correlates with activation of multiple cortical and subcortical regions. *Gastroenterology* (2001) 120(2):369–76. doi: 10.1053/gast.2001.21201
20. Lu CL, Wu YT, Yeh TC, Chen LF, Chang FY, Lee SD, et al. Neuronal correlates of gastric pain induced by fundus distension: a 3T-fMRI study. *Neurogastroenterol Motil* (2004) 16(5):575–87. doi: 10.1111/j.1365-2982.2004.00562.x
21. Stephan E, Pardo JV, Faris PL, Hartman BK, Kim SW, Ivanov EH, et al. Functional neuroimaging of gastric distention. *J Gastrointest Surg* (2003) 7 (6):740–9. doi: 10.1016/S1091-255X(03)00071-4
22. Mayer EA, Naliboff BD, Craig AD. Neuroimaging of the brain-gut axis: from basic understanding to treatment of functional GI disorders. *Gastroenterology* (2006) 131(6):1925–42. doi: 10.1053/j.gastro.2006.10.026
23. Jones MP, Crowell M, Olden K, Creed F. Functional Gastrointestinal Disorders: An Update for the psychiatrist. *Psychosomatics* (2007) 48(2):93–102. doi: 10.1176/appi.psy.48.2.93
24. Van Oudenhove L, Demyttenaere K, Tack J, Aziz Q. Central nervous system

involvement in functional gastrointestinal disorders. *Best Pract Res Clin Gastroenterol* (2004) 18(4):663–80. doi: 10.1016/j.bpg.2004.04.010

25. Farmer AD, Qasim Aziz Q. Mechanisms of visceral pain in health and functional gastrointestinal disorders. *Scandinavian J Pain* (2014) 5(2):51–60. doi: 10.1016/j.sjpain.2014.01.002

26. Kano M, Dupont P, Fukudo S. Understanding neurogastroenterology from neuroimaging perspective: a comprehensive review of functional and structural brain imaging in functional gastrointestinal disorders. *J Neurogastroenterol Motil* (2018) 24(4):512–27. doi: 10.5056/jnm18072

27. Farmer MA, Baliki MN, Apkarian AV. A dynamic network perpective od chronic pain. *Neurosci Lett* (2012) 520(2):197–203. doi: 10.1016/j.neulet.2012.05.001

28. Qi R, Ke J, Schoepf UJ, Varga-Szemes A, Milliken CM, Liu C, et al. Topological Reorganization of the default mode network in irritable bowel syndrome. *Mol Neurobiol* (2016) 53(10):6585–93. doi: 10.1007/s12035-015-9558-7

29. Liu P, Li R, Bao C, Wei Y, Fan Y, Liu Y, et al. Altered topological patterns of brain functional networks in Crohn's disease. *Brain Imaging Behav* (2018) 12 (5):1466–78. doi: 10.1007/s11682-017-9814-8

30. Fan W, Zhang S, Hu J, Liu B, Wen L, Gong M, et al. Aberrant Brain Function in active-stage ulcerative colitis patients: a resting-state functional MRI study. *Front Hum Neurosci* (2019) Apr 313:107. doi: 10.3389/fnhum.2019.00107

31. Qin P, Northoff G. How is our self related to midline regions and the default-mode network? *Neuroimage* (2011) 57(3):1221–33. doi: 10.1016/j.neuroimage.2011.05.028

32. Beckmann CF, DeLuca M, Devlin JT, Smith M. Investigations into resting-state connectivity using independent component analysis. *Philos Trans R Soc Lond B Biol Sci* (2005) 360(1457):1001–13. doi: 10.1098/rstb.2005.1634

33. Ma L, Wang B, Chen X, Xiong J. Detecting functional connectivity in the resting brain: a comparison between ICA and CCA. *Magn Reson Imaging* (2007) 25(1):47–56. doi: 10.1016/j.mri.2006.09.032

34. Talley NJ, Choung RS. Whither dyspepsia? A historical perspective of functional dyspepsia, and concepts of pathogenesis and therapy in 2009. *J Gastroenterol Hepatol* (2009) 24 Suppl 3:S20–8. doi: 10.1111/j.1440-1746.2009.06067.x

35. De la Roca-Chiapas JM, Solís-Ortiz S, Fajardo-Araujo M, Sosa M, Córdova-Fraga T, Rosa-Zarate A. Stress profile, coping style, anxiety, depression, and gastric emptying as predictors of functional dyspepsia: A case-control study. *J Psychosom Res* (2010) 68(1):73–81. doi: 10.1016/j.jpsychores.2009.05.013

36. Olafsdottir LB, Gudjonsson H, Jonsdottir HH, Thjodleifsson B. Stability of the irritable bowel syndrome and subgroups as measured by three diagnostic criteria – a 10-year follow-up study. *Aliment Pharmacol Ther* (2010) 32 (5):670–80. doi: 10.1111/j.1365-2036.2010.04388.x

37. Koloski NA, Jones M, Talley NJ. Commentary: Psychological disorders linked to functional dyspepsia. *Aliment Pharmacol Ther* (2012) 36(11-12):1099–100. doi: 10.1111/apt.12079

38. Chang JY, Locke G, McNally MA, Halder SL, Schleck CD, Zinsmeister AR, et al. Impact of functional gastrointestinal disorders on survival in the community. *Am J Gastroenterol* (2010) 105(4):822–32. doi: 10.1038/ajg.2010.40

39. Phan KL, Wager T, Taylor SF, Liberzon I. Functional neuroanatomy of emotion: a meta analysis of emotion activation studies in PET and fMRI. *Neuroimage* (2002) 16(2):331–48. doi: 10.1006/nimg.2002.1087

40. Price DD, Craggs J, Verne GN, Perlstein WM, Robinson ME. Placebo analgesia is accompanied by large reductions in pain-related brain activity in irritable bowel syndrome patients. *Pain* (2007) 127(1-2):63–72. doi: 10.1016/j.pain.2006.08.001

41. Ringel Y, Drossman DA, Leserman JL, Suyenobu BY, Wilber K, Lin W, et al. Effect of abuse history on pain reports and brain responses to aversive visceral stimulation: an FMRI study. *Gastroenterology* (2008) 134(2):396–404. doi: 10.1053/j.gastro.2007.11.011

42. Song GH, Venkatraman V, Ho KY, Chee MW, Yeoh KG, Wilder-Smith CH. Cortical effects of anticipation and endogenous modulation of visceral pain assessed by functional brain MRI in irritable bowel syndrome patients and healthy controls. *Pain* (2006) 126(1-3):79–90. doi: 10.1016/j.pain.2006.06.017

43. Liu P, Qin W, Wang J, Zeng F, Zhou G, Wen H, et al. Identifying Neural Patterns of Functional Dyspepsia Using Multivariate Pattern Analysis: A Resting-State fMRI Study. *PloS One* (2013) 8(7):e68205. doi: 10.1371/journal.pone.0068205

44. Mayer EA, Berman S, Suyenobu B, Labus J, Mandelkern MA, Naliboff BD, et al. Differences in brain responses to visceral pain between patients with bowel syndrome and ulcerative colitis. *Pain* (2005) 115:398–409. doi: 10.1016/j.pain.2005.03.023

45. Bubb EJ, Metzler-Baddeley C, Aggleton JP. The cingulum bundle: Anatomy, function, and dysfunction. *Neurosci Biobehav Rev* (2018) 92:104–27. doi: 10.1016/j.neubiorev.2018.05.008

46. Beckmann M, Johansen-Berg H, Rushworth MFS. Connectivity-based parcellation of human cingulate cortex and its relation to functional specialization. *J Neurosci* (2009) 29(4):1175–90. doi: 10.1523/JNEUROSCI.3328-08.2009

47. Cohen RA, Kaplan RF, Zuffante P, Moser DJ, Jenkins MA, Salloway S, et al. Alteration of Intention and Self-Initiated Action Associated With Bilateral Anterior Cingulotomy. *J Neuropsychiatry Clin Neurosci* (1999) 11(4):444–53. doi: 10.1176/jnp.11.4.444

48. Apkarian AV, Hashmi JA, Baliki MN. Pain and the brain: Specificity and plasticity of the brain in clinical chronic pain. *Pain* (2011) 152(3 Suppl):S49–64. doi: 10.1016/j.pain.2010.11.010

49. Lima CF, Krishnan S, Scott SK. Roles of Supplementary Motor Areas in Auditory Processing and Auditory Imagery. *Trends Neurosci* (2016) 39 (8):527–42. doi: 10.1016/j.tins.2016.06.003

50. Van Oudenhove L, Aziz Q. Recent insights on central processing and psychological processes in functional gastrointestinal disorders. *Dig Liver Dis* (2009) 41(11):781–7. doi: 10.1016/j.dld.2009.07.004

Permissions

The contributors of this book come from diverse backgrounds, making this book a truly international effort. This book will bring forth new frontiers with its revolutionizing research information and detailed analysis of the nascent developments around the world.

We would like to thank all the contributing authors for lending their expertise to make the book truly unique. They have played a crucial role in the development of this book. Without their invaluable contributions this book wouldn't have been possible. They have made vital efforts to compile up to date information on the varied aspects of this subject to make this book a valuable addition to the collection of many professionals and students.

This book was conceptualized with the vision of imparting up-to-date information and advanced data in this field. To ensure the same, a matchless editorial board was set up. Every individual on the board went through rigorous rounds of assessment to prove their worth. After which they invested a large part of their time researching and compiling the most relevant data for our readers.

The editorial board has been involved in producing this book since its inception. They have spent rigorous hours researching and exploring the diverse topics which have resulted in the successful publishing of this book. They have passed on their knowledge of decades through this book. To expedite this challenging task, the publisher supported the team at every step. A small team of assistant editors was also appointed to further simplify the editing procedure and attain best results for the readers.

Apart from the editorial board, the designing team has also invested a significant amount of their time in understanding the subject and creating the most relevant covers. They scrutinized every image to scout for the most suitable representation of the subject and create an appropriate cover for the book.

The publishing team has been an ardent support to the editorial, designing and production team. Their endless efforts to recruit the best for this project, has resulted in the accomplishment of this book. They are a veteran in the field of academics and their pool of knowledge is as vast as their experience in printing. Their expertise and guidance has proved useful at every step. Their uncompromising quality standards have made this book an exceptional effort. Their encouragement from time to time has been an inspiration for everyone.

The publisher and the editorial board hope that this book will prove to be a valuable piece of knowledge for researchers, students, practitioners and scholars across the globe.

List of Contributors

Jessica Aigbologa
APC Microbiome Ireland, Cork, Ireland

Maeve Connolly
Department of Physiology, University College Cork, Cork, Ireland

Julliette M. Buckley
Department of Surgery, University College Cork, Cork, Ireland
Mater Private Hospital, Cork, Ireland

Dervla O'Malley
APC Microbiome Ireland, Cork, Ireland
Department of Physiology, University College Cork, Cork, Ireland

Thomas Jan Konturek
Division of Gastroenterology, Loyola University Medical Center, Stritch School of Medicine, Maywood, IL, United States
Department of Internal Medicine, Institute of Neurogastroenterology, Martin Luther Hospital, Johannesstift Diakonie, Berlin, Germany

Cristina Martinez
Lleida Institute for Biomedical Research Dr. Pifarré Foundation (IRBLleida), Lleida, Spain
Department of Human Molecular Genetics, University Hospital Heidelberg, Heidelberg, Germany

Beate Niesler
Department of Human Molecular Genetics, University Hospital Heidelberg, Heidelberg, Germany
nCounter Core Facility Heidelberg, Institute of Human Genetics, Heidelberg, Germany

Ivo van der Voort
Department of Internal Medicine, Institute of Neurogastroenterology, Martin Luther Hospital, Johannesstift Diakonie, Berlin, Germany
Department of Internal Medicine and Gastroenterology, Berlin Jewish Hospital, Berlin, Germany

Hubert Mönnikes
Department of Internal Medicine, Institute of Neurogastroenterology, Martin Luther Hospital, Johannesstift Diakonie, Berlin, Germany

Miriam Goebel-Stengel
Department of Internal Medicine, Institute of Neurogastroenterology, Martin Luther Hospital, Johannesstift Diakonie, Berlin, Germany
Department of Psychosomatic Medicine, University Hospital Tübingen, Tübingen, Germany
Department of Internal Medicine and Gastroenterology, Helios Clinic Rottweil, Rottweil, Germany

Dominik Langgartner, Till S. Böbel, Sascha B. Hackl and Stefan O. Reber
Laboratory for Molecular Psychosomatics, Department of Psychosomatic Medicine and Psychotherapy, University of Ulm, Ulm, Germany

Cristian A. Zambrano, Jared D. Heinze and Christopher E. Stamper
Department of Integrative Physiology, University of Colorado Boulder, Boulder, CO, United States

Marc N. Jarczok, Harald Gündel and Christiane Waller
Department of Psychosomatic Medicine and Psychotherapy, University of Ulm, Ulm, Germany

Nicolas Rohleder
Department of Psychology, Friedrich-Alexander University, Erlangen, Germany

Graham A. Rook
Center for Clinical Microbiology, University College London (UCL), London, United Kingdom

Christopher A. Lowry
Department of Integrative Physiology, University of Colorado Boulder, Boulder, CO, United States
Center for Neuroscience and Center for Microbial Exploration, University of Colorado Boulder, Boulder, CO, United States
Department of Physical Medicine and Rehabilitation and Center for Neuroscience, University of Colorado Anschutz Medical Campus, Aurora, CO, United States
Veterans Health Administration, Rocky Mountain Mental Illness Research Education and Clinical Center (MIRECC), The Rocky Mountain Regional Medical Center (RMRMC), Aurora, CO, United States
Military and Veteran Microbiome: Consortium for Research and Education (MVMCoRE), Aurora, CO, United States
inVIVO Planetary Health, Worldwide Universities Network (WUN), West New York, NJ, United States

Alison Accarie
Department of Chronic Diseases, Metabolism and Ageing (ChroMetA), Translational Research Center for Gastrointestinal Disorders (TARGID), KU Leuven, Leuven, Belgium

Tim Vanuytsel
Department of Chronic Diseases, Metabolism and Ageing (ChroMetA), Translational Research Center for Gastrointestinal Disorders (TARGID), KU Leuven, Leuven, Belgium
Department of Gastroenterology and Hepatology, University Hospitals Leuven, Leuven, Belgium

Larissa Hetterich
Department of Psychosomatic Medicine and Psychotherapy, University Hospital Tübingen, Tübingen, Germany

Andreas Stengel
Department of Psychosomatic Medicine and Psychotherapy, University Hospital Tübingen, Tübingen, Germany
Department for Psychosomatic Medicine—Germany, Charité Center for Internal Medicine and Dermatology, Corporate Member of Freie Universität Berlin, Berlin Institute of Health, Charité - Universitätsmedizin Berlin, Humboldt-Universität zu Berlin, Berlin, Germany

Lauren P. Manning and Jessica R. Biesiekierski
Department of Rehabilitation, Nutrition and Sport, La Trobe University, Melbourne, VIC, Australia

C. K. Yao
Department of Gastroenterology, Central Clinical School, Monash University & Alfred Health, Melbourne, VIC, Australia

Franziska Labrenz, Sopiko Knuf-Rtveliashvili and Sigrid Elsenbruch
Institute of Medical Psychology & Behavioral Immunobiology, University Hospital Essen, University of Duisburg-Essen, Essen, Germany

Paul Enck and Sibylle Klosterhalfen
Department of Internal Medicine VI: Psychosomatic Medicine and Psychotherapy, University Hospital Tübingen, Tübingen, Germany

Karen Van den Houte, Emidio Scarpellini, Wout Verbeure, Hideki Mori, Jolien Schol, Imke Masuy, Florencia Carbone and Jan Tack
Translational Research Center for Gastrointestinal Diseases, University of Leuven, Leuven, Belgium

Swapna Mahurkar-Joshi and Lin Chang
G. Oppenheimer Center for Neurobiology of Stress and Resilience, Division of Digestive Diseases, Department of Medicine at UCLA, Los Angeles, CA, United States

Adriane Icenhour, Till Roderigo and Sven Benson
Institute of Medical Psychology and Behavioral Immunobiology, University Hospital Essen, University of Duisburg-Essen, Essen, Germany

Ann-Katrin Kraeuter
Laboratory of Psychiatric Neuroscience, Centre for Molecular Therapeutics, James Cook University, Townsville, QLD, Australia
Australian Institute of Tropical Health and Medicine, James Cook University, Townsville, QLD, Australia, Faculty of Health and Life Sciences, Psychology, Northumbria University, Newcastle upon Tyne, United Kingdom

Riana Phillips and Zoltán Sarnyai
Laboratory of Psychiatric Neuroscience, Centre for Molecular Therapeutics, James Cook University, Townsville, QLD, Australia
Australian Institute of Tropical Health and Medicine, James Cook University, Townsville, QLD, Australia

Henri Duboc
Université de Paris, Paris, France
AP-HP, Gastroenterology Unit, Hopital Louis Mourier, Colombes, France
INSERM UMR 1149, Université de Paris, Paris, France

Sofya Latrache and Benoit Coffin
Université de Paris, Paris, France
AP-HP, Gastroenterology Unit, Hopital Louis Mourier, Colombes, France

Nicoleta Nebunu
AP-HP, Gastroenterology Unit, Hopital Louis Mourier, Colombes, France

Yong Sung Kim
Wonkwang Digestive Disease Research Institute, Gut and Food Healthcare, Wonkwang University School of Medicine, Iksan, South Korea
Good Breath Clinic, Gunpo, South Korea

Jung-Wook Kim
Department of Gastroenterology, Kyung Hee University College of Medicine, Seoul, South Korea

Na-Yeon Ha
Department of Clinical Korean Medicine, College of Korean Medicine, Graduate School, Kyung Hee University, Seoul, South Korea
Department of Gastroenterology, College of Korean Medicine, Kyung Hee University, Seoul, South Korea

Jinsung Kim
Department of Gastroenterology, College of Korean Medicine, Kyung Hee University, Seoul, South Korea

Han Seung Ryu
Wonkwang Digestive Disease Research Institute, Gut and Food Healthcare, Wonkwang University School of Medicine, Iksan, South Korea
Brain-Gut Stress Clinic, Division of Gastroenterology, Wonkwang University Hospital, Iksan, South Korea

Chloé Melchior and Philippe Ducrotté
INSERM U1073, UNIROUEN, Normandie University, Rouen, France
Department of Gastroenterology, Rouen University Hospital, Rouen, France

Charlotte Desprez and Guillaume Gourcerol
INSERM U1073, UNIROUEN, Normandie University, Rouen, France
Department of Physiology, Rouen University Hospital, Rouen, France

Ghassan Riachi
Department of Gastroenterology, Rouen University Hospital, Rouen, France

Anne-Marie Leroi
INSERM U1073, UNIROUEN, Normandie University, Rouen, France
Department of Physiology, Rouen University Hospital, Rouen, France
INSERM CIC-CRB 1404, Rouen University Hospital, Rouen, France

Pierre Déchelotte and Najate Achamrah
INSERM U1073, UNIROUEN, Normandie University, Rouen, France
Department of Nutrition, Rouen University Hospital, Rouen, France

Marie-Pierre Tavolacci
INSERM U1073, UNIROUEN, Normandie University, Rouen, France
INSERM CIC-CRB 1404, Rouen University Hospital, Rouen, France

Will Takakura
Department of Medicine, Medically Associated Science and Technology (MAST) Program, Cedars-Sinai Medical Center, Los Angeles, CA, United States

Mark Pimentel
Department of Medicine, Medically Associated Science and Technology (MAST) Program, Cedars-Sinai Medical Center, Los Angeles, CA, United States
Department of Medicine, Division of Digestive and Liver Diseases, Cedars-Sinai Medical Center, Los Angeles, CA, United States

Yuanjun Dong, David Baumeister, Sabrina Berens, Wolfgang Eich and Jonas Tesarz
Department of General Internal Medicine and Psychosomatics, University Hospital Heidelberg, Heidelberg, Germany

Katarzyna Skrobisz
Department of Radiology, Medical University of Gdansk, Gdansk, Poland

Grazyna Piotrowicz
Department of Gastroenterology, Self- Dependent Health Care Unit of Ministry of Interior, Gdansk, Poland

Patrycja Naumczyk
Institute of Psychology, University of Gdansk, Gdansk, Poland

Agnieszka Sabisz, Karolina Markiet and Edyta Szurowska
II Department of Radiology, Medical University of Gdansk, Gdansk, Poland

Grazyna Rydzewska
Central Clinical Hospital of the Ministry of Interior, Warsaw, Poland

Index

Printed in the USA
CPSIA information can be obtained
at www.ICGtesting.com
JSHW062237071123
51533JS00031B/126